# Cleft Lip and Palate

## For Clinicians by Clinicians

Michael P. Cannito and Deanie Vogel, Series Editors

This book, *Cleft Lip and Palate: Interdisciplinary Issues and Treatment,* is the second edition of the seventh volume in the For Clinicians by Clinicians series of texts on the diagnosis and clinical management of speech, language, voice, and swallowing disorders. Each text provides a contemporary perspective on one major disorder or clinical area and is designed for use in clinical methodology courses, in continuing education programs, and as a clinical practice resource. Authors have been selected who represent a broad spectrum of clinical interests and theoretical positions and who hold the common belief that their viewpoints, experiences, and successes should be shared in order to provide a forum for clinicians by clinicians.

The idea for this series came from Dr. Harris Winitz, who served as editor of the series until 1997. During Winitz's tenure as series editor, many important titles were added to the series, including the following volumes: *Treating Language Disorders, Treating Articulation Disorders, Case Studies in Aphasia Rehabilitation, Treating Cerebral Palsy, Alaryngeal Speech Rehabilitation, Treating Disordered Speech Motor Control, Cleft Palate,* and *Language Interventions: Beyond the Primary Grades.*

The last five additions to the series—*Aging and Communication, Evaluation of Dysphagia in Adults, Vocal Rehabilitation for Medical Speech-Language Pathology,* and *Early Childhood Stuttering*—have been guided by the current series coeditors, Michael P. Cannito and Deanie Vogel. Their intent is to continue the rich tradition of this important series that was established many years ago by Dr. Winitz.

# Cleft Lip and Palate

## Interdisciplinary Issues and Treatment

SECOND EDITION

Edited by

**Karlind T. Moller**

**and**

**Leslie E. Glaze**

pro·ed
An International Publisher
8700 Shoal Creek Boulevard
Austin, Texas 78757-6897
800/897-3202 Fax 800/397-7633
www.proedinc.com

An International Publisher

© 2001, 2009 by PRO-ED, Inc.
8700 Shoal Creek Boulevard
Austin, Texas 78757-6897
800/897-3202 Fax 800/397-7633
www.proedinc.com



**Library of Congress Cataloging-in-Publication Data**

Cleft lip and palate : interdisciplinary issues and treatment / edited by Karlind T. Moller and Leslie E. Glaze.—2nd ed.
p. ; cm.—(For clinicians by clinicians)
Includes bibliographical references and indexes.
ISBN-13: 978-1-4164-0368-5
1. Cleft palate. 2. Cleft lip. 3. Cleft palate children—Rehabilitation. I. Moller, Karlind T. II. Glaze, Leslie E. III. Series.
[DNLM: 1. Cleft Palate. 2. Cleft Lip. 3. Continuity of Patient Care. 4. Patient Care Team. WV 440 C6238 2008]
RD525.C54 2008
617.5'225—dc22

2007039718

Art Director: Jason Crosier
Designer: Vicki DePountis
This book is designed in Minion and Charlotte.

Printed in the United States of America

1 2 3 4 5 6 7 8 9 10 17 16 15 14 13 12 11 10 09 08

# Contents

# Contributors

**Cassandra L. Aspinall, MSW, LICSW**
Children's Hospital and Regional Medical Center, Craniofacial Center
University of Washington
Seattle, WA

**Adriane L. Baylis, PhD**
Children's Hospital of Wisconsin
Milwaukee, WI

**Richard R. Bevis, DDS, PhD**
School of Dentistry, Department of Developmental and Surgical Sciences
Cleft Palate/Craniofacial Clinics
University of Minnesota
Minneapolis, MN

**Mary L. Breen, RN, MS**
Craniofacial and Reconstructive Plastic Surgery Center
Dell Children's Medical Center of Central Texas
Austin, TX

**Marie-Claire Buckley, MD**
Division of Plastic and Reconstructive Surgery
University of Minnesota, Department of Surgery
Minneapolis, MN

**Jane E. Carlstrom, AuD**
Department of Speech-Language-Hearing Sciences
University of Minnesota
Minneapolis, MN

**Kathy L. Chapman, PhD**
Department of Communication Sciences and Disorders
University of Utah
Salt Lake City, UT

**David H. Charles, DDS, MS**
University Hospital
Division of Prosthodontics
Faculty of Medicine and Dentistry
Oral Facial Rehabilitation Unit
University of Western Ontario
London, Ontario, Canada

**Patricia D. Chibbaro, RN, MS, CPNP**
Institute of Reconstructive Plastic Surgery
New York University Medical Center
New York, NY

**Michele J. Eliason, PhD**
Institute for Health and Aging
University of California–San Francisco
San Francisco, CA

**Leslie E. Glaze, PhD**
Department of Speech-Language-Hearing Sciences
University of Minnesota
Minneapolis, MN

**Robert J. Gorlin, DDS, MS**
(Deceased) Previous affiliation:
School of Dentistry, Department of Diagnostic and Biological Sciences
Division of Oral Pathology
University of Minnesota
Minneapolis, MN

**Virginia A. Hinton, PhD**
Department of Communication Sciences and Disorders
School of Health and Human Performance
University of North Carolina–Greensboro
Greensboro, NC

**Gerrilyn M. Hopper, MHSc, RD, CD**
Research Nutritionist, Fred Hutchinson Cancer Research Center
Women's Health Initiative
Seattle, WA

**David L. Jones, PhD**
Division of Communication Disorders
University of Wyoming
Laramie, WY

**George H. Landis, MD**
School of Dentistry, Cleft Palate-Craniofacial Program
University of Minnesota
Minneapolis, MN

**Herbert A. Leeper, Jr., PhD**
(Deceased) Previous affiliation:
Department of Communication Disorders
University of Western Ontario
London, Ontario, Canada

**Karlind T. Moller, PhD**
School of Dentistry, Department of Developmental and Surgical Sciences
University of Minnesota
Minneapolis, MN

**Jerald B. Moon, PhD**
Department of Speech Pathology and Audiology
University of Iowa
Iowa City, IA

**Peggy B. Nelson, PhD**
Department of Speech-Language-Hearing Sciences
University of Minnesota
Minneapolis, MN

**Lynn C. Richman, PhD**
Department of Pediatrics
University of Iowa Hospitals
Iowa City, IA

**Earl J. Seaver, PhD**
Division of Communication Disorders
Northern Illinois University
DeKalb, IL

**Helen M. Sharp, PhD**
Department of Speech Pathology and Audiology
Western Michigan University
Kalamazoo, MI

**James D. Sidman, MD**
Children's Hospitals and Clinics of Minnesota
Department of Otolaryngology
University of Minnesota

**Paul S. Sills, DDS**
(Deceased) Previous affiliation:
Faculty of Dentistry
Division of Removable Prosthodontics
University of Western Ontario
London, Ontario, Canada

**James Q. Swift, DDS**
University of Minnesota
Division of Oral and Maxillofacial Surgery
School of Dentistry, Developmental and Surgical Sciences
Minneapolis, MN

**Judith E. Trost-Cardamone, PhD**
Department of Communication Disorders and Sciences
California State University at Northridge
Northridge, CA

**Bryan J. Williams, DDS, MSD, MEd**
Department of Dental Medicine
Seattle Children's Hospital and University of Washington Craniofacial Center
Seattle, WA

# Preface to the Second Edition

As we contemplated the additions and modifications we planned for this second edition, we prepared ourselves by reviewing the preface to the first edition. We were impressed that the objectives remain consistent, despite the many changes in this current edition. This book remains, first and foremost, an exposition of interdisciplinary knowledge and experience in the care of cleft palate and craniofacial anomalies. In the preface to the first edition, we spoke about the importance of clinical outcome, convinced that successful, indeed optimal, outcome was highly dependent upon the interdisciplinary approach. We remain convinced!

We believe that our best clinical work is grounded in research. This is a clinical text by the very nature of the series—*For Clinicians, by Clinicians*—yet we intend for it to be an important and useful reference that explores in depth what we know, how we know it, what we still need to accomplish, and what future investigations will advance our knowledge. That is still true!

Although speech-language pathologists and audiologists are anticipated to be our primary readers, this edition will benefit professionals from a wide variety of disciplines (medicine, dentistry, surgery, psychology, social work, etc.) who are curious about or directly involved with interdisciplinary enterprise. Successful interdisciplinary activity demands that all participants be well informed, have mutual respect for each discipline and each other, and appreciate how each can best contribute.

What have we done to "grow" this second edition? There are several new chapters to help the reader appreciate a more complete range of disciplines involved on interdisciplinary care teams. Best practice involves not only the gifted and caring surgeon, but also a host of professionals diagnosing, evaluating, planning, and treating as the child matures physically and behaviorally. Because interdisciplinary teamwork involves so many disciplines from birth to adulthood, we added the following chapters: "Social

Work: Assessing Family Issues and Burdens of Care" (Aspinall), "Ethical Issues in the Care of Patients with Cleft Palate and Craniofacial Anomalies" (Sharp), "Transcultural Care of Patients with Cleft Palate and Craniofacial Anomalies" (Hinton), "Nursing Care, Feeding, and Nutrition in the First Year" (Breen, Chibbaro, and Hopper), and "Pediatric Otolaryngology: Management of the Ear, Nose, Throat, and Airway" (Sidman).

We listened to our students. Although their judgments about the first edition were clearly favorable, the most frequent suggestions were to add a chapter on anatomy and physiology of the craniofacial complex and the velopharyngeal closure mechanism, and a chapter focusing on language development in children with cleft palate. We agreed and added "Anatomy and Physiology of the Normal and Cleft Palate Speech Mechanism" (Jones and Seaver) and "Speech and Language of Children with Cleft Palate: Interactions and Influences" (Chapman). Other chapters underwent major updating and revisions, frequently by different authors from those who contributed to the previous edition. As editors, we have attempted to organize sections more logically and to cross-reference the chapters liberally.

We honestly applaud ourselves for recruiting an absolutely outstanding and impressive group of contributors for this edition. The reader need only glance at the literature or at national and international conferences to recognize and appreciate the contributors to this book. They are all skilled clinicians and productive scholars who are relentlessly committed to the interdisciplinary approach. We are so grateful for their willingness to share their expertise and perspective.

There are so many other people to thank for this effort:

- To our patients and families who are constantly teaching us about the importance and value of teamwork and patient-centered care—we are indebted!
- To our predecessors and our own mentors who saw the wisdom, potential, and caveats of interdisciplinary care for persons with cleft and craniofacial conditions—we thank you for your vision, work, and guidance!
- To our students, who challenge us with curiosity and insights, delight us with your intelligence and enthusiasm, and teach us new lessons as well.
- To our own families, who encourage us to have patience and worry less and who shared our conviction that what we were trying to accomplish was worthwhile—we are grateful for your support and we love you!

We were shocked and dismayed with the sudden death of Herbert A. (Andy) Leeper, Jr., primary author of the chapter on prosthodontic management. Andy was excited about this second edition and was actively working on a revision at his untimely death in 2001. Before this edition went into production, we were saddened to learn about the death of Paul S. Sills, a coauthor of the same chapter. Their collaborator David Charles and we agreed unanimously to retain Andy's first author listing for the chapter. Most recently, in August 2006, we mourned the loss of our colleague and friend Robert Gorlin, a most respected and distinguished contributor to the chapter on identification and delineation of craniofacial syndromes. We will certainly miss their presence among us, but so appreciate their excellent contributions to this book.

Finally, but very importantly, we acknowledge and fondly remember my (KM) coeditor for the first edition, Clark D. Starr. I continue to be inspired by his mentorship, friendship, and influence for over 40 years. Clark died in 1999. I know he would be delighted to know that Leslie joined me as coeditor for this second edition.

We are privileged to have found a specialty that brings us such professional satisfaction and personal reward, through our endless opportunities to learn, our cherished collaborations with interdisciplinary colleagues, and our zeal for positive clinical outcomes. Our hope is that you, our readers, detect that same satisfaction within these pages.

*Karlind T. Moller*
*Leslie E. Glaze*

# Preface to the First Edition

Some years ago, Harris Winitz approached us to consider developing a text for clinicians, by clinicians, in the area of cleft lip and palate. Collectively, we have had a strong clinical interest in persons with cleft palate for almost 70 years. *Sustaining* interest for this long has not been difficult. In many ways, cleft lip and palate is one of the most rewarding disorders with which to be involved. Clearly, it is an area where we, as speech and language pathologists, have much to offer and, in many instances, what we say has a significant impact on what happens to our patients—they may or may not have surgery based on our evaluation of what they can or cannot do with their present speech mechanism. We have come to appreciate the true value of working with other medical and dental specialists focusing on a common goal. That goal is a successful outcome—acceptable appearance, dental-facial form and function, communicative ability, and psychosocial skills.

Clinical outcome is something all of us will be hearing much more about as we approach the 21st century. We firmly believe that successful and, indeed, optimal outcome for persons with cleft lip and palate is highly dependent upon the interdisciplinary approach. That is what this book is all about.

Although the primary readership of this book is anticipated to be speech-language pathologists and audiologists, we believe that medical, dental, and other specialists involved in cleft palate management will benefit because of the interdisciplinary nature of the disorder. Additionally, speech-language pathologists should be well informed and knowledgeable, not only about their own discipline as it applies to cleft lip and palate management, but about other professionals who work with them in interdisciplinary diagnosis and treatment planning. For an interdisciplinary team to be successful, there needs to be a mutual respect among team members and for their specialty areas, with a good understanding of what each can and cannot do. The following chapters are written by professionals trained in their specialties so that the readers can appreciate the nature of their training and the issues and procedures involved in cleft palate management. Indeed, we requested the authors of several chapters to specify the training required for their specialties. Although this is a clinical text, we are persuaded that what we do well clinically is grounded in research. Therefore, this book is intended to be a strong research reference to explore in depth what we currently know, what investigative procedures and results have led to our knowledge base, and what we still need to accomplish. Although much of the content of this text could be variously applied to other craniofacial disorders, the clear focus is cleft lip and palate. It is assumed that readers of this text will have some knowledge of the anatomy and physiology of the speech and hearing mechanism.

It is not possible to thank all of the people who have influenced and contributed to this venture. We certainly thank Harris Winitz, who first approached us too many years ago. Then it was our responsibility to contact persons in the various disciplines to share their expertise and perspective on cleft lip and palate management. We believe that we have obtained highly skilled clinicians with the appreciation for research methodology, and we thank them for their contributions. In an edited text with multiple authorship, it is difficult to blend all of the pieces (chapters) masterfully; however, the common thread in the fabric is the patient with cleft lip and palate. To those patients and their families, we thank you for all you have taught us. And this book is certainly dedicated to people like Eugene T. McDonald, who not only saw the wisdom of interdisciplinary care, but who, by their example, helped many to see.

Importantly, for the sharing of our time and for understanding that we were doing something worthwhile, we sincerely thank our own families. Their encouragement and gentle but sometimes firm prodding got the job done.

*KTM*
*CDS*

# PART I

# Interdisciplinary Care: Professional Team, Patient, and Family Issues

# CHAPTER 1

# Interdisciplinary Team Approach

## Issues and Procedures

*Karlind T. Moller*

Moller clearly advocates for interdisciplinary care for persons with cleft lip and cleft palate and other craniofacial disorders because these conditions affect appearance, dental function, and speech and hearing. He reviews why and how teams were first formed, as well as contemporary team structure and function. Issues relating to the value and quality of team function and the future of the interdisciplinary approach are also discussed.

1. Moller states that knowledge of the cleft allows for several assumptions regarding management. What are these assumptions, and why is it important for parents/caregivers to know about them early?
2. Define an interdisciplinary team. Distinguish between multidisciplinary and interdisciplinary teams.
3. What factors were influential in the early formation of interdisciplinary teams, and what was the caveat about specialization at that time?
4. What does Moller mean by the "desirable" team as opposed to the "core" team?
5. Moller lists several functions of organized teams. Discuss one and defend its importance as it relates to other team functions.
6. For the interdisciplinary team approach to continue to be successful, will teams need to be "different" in the future?
7. What external factors does Moller believe will impact the future of teams?

The following excerpt from the preamble of the constitution of the American Cleft Palate-Craniofacial Association (2005) points out the range of concerns and the potential impact on the quality of life for persons with cleft palate:

> We wish to encourage by every appropriate method and device the improvement of scientific clinical services to persons with cleft lip/palate and other craniofacial anomalies in order that they may achieve a more adequate physical, emotional, social, educational, and vocational adjustment. (p. xix)

The constitution also includes a mission statement: "to optimize interdisciplinary care of persons affected by cleft palate and other craniofacial anomalies" (p. xix). Furthermore, the following values are listed in order to accomplish the mission: the well-being of patients and families; the development and dissemination of knowledge; excellence in clinical care; interdisciplinary respect and collaboration; and professional integrity. These statements and values clearly suggest that the concerns for and problems of persons with cleft lip and palate and other craniofacial disorders are multidimensional and that excellence of treatment requires interdisciplinary attention and cooperation.

It is not uncommon for a person with a cleft palate or another craniofacial anomaly to be evaluated and/or treated during the growing years by as many as 10–20 medical, dental, speech, hearing, and other behavioral and social specialists. Periodic evaluations and treatment by these specialists will take many years and require family resources of time, energy, and finances. That is the hard news; the good news is that clefts of the lip and/or palate are very treatable. With the cooperative efforts of the patient and family and multiple specialists, acceptable appearance, communication, social skills, and oral function are very realistic outcomes. However, successful treatment does not merely happen. This chapter focuses on the approach I believe has the best chance of ensuring success—the interdisciplinary approach. Although much of the information is applicable to persons with a variety of craniofacial anomalies, the focus in this text is on cleft lip and palate. First, some aspects of the nature of clefting and the assumptions, biases, and definitions pertaining to interdisciplinary care are important to discuss.

## Nature of Clefting and Assumptions About Treatment

Clefts of the lip and/or palate are among the most frequent congenital anomalies. In fact, these clefts are now the most prevalent birth defect in the United States, affecting 6,800 infants each year (Centers for Disease Control, 2006). The incidence of clefting of some kind in the Caucasian population is approximately 1 in 600 births; it is higher in the American Indian and Asian groups and lower in the African American groups.

Not all clefts are alike. Clefts can involve only the lip and alveolar ridge (primary palate), only the hard and soft palate (secondary palate), or both the primary and secondary palates. Clefts involving the primary palate, the secondary palate, or both vary in severity. Clefts of the lip may not extend to the floor of the nostril, may not involve all of the primary palate or secondary palate, and may occur on one or both sides. Some clefts, such as submucous cleft palate, may be difficult to detect. More detailed information about the embryological developmental aspects and types of clefting is included in Chapter 5 by Gorlin and Baylis.

Considering the heterogeneous nature of clefting, treatment needs to be planned in accordance with the specific problems and needs of each patient. Because cleft lip and palate can be seen, felt, and heard (Lis, Pruzansky, Koepp-Baker, & Kobes, 1956), it is a somewhat unique disorder. It is, or should be for the most part, identifiable at birth.

When cleft lip or palate is detected at birth, several assumptions can be made relative to treatment. First, there will be concerns—not necessarily problems—with appearance, dental and jaw relationships, speech and hearing, and the potential these have to affect psychosocial adjustment.

Second, care of cleft lip and palate will be long term. Treatment will begin immediately after birth and may extend into late adolescence before final treatment, directly related to the cleft, is completed. Medical disciplines such as pediatrics, reconstructive surgery, and otolaryngology (ear, nose, and throat) are most typically involved from a very early age; however, assessment and counseling services from professionals in genetics, psychology, social work, speech-language pathology, audiology, preventive dentistry, and other dental specialties are also very appropriate, important, and strongly encouraged. As the child grows and matures physically and behaviorally, treatment priorities may shift among specialists, but each discipline contributes throughout the growing years.

Third, appropriate treatment for any child with cleft lip or palate must be closely aligned with physical and behavioral growth and development. State-of-the-art knowledge dictates times when certain treatment is most appropriate and times when it is not. For example, speech development and proficiency (behavior aspects) as well as facial growth and development (physical aspects) directly influence the timing of certain physical management procedures.

Fourth, the patient and the family/caregivers need to be well informed and actively involved in the treatment program. The patient and the family must decide to comply and proceed with a specific treatment plan. Patients and families who have not been well informed, have been misinformed, or do not understand the rationale for certain treatments tend to be less actively involved in and less compliant with treatment recommendations. The result is compromised outcome.

The foregoing may lead the reader to believe that optimal cleft palate management is rather painstaking, is arduous, and perhaps does not occur very often. Quite the contrary! However, professionals and parents/caregivers must recognize and accept these assumptions and have a solid understanding of the disorder. When the treatment is well planned and coordinated, with each phase of treatment associated with growth and development, persons with cleft lip and palate are very likely to achieve their physical, educational, social, and vocational potentials.

## The Interdisciplinary Approach—Biases and Definitions

Clinicians need to accept that cleft lip and palate is a multifaceted, complex disorder requiring several disciplines and that an approach or system is necessary to achieve the best possible outcome. For many years, specialists involved with cleft palate habilitation have recognized that no one person has the expertise to address the range of concerns for persons with cleft palate. The contributors to this book share the strong bias that the interdisciplinary team approach is the best, most effective, and most efficient way to achieve optimal facial appearance and function, dental and occlusal form and function, and communication and psychosocial skills.

Various authors have espoused the benefits and recognized the potential limitations and problems of the interdisciplinary approach in cleft lip and palate management (Bzoch, 2004; Kummer, 2001; Lillywhite, 1957; Moller & Starr, 1993; Pannbacker & Scheuerle, 1993; Peterson-Falzone, Hardin-Jones, & Karnell, 2002; Sharp, 1995; Shprintzen, 1995; Sidman, 1995; Strauss, 1997, 1998, 1999; Strauss & Ellis, 1996). All have concluded, however, that the cooperative and integrative efforts of several specialists, over many years, are the best way to achieve the optimal result. Dynamics of team activities and characteristics that contribute to positive and negative team function are discussed later in this chapter.

Several adjectives have been used in conjunction with *teams: interdisciplinary, multidisciplinary, intradisciplinary, interprofessional, intraprofessional, transprofessional,* and *transdisciplinary.* Shprintzen (1995) described the transdisciplinary team as one in which multiple examinations and team conferencing occur and participating specialists learn about each other's disciplines. As I discuss later, team members' motivations to learn constitute an important characteristic of a high-quality interdisciplinary team. I have difficulty envisioning a well-functioning interdisciplinary team where important learning does not occur.

Nackashi and Dixon-Wood (1989), Strauss and Ellis (1996), and Strauss (1999) addressed intradisciplinary, multidisciplinary, and interdisciplinary teams. They suggested that *intradisciplinary* connotes similar specialists within a narrow or single discipline, *multidisciplinary* refers to varied specialists assessing patients independently, and *interdisciplinary* implies more collaboration with other team members. Indeed, I am convinced that it is the face-to-face sharing of information, open communication, and discussion, followed by development of an appropriate and prioritized treatment plan, that is the hallmark of optimal team activity for patients with clefts and craniofacial disorders.

Although specialists can argue about semantic differences and preferences, the professions involved in cleft palate management are clearly between (*inter-*) and not within (*intra-*) disciplinary boundaries. Just as clear is the fact that several disciplines are required. Koepp-Baker (1979), over 25 years ago, eloquently distinguished between multidisciplinary teams and interdisciplinary teams:

> We have come to regard the word multidisciplinary as reflecting the quality of immaturity. The proper adjective describing the mature and effective team, as we conceive it, is interdisciplinary. It better suggests the attributes of the interpersonal and interprofessional intervention that distinguishes this form of human enterprise. (p. 61)

Because the various treatments required for the patient are closely related and interdependent, that element of person-to-person interaction is necessary if the team concept is to be worthwhile and productive and is to yield optimal outcome. Therefore, we consider *interdisciplinary* to be the most desirable term, and it will be used in this text.

Writers addressing interdisciplinary care in general (Ducanis & Golin, 1979; Margolis & Fiorelli, 1984; Valletutti & Christoplos, 1977) stress that a team is not merely a collection of people and input, but a system to make collaboration effective in best meeting the needs of the patient. Team care is the antithesis of fragmented care. The team needs to operate as one unit with the specified goal of providing the best care for the patient. Indeed, the effective team cannot deviate from being totally patient centered. Ducanis and Golin (1979) succinctly defined an interdisciplinary team as "a functioning unit composed of individuals with varied and specialized training, who coordinate activities to provide services to a client or group of clients" (p. 3).

Herbert Cooper (1979), an orthodontist and strong advocate for interdisciplinary care for persons with cleft lip and palate, commented on the importance of team effort with patient focus:

> Individualism and initiative are to be respected, but a team can succeed only with smooth cooperation by men and women who, while feeling free and independent, are willing to do what is expected of them without friction. They must be motivated to act in the greatest interest of the patient, and in my opinion, the only way to make this philosophy work is to follow the three "C's"—communication, cooperation, and coordination of effort. (p. 9)

Morris (1980) defined the interdisciplinary team by the function performed: "to bring to bear, on the problem-solving process, for the patient, the expertise of relevant science, basic and clinical in an effective and efficient and practical manner" (p. 106).

Many words can describe what an effective team is supposed to do: *communicate, discuss, collaborate, integrate, synthesize, recommend, coordinate, prioritize, cooperate, follow up*, and surely several more. All of these tasks are a part of interdisciplinary function; however, not all teams do equally well with all activities. Better functioning and more mature and effective teams perform more of these tasks successfully. Assembling a certain number of people into a team for some purpose initially may allow for discussion and some level of communication, but it certainly does not ensure coordination, cooperation, or integration. Communication is perhaps the key element to "jump-start" effective interdisciplinary care. Certainly, difficulty in communication among team members and with patients and families is no new revelation (Halfond, 1961; Koepp-Baker, 1952; Lillywhite, 1957; Nackashi & Dixon-Wood, 1989; Strauss, 1999). Valletutti and Christoplos (1977), in discussing interdisciplinary approaches to human services, pointed out that communication is prerequisite to cooperation. They stated,

> Sharing interdisciplinary information is an initial step toward providing a mechanism through which the collective wisdom of individual team members may be marshaled for the purpose of arriving at the most logical, productive, efficient means to remediate the difficulties that clients experience. (p. 1)

In summary, interdisciplinary management for persons with cleft palate requires a cooperative effort to effectively identify the concerns; to recommend, prioritize, and coordinate the treatment plan; and to follow up on treatment objectives. Clearly, the range of concerns that exist for a patient with cleft lip and palate are best addressed by the interdisciplinary approach.

## History and Development of Teams

The advent of health care teams as we know them today dates back to the 1920s. Around that time, there was considerable interest in and movement toward medical specialization. This resulted in much discussion about the potential dangers of specialization if findings and treatments were not satisfactorily coordinated (Barker, 1922).

According to Ducanis and Golin (1979), establishment of teams was influenced by three major factors: (1) the importance of treating the "whole" client, (2) the needs of the organization, and (3) external mandates. Participants in the White House Conference of 1930 espoused the philosophy that treatment of patients must include the whole person and not an isolated part. At the same time, with the increasing trend toward medical and dental specialization, specialty consultations and interdisciplinary coordination of effort became necessary within organizations, rather than fragmented care. At least theoretically, the interdisciplinary team offered a way of organizing personnel, to enhance communication and exchange information concerning clients and patients. In more recent years, external mandates by third-party payors, governmental agencies, and others have demanded professional accountability and improvement in the quality of care. Currently, the team concept is applied to many health areas, as well as educational, vocational, and social programs.

Health care teams have long been a part of rehabilitation services. Whitehouse (1951), a rehabilitative specialist, emphasized the importance of treating the whole person and the importance of teamwork: "Fundamentally, no treatment is medical, social, psychological, vocational—all treatment is total" (p. 45). The team concept for diagnosis and treatment of patients with cleft lip and palate, which surfaced in the 1930s, was likely influenced by similar factors. The first functioning cleft palate team was reported to be in the shared office of James Maby, a maxillofacial surgeon, and Albert MacDougal, an orthodontist (R. Kersten, personal communication, 1970).

Cooper, the orthodontist mentioned previously, was a leading and vocal proponent for the team concept for patients with cleft lip and palate. In 1938, he established the first clinic devoted to interdisciplinary diagnosis and treatment for patients with clefts in Lancaster, Pennsylvania. Cooper (1953, 1979) lobbied for federal support for these patients for several years and pointed out that the National Society for Crippled Children and Adults, which was established in 1919, did not consider patients with cleft lip and palate to be eligible for services. Eligibility was primary for patients with orthopedic problems. Cooper spoke convincingly that patients with cleft palate could be considered "facially crippled." As a result of Cooper's work, most states for many years provided services and financial assistance of some kind for cleft lip and palate and craniofacial disorders as part of what was formerly called Crippled Children's Services and administered federally through the Maternal and Child Health Program.

The interdisciplinary approach for persons with cleft palate became more prevalent yearly, and in 1943, the Academy of Cleft Palate Prosthesis was established. A significant factor in the emergence and subsequent growth of interdisciplinary cleft palate teams was the increasing interest in and recognition of the effect of surgical procedures on facial and dental growth and development. The interconnectedness of surgical repair, facial growth and development, and speech function made cleft lip and palate a natural for the team approach. The name of the professional organization was changed to the American Association for Cleft Palate Rehabilitation in 1949, the American Cleft Palate Association (ACPA) in 1961, and the American Cleft Palate-Craniofacial Association in 1988. In 1955, the association listed 44 teams. As of 2007, there were 211 teams in the United States and Canada and an additional 42 teams from other countries (American Cleft Palate-Craniofacial Association, 2007). Current (2007) membership is over 2,600, representing 33 different disciplines and over 60 different countries. The interested reader is referred to a history of the first 36 years of the American Cleft Palate Association (Wells, 1979). Although the number of organized teams, professional specialists represented, and membership has grown rapidly over the years for cleft and craniofacial care, there has been minimal evaluation and study of teams as a health service for cleft and craniofacial care (Strauss, 1999). Over the last quarter century, remarkable changes have occurred, and continue to occur, in state and national health services and coverage for care.

It is significant that in June 1987, a report by the Surgeon General of the United States called for comprehensive, coordinated care provided by health care systems for children with specific health needs. The ACPA believed it important to provide leadership in establishing criteria for care in response to public funding, health insurance, and managed care forces. Subsequently, the Maternal and Child Health Bureau provided funding to the ACPA for the purpose of recommending practices in the care of children with craniofacial anomalies. A consensus conference was convened in 1991, bringing together experienced multidisciplinary specialists in diagnosis and treatment of craniofacial anomalies, patients and their families, persons with multicultural interests, and representatives from governmental agencies. Resolutions and recommendations were included in a parameters-of-practice document on which at least 75% of the participants agreed. This was followed by a widespread peer review process, committee review and revision, and ratification by conference participants. The *Parameters for Evaluation and Treatment of Patients with Cleft Lip/Palate or Other Craniofacial Anomalies* was approved by the ACPA Executive Committee in 1992, published by the association in 1993, and revised in 2000 and 2004. The 10 fundamental principles reported in the document clearly depend on interdisciplinary enterprise. In fact, the first principle states, "Management of patients with craniofacial anomalies is best provided by an interdisciplinary team of specialists" (p. 5). This document is important because it specifies a standard of care for optimal outcome, useful for patients and families, health care providers, third-party payors, and other funding and governmental agencies. The document also specifies timely review guided by advances in technology and research.

Additionally, and again in proactive response to external health system forces and anticipated mandates, the ACPA worked to establish basic standards for organized teams in the 1990s. A comprehensive questionnaire was sent to all cleft and craniofacial teams listed in the ACPA's *Membership-Team Directory* in 1991. The purpose was to survey team organization, team service, and quality assurance procedures. The response rate was very high (94%). As Strauss and Ellis (1996) noted, this survey provided a starting place for health services research and allowed individual teams to compare their characteristics with other teams.

Strauss (1998) and the ACPA Team Standards Committee reported on the standards of care and the criteria for categorization of teams listed in the *Membership-Team Directory.* Questionnaires were sent to team directors in 1996. The response rate was over 83%. Team categorization was determined on the basis of responses (self-rating process) delineating criteria that permitted directory listing as a cleft palate team, craniofacial team, or both, as well as special categories of teams including evaluation and treatment review only team, interim (developing) team, and low population density team or geographically listed team. Based on the results of the team self-assessment, 84% of the teams listed in the directory were either cleft palate teams or craniofacial teams. As Strauss (1998) pointed out, the self-assessment methodology provided the opportunity for teams to evaluate their role in care delivery and address areas of noncompliance. The findings also have implications for the future of team care and health policy. In summary, it appears clear that the interdisciplinary approach is alive and well, and that the professional association has grown rapidly, has been responsive to external forces and mandates, and faces opportunities and challenges for the future.

# Structure and Function of Interdisciplinary Teams

## Structure

The structure of teams and the manner in which teams organize themselves vary considerably. Decisions regarding who serves, who leads, and what format the operation and procedures should take depend in large part on the team's primary role and the physical setting in which the team operates. The optimal setting for team activities and meetings should be based on the diagnostic and treatment needs of the patient population served. For persons with cleft lip and palate and other craniofacial anomalies, that setting should ideally be a medical and/or dental facility. In certain geographic areas, however, this is not possible, and teams need to meet in less optimal facilities.

Morris (1980) listed several factors that determine any health team's structure: an identifiable common objective, a workable administrative system, a basis for regular team activities, and an atmosphere of respect among members and for the system. Cooper (1979) emphasized that the varying structure of teams depends on goals and function. He stated,

> There is the "vertical" team in which the decisions and the instructions originate at the top, with one person; the other members merely carry out their assigned duties. This works well on the football field where the goal is a straight white line. In a clinic addressing itself to the complex shifting in ramifications of cleft lip and palate, however, it is our experience that a more even distribution of input, a wider sharing of ideas and opinions, among team members, achieves a better result. (p. 9)

Strauss (1999) reviewed literature focusing on craniofacial team organization and described team structure as being hierarchical (leader centered) or egalitarian (fraternally oriented). In the former, authority lies with the team leader, and in the latter, authority is allocated to all members. I personally believe that true and effective interdisciplinary activity demands that all members have equal participation and decision-making authority. Any less diminishes the multifaceted aspects of the disorder. That is to say, because clefting and craniofacial anomalies involve appearance, speech and hearing, dental and occlusal, and psychosocial issues, all team members need to share equally in making decisions.

Although a team may assume a variety of organizational configurations, the focus on cleft lip and palate and other craniofacial disorders requires information and opinions from several specialty areas and a sharing and discussion of that information to contribute to the optimal treatment for the patient. Ultimately, the contribution of the team approach to patient management must be greater and better than the sum of its parts.

## Team Composition

Although for many years there was reasonable justification for a surgeon, dentist, and speech-language pathologist to constitute a core team, the inclusion of representatives from several other disciplines results in a more desirable team. As previously discussed, criteria have been established for basic standards on what constitutes a cleft or craniofacial team (see Strauss, 1998). What constitutes the "desirable" team in terms of size and representation depends on the constellation of concerns of the particular clinical disorder or population. A team focusing on cleft lip and palate often includes a medical and surgical component, which consists of reconstructive surgery, otolaryngology, pediatrics, nursing, and radiology; a dental component, comprising orthodontics, pediatric or family dentistry, prosthodontics, oral and maxillofacial surgery, and dental hygiene; a speech and hearing component, consisting of speech and language pathology and audiology; a psychosocial component, consisting of psychology and social work; and a genetic component, consisting of genetics and genetic counseling. Although not all specialists in each component may be represented at all visits or with every patient, each component is usually represented or readily available for most teams. Team representation would be similar for patients with disorders involving craniofacial structures, but with the addition of at least neurosurgery and ophthalmology.

Personnel decisions about who can and should serve on a particular team can present interesting challenges, and team leaders, members, and administrators frequently follow no predetermined plan or procedure. Sageser (2000) advocated for establishment of a team membership committee that selects new members utilizing established criteria, maintains high professional standards, and regulates participation.

All teams need a leader or an identifiable person to direct and coordinate the team activities, lead the interdisciplinary conference, seek information, facilitate communication and discussion, summarize recommendations of the interdisciplinary team conference, and communicate findings to parents, patients, and the professional community. Margolis and Fiorelli (1984) described an interdisciplinary team leader as an "impartial facilitator" focusing on efficiency of team function. The key is the leader's function, not necessarily his or her professional background or personal style. The leader must serve to ensure that the best service will be provided to the patient. In my view, all conflicts that might arise in team discussion and care can be resolved if indeed all participants are reminded of the sentinel question, "What is the best thing to do for this patient at his or her particular stage of physical and behavioral growth and development?"

Although some teams may favor a change in leadership as the treatment focus changes with the patient's growth and development, I believe there is value in having the same person assume the various leadership functions for an extended time period. In this way, the consumers of the team care product (patient, parent/caregiver, and care provider) experience the stability and assurance of communicating with one person who has knowledge about the history of care. Surgeons are frequently the team leaders; however, teams can be led effectively by persons in any of the participating disciplines. Valletutti and Christoplos (1977) argued that no single profession should assume constant hegemony over any team and that change in leadership should correlate with the patient's changing needs and with the team setting. However, they also noted that leadership function involves execution of the team's decision and reception of the team's advice. Furthermore, it is frequently this person who communicates and interprets the team's findings and recommendations to the patient and/or family. They stated,

> Unless a special rapport exists, successful implementation may be severely threatened. It is no small task to identify and establish the modus operandi for selecting the effective leader(s) to structure organizational pattern, to develop operating rules of the team, and to provide the most effective communication with the client. (p. 11)

## Team Operation and Procedures

The interdisciplinary team approach for persons with cleft lip and palate and other craniofacial anomalies essentially involves referring and identifying patients, scheduling appointments, documenting results of evaluations, and distributing interdisciplinary reports. In addition, for any scheduled appointment, team activity requires interdisciplinary examinations, interdisciplinary conferencing to determine appropriate treatment recommendations, and a sharing of that information with the patient and family. These activities are necessary for any team. Specific procedures utilized to perform these activities, however, vary from team to team and from clinic to clinic. Again, the variability often depends on specific team function and physical setting. For example, a setting such as a large university medical-dental complex may have sophisticated equipment for imaging the dental and craniofacial structures and oral and speech physiology, and for evaluating the speech signal and speech aerodynamics. Therefore, team operation and procedures in this setting involve time to obtain and review this information for interdisciplinary patient examinations and conferencing. In a setting where little, if any, of this equipment is available, patient examinations are more cursory and based on visual and perceptual clinical judgments. In this situation, referral to another facility, perhaps regional, is frequently required for needed diagnostic imaging and instrumental assessments.

The manner in which patients are examined by teams may differ. Some patients are examined by all team members at the same time and in the same room. Subsequently, an interdisciplinary conference is held to determine the appropriate treatment plan. The patient and family may or may not be present at this meeting. If they are not present, usually the team leader, coordinator, social worker, or someone else shares the findings and recommendations with the patient and family. In other settings, patients are examined individually by the team members and, although some interdisciplinary consultation and discussion may occur during that time, full discussion of observations occurs after all the individual examinations have been completed. Unfortunately, in some clinics, not all team members participate in the interdisciplinary conference. Following the individual examinations, these specialists record or write their findings and recommendations for the patient's report but do not (or cannot) attend the interdisciplinary conference. I firmly believe the "heart" of the interdisciplinary approach, however, requires that *all* members of the team engage in face-to-face sharing, discuss and interpret findings, determine patients' needs, inquire about observations, examine the priorities of treatment, and decide on a coordinated treatment plan. This works best for the patient when all members are present and actively participating in a meeting.

## Function

As previously noted, the structure of a given team is dependent on its function. The primary functions of interdisciplinary teams are (1) to provide consultation regarding treatment and/or (2) to prescribe and carry out the treatment. In the first situation, the team members examine and evaluate patients and, through interdisciplinary discussion, recommend a treatment plan. Final decisions are at the discretion of the patient and family and the direct treatment providers. In the second situation, the interdisciplinary team members are the providers; that is, the diagnosis and evaluation team is the treatment team. This is an important distinction and, of course, related directly to how clinics and teams obtain their patients. The professional referring a patient to a team needs to understand the function of a particular clinic or team: to consult regarding treatment of the professional's patient (Situation 1) or to evaluate *and* treat the patient (Situation 2).

Valletutti and Christoplos (1977) discussed the implications of these primary team functions and noted that responsibility of the direct provider, not the team, is crucial in Situation 1, whereas accountability for the treatment outcome rests with the team in Situation 2. Thus, the team functions are similar but for different purposes. The most important function of any team is to provide the best possible service to the patient. To fulfill that purpose, the team organized with a focus on cleft lip and palate and other craniofacial anomalies has several important and related functions:

1. Diagnosis and evaluation
2. Discussion of findings
3. Treatment planning
4. Communication with patient and family
5. Communication with care providers
6. Facilitation and coordination
7. Follow-up on treatment

## Diagnosis and Evaluation

Optimal team function and service requires accurate diagnosis and complete evaluation of the patient's status at his or her stage of growth and development. The information gathering function must be carried out by all team members before they can adequately contribute to interdisciplinary discussion. Information gathering, or data collection as described by Ducanis and Golin (1979), involves thorough review of available information about the patient, based on observation and examination according to each discipline's clinical protocol and perspective, identification of the patient's problems and concerns, and judgment of the patient's treatment needs from a growth and development standpoint. Quantitative and qualitative results of certain physical, physiological, or psychosocial assessments may be available for the patient or performed at the time of the examination. Again, the techniques and methods available for these assessments depend on the team's physical facility. In some instances, the diagnosis and evaluation phase may consist only of clinical observation and on-site examination of the patient.

### Discussion of Findings

Following the information gathering, the team discusses the findings in an interdisciplinary conference. Although some interdisciplinary discussion occurs when two or more members are examining the patient, the opportunity for full team discussion of each specialist's observations, examination results, problems and concerns, and treatment needs is necessary. What occurs in the interdisciplinary discussion of findings can be described variously as sharing, collaborating, learning, convincing, checking, compromising, and so forth. However, it is critical in this phase for the discussion to be, as Koepp-Baker (1979) stated, a "free and open communication." The outcome of discussion should result in an *integration* of the information gathered in order to most efficiently and effectively establish treatment plans. Integration involves interpretation and reporting of the findings so that they are understandable to all team members.

### Treatment Planning

Once the team has sufficiently discussed the findings and integrated the information, the team establishes the treatment plan for the patient. Ducanis and Golin (1979) noted that treatment planning must involve evaluation of the options. For persons with cleft lip and palate and other craniofacial anomalies, evaluation of options must include determining the best or most ideal treatment option; however, alternative approaches, perhaps less than ideal, need to be considered. Indeed, the optimal outcomes may be accomplished with more than a single approach. An example is the treatment of excessive hypernasality due to an inadequate velopharyngeal closure mechanism. Based on all diagnostic information available, the patient may be an excellent candidate for a surgical procedure such as a pharyngeal flap, but also an excellent candidate for construction of a speech prosthesis. Each treatment has advantages and disadvantages that the patient and the family need to fully understand before making a decision. Additionally, the team must be fully informed about and sensitive to family and social situations that constitute "burdens of care," as discussed by Aspinall in Chapter 2.

The treatment planning function for patients with cleft lip and palate involves *prioritizing* treatment plans. Prioritization of treatment, both short term and long term, can be accomplished effectively with full interdisciplinary participation. For example, surgical repair of the alveolar cleft, orthodontic treatment, speech articulation treatment, and restorative dental care may all be strongly indicated for a 9-year-old patient. A key to the best treatment plan is the priority, or desired order, of those treatments. Initiating speech treatment may depend on the timing and extensiveness of orthodontic treatment. Orthodontic cross-bite correction (upper arch expansion) may be desirable before the alveolar cleft is repaired; however, it may be that orthodontic treatment cannot be initiated until the dental restorative work has been completed and oral and dental health have been improved. Therefore, the most appropriate treatment plan may require (1) establishing immediate dental care and home program of oral hygiene, (2) initiating a phase of orthodontic treatment to correct the cross bite, (3) proceeding with repair of the alveolar cleft when orthodontic treatment is completed, and (4) deferring active speech treatment for articulation until bone grafting has been completed. With optimal facilitation, cooperation, and coordination, it may be possible that speech treatment could be initiated in approximately 9–12 months.

The treatment planning function directly implies decision making. With all pertinent information gathered, discussed, and integrated, the guiding question for the clinical decision making regarding the treatment plan is, What is the optimal treatment for this patient at this time and for the future? The patient must be at the "heart" and center of all that occurs.

## Communication with Patient and Family

The team's optimal treatment plan will likely be less successful and indeed compromised if it is not effectively communicated to the patient and family. Although the team may have agreed on a treatment plan, the patient and family must ultimately comply with the plan and, furthermore, actively proceed with the plan. Therefore, an important team function is to communicate the findings, recommendations, and decisions in an understandable manner. It is reasonable to assume that the degree to which patients and families pursue team recommendations is related to communication among teams, care providers, and patients and families. Studies have been sparse on compliance with team recommendations by patients with cleft lip and palate and their families. However, Paynter, Jordan, and Finch (1990) investigated the degree of compliance with interdisciplinary team recommendations over an 8-year period. They obtained responses from the most appropriate person who could provide that information.

They found a range of compliance from 0% to 100%, with a mean of 64%. In their analysis, they classified only 17% as full compliers, 78% as partial compliers, and 5% as noncompliers. Obviously, there was considerable variability. No factors were found to be significantly related to compliance. In this study and others carried out regarding patient and family compliance (Topic, 1987; Westra, 1982), patient and family *understanding* of the treatment recommendations was not assessed.

Paynter, Edmonson, and Jordan (1991) compared the information that parents and children with cleft palate *demonstrated* about team recommendations made. (The authors were careful not to use the word *understanding* because of the difficulty in interpretation.) They found that parents demonstrated accurate information about the team recommendations at an 80% level, whereas the children demonstrated a 67% level of accuracy. Interestingly, parents were able to estimate their children's responses quite accurately. In a subsequent report, Paynter, Wilson, and Jordan (1993) noted improved patient compliance when steps were taken by the team to improve patient compliance with team recommendations and to identify variables that interfered with compliance. In this study, the authors found mean compliance rates of 82% compared to 64% reported in the 1990 study.

A survey conducted by Pannbacker and Scheuerle (1993) assessed the extent to which parents were and desired to be involved in treatment decisions. Of these parents, 57% reported satisfaction with their involvement in treatment decisions, 36% wished for more involvement, and only 7% wished for less involvement.

The above studies, I believe, demonstrate the importance of effective communication of team findings and recommendations to optimize the patient's and family's understanding of the rationale for treatment and their role in making final decisions to proceed with treatment. It is important to recognize that team recommendations and decisions are made collectively and may present ethical issues. Sharp (1995) discussed the processes of team decision making and presented a model for clinical and ethical decision making. Issues about clinical indications for treatment, timing of treatment, patient preferences, and informed consent are discussed by Sharp in Chapter 3.

## Communication with Care Providers

The interdisciplinary team needs to communicate the findings, recommendations, and treatment plan to persons involved with the patient's welfare and persons providing direct care. As previously discussed, the consultative team may not comprise any of the patient's direct providers. In this case, because final decisions to carry out treatments rest with the family and specific care providers, communication is an important and necessary team function. Usually, a team distributes a clinic report and/or letter to all appropriate providers, agencies, and payors.

### Facilitation and Coordination

Team functions of facilitation and coordination may occur during the interdisciplinary conference or after the conference. These functions relate directly to the often-cited advantages of the team approach—efficiency and effectiveness. For example, a patient requires surgical revision of the nose (perhaps at 16–18 years of age), removal of the wisdom teeth, and exploratory middle ear surgery. All these procedures can be done at the same time, thus avoiding multiple hospitalizations, administrations of anesthesia, and outpatient visits. This facilitation and coordination of treatment is most likely to occur with the interdisciplinary team approach.

### Follow-up on Treatment

It should be quite obvious that interdisciplinary team care for persons with cleft lip and palate is not a one-time event. Treatment is long term and associated with physical and behavioral growth and development. Follow-up, or follow-through (Koepp-Baker, 1979), is an integral function of the team. In this activity, the team can document and measure patient progress toward optimal outcome. Patient records consisting of speech recordings, audiometric data, photographs and a radiographs, speech physiological data, psychosocial and growth and development information, and so forth, can be evaluated and compared. Through the team function of follow-up, treatment can proceed in the right direction—one step at a time—most effectively and efficiently.

Although not listed as a specific team function, research and education are other important functions of interdisciplinary teams. Interdisciplinary teams in academic institutions and/or medical-dental environments can serve as a rich resource for training future members of health care teams and providers of care for persons with cleft lip and palate and other craniofacial anomalies. Furthermore, data obtained through patient observation and examination over many years can be fertile ground for research activities. Systematic, detailed, and standardized documentation by all specialties can contribute to better understanding of the effect of certain treatments that ultimately lead to improved care.

# Interdisciplinary Team Issues

To this point, I have considered some assumptions and biases about interdisciplinary management, reviewed historical development of teams, and discussed team structure and function. It should be no surprise that some teams flourish more than others and, by a variety of criteria, are more effective. Although interdisciplinary teams with satisfactory structure and defined goals and functions *can* provide the best and most effective and efficient management, not all teams are as "successful" as others. Several issues can be explored regarding interdisciplinary team management for persons with cleft lip and palate and other craniofacial disorders; however, discussion here is limited to issues related to team value, team quality, and team future.

## Team Value

Reasonable questions and issues have been raised over many years about the advantages and, in fact, need for interdisciplinary teams. As mentioned previously, Barker (1922) cautioned about the dangers of increasing specialization without adequate coordination and integration. Curtin (1962) asked several questions about cleft palate teams: Does a team of specialists threaten the time-honored and personal doctor-patient relationship? Do teams tend to submerge and inhibit individual initiative? Is the team approach an efficient method of providing health services? However, despite asking the hard questions, Curtin concluded, "We can no longer thrive in the backwoods of individual specialties, but need to join with the allied disciplines in an effort to increase our understanding of all dimensions of the patient's needs and to improve standards of care" (p. 292). Others have raised questions and cited certain difficulties with team care (Halfond, 1961; Kummer, 2001; Lillywhite, 1957; Patterson, 1959; Sidman, 1995); however, all have concluded that there is decided value in the interdisciplinary approach.

Support for the value of interdisciplinary cleft palate and craniofacial care is not hard to find. The specialization versus holistic controversy seems nicely resolved with effective interdisciplinary management. Although a good deal of person power, time, and energy are required in interdisciplinary activity, Valletutti and Christoplos (1977) pointed out that teams provide a check against hasty decisions made by individuals who do not face peer accountability. They also pointed out that, at the same time, teams sometimes stifle creativity and unorthodox approaches to solving problems. I personally believe the latter does not need to be true: Creativity *can* and, in fact, *should* flourish on teams while checks and balances are maintained. In a very real sense, teams can offer the best of both worlds—the best treatment may be cutting-edge and innovative, but also be most appropriate and practical. As discussed previously, the 1991 consensus conference of the ACPA clearly advocated for the team approach.

Although there appears to be overwhelming anecdotal support for interdisciplinary activity—not only in cleft palate and craniofacial disorders, but in a variety of medical-dental, social, educational, and vocational areas—there is no scientific evidence at this time for concluding it is the best approach. According to Whitehouse (1965), "Team work as a method has been so logically appealing and so seemingly an obvious solution to the 'whole man' commitment as well as to the issue of specialization, that the practice has developed without examination of the premises" (p. 16). Valletutti and Christoplos (1977) noted that there are no guidelines for patients to determine whether the team effort is more beneficial than individual effort. There are no "hard data" regarding comparative effects of team versus individual effort. In the absence of clear support, decisions are left to chance or to the inclinations and sophistication of the patient and to persons, agencies, and third-party payors referring patients.

Ducanis and Golin (1979) summarized some of the limited research concerning evaluation of team effectiveness. Other than the previously mentioned studies of patient compliance, no controlled or comparative studies have investigated the effectiveness of cleft palate or craniofacial teams. Ducanis and Golin (1979) raised some interesting evaluation issues in investigating team effectiveness, including what to evaluate and how to measure "effectiveness" or "success." Research issues about team systems might involve relationships among team variables such as structural aspects, function, and outcome. Strauss and Ellis (1996) stated, "As organizations, cleft/craniofacial teams have received little study as a health service" (p. 130).

Questions such as "Does therapy work?" or "Is treatment approach A more effective than treatment approach B?" are not easy to answer in the scientific sense. Siegel (1987) commented that these questions may not be appropriate for research. He wrote that research on clinical outcome is confounded by so many variables that cannot be controlled that any conclusions are rendered meaningless. Siegel stated that science is a "very powerful tool for answering the questions it was designed to answer, but there are realms where science is not the most effective approach to elucidating and solving problems" (p. 311). Perhaps, as he suggested, the issue is not whether therapy or a therapy approach works, but whether the benefits exceed the cost, and these are questions of values. Kent (1990) argued that it is indeed appropriate to ask whether one treatment approach is more effective than another and that answers are possible only through therapeutic outcome research. He stated that outcome research is needed to determine how treatment can be more efficient and effective. Kent clearly felt that clinical service issues should not be dissociated from research. More recently, in a state-of-the-art paper on delivery of craniofacial health services, Strauss (1999) recognized the importance of the scientific study of cleft and craniofacial teams as organizations but acknowledged that little research has been done and that there are inherent barriers to investigating team versus nonteam benefits. He stated that one barrier to constructing comparative research studies relates to the systematic differences between patients who seek team care and those who do not. Teams are more likely than solo, community-based clinicians to attract patients with more complex biological and/or social needs. Furthermore, according to Strauss it is difficult to identify study samples of persons being cared for outside the team context (p. 192).

More on patient outcome appears later in this chapter; however, the primary test or measure of team value and success in cleft lip and palate and other craniofacial disorders must be some measure of outcome. The success of the team approach needs to be evaluated in terms of all factors that eventually contribute to outcome—clinical service, research, and education.

## Team Quality

What are the characteristics of the excellent team? Why are some teams more "effective," "successful," "smooth running," and "healthy" than others? Although these are subjective descriptions, nobody would argue with the notion that some teams seem to function more efficiently and effectively than others. Certainly, aspects of organizational structure and function are important, but team dynamics and personal interaction also contribute significantly to team quality and health. Valletutti and Christoplos (1977) stated that efficiency is meaningless without effectiveness.

Koepp-Baker (1979) postulated that outcomes of group interaction to make effective decisions and solve problems are contingent on meeting two conditions: the *quality* of the decision based on the objective information available and the *acceptability* of the decision based on human feelings, attitudes, and biases. Clearly, the interdisciplinary approach to determining treatment in craniofacial disorders involves *people* making clinical decisions. We are not yet near the situation where bits of information can be fed into a computer that ultimately prints out the most appropriate treatment. There are simply too many important bits of information, some of which are not quantifiable and some of which are people-generated judgments based on quantitative as well as qualitative information.

Whitehouse (1965) described teamwork as a dynamic system. He pointed out that the successful team

> is effective not primarily because of the quality of its individual components but to the extent to which each component is complementary to, contributes to, and mutually enhances each other so that the main purposes and goals may be achieved. (p. 17)

## Personal Characteristics of Team Members

Interdisciplinary teams consist of people with varying perspectives, training, experience, and, indeed, personality. A myriad of personal characteristics—both positive and negative—contribute to team quality. The following represent, in my judgment, some of the more important ones:

1. *Interest in the patient and the disorder*—Strong interest in contributing to the welfare of patients with cleft lip and palate and craniofacial disorders is essential. The patient must be the highest priority! Team members must view team participation as contribution to the whole patient, not to isolated parts.
2. *Willingness to share openly*—Team recommendations and decisions are based on complete information and input from all specialists involved. There needs to be full and open communication of findings and judgments.
3. *Mutual respect*—Each team member must have respect for each other member as a person, as well as for each discipline. Team

members need a good understanding of what each discipline can and cannot do.

4. *Equal partnership*—There should be a feeling or perception that all members contribute equally to the team function. All members need to be confident in themselves as professionals and be convinced that their profession contributes to the whole. Equal partnership in team function is critical because it "encourages freedom to grow, gives opportunity for open presentation of opinions, tends to educate each member of the group, develops mature responsibility, and strengthens pride in professional integrity" (Whitehouse, 1951, p. 52).
5. *Motivation to learn*—A characteristic of persons associated with high-quality teams is the desire to learn from each other about the disorder and to remain knowledgeable about new findings in their respective disciplines. Team members should not be satisfied with current techniques for evaluation and management, but should continually update their knowledge and understanding. Certainly, contributing new information through research enhances team quality and health.

Margolis and Fiorelli (1984) suggested four constructs useful for enhancing cooperation among members of teams: (1) understanding the unique perceptual field of each discipline, (2) reducing interdisciplinary defensiveness, (3) collaboratively developing ideas, and (4) encouraging two-way rather than one-way communication. Clearly, optimal cooperation and communication are at the heart of high-quality teams.

Successful teams communicate results to appropriate persons effectively and efficiently. Immediate feedback to the patient and family, direct care providers, appropriate agencies, and third-party payors is critical. When there is open communication among the patient and family, interdisciplinary team, and care providers outside the team, the interdisciplinary approach can be very successful.

Can the quality of team care be measured? Ingelhart (1996) clearly recognized that the science of quality assessment is in its infancy and that attempts to measure quality through an accreditation process are "fledgling" ones and influenced primarily by the purchasers of health care. Ultimately, it seems to me that the measure of quality must be associated with how the outcome is measured, and this will be addressed later in this chapter.

## Interdisciplinary Problems and Cautionary Notes

It should be clear at this point that effective team function does not merely happen with the formation of a team. Over the years, writers have commented on certain problems of the interdisciplinary approach. Whitehouse (1951) pointed out that just because a group of persons admits interest in a problem does not guarantee cooperation and efficiency. He discussed several factors that inhibit what teamwork attempts to accomplish: (1) Professionals are not necessarily cooperative persons, (2) some professionals are unwilling to admit that others can accomplish a goal more effectively and efficiently, and (3) the team's goals may be too high and not practically obtainable.

Team evaluation and treatment planning for persons with cleft lip and palate may confuse the patient and family because a variety of opinions and treatment possibilities are inherent in the process. Indeed, determining various options is one of the functions of the interdisciplinary approach. Inadequate communication within the team (Lillywhite, 1957), as well as between the family and the team (Spriestersbach, 1973), can be a potential major problem. Spriestersbach (1973) noted that patients and families do not always understand all the information, do not always know what they want to know, are afraid to ask "silly" questions, and are confused by the "conflicting" advice from experts on the team. The antidote for this situation is more effective communication by the team leader or coordinator to summarize to the patient and family the team's discussion, differences, conclusions, and decisions. Thus, the team enterprise is not merely a listing of things that each specialist considers appropriate from his or her area of expertise, but must be a unified and cohesive plan developed by all the specialists.

Another frequently cited complaint is that teams can appear impersonal to patients and families. Again, teams need to take precautions to prevent this impression from occurring. Families can have an important impact on decisions made and treatment pursued, but some families wish to be more involved than others (Pannbacker & Scheuerle, 1993). At least one team member—someone with whom the family feels comfortable—needs to be identified as the effective communicator with the patient and family. Typically, that person is the leader or coordinator, but any member of the team can serve this function.

The patient and family must perceive the team's recommendations as a well-integrated whole, not as unrelated parts. Again, no treatment is medical, social, psychologic, or vocational—all treatment is total

(Whitehouse, 1951). Similarly, no treatment is related solely to oral surgery, orthodontics, speech, or otology. Campbell and Gooch (1988) suggested that interdisciplinary course instruction "should look seamless to the students" (p. 8). Similarly, interdisciplinary treatment should look seamless to the patient. Patients need to view the team as one large provider. Distinct professional boundaries should not be obvious.

Although team operation and procedure can be cumbersome and may appear to lack efficiency at times, teams enable the patient to see, and have the opportunity to consult with, several professionals at one visit. An added bonus is that those professionals can communicate with each other to make appropriate and specific interdisciplinary recommendations.

Interdisciplinary activity is clearly more time-consuming than one individual making a decision; however, if that one professional attempted to obtain information from all appropriate specialists, the time and energy required would be greater than with established interdisciplinary procedures. Margolis and Fiorelli (1984) cautioned that some "view team meetings as isolated time-bound entities rather than as products of, and contributing to, an ongoing rehabilitative and interpersonal process" (p. 13).

Another potential problem with interdisciplinary team activity is lack of patient focus. At times, team members can get caught up with their own activities and concerns, leading to professional overlap of treatment, which can then result in defensive behavior. The focus in such cases becomes more directed at the team members themselves rather than the patient. Clearly, there are recommended treatments for patients where there is common interest, skill, and scope of practice by more than one member or clinical discipline. With varying geographic areas, institutional settings, or specific team practice history, "turf wars" can occur. Strauss and Ellis (1996) addressed "team ideology" and pointed out that too much emphasis on process (a within-team focus) can create problems, whereas emphasis on outcome is more patient oriented and better meets the needs of the patient. Strauss (1999) also discussed situations in which interprofessional tension occurs, such as when multiple surgical specialists are all trained and capable in performing a particular surgery. He noted that these "conflicts have the potential for being destructive to the team process and continuity of patient care" (p. 191). Although I agree that tensions can and do occur, the remedy is in the team members' perceptions that the patients' needs are first priority. Team characteristics and personal attributes of the team members, as previously discussed, are paramount in alleviating this problem.

Koepp-Baker (1979) noted that team procedures can become routine and pedestrian behavior, resulting in a feeling of weariness or dissatisfaction on the part of some members. He suggested that research and continued education are corrective measures for boredom. Each interdisciplinary conference can and should be an educational experience; the desire to inform and be informed must be prevalent on teams.

## Team Future

What is the future of interdisciplinary teams? Will the importance and impact of team management for persons with cleft lip and palate and other craniofacial anomalies increase? The factors discussed early in this chapter contributing to the development and formation of interdisciplinary teams continue to exist—the concept about caring for the whole person, the needs of the organization (specialization), and external mandates (Ducanis & Golin, 1979). Indeed, it is likely that increased numbers of specialists will be providing care for each patient with a particular craniofacial disorder. Furthermore, there is increasing demand for professionals to deliver the highest standards of care, as efficiently and economically as possible. This demand comes from several sources: consumers of services (patients and families), referral sources (private practitioners, professional groups, agencies), and third-party payors.

The concept of establishing regional centers for cleft palate and craniofacial evaluation and treatment, based on criteria determined by others, likely will continue to be debated along with new established ACPA criteria and standards. Brown and Cohen (1990) discussed a 10-year experience in New Jersey. Three centers were selected to provide interdisciplinary diagnostic services and treatment to persons with cleft lip and palate and/or associated craniofacial anomalies and/or velopharyngeal problems, "thus bringing to an end the isolated, independent approach of earlier years with its lack of beneficial cost-effectiveness and quality control" (p. 2). The specific guidelines and criteria that had to be met were established by the state before the centers were selected. Brown and Cohen reported that regionalization and creation of state standards with this contractual system for providing service have significantly reduced the cost of the care. They also believed that quality of care is improved when specialized care is provided in a limited number of centers. Although cost-effective, quality service is a laudable goal, an important issue is who sets the standards. Shprintzen (1990), referring to the New Jersey government sanction formula, questioned whether it is ethical for the state to determine the standards and raised issues of patient and provider rights.

Certainly, patients with clefts and their families want to receive the best care, and interdisciplinary professionals want to provide the best care. Remember the mission statement of the ACPA (2005): "to optimize interdisciplinary care." Remember the first principle of the Parameters of Care document (1993, 2000, 2004): "Management of patients with craniofacial anomalies is best provided by an interdisciplinary team of specialists." We as practitioners cannot be content to simply verbalize the above statements. We must recognize and appreciate the external forces that will affect the future of teams. In my view, two of the most important include (1) evidence that team care results in the best possible (optimal) outcome and (2) appropriate third-party reimbursement for interdisciplinary diagnosis, evaluation, and treatment. These forces, discussed in the following paragraphs, are not mutually exclusive.

## Optimal Outcome

Strauss (1999) stated, "The health outcomes of craniofacial team management have not yet been established in the research literature, though clinicians and administrators report many advantages of team-based care over fragmented community-based, multidisciplinary care" (p. 190). As discussed previously, there are inherent difficulties and limitations in the design and implementation of research to scientifically determine the outcome and benefits of team care, given the myriad of variables that are difficult if not impossible to control (Kent, 1990; Siegel, 1987; Strauss, 1999). However, this does not mean that professionals should not continue to search for what constitutes high-quality, efficient, and effective team function that leads to optimal outcome for the patient. Indeed, there is no universal agreement about just what optimal outcome is and how outcome can best be measured. The Parameters of Care document (1993, 2000, 2004) is a good start to establishing basic team practices and longitudinal assessments, but it does not address how outcome ultimately is to be measured. Outcome, by some definitions, is the criteria by which any therapy or treatment is measured. In recent years, there has been an increased call and attention to outcome research. Databases have been developed and utilized by individual centers and on a national level for the ultimate purpose of assessing clinical outcome and establishing standards of care.

Morris, Jakobi, and Harrington (1978) reported the results of two conferences conducted to identify standards of care for cleft lip and palate management. They cited several reasons why standards of care are needed: significant advances in treatment over time, the need for treatment goals and results to be evaluated and assessed, the fact that many practitioners are legally qualified to provide services but have little experience or knowledge about the disorder, and the variability of the disorder and its effects on patients and families.

According to Paul Ellwood (1990), president and chair of the Board of InterStudy, a nonprofit research group dealing with health care issues, it is important to determine precisely what outcome is desirable. For example, in heart bypass surgery, is the outcome an issue of life versus death or pain versus no pain? What is the desired outcome in the treatment of persons with cleft lip and palate: acceptable appearance, dental function, and communication skills, or possibly career success? And how are these outcomes to be measured? Ellwood challenged practitioners with a concept called "outcomes management"—the effect of treatment on patients' "well-being." This concept is based on continuous clinical trials, with no one person, group, or category excluded. He stated that outcomes management must be based on sound epidemiological principles, not merely casual observation, to determine the impact of treatment on quality of life. Practitioners need to refocus on how outcome can be assessed in a standard fashion: Can a protocol be developed on how to describe patients and specific desirable outcomes? Ellwood concluded, perhaps correctly, that practitioners need to be assured that what they are doing in health care produces a beneficial effect. Interestingly, he identified interdisciplinary management for persons with cleft lip and palate as an example of pursuing the appropriate thing for many years.

Ellwood (1988) stated that the outcomes management concept allows patients and families to be more involved in decision making for their care in conjunction with their providers and health maintenance organizations (HMOs). However, for this to be effective, "powerful" databases need to be generated where one of the very important bits of data is quality-of-life (well-being) information. Furthermore, he opined that there is a need to identify and measure "functional outcomes" and that the "most controversial element in the outcomes management concept is the starting point—the increasing reliance on standards or assessments for medical intervention" (p. 1553).

Epstein (1990) cautioned that although the outcomes management concept, as defined by Ellwood, is appropriate and "good," we as professionals need to move slowly and perhaps modify our expectations about what the goals of outcomes management can accomplish. In my judgment, we clearly need to focus more on patient quality-of-life outcomes in cleft and craniofacial care. We spend considerable time defining the "standards and guidelines" for our patients' communication, facial appearance, and functional and aesthetic dental relationships, but clearly devote less time to seeking information directly from our patients about their well-being. We all need to work harder to heed this principle from the ACPA Parameters document (1993, 2000, 2004): "Evaluation of treatment outcomes must take into account the *satisfaction* and psychosocial well-being of the patient as well as effects on growth, function, and appearance" [italics added].

### Reimbursement for Services

Reimbursement for treatment and, indeed, for interdisciplinary diagnosis, evaluation, and treatment planning services will also have a significant impact on the future of teams. As discussed above, third-party payors first need to be convinced of the economic wisdom of comprehensive coordinated team care for persons with clefts and craniofacial disorders. As Strauss (1999) stated, "decisions about funding of team-based care will be made based on evidence that cost-conscious *and* comprehensive treatment can most effectively be provided through the cleft/craniofacial team" (p. 194). However, the amount and distribution of dollar resources provided for the required surgical, dental, speech and hearing, and other therapies will continue to be a major issue. Strauss (1994) addressed several health policy and resource allocation concerns in the ever-changing national health delivery systems. Managed care networks seem particularly resistant to reimbursing multispecialty care. I have taken great delight in personally visiting with third-party payors and extending invitations to their policy makers to attend interdisciplinary conferences and to carefully peruse and read interdisciplinary team reports for their members. It requires no genius to conclude that there is economic advantage in performing three to four surgical procedures with one hospitalization and anesthesia, as recommended by an interdisciplinary team. Quite frankly, I would think third-party payors would want to mandate periodic interdisciplinary team diagnosis, evaluation, and treatment planning, because it can be so cost-effective for them.

It is very curious and frustrating to me that there is no Current Procedural Terminology (CPT) code for comprehensive interdisciplinary diagnosis, evaluation, and treatment planning services. The CPT is a listing of codes and descriptions for procedures, services, and supplies published by the American Medical Association. These codes are frequently used to bill insurance carriers for diagnosis codes (*ICD-9-CM*, 2006). It appears possible for a surgeon to use CPT codes, perform multiple surgeries at various and perhaps somewhat capricious times, and receive reimbursement. I believe interdisciplinary evaluation and treatment planning is critical for appropriate and timely treatment, whether that treatment is center based or community based. Although the process involved in establishing a CPT code is not simple, I believe professionals involved in cleft lip and palate and other craniofacial disorders should continue to pursue appropriate coding.

For several years, the ACPA has aggressively explored the means to establish a CPT code for interdisciplinary evaluation and treatment planning activity. If accurate diagnosis, interdisciplinary evaluation, and treatment planning and coordination are truly important, then there should be a code or uniform description of that service that can be used for reimbursement. In his keynote address to the 2004 ACPA annual meeting in Chicago, Michael Maves, executive vice president and chief executive officer of the American Medical Association, expressed encouragement and support for pursuing this activity. Dr. Maves correctly pointed out that typical CPT reimbursement has historically focused on *individual* services, by individual providers, for individual patients. He noted that team care (as discussed in this chapter) for persons with clefts fulfills a critical need—convenience, coordination, and compassion. Maves noted further that there are some "team" codes currently in effect (end-stage renal disease, neonatal and pediatric critical care) and others have been proposed (comprehensive cancer care, comprehensive geriatric care).

With the partnership of ACPA and the American Speech-Language-Hearing Association (ASHA), an important step was recently accomplished toward CPT coding for speech-language pathologists' and audiologists' participation in medical team conferencing. Beginning in 2008, two new CPT codes were available for medical team conferencing by a non-physician qualified health care professional, such as speech-language pathologists and audiologists. One code (99366) could be used with an interdisciplinary team of health care professionals, face-to-face *with* patient and/or family for 30 minutes or more, and another (99368) for similar activity, but *without* patient or family present. Although this is clearly a positive step forward, there still remains no *one* code for collective activity of the interdisciplinary team. Our profession continues to strongly advocate for coding options that accurately and appropriately reflect the valuable contributions of interdisciplinary team assessment and management.

## Final Thoughts

Education and training about the interdisciplinary approach—the issues, opportunities, and future challenges—must be a priority. There should be increased emphasis on education of professionals in the interdisciplinary process at the undergraduate, graduate, and professional continuing education levels. Furthermore, workshops, symposia, and conferences are helpful for persons currently serving on interdisciplinary teams. Clark Starr, my mentor and coeditor of the first edition of this book, frequently said it is only fair to critique an approach after you have experienced it, observed it, or participated in it. For those readers who have not had the professional opportunity, or who have chosen not to, I strongly encourage you to observe and hopefully participate in interdisciplinary activity.

The following chapters of this text are written by experienced professionals who are committed to the interdisciplinary approach. This book is intended to give the reader knowledge about the disciplines involved, their procedures, and the multiple medical, surgical, dental, speech, language, hearing, psychosocial, cultural, family, and ethical issues that impact management of cleft lip and palate and other craniofacial disorders. This chapter closes with a statement made by L. F. Barker in 1922 to his New York State medical colleagues. The interdisciplinary message is relevant today, and will be for a long time to come.

> The conception of a diagnostic survey of a patient as a whole (with full consideration of all the somatic, psychic, and social elements concerned), though relatively new, is rapidly growing in appreciation in the minds as well as in those of the producers of medical services. All are coming to recognize the dangers of an ever-increasing medical specialization that does not provide for proper coordination of the activities of the specialists and the suitable integration of the results of their work; only through such coordination and integration can unified diagnostic conclusions be safely arrived at, conclusions on which a comprehensive therapeutic regimen dare be based and executed. (p. 777)

# References


American Cleft Palate-Craniofacial Association. (1993). *Parameters for evaluation and treatment of patients with cleft lip/palate or other craniofacial anomalies.* (Revised 2000 and 2004). 2004 revision retrieved September 13, 2007, from www.acpa-cpf .org/teamcare

American Cleft Palate-Craniofacial Association. (2005–2006). *Membership-team directory.* Chapel Hill, NC: Author.

Barker, L. F. (1922, March 18). The specialist and the general practitioner in relation to team-work in medical practice. *Journal of the American Medical Association, 78,* 773–779.

Brown, A. S., & Cohen, M. A. (1990). The New Jersey experience. *Cleft Palate Journal, 27,* 1–2.

Bzoch, K. R. (2004). *Communicative disorders related to cleft palate* (5th ed.). Austin, TX: PRO-ED.

Campbell, W. E., & Gooch, V. (1988). Philosophical biology or biological philosophy? In V. Turdik (Ed.), *Focus on teaching and learning* (Vol. 3, No. 3). Minneapolis: University of Minnesota, Office of Educational Development Program.

Centers for Disease Control. (2006, January 6). Improved national prevalence estimates for 18 selected major birth defects—United States, 1999–2001. *MMWR Weekly, 54*(51 & 52), 1301–1305. Retrieved September 13, 2007, from www.cdc.gov

Cooper, H. K. (1953). Integration of services in the treatment of cleft lip and palate. *Journal of the American Dental Association, 47,* 27–32.

Cooper, H. K. (1979). Historical perspectives and philosophy of treatment. In H. K. Cooper, R. L. Harding, W. M. Krogman, M. Mazaheri, & R. T. Millard (Eds.), *Cleft palate and cleft lip: A team approach to clinical management and rehabilitation of the patient.* Philadelphia: Saunders.

Curtin, J. W. (1962). A surgeon's evaluation of the cleft palate team. *Plastic and Reconstructive Surgery, 29,* 289–292.

Ducanis, A. J., & Golin, A. K. (1979). *The interdisciplinary health care team.* Germantown, MD: Aspen Systems.

Ellwood, P. M. (1988). Outcomes management: A technology of patient experience. *New England Journal of Medicine, 318,* 1549–1556.

Ellwood, P. (1990). *Patient outcome research: Trends in the 90's.* Invited presentation to the American Cleft Palate-Craniofacial Association, St. Louis, MO.

Epstein, A. M. (1990). The outcomes movement: Will it get us where we want to go? *New England Journal of Medicine, 323,* 266–270.

Halfond, M. M. (1961). *The team approach—cum grano salis.* Abstract of paper presented at the American Association for Cleft Palate Rehabilitation, Montreal, ON.

*ICD-9-CM* (9th rev.). (2008). Downers Grove, IL: PMIC.

Ingelhart, J. K. (1996). The National Committee for Quality Assurance. *New England Journal of Medicine, 335,* 995–999.

Kent, R. D. (1990). Fragmentation of clinical service and clinical science in communicative disorders. *National Student Speech Language Hearing Association Journal, 17,* 4–16.

Koepp-Baker, H. (1952, October 4–8). Presidential address, American Association for Cleft Palate Rehabilitation. *Cleft Palate Bulletin, 2*(4).

Koepp-Baker, H. (1979). The craniofacial team. In K. R. Bzoch (Ed.), *Communicative disorders related to cleft lip and palate.* Boston: Little, Brown.

Kummer, A. W. (2001). *Cleft palate and craniofacial anomalies.* San Diego, CA: Singular.

Lillywhite, H. (1957). Communication problems in the cleft palate rehabilitation team. *Cleft Palate Bulletin, 7,* 8–10.

Lis, E. F., Pruzansky, S., Koepp-Baker, H., & Kobes, H. (1956). Cleft lip and cleft palate: Perspectives in management. *Pediatric Clinics of North America, 3*(4), 995–1028.

Margolis, H., & Fiorelli, J. S. (1984). An applied approach to facilitating interdisciplinary teamwork. *Journal of Rehabilitation, 50,* 13–17.

Moller, K. T., & Starr, C. D. (1993). *Cleft palate: Interdisciplinary issues and treatment.* Austin, TX: PRO-ED.

Morris, H. L. (1980). The structure and function of interdisciplinary health teams. In C. F. Salinas & R. J. Jorgenson (Eds.), *Dentistry in the interdisciplinary treatment of genetic diseases* (Birth Defects: Original Article Series, Vol. 16, No. 5). New York: Alan R. Lis.

Morris, H. L., Jakobi, P., & Harrington, D. (1978). Objectives and criteria for management of cleft lip and palate and the delivery of management services. *Cleft Palate Journal, 15,* 1–5.

Nackashi, J. A., & Dixon-Wood, V. L. (1989). The craniofacial team: Medical supervision and coordination. In K. R. Bzoch (Ed.), *Communicative disorders related to cleft lip and palate.* Austin, TX: PRO-ED.

Pannbacker, M., & Scheuerle, J. (1993). Parents' attitudes toward family involvement in cleft palate treatment. *Cleft Palate-Craniofacial Journal, 30,* 87–89.

Patterson, C. H. (1959). Is the team concept obsolete? *Journal of Rehabilitation, 25,* 9–10.

Paynter, E. T., Edmonson, T. W., & Jordan, W. J. (1991). Accuracy of information reported by parents and children evaluated by a cleft palate team. *Cleft Palate-Craniofacial Journal, 28,* 329–337.

Paynter, E. T., Jordan, W. J., & Finch, D. L. (1990). Patient compliance with cleft palate team regimens. *Journal of Speech and Hearing Disorders, 55,* 740–750.

Paynter, E. T., Wilson, B. M., & Jordan, W. J. (1993). Improved patient compliance with cleft palate team regimens. *Cleft Palate-Craniofacial Journal, 30,* 292–301.

Peterson-Falzone, S. J., Hardin-Jones, M. A., & Karnell, M. P. (2002). *Cleft palate speech.* St. Louis, MO: Mosby.

Sageser, I. H. (2000). *The approach to craniofacial team membership: Who should be a member?* Paper presented at the American Cleft Palate-Craniofacial Meeting, Seattle, WA.

Sharp, H. M. (1995). Ethical decision-making in interdisciplinary team care. *Cleft Palate-Craniofacial Journal, 32,* 495–499.

Shprintzen, R. J. (1990). Editorial: Who sets the standards. *Cleft Palate Journal, 27,* 92–93.

Shprintzen, R. J. (1995). A new perspective on clefting. In R. J. Bardach (Eds.), *Cleft palate speech management—A multidisciplinary approach.* St. Louis, MO: Mosby.

Sidman, J. D. (1995). The team approach to cleft and craniofacial disorders: The down side (Editorial). *Cleft Palate-Craniofacial Journal, 32,* 363.

Siegel, G. M. (1987). The limits of science in communication disorders. *Journal of Speech and Hearing Disorders, 52,* 306–312.

Spriestersbach, D. C. (1973). *Psychosocial aspects of the cleft palate problem* (Vol. 1). Iowa City: University of Iowa Press.

Strauss, R. P. (1994). Health policy and craniofacial care: Issues in resource allocation. *Cleft Palate-Craniofacial Journal, 31,* 78–80.

Strauss, R. P. (1997). Social and psychological perspectives on cleft lip and palate. In K. R. Bzoch (Ed.), *Communicative disorders related to cleft palate.* Austin, TX: PRO-ED.

Strauss, R. P. (1998). Cleft Palate and Craniofacial Teams in the United States and Canada: A national survey of team organization and standards of care. *Cleft Palate-Craniofacial Journal, 35,* 473–480.

Strauss, R. P. (1999). The organization and delivery of craniofacial health services: The state of the art. *Cleft Palate-Craniofacial Journal, 36,* 189–195.

Strauss, R. P., & Ellis, J. H. P. (1996). Comprehensive team management. In T. A. Turvey, K. W. L. Vig, & R. J. Fonseca (Eds.), *Facial clefts and craniosynostosis: Principles and management.* Philadelphia: Saunders.

Topic, M. (1987). *A study of compliance of patients/families seen in a cleft palate clinic.* Unpublished master's thesis, University of Minnesota, Minneapolis.

Valletutti, P. J., & Christoplos, F. (1977). *Interdisciplinary approaches to human services.* Baltimore: University Park Press.

Wells, C. (1979). The American Cleft Palate Association: Its first 36 years. *Cleft Palate Journal, 16,* 86–123.

Westra, S. E. (1982). *Velopharyngeal insufficiency: Treatment recommendations, treatment implementations, and effects on speech in a selected cleft palate population.* Unpublished master's thesis, University of Minnesota, Minneapolis.

Whitehouse, F. A. (1951). Teamwork—A democracy of professions. *Exceptional Children, 18,* 45–52.

Whitehouse, F. A. (1965). Teamwork as a dynamic system. *Cleft Palate Journal, 2,* 16–27.

# CHAPTER 2

# Social Work

## Assessing Family Issues and Burdens of Care

*Cassandra L. Aspinall*

As a social worker, Aspinall advocates for the patient's and family's understanding of an interdisciplinary treatment plan *and* the interdisciplinary team's understanding of the patient and family. Consideration of the patient's and family's culture, education, medical/dental experience, socioeconomic resources, and family values can have a significant impact on compliance with optimal treatment plans. Aspinall provides a history of medical social work and special indications for social work expertise and input in the current health care system. She delineates important areas of patient and family inquiry of service and timing of assessment that may contribute to burdens of care.

1. Aspinall describes the health care environment as a complex setting with many competing priorities. What does she mean by that?
2. Why does Aspinall say that the social worker on the cleft and craniofacial teams may be the "most welcome and controversial" member?
3. What does Aspinall say about biopsychosocial theory and its relation to the importance of early baseline assessment of the patient and family?
4. Aspinall lists a number of areas that she considers important to review in a social work baseline assessment. Do you believe some are more important than others? If so, which ones(s)?
5. What does Aspinall say about adjusting social work assessment for adolescents with cleft and craniofacial disorders?
6. What does Aspinall say is important for the patient to understand after "graduating" from a "pediatric setting"?

An understanding of the impact of medical diagnosis and treatment on patients and families is of growing importance and interest. At the same time, the specialization and technical nature of medicine continue to increase while resources (particularly time and money) seem to be on the decrease. From the perspectives of both patient and provider, it is critical to determine up front how a medical diagnosis and its treatment will affect everyone's day-to-day life. In the most basic sense, this is the specific task of a social work professional in the health care setting.

## History of Medical Social Work

Medical social work was developed in the context of immense social changes in the early 1900s (Fort Cowles, 2003). At this time, public health issues such as disease and sanitation were of concern. Keeping the public safe meant getting a handle on the spread of germs and promoting public hygiene. This effort was complicated by the influx of immigrants into America; it became increasingly difficult to balance the protection of public health with the development of human rights protections in such a diverse population. In addition, there were growing worries about how to make certain that women and children were well cared for in the health care community. Identifying both what patients understood and what they wanted in terms of treatment was critical to controlling epidemics and delivering public health services. These were the roots of social work's commitment to patient advocacy, safety, and empowerment, with a particular focus on eliminating bias or prejudice in the delivery of care.

It was during this time that social work established its important role in health care delivery. In addition to working with patients and families in the hospitals where they were treated, social workers went into the communities where families lived to find out how best to meet their needs and their neighbors' needs. A standard for educating social workers to provide a thorough and professional service to both families and health care institutions was developed and is under constant revision. Adjustments must be made to adapt to what is learned from research and what is learned from patients and families themselves.

The current delivery of social work services can best be understood by reviewing the preamble to the profession's Code of Ethics, which was adopted by the National Association of Social Workers (NASW) in 1996:

> To enhance human well-being and help meet the basic human needs of all people, with particular attention to the needs and empowerment of people who are vulnerable, oppressed, and living in poverty. A historic and defining feature of social work is the profession's focus on individual well-being in a social context and the well-being of society. Fundamental to social work is attention to the environmental forces that create, contribute to, and address problems in living. (NASW, 1999)

Social workers help to achieve these goals by utilizing their training in social theory, community organization, and research. Empowering clients by identifying their strengths while also holding systems accountable is part of the balance that is carefully assessed and supported. To achieve this balance, social workers focus on in-depth study of a variety of important content areas: They need to be well grounded in the needs of the specific client population and problem area; be aware of the particulars of their organizational setting; stay updated regarding the characteristics of their community and the resources that are available within it; have the ability to utilize specific intervention modalities; and look toward the application of research, evaluation, and documentation in the interests of updating their practice and advancing the needs of their clientele (Fort Cowles, 2003).

Many medical diagnostic specialty areas recognize the important role of social workers in developing effective medical care plans that take into consideration psychosocial parameters. Assessing psychosocial needs up front and tracking them throughout treatment regimens have been described as helpful for such wide-ranging diagnoses as cancer and rare genetic conditions (Bryant, Heiney, Henslee-Downey, & Cornwell, 1997; Jackson, Tsantefski, Goodman, Johnson, & Rosenfeld, 2003).

The health care environment is a complex setting with many competing priorities. Patients hope to access the best care in a way that will be the least disruptive and stressful while providing the greatest possible benefits to health and well-being. Although medical team members also strive for these goals, they must also provide care that is efficient and promotes the goals of the institution they work in. Many providers must also consider the requirements and goals of an academic system. Delivering care while working to satisfy a variety of priorities can make it difficult to maintain a focus on the patient, his or her family, and the community. As mentioned earlier, a social worker is bound by the profession's ethical code to do exactly this (Fort Cowles, 2003).

One important difference between the social worker and other professionals in a medical setting is the social worker's emphasis on the patient's and family's strengths and assumed resilience. Resilience has been promoted as an important theoretical shift in the care of patients with craniofacial conditions (Strauss, 2001). Medicine—based on cultural and historical practices and (some would say) due to necessity—starts with a search for pathology so that a problem can be identified and treatment can be planned. Clearly these two perspectives need to be combined. The job of a social worker is to work early on with the patient and family to identify their strengths and understand their background while assessing the impact of the diagnosis or medical pathology, and then to facilitate a thorough process of communication.

To fulfill their professional obligation, social workers utilize many types of psychosocial evaluation and treatment. Using a systems model of assessment, the social worker in the health care setting helps to analyze and coordinate care from a patient and family perspective. This approach to assessment, which is often referred to as biopsychosocial, integrates holistic care, cultural sensitivity, awareness of mental health, promotion of positive health behaviors, evaluation of illness behaviors, and a focus on client empowerment and identification of social support (Fort Cowles, 2003).

Yuen, Skibinski, and Pardeck (2003) provided another framework that is useful in understanding how a social worker conceptualizes the integration of the patient and family into the care plan. These authors promote the use of the term "family health social work practice" and see the goal of intervention as being achieving an overall state of family health. This can be achieved by understanding that "family health is manifested by the development of and continuous interaction among the economic, physical, mental, emotional, social, cultural and spiritual dimensions of the family that result in its holistic well-being as well as that of its beings" (Yuen et al., 2003, p. 205).

## Indications for Social Work in the Current Health Care System

In the current health care delivery system, many important obligations must be met to make sure that treatments are provided in an individually respectful manner that also takes into consideration the systemic impacts across the broader environment. A primary obligation for the social work profession is to deliver care that is both family centered and culturally sensitive.

In a traditional hospital care delivery pattern, patients and families are expected to adapt their lives to the health care environment. Initiatives in hospitals today are aimed at a "bidirectional" approach to child health, in which medical settings such as hospitals will also adapt their operations to the meet the needs of the patient. Such a change will require more than just philosophical agreement. Health care institutions will need to demonstrate concentrated efforts to make such changes (Hanson & Lynch, 2004).

Additionally, concerns about access to health care and the problems with health care delivery to patients from diverse ethnic and cultural backgrounds have led to the development of national standards for the delivery of culturally appropriate services. At the same time, concerns about the disparities in health care are being heard and investigated with clearer and more direct research approaches (Spector, 2004). Social workers can be an important resource to medical institutions and families who agree that providing both family-centered and culturally appropriate care is of primary importance.

It is also important for professionals to remember that pediatric patients are considered a vulnerable population, and both law and professional ethics mandate that children should be protected from harm. There are times when concerns about child safety in a medical setting need to be acknowledged and addressed. The spectrum of concerns is broad and includes everything from the impact of noncompliance and neglect (Krener & Adelman, 1988; Menahem & Halasz, 2000) to concerns about overtreatment and pediatric falsification syndrome (formerly Munchausen's syndrome by proxy) (Libow, 2000; Stutts, Hickey, & Kasdan, 2003). Social workers' expertise and baseline assessment skills will provide an opportunity for proactive interventions, along with early intervention and team education and support.

## Social Work in the Craniofacial Care Team

On the craniofacial care team, a social worker can be an indispensable resource for helping the family and patient to better understand the medical treatment plan while also helping the medical treatment team better understand the patient and family. Getting an accurate picture of how to deliver the most appropriate and respectful care is complicated by the diversity of patients and treatment teams. It is critical to consider the effects of such things as culture, education, previous medical experience, socioeconomic resources, and family values when medical care decisions are made and plans are based on those decisions. This is no small task and is greatly helped by involving a psychosocial care provider such as a social worker to find out more about both patients and teams.

All medical diagnoses require adjustment and management. In some cases the care needs are acute and time limited, and in others the needs can be chronic and care may be needed over a lifetime. It is now understood that helping children and families cope with the impacts of chronic illness, including the psychological impact (Goodman, 2001), is important. For those individuals born with craniofacial conditions, there are often particular areas of adjustment that require assessment and attention. These areas include (but are not limited to) the impact of facial difference on the individual's adjustment and resulting self-esteem (Broder, Smith, & Strauss, 1992; Pertschuk & Whitaker, 1982; Pope & Ward, 1997), the stress of considering and participating in surgery as a treatment modality, and the inconsistent funding of treatments that focus on care of the teeth and jaw as well as ongoing speech and hearing therapies (Strauss, 1994, 1995). Without adequate assessment of these areas, weighing the benefits and burdens of care options can be flawed. In many situations, concrete burdens will vary tremendously and benefits can be uncertain. Therefore, making decisions and plans must be done carefully and thoroughly.

As described earlier, social workers are expertly trained in assessing the complexities of a variety of systems. Such assessments help teams to more fully appreciate the variables that interact in the care of each patient. Beyond what is learned in clinical conversations that other team members have with families, social workers are trained to identify important nuances across and throughout a full social assessment. The social worker is specifically trained to help the family identify their strengths, to figure out how to access outside resources, and to check for biases in how patients are treated. The social worker must also take the responsibility to communicate any concerns directly to the team or to the family. Protecting and advocating for the most vulnerable patients while also looking out for system flaws and biases is an important but complex job description. Having this politically charged position may make a social worker both the most welcome and the most controversial member of a team.

On a craniofacial team, a social worker can provide a variety of services and is often categorized as a mental health professional. However, many health care providers may not be familiar with the role of social workers from firsthand experience. Documentation from the American Cleft Palate-Craniofacial Association (ACPA) indicates that many teams do not yet include a mental health provider on their rosters or provide psychosocial services. Strauss and the ACPA Team Standards Committee (1998) surveyed teams regarding areas of noncompliance. Psychosocial resources and services represented the area of greatest deficit: 34% of teams did not have a mental health practitioner, and 26% did not document the patient's social and family history. "The areas of noncompliance were striking and suggest the need for specific efforts to assure the availability of psychological and social services to team patients" (Strauss & ACPA Team Standards Committee, 1998, p. 476).

## Areas and Timing of Social Work Assessment

Regardless of the patient's age, the social worker should perform a thorough *baseline psychosocial assessment.* Clearly, there are some important differences in exactly how a social worker interfaces with a patient and family depending on how old the patient is. However, there are some basic components of an introductory assessment. In addition to reviewing the important things to cover in a first assessment, I provide information about evaluations done for the following reasons: prenatal and newborn assessments, surgical decision making, surgical planning, and adolescent transition.

### Baseline Assessment

As mentioned earlier, there are many theoretical frameworks that provide a rationale for the importance of careful collection of information about a variety of family and patient issues. According to biopsychosocial theory,

> primary health care is rooted in the belief that health status is the result of a complex interaction of biological, psychological, social, cultural and physical environmental factors. Consequently, good health will never result from simply seeking medical intervention from any one of an array of specialist physicians, depending on the particular health problems one has already developed. Rather, the biopsychosocial model

> holds that health status is the result of genetic inheritance, learned behavior, cultural influences, the quality of the physical environment, socioeconomic status, one's age and sex, the amount of stress experienced, coping mechanisms, diet, exercise, avoidance of intake of dangerous drugs, social supports, sense of empowerment, and access to medical care especially at the primary level. (Fort Cowles, 2003, p. 102)

It is best practice to obtain such an early, thorough psychosocial assessment as part of a craniofacial team evaluation. When this information is available up front, the additional tasks and impact on existing coping strategies can be better understood and supported.

The following general categories should be reviewed by the social worker in the completion of a baseline assessment: impact and understanding of the diagnosis, social supports, partnering relationships, concrete resources, financial resources, previous history with hospitals and/or medical treatments, coping history, health and safety issues, and interactions with others.

***Impact and Understanding of the Diagnosis.*** Before developing a recommended treatment plan, the team needs to determine what the patient and family understand about the diagnosis and how they describe its impact on the family as a whole and on each member of the family. Craniofacial diagnoses are complex, and there may be many levels of misunderstanding and guilt about how they happened. By asking the family (and the patient, if old enough) what they understand about the condition's origin, the social worker can learn much about what they have already learned and how they have interpreted that information. Follow-up questions about how dealing with this medical condition has impacted the family's life will indicate how family members have coped and whether additional resources are needed to decrease negative impacts. The social worker also needs to ask about the positive changes or life events that a family may see as connected with the diagnosis.

Strauss (2001) suggested some basic steps that professionals need to take in order to see patients in a more positive light while also providing a more hopeful picture to families. Two of these steps are specifically related to counseling and assessing patients. First, it is important to intentionally create an environment of optimism and positive expectation for families and patients by mindfully conducting evaluations that are both accurate and positive. A focus on the contributions that a person can make in the context of his or her diagnosis rather than emphasizing the potential difficulties and pain provides an important balance to the overall possibilities that can be expected. Second, the social worker should ask patients and families about the things that are going right for them rather than focusing only on what is going wrong. Then discussions can be about building on what is going well and about treatments other than those that are focused on surgical or physical change. Discussing internal strengths rather than focusing only on external qualities sends a message that a balance is important in the establishment of self-esteem. This is part of a well-recognized psychological process where an individual's sense of control over life includes perceptions of both external and internal control points (Rotter, 1971). In the context of craniofacial care, it is important to explore how patients can influence how they experience life based on what they think of themselves combined with what they know about what others think.

*Social Supports.* The positive impacts that social supports have on health have been established for quite some time (Kaplan, Cassel, & Gore, 1977). Therefore, the social worker should determine who is involved with the patient, including who lives in the home and who is available from the community (e.g., friends, family, coworkers, church members). Finding out how much others help and in what ways is also critical. It is important not to make overly negative or positive assumptions about who is doing what. Getting a sense for any recent changes in support is key as well.

*Partnering Relationships.* It is important to ask specifically about the role of each parent, both socially and legally. The family takes on many permutations these days, and especially when dealing with a diagnosis that may involve the use of surgical treatment, it is critical to know who is considered a patient's legal guardian.

*Concrete Resources.* When a family is faced with coping with increased needs of one of their members, the social worker needs to determine what their situation is for shelter, safety, transportation, and nutrition. As was first described by Maslow (1943), there are basic needs that must be met in order for an individual to be able to develop self-esteem and motivation. If these basic needs are not being met, then the strain of having to make adjustments in the context of a new medical diagnosis will place additional stress on the patient and family. Understanding what gaps or concerns families have in the area of concrete resources is critical.

*Financial Resources.* The social worker needs to gain a sense of the family's financial situation. It is particularly important to ask questions about employment and to determine whether family members have access to health care and have a supportive workplace. It is also worthwhile to find out if current employment status will change based on the patient's medical needs and if this issue presents additional concern to the family. It may be especially hard for parents to talk about needing to put off promotions or plans for education because of another family member's health care needs; however, the opportunity to discuss these stressors can be immensely supportive to families. Research indicates that both patients and doctors are interested in getting this information out into the open (Alexander, Casalino, & Meltzer, 2003).

*Previous History with Hospitals and/or Medical Treatments.* When a family takes a member for assessment, they almost always carry with them what they have learned from their previous personal, familial, or work-related health care experiences. This history can work both for them and against them, depending on their experience. Prior experiences, whether good, bad, or indifferent, will almost certainly affect future expectations. This may be especially true when another family member carries the same diagnosis as the patient.

*Coping History.* Finding out how patients and families have previously coped under stress can be invaluable to helping them in a new and different situation. It will be easier to support those who have developed positive coping strategies if the team knows up front what the patients and families need. For patients and families who struggle with negative or destructive coping strategies, early awareness of such problems will increase the likelihood that a supportive intervention can be offered to head off trouble. Finding out after the fact that help could have prevented the disruption of a care plan not only is unhelpful but also can be dangerous to the patient.

*Health and Safety Issues.* Teams should also screen families regarding public health issues such as domestic violence, mental health problems, gun violence, substance abuse, and child abuse and neglect. Although asking questions about these areas can be uncomfortable for both patient and practitioner, the benefits of finding out about these problems far outweigh the temporary burden of discomfort. Many health care providers report a lack of training in areas such as domestic violence, and this adds to their discomfort (Lapidus et al., 2002). Therefore, a psychosocial provider such as a social worker may find it easier to ask such questions. In addition, when screening reveals either a current or past concern, the social worker can provide orientation to other team members and discuss interventions with families.

*Interactions with Others.* Patients with craniofacial disorders and their family members may experience discomfort when interacting with other people. Especially because craniofacial conditions are visible, those who are affected do not get to choose the timing of disclosing their diagnosis. Short of deciding not to interact with other people, patients and family members are faced with the likely prospect that they will be asked questions about their condition. The condition may also elicit discomfort from others. Natural curiosity can lead to a change in interactions with both known and unknown people. Sometimes a patient's behavior may be negatively affected by such uncomfortable situations (Richman, Holmes, & Eliason, 1985). For all of these reasons, it is very important to get a sense from a patient and family about how they are doing with such situations.

Comfort in dealing with interpersonal interactions and in discussing them is key to being able to focus on the nonmedical or nondiagnostic aspects of one's life. Without having this discussion with patients, families and teams may attribute qualities of appearance to the qualities of relationships specifically and life in general. Assessment of these issues is central to developing treatment plans. For example, if a patient feels good about herself but bad about the way she is being treated, then what sorts of interventions would be most effective? Should a patient's appearance be changed to reduce the attention from others? Or should the attitudes of others be changed to make them less reactive to facial differences?

## Prenatal and Newborn Assessments

Parents may find it difficult to mentally prepare for the birth of an infant with a cleft or craniofacial disorder or to adjust to the unexpected birth of a child with a cleft or craniofacial disorder. The intensity of their feelings requires some additional areas of assessment that are worthy of noting separately from those discussed previously in relation to the standard assessment. Prenatal assessments can challenge support systems because the actual needs cannot be identified until after delivery. For this reason, there has been interest in the literature about the reaction to such a situation (Aspinall, 2002).

Two important areas of concern when counseling families either before or after delivery are possible loss issues related to feeding challenges and guilt about causation of the birth defect. When there are problems with infant feeding related to the presence of a cleft or craniofacial disorder, it is important for the social worker to check in with mothers about the emotional impact of this change. It is very helpful to normalize these feelings when meeting with parents in the early days following birth.

Guilt around the presence of a congenital abnormality can come from many sources, but parents often express worry about possible prenatal exposure to some dangerous substance or concerns about a known or unknown genetic diagnosis. Asking parents to explain their child's problem can be very helpful toward finding out whether they harbor any hidden guilt. It is important to encourage such discussion because parents often feel "silly" for the explanations they have considered and find it helpful to discuss them. It takes some time for parents to fully accept their child's diagnosis. Part of this process is realizing that science cannot explain everything that happens.

## Surgical Decision Making

Helping patients and families evaluate whether it would be beneficial to consent to surgical treatment involves specific attention to several additional assessment areas: identifying the goals of the treatment, reviewing the understanding of the benefits and burdens of the treatment from the perspectives of both the legal decision makers (usually the parents when working with children) and minor patients, and getting clear disclosure from team members about the treatment's direct impacts (e.g., pain, missing regularly scheduled activities) and indirect impacts (e.g., financial costs, time away from work for caretakers).

## Surgical Planning

Along with nursing, social work plays an important role in helping families and patients prepare for surgical treatments. The varieties of tasks that require coordination are well outlined in an article by Chibbaro (1999). Because of the time that parents and patients must be away from work and school, communication with both environments is important. In most cases, with the appropriate submission of letters, students can access in-home tutoring and parents' jobs can be protected because of the Family and Medical Leave Act of 1993. Letters written to schools can also include information regarding any activity or dietary restrictions so that the patient's return to school will be easier.

Emotional preparation for surgery is another important area for assessment. Parents and children may both be anxious about the process of anesthesia and hospitalization. Referrals to Child Life Specialists who can develop plans with families specifically targeted toward the comfort of children in the context of hospital treatments can be very beneficial. Combining Child Life Specialist consultation with supportive counseling for parents not only makes things easier for a particular surgery but also provides education for the future.

## Adolescent Transition

In the care of patients throughout their childhood, the developmental stage of adolescence demands particular attention when it comes to adjusting the psychosocial assessment to fully address the issues. In adolescence there are many parallel priorities that must be clearly described. Currently, researchers are trying to learn more about what things adolescents feel influence their quality of life (Edwards, Huebner, Connell, & Patrick, 2002). This research reflects an interest in understanding this group better and in developing interventions that are more effective.

The craniofacial team needs to make sure that medical and surgical plans are reviewed for completeness so that once a patient "graduates" from a pediatric setting, he or she has finished as much care as possible. When care needs remain, it is important for the patient to have a clear sense of what still needs to be done. In the process of reviewing where the patient is in terms of habilitation of his or her medical needs, the craniofacial team can make sure that the patient is fully updated about his or her diagnosis and treatment history. This is an important step in making sure that patients can successfully advocate for themselves in the adult setting.

As team members are combining their efforts to make certain that patients have a clear understanding of the medical issues, social workers can review behavioral, social, and life planning issues with these patients. Social work assessment is focused on getting answers to questions about the patient's plans for the future, involvement in any risk-taking behaviors, platonic and romantic relationships, and understanding of his or her treatment and diagnosis. This information helps to clarify what individual patients may need before team-based pediatric care is considered complete. It may also be possible to direct patients to a variety of resources in the community to assist in further evaluation of vocational or mental health concerns.

## Summary

A patient with a craniofacial condition who participates in a team evaluation needs assistance beyond receiving medical recommendations. A care plan needs to take into account a patient's preferences, background, and values. In the context of such information and with the skillful guidance of a trained social worker, patients and teams can work carefully toward the development of a plan that optimizes the benefits of care while minimizing the burdens. Working on a multidisciplinary team, a social worker provides a unique point of view that focuses on the resilience of patients while simultaneously assessing the limits of surrounding systems and tracking the vulnerability of patients.

## References

Alexander, G., Casalino, L. P., & Meltzer, D. O. (2003). Patient-physician communication about out-of-pocket costs. *Journal of the American Medical Association, 290,* 953–958.

Aspinall, C. L. (2002). Dealing with the prenatal diagnosis of clefting: A parent's perspective. *Cleft Palate-Craniofacial Journal, 39,* 183–187.

Broder, H. L., Smith, F. B., & Strauss, R. P. (1992). Habilitation of patients with clefts: Parent and child ratings of satisfaction. *Cleft Palate-Craniofacial Journal, 29,* 262–267.

Bryant, L. H., Heiney, S. P., Henslee-Downey, P. J., & Cornwell, P. (1997). Proactive psychosocial care of blood or marrow transplant patients. *Cancer Practice, 5,* 234–240.

Chibbaro, P. D. (1999). Living with craniofacial microsomia: Support for the patient and family. *Cleft Palate-Craniofacial Journal, 36,* 40–42.

Edwards, T. C., Huebner, C. D., Connell, F. A., & Patrick, D. L. (2002). Adolescent quality of life: Part 1. Conceptual and measurement model. *Journal of Adolescence, 25,* 275–286.

Family and Medical Leave Act of 1993, 29 U.S.C. § 28.

Fort Cowles, L. A. (2003). *Social work in the health care field: A care perspective* (2nd ed.). New York: Haworth Social Work Practice Press.

Goodman, R. F. (2001). Children with a chronic illness: The interface of medicine and mental health. *Child Study Center Letter, 5*(4), 1–5.

Hanson, M. J., & Lynch, E. W. (2004). *Understanding families: Approaches to diversity, disability and risk.* East Peoria, IL: Versa Press.

Jackson, A. C., Tsantefski, M., Goodman, H., Johnson, B., & Rosenfeld, J. (2003). The psychosocial impacts on families of low-incidence, complex conditions in children: The case of craniopharyngioma. *Social Work in Health Care, 38*(1), 81–107.

Kaplan, B. H., Cassel, J. H., & Gore, S. (1977). Social support and health. *Medical Care, 15,* 47–58.

Krener, P., & Adelman, R. (1988). Parent salvage and parent sabotage in the care of chronically ill children. *American Journal for the Diseases of Children, 142,* 945–951.

Lapidus, G., Beaulieu-Cooke, M., Gelven, E., Sherman, K., Duncan., M., & Banco, L. (2002). A statewide survey of domestic violence screening behaviors among pediatricians and family physicians. *Archives of Pediatrics and Adolescent Medicine, 156,* 332–336.

Libow, J. A. (2000). Child and adolescent illness falsification. *Pediatrics, 105,* 336–342.

Maslow, A. H. (1943). A theory of human motivation. *Psychological Review, 50,* 370–396.

Menahem, S., & Halasz, G. (2000). Parental non-compliance—A paediatric dilemma: A medical and psychodynamic perspective. *Child Care, Health and Development, 26*(1), 61–72.

National Association of Social Workers. (1999). *Code of ethics of the National Association of Social Workers.* Retrieved March 26, 2007, from www.socialworkers.org/pubs/code/code.asp

Pertschuk, M. J., & Whitaker, L. A. (1982). Social and psychological effects of craniofacial deformity and surgical reconstruction. *Clinics in Plastic Surgery, 9,* 297–306.

Pope, A. W., & Ward, J. (1997). Self-perceived facial appearance and psychosocial adjustment in preadolescents with craniofacial anomalies. *Cleft Palate-Craniofacial Journal, 34,* 396–401.

Richman, L. C., Holmes, C. S., & Eliason, M. J. (1985). Adolescents with cleft lip and palate: Self-perceptions of appearance and behavior related to personality adjustment. *Cleft Palate-Craniofacial Journal, 22,* 93–96.

Rotter, J. B. (1971). External control and internal control. *Psychology Today, 5*(1), 37–42, 58–59.

Spector, R. E. (2004). *Cultural diversity in health and illness.* Old Tappan, NJ: Pearson Education.

Strauss, R. P. (1994). Health policy and craniofacial care: Issues in resource allocation. *Cleft Palate-Craniofacial Journal, 31,* 78–80.

Strauss, R. P. (1995). Resource allocation, health policy, and rationing craniofacial care. *Cleft Palate-Craniofacial Journal, 32,* 515–519.

Strauss, R. P. (2001). "Only skin deep": Health, resilience, and craniofacial care. *Cleft Palate-Craniofacial Journal, 38,* 226–230.

Strauss, R. P., & The American Cleft Palate-Craniofacial Association Team Standards Committee. (1998). Cleft palate and craniofacial teams in the United States and Canada: A national survey of team organization and standards of care. *Cleft Palate-Craniofacial Journal, 35,* 473–480.

Stutts, J. T., Hickey, S. E., & Kasdan, M. L. (2003). Malingering by proxy: A form of pediatric condition falsification. *Developmental and Behavioral Pediatrics, 24,* 276–278.

Yuen, F. K., Skibinski, G. J., & Pardeck, J. T. (2003). *Family health social work practice: A knowledge and skills casebook.* New York: Haworth Social Work Practice Press.

# CHAPTER 3

# Ethical Issues in the Care of Patients with Cleft Palate and Craniofacial Anomalies

*Helen M. Sharp*

Sharp discusses important ethical issues that surface in the treatment of children with cleft lip and palate or other craniofacial anomalies, particularly with regard to decisions made by parents on behalf of their children and by the children themselves. In addition, Sharp identifies how interdisciplinary care presents some special ethical considerations and how technological advancements in prenatal diagnosis raise new ethical questions.

1. Sharp notes that the best interest standard is often applied to decisions for children or adults whose wishes are unknown. What are the limitations of using the best interest standard?
2. Why does Sharp believe it is important for clinicians to be aware of their own beliefs and biases before offering prenatal counseling to a family?
3. What does Sharp believe is the value of including children and adolescents in making decisions about their own care? What are the risks?
4. Sharp discusses the main differences between the goals of clinical care and the goals of research. Describe them.

Ethical issues arise in the care of patients across all clinical settings. The field of ethics, as a branch of philosophy, relates to the study of how morals or values are balanced in particular circumstances (Beauchamp

& Childress, 2001). Clinical ethics applies ethical theories to analyzing and resolving practical problems in the care of patients (Jonsen, Siegler, & Winslade, 1998). This chapter highlights some of the ethical issues that arise in the care of children and adolescents with cleft lip and palate or other craniofacial anomalies and their families. Because the majority of patients seen in a cleft palate or craniofacial clinic are under 18 years of age, the discussion focuses on issues affecting the care of children, such as the role of parents as decision makers for their children and the role of children and adolescents in making decisions about their own health care.

The majority of care for children with cleft and craniofacial conditions is provided by interdisciplinary teams. In 1996, the American Cleft Palate-Craniofacial Association (ACPA) identified 296 interdisciplinary cleft palate or craniofacial teams in North America (Strauss & ACPA, 1998). Interdisciplinary team care alters the traditional doctor-patient relationship, which is the focus of much of the literature in clinical ethics. Therefore, special ethical considerations of interdisciplinary team care are also explored in this chapter.

The care of patients with congenital anomalies often requires adaptation of clinical, medical, dental, and surgical approaches to treatment. The implementation of innovative or untested treatments raises important ethical questions about the distinctions between research and clinical care. Cases are used to illustrate some of the issues and form a basis from which to discuss possible resolutions. The issues and cases are constructed from clinical experience, but the names and specifics of the cases are fictionalized.

## Parents as Decision Makers for Their Children

Infants and young children are unable to participate in decision making about their care; therefore, parents and clinicians usually work together to make informed decisions by weighing the benefits and burdens of treatment and assessing what will serve a child's best interests. The best interest standard is consistent with a primary ethical principle of beneficence or maximizing the patient's welfare (Beauchamp & Childress, 2001). However, deciding what is "best" for another person may present dilemmas for clinicians and families because people's tolerance for risk or burden of intervention varies, as do individuals' values for the benefits achieved (Elliott & Elliott, 1991; Slevin et al., 1990). Estimates of others' suffering or "burden" are questionable and may pose a risk for under- or overtreatment of people who cannot participate in decision making for themselves (Elliot & Elliot, 1991). Studies show that caregivers' estimates of patients' quality of life are uniformly lower than the patients' own ratings across a variety of disabilities (Pearlman & Uhlmann, 1988). Nonetheless, decisions for children are usually limited to adults' perceptions of the balance between the burden and the relative benefit because a child's current and future preferences cannot be determined. In most circumstances, parents are considered the most appropriate people to make best interest judgments as surrogate decision makers for their children (Holder, 1983). The widespread use of ultrasound and other prenatal testing means that parental responsibilities now extend to exceptionally difficult decisions about the "best interests" of the unborn.

## Prenatal Decisions About Cleft and Craniofacial Conditions

### Case Study 1

Joanne and Paul Benson are expecting their second child. A routine ultrasound conducted at 18-weeks gestation detected a unilateral cleft lip in an otherwise healthy fetus. Further testing was recommended, and the amniocentesis yielded normal chromosomes for a female fetus. The Bensons met with a genetic counselor in conjunction with the follow-up testing. Joanne calls the Cleft Palate Clinic to make an appointment for a team consultation to help them prepare for their daughter's birth.

Knowledge of fetal health early in the pregnancy raises profound questions about parental responsibilities, regardless of the decision the parents make. When prospective parents learn that the fetus has a cleft, they mourn the loss of a "perfect" baby (M. C. Jones, 2002). A finding of a cleft or other facial anomaly typically leads to more definitive assessments, such as chromosomal analysis and genetic counseling. Even when major associated syndromes are "ruled out," current estimates suggest that about 12% of fetuses have other associated anomalies that cannot be detected prenatally (M. C. Jones, 2002). The chance that an associated syndrome will be detected postnatally makes prenatal counseling challenging because syndromes are known to affect short-term and long-term outcomes. Therefore, prospective parents, such as the Bensons, face uncertainty about the implications of the cleft and the wide range of possible outcomes that could be associated with the finding of a cleft lip or palate on ultrasound.

Knowledge that the fetus is healthy is a source of comfort and reassurance to expectant parents (Aspinall, 2002). Proponents of prenatal testing suggest that infants, parents, and their physicians may benefit because they are better able to prepare for the infant's birth. The benefit of early detection, however, must be balanced against the stress of discovering a fetal anomaly (Aspinall, 2002). Although prenatal diagnosis is often credited with improving prenatal care, the testing does not prevent congenital anomalies or lead to changes in treatment planning because prenatal therapy is not available or effective for most conditions that can be detected prenatally (Parens & Asch, 1999). Fetal surgery has been tried with limited success for conditions that are associated with high mortality rates postnatally, such as diaphragmatic hernia (Wagner & Harrison, 2002). Fetal surgery is thought to offer the possibility of scarless healing, and its use has been explored for cleft lip repair in animal models (Canady, Landas, Morris, & Thompson, 1994; Evans, Oberg, Kirsch, Zhu, & Hardesty, 1995; Mast, Diegelmann, Krummel, & Cohen, 1992). However, advances in the application of fetal surgery for conditions that can be treated postnatally continue to be limited by the problem of preterm labor and premature birth as a result of the surgery (Harrison, 1996; Wagner & Harrison, 2002), raising substantial questions about acceptable levels of risk to both mother and child. Also, many conditions that are detected with prenatal testing are not correctable with surgery or medical interventions.

Although not necessarily intended, the process of prenatal testing can convey to parents that they are required to make a conscious choice about whether to continue or terminate the pregnancy, if the testing reveals a disorder. For example, finding certain fetal anomalies, such as Down syndrome, is highly associated with the termination of the pregnancy (Mansfield, Hopfer, & Marteau, 1999). Prospective parents' general rights to terminate a pregnancy raise a host of moral, political, and societal issues that are well beyond the scope of this chapter. The discussion here relates only to parents' decisions to terminate a singular pregnancy, because of a specific characteristic or risk (Parens & Asch, 1999). This issue is raised here to heighten clinicians' awareness of their own beliefs and biases about the termination of pregnancies, specifically when the decision is based on a diagnosis that the clinician treats as a matter of routine.

Decisions whether to continue or terminate a pregnancy based on a prenatal diagnosis of a cleft vary widely. A series of 24 families followed in Israel revealed that 23 families elected to terminate the pregnancy based on transvaginal ultrasound images that revealed the presence of a cleft (Blumenfeld, Blumenfeld, & Bronshtein, 1999a). Data from one site in the United States revealed a lower rate of termination, with 2 of 8 families (25%) electing to terminate pregnancies (M. C. Jones, 1999). A review of 9 reports revealed a broad range of parental decisions—from 0% to 92%—to terminate pregnancies, with a total across reports of 21 terminations in 174 identified pregnancies (12%) (Johnson & Sandy, 2003). Although not well understood, the decision whether to continue or terminate a pregnancy upon learning that the fetus has a congenital anomaly appears to be influenced by timing of detection in the pregnancy, perceived burden, family needs, cultural and religious values, availability of genetic counseling, maternal age, and history of previous terminations (Britt et al., 2000; M. C. Jones, 1999). The decision to terminate a pregnancy that was otherwise wanted is painful, but the decision to carry the pregnancy to term also carries potential social and emotional burdens. Parents may worry about stigmatization because of the potential for others to ascribe blame for their informed decision to have a child with a disability or medical condition (Strauss, 2002; Walker, 2004).

Prospective parents are increasingly likely to arrange a consultation with members of a cleft and craniofacial care team (Matthews, 2002; Matthews, Cohen, Viglione, & Brown, 1998; Strauss, 2002). Matthews (2002) found that 85% of plastic and reconstructive surgeons affiliated with cleft palate or craniofacial teams who responded to a survey regarding prenatal diagnosis reported counseling at least one family, and most offered prenatal consultation routinely. Although genetic counselors strive for nondirective, neutral counseling (Saal, 2002), professionals who work with children with clefts have expressed alarm at the relatively high rates of pregnancy terminations (Eiserman & Strauss, 1999). The presence of a cleft lip or cleft lip and palate may be considered a relatively minor anomaly by clinicians who routinely provide care for infants, children, and teens. However, clinicians must recognize the influence of their own values, biases, and sense of discomfort when families seek information to help decide whether to continue their pregnancy (Matthews, 2002). Parents should be encouraged to seek information from many sources, including genetic counselors and members of the cleft and craniofacial team. Clinicians should be sensitive to the possibility of overwhelming parents with information. M. C. Jones (2002) suggested prioritizing information about the immediate postpartum period, such as feeding and initial surgical procedures, along with common concerns about pain, speech, and self-esteem. Parents of children with similar conditions can also be a useful source of information for expectant families (Blumenfeld, Blumenfeld, & Bronshtein, 1999b), although M. C. Jones (2002) cautions that meeting a child with a cleft can "personalize" a fetus and make decision making more difficult. Clinicians who refer prospective parents to another family should seek permission to release names and contact information and should recognize the biases introduced by selecting a particular (usually well-functioning) family to provide additional information. Online resources and an international network for family support can be accessed through the Cleft Palate Foundation (www.cleftline.org).

## Parents' Refusal of Recommended Treatment

### Case Study 2

Manuel was born at the local community hospital and has a complete unilateral cleft lip and palate. The cleft team nurse, pediatrician, and geneticist all assessed Manuel in the neonatal period and consulted with the family about feeding. The parents understand a lot of English but depend on a translator to ask questions and clarify instructions. They have followed through with all of the team's recommendations to date, attended all appointments, and appear to be doing well emotionally. Manuel is growing well and the cleft appears to be an isolated congenital anomaly, not associated with a syndrome.

When Manuel is 6 weeks of age, he and his parents attend the cleft palate clinic for a weight check and for consultation and education with the surgeon and speech-language pathologist. The parents ask all the team members a lot of questions about the plans for surgery. They specifically ask the pediatrician, speech-language pathologist, and plastic and reconstructive surgeon to explain what would happen if Manuel did not have surgery on his lip or palate. At the end of their appointment, they tell the clinic coordinator that they will not need next month's appointment in plastic surgery to schedule the lip repair, because they do not plan to have the cleft lip or palate repaired.

When a family decides not to follow the recommendations of a professional or a team, the health professionals may be puzzled or even angry (Berg, Appelbaum, Lidz, & Parker, 2001). Repairs of cleft lip and palate are considered routine procedures, especially for members of a cleft and craniofacial team. However, these are major surgeries from the perspective of the family. Families make decisions based on past experience, financial factors, cultural and religious traditions, and personal preferences. These factors weigh into the calculation of the risks versus benefits of a given treatment for that family. For example, McDermott (2000) reported an exchange with a craniofacial clinic coordinator as follows:

> We have a patient here, a young man with Apert syndrome. He was born in Connecticut to a devout Russian Orthodox family. The parents brought him to the clinic when he was a baby and we explained what could be done, they thanked us and said "We love him the way he is. This is how God made him." They refused surgery for the skull, even to separate his fingers. Love would be enough. (p. 211)

Parents are widely regarded as the appropriate decision makers for their children. While parents are usually invited to give permission for medical treatment, their rights to refuse treatment may be restricted (Lo, 2000). If the proposed treatment has an expected benefit and low risk, as in the administration of antibiotics or a blood transfusion, then parents' rights to refuse the treatment are more likely to be overridden (Lo, 2000). Beauchamp (2003) argued that clinicians have a moral duty to implement life-sustaining treatment over the parents' objection, as in a blood transfusion for a young child of parents who are Jehovah's Witnesses. Clinicians and the state government hold a responsibility to protect children and other vulnerable populations from abuse and neglect (reviewed in Beauchamp, 2003; Lo, 2000). However, parents maintain considerable latitude for decisions regarding elective procedures (Lo, 2000).

Most cleft and craniofacial procedures are considered elective, although a lack of intervention can have serious consequences for the child's ability to function. There is very little case law or guidance about how parental refusals of elective treatments that enhance a child's function and quality of life should be handled. These cases are rare, but when parents refuse treatment, health professionals' obligations to respect the family's choices are often in deep conflict with their duty to benefit the child. Many institutions have an ethics consultant or ethics committee available to consult with clinicians about specific cases, such as the refusal of cleft lip and palate repair by Manuel's parents.

### Case Study 2 (*continued*)

The team invites a clinical ethics consultant to discuss Manuel's case with them. Initially, the team and ethics consultant are concerned that the parents misunderstood the risks of surgery or that the team misunderstands the family's culture or beliefs. However, when the ethics consultant meets with the family, Manuel's mother reveals that her sister's infant also had a cleft and died during surgery for a cardiac condition. This information helps the team understand that Manuel's parents are focused on understanding the risks of cleft surgery. For them, Manuel's life is more important than his appearance or his speech. Following further discussions directed at addressing the parents' concerns about the risks of surgery for cleft lip and palate for Manuel, the parents agree to surgery.

## Parents' Request for Treatment That the Team Considers Inappropriate or Futile

### Case Study 3

Michael is 16 months old. He was diagnosed shortly after birth with a holoprosencephaly disorder and microcephaly (see K. L. Jones, 1997). He has an unrepaired midline cleft lip and palate, with an absent philtrum. His parents were informed that many infants with this condition die in infancy and were therefore counseled not to pursue surgery. The family received some training in feeding Michael, and he has grown and gained weight. There is little evidence of cognitive function in this young child, and his parents seem to recognize this.

The parents make an appointment to see the cleft lip and palate team because they would like Michael's lip to be repaired. During the interview with the social worker, the parents express sadness over Michael's lack of development. They appear to understand that repairing his cleft lip will not "fix" Michael's problems, but they are anxious for him to appear as normal as possible for his sake and hope to reduce the curious looks and questions from strangers that bother them and Michael's three siblings.

When the plastic and reconstructive surgeon meets with the family, the parents are ready to schedule the procedure. The surgeon had an experience with a child with holoprosencephaly during her fellowship program; that child had a lip repair, stopped eating, developed significant airway problems, and died a month after surgery. The surgeon presents the serious risks, and the family continues to request surgery.

---

Michael's parents request surgical repair of a cleft lip although they know that Michael is unlikely to experience direct benefit from the procedure. Their request is likely to be met with concern from the cleft team about "cost-effectiveness" and probable outcome, including a relatively high risk that Michael will be harmed by the surgery. The parents frame their request in terms of the overall interests of their family—to reduce staring and questions and to increase the normalcy of their lives. The fact that Michael is alive speaks to the care they offer him every day.

Some might argue that any surgery for an infant with such limited life expectancy and a low probability of being aware of or able to experience a "quality of life," falls into the class of futile interventions. Although the concept of futility has been debated (Helft, Siegler, & Lantos, 2000), cases such as Michael's force health care professionals to confront whether the intervention provides any measurable benefit for the patient. This case also raises the question, "Who is the patient?" Is it appropriate to perform treatment that is unlikely to provide direct benefit to the patient but will most likely benefit his family? There are no easy answers to these questions. Many teams draw a line between performing cleft lip surgery and palatal surgery. Michael is feeding well and gaining weight, so theoretically the primary goal of palate repair would be to provide the structures for speech production. However, because Michael is unlikely to speak, there is little justification for closing his palate at this time. However, lip repair would provide a cosmetic benefit to the family, and the compassionate benefit is adequate justification for many teams to conduct the lip repair.

## Role of Children and Adolescents in Decision Making

### Case Study 4

Laura is 9 years old. She has a repaired unilateral cleft lip and palate with significant midface retrusion. Laura is very likely to require a midface advancement in the future. When the surgeons mention this to her, she asks whether the surgery could be done this summer because she is teased a lot about her appearance and she is scheduled to start at a new school next fall. The team usually performs orthognathic procedures once facial growth is complete, at about age 15 or 16 years, in order to reduce the chance of needing to repeat the procedure. The surgeons prefer to wait another 5 years or so before considering this procedure. Laura's parents are concerned about Laura's social development and about multiple surgeries and are undecided about what to do. Laura says she is willing to have two surgeries, if they can do one soon.

Although parents have the legal authority to consent to medical treatment until children are 18, older children and adolescents often participate in decisions about their own care and provide an informal agreement or assent to planned assessment or interventions. Teams should show respect for children's ideas and concerns and allow them the opportunity to express themselves. When clinicians include children or adolescents in decisions about their own care, they demonstrate respect for the person, foster trust with medical professionals, and increase the child's participation in shared decision making, despite the legal limitations to giving fully informed consent (American Academy of Pediatrics [AAP] Committee on Bioethics, 1995). Adolescents often have the cognitive capacity to participate in clinical decision making (AAP, 1995; Weir & Peters, 1997). Weir and Peters (1997) suggest that adolescents with chronic conditions are likely to hold well-informed opinions about their own care.

The inclusion of children and adolescents in the shared decision-making process raises immediate questions about how health care professionals should respond to disagreements within the family; for example, when the parents consent to treatment but an adolescent refuses to assent. The adolescent's reasons for refusal should be explored and addressed. Treatment decisions can often be delayed or a trial of treatment offered to allow a better informed decision. At times, it can help to give an adolescent time to talk with clinicians without the parents present. There are no easy answers to such conflicts, but these cases should be handled individually, with careful attention to the risks and benefits of the treatment and the urgency of the decision. For instance, teens may have a greater role in refusing non-life-threatening treatments, such as speech therapy or orthodontics, particularly where their cooperation is essential to the success of the treatment and a delay will not pose significant risks (AAP, 1995). On the other hand, a teen's refusal of chemotherapy for cancer treatment is likely to be cause for more rigorous negotiation (Ross, 1998). Perhaps more difficult are situations, such as Laura's, where an adolescent seeks elective treatment, but the parents do not agree. Since elective procedures can often be delayed without harm to the patient, education, discussion, and sometimes psychosocial support can often provide ways to resolve these difficult conflicts.

## Interdisciplinary Team Care

### Case Study 5

Jacob is 3 years old and has a repaired unilateral cleft lip and palate. He has no known syndrome, but his behavior in the clinic and the parents' reports raise questions about whether he may have attention-deficit/hyperactivity disorder. He has a residual oronasal fistula in the middle of his hard palate that leaks during eating and speech. Jacob had a number of sinus infections in the past year. In the clinic, the speech-language pathologist occludes the fistula with bubble gum and notes that Jacob's resonance is improved and audible nasal emission is markedly reduced.

The speech-language pathologist recommends that the fistula be closed to assist Jacob in learning alveolar sounds and fricatives. The pediatric dentist sees the patient and recommends a palatal appliance but acknowledges that maintaining a temporary appliance may be challenging in this youngster. The oral surgeon and plastic surgeon both recommend waiting another year or two to repair the fistula at the same time as the planned bone graft.

---

Although health care delivery is moving toward increased use of team models, ethical decision-making theories and models continue to focus on the relationship between a single practitioner and a single patient. Decision making changes when multiple clinicians must reach agreements while retaining individual responsibility for the patient's welfare. While team care offers strengths, there are also potential problems related to interprofessional conflict and the potential for a group of professionals to overwhelm a patient or family.

The team's function and the nature of the interaction between team members evolve over time from independent professionals each offering their own expertise and service to a synthesized, flexible, patient-centered approach (Lowe & Herranen, 1981). When a team is functioning well, the process of discussing and considering multiple points of view can improve the quality of decision making. However, when teams are in conflict, individual agendas and defending one's own area of practice or expertise can interfere with achieving care that meets the patient's needs (Lowe & Herranen, 1981).

The interactions between professionals open the potential for differences of opinion that stem from differing treatment philosophies or personal-professional moral positions. Teams approach conflicts differently—some with humor, some with outright anger—but it appears that a team's style for resolving conflicts relates to the stage of the team's development (see Lowe & Herranen, 1981).

Spielman (1993) summarized approaches to resolving conflicts with patients that also apply to conflicts within a team structure. Spielman hypothesized that conflict is resolved by one of five approaches: avoidance, accommodation, coercion, compromise, or collaboration. She also proposed that the approach to resolution is influenced by the time available, the degree of moral certainty about the problem, the strength of commitment to the relationship, and the cost-benefit of finding a resolution. For example, Spielman's model suggests that a pediatrician is more likely to accommodate a parent's request for an unnecessary antibiotic prescription when the physician is rushed, is uncertain about the actual diagnosis, and has a minimal relationship with the family. This analogy applies across professional relationships: Because team members must continue to work with one another, there is an inherent motivation to compromise or find collaborative solutions to disagreements.

Teams also employ strategies for handling conflict of delaying the decision and using mediation. For instance, some teams defer treatment planning for particularly complex cases until a designated "difficult case conference" can be convened. A short delay also allows the clinicians to clarify their positions, gather more information from the literature, and obtain necessary medical tests, all of which aid decision making. Furthermore, time away from a conflict (or potential conflict) tends to decrease reactive responses, thereby improving interprofessional relationships. A delay may be difficult for the family, if they expect a definitive treatment plan during their visit. The team should explain that time is needed to gather information and give the family a time frame within which the team meeting will occur. Follow-up communication, by telephone or in writing, should be prompt after the team has an opportunity to reach a decision or to develop a series of options.

One danger of team care is that the members of the team might focus inward in resolving disagreements with each other (Lowe & Herranen, 1981). Team members may feel obligated to resolve conflicts within the team first so they can present a cohesive plan to families. However, the patient and family should not be marginalized in the decision-making process. When there is more than one reasonable option, the patient or parents should be informed about all the estimated risks, benefits, and costs of each option. While families vary with respect to their tolerance for uncertainty and desire to know about multiple approaches, clinicians should continue to uphold the partnership between the professionals and families in achieving shared, informed decision making.

### Case Study 5 (*continued*)

The speech-language pathologist meets with Jacob's parents to review the team's findings and to discuss treatment options. The options—a palatal appliance to obturate the fistula temporarily or surgical closure of the fistula with early bone grafting—are presented to the family. The parents participate in a discussion of the advantages and disadvantages of both options and elect to try a removable appliance with pediatric dentistry. The team and family agree that if the appliance does not work well for Jacob, they will re-evaluate and plan for surgical repair.

## Innovation and Untested Treatment

The complex needs of infants, children, adolescents, and adults with craniofacial anomalies require adaptation and modifications of techniques in nearly every case. Surgical techniques are the focus of many discussions about the risks of implementing new treatment solutions (Iserson & Chiasson, 2002; McKneally, 1999; Shaw, Mandall, & Mattick, 2002). Presumably, untested surgeries present increased physical risks to patients, whereas ineffective behavioral interventions, such as speech therapy, relate to less tangible risks. From an ethics perspective, however, all potential risks should be considered and presented to the patient and family regardless of the nature of the procedure.

The application of untested techniques raises important ethical questions about where to draw the line between experimental treatment and innovative clinical care. Research is usually distinguished from clinical care based on the underlying goals of these endeavors. Clinical tasks are conducted with the goal of improving the patient's welfare, while research contributes to generalizable knowledge but may not provide direct benefit to the participant. Innovative procedures are usually developed and offered with the intent to provide direct benefit to a patient, but the learning associated with implementing a novel approach also contributes to generalizable knowledge. Therefore, innovation blurs the line between clinical and research practices. Labeling a clinical procedure "research" has practical implications with regard to regulations and oversight that differ from typical clinical care in most countries.

Untested approaches to patient care should be subject to more stringent standards for informed and voluntary consent from patient-participants than are required in most clinical settings. Some institutions will continue to rely on their institutional review boards (IRBs), or equivalent, to provide oversight for "experimental" procedures, whereas others may develop separate, sophisticated monitoring and consent processes specific to innovative treatments that are intended to provide direct benefit to the patient. The language used in the consent process should be selected with care. McKneally (1999) cautioned that the term *innovative* connotes positive progress but fails to denote the real risks involved in what he terms "nonvalidated" procedures.

Finding the precise point of distinction between research and novel approaches to treatment is less important than ensuring that the patients and families have a good understanding of the nature and certainty of the proposed intervention (Fost, 1998). If a patient and family give fully informed consent for a procedure they know is untested or has not been tried in this circumstance, then some of the clinician's ethical obligations are met. Some innovative therapies are implemented as research protocols; however, McKneally and Daar (2003) suggested that the IRB model is often cumbersome for testing clinical procedures. They advocated for a variation on the research review model, as follows:

- The potential risks must be discussed in more detail than is required in clinical care.
- The participants must know that they can choose a more standard treatment approach.
- The rationale and plan should be approved by the chief of surgery and two members of the appropriate surgical service.
- The consent form and consent process should be reviewed by the IRB.
- Institutions should form a task force, or innovations committee, comprised of community members and institutional stakeholders to review the outcomes, the adverse events, and the resource and financial implications of the procedure.

Negative findings and complications should be disseminated (McKneally & Daar, 2003). Variations of this model have been used to monitor consent and the application of particularly invasive, risky, or controversial procedures such as fetal surgeries for life-threatening conditions (Harrison,

1996). Regardless of the oversight mechanism, Iserson and Chiasson (2002) emphasized that the ultimate responsibility rests with the individual clinician who decides whether and how to implement new or modified procedures.

## Summary

Ethical issues arise in the care and treatment of infants, children, and adolescents with clefts or other craniofacial anomalies. Parents and clinicians are obligated to act in the best interests of the child, but at times it is difficult to determine what course of treatment will best serve a given child. Parents' decisions are made amid multiple (sometimes competing) considerations for their family's needs, cultural background, spiritual beliefs, financial resources, and personal experiences. Speech-language pathologists, dentists, surgeons, and other members of the interdisciplinary team should recognize the influence of their own beliefs and experiences in order to counsel families about treatment decisions in the context of various influences on clinical decision making. Clinicians should inform children and adolescents to the extent that the youngsters are capable of understanding and should encourage their participation in decision making. The study of comprehensive outcomes for children with clefts and other craniofacial anomalies is critical to clinicians' ability to provide accurate and effective counseling to patients and their families.

Technological advances, such as improvement in prenatal diagnosis, will continue to raise difficult questions about the role of the cleft and craniofacial team in prenatal counseling and possible future fetal therapies. Clinicians and teams should continue to exercise judgment in the implementation of new techniques that blur the lines between research and therapy. As new ethical issues arise, cleft and craniofacial teams should continue to work together with patients and their families to find solutions that uphold central ethical values.

## Acknowledgments

I thank Robert Orr, Ron Strauss, and Margie Wells-Friedman for their role in constructing several of the cases included in this chapter. Drs. Strauss and Orr have shaped my thinking about the ethical issues in the care of patients with cleft and craniofacial conditions, and much of the discussion here reflects my interpretation of our shared discussions of these issues over many years.

## References


American Academy of Pediatrics Committee on Bioethics. (1995). Informed consent, parental permission, and assent in pediatric practice. *Pediatrics, 9,* 314–317.

Aspinall, C. L. (2002). Dealing with the prenatal diagnosis of clefting: A parent's perspective. *Cleft Palate-Craniofacial Journal, 39,* 183–187.

Beauchamp, T. L. (2003). Methods and principles in biomedical ethics. *Journal of Medical Ethics, 29,* 269–274.

Beauchamp, T. L., & Childress, J. F. (2001). *Principles of biomedical ethics* (5th ed.). New York: Oxford University Press.

Berg, J. W., Appelbaum, P. S., Lidz, C. W., & Parker, L. S. (2001). *Informed consent: Legal theory and clinical practice.* New York: Oxford.

Blumenfeld, Z., Blumenfeld, I., & Bronshtein, M. (1999a). The early prenatal diagnosis of cleft lip and the decision-making process. *Cleft Palate-Craniofacial Journal, 36,* 105–107.

Blumenfeld, Z., Blumenfeld, I., & Bronshtein, M. (1999b). Response to commentary on "The early prenatal diagnosis of cleft lip and the decision-making process." *Cleft Palate-Craniofacial Journal, 36,* 544–545.

Britt, D. W., Risinger, S. T., Miller, V., Mans, M. K., Krivchenia, E. L., & Evans, M. I. (2000). Determinants of parental decisions after the prenatal diagnosis of Down syndrome: Bringing in context. *American Journal of Medical Genetics, 93,* 410–416.

Canady, J. W., Landas, S. K., Morris, H., & Thompson, S. A. (1994). In utero cleft palate repair in the ovine model. *Cleft Palate-Craniofacial Journal, 31,* 37–44.

Eiserman, W., & Strauss, R. P. (1999). Commentary on Blumenfeld Z, Blumenfeld I, and Bronshtein M. The early prenatal diagnosis of cleft lip and the decision-making process (Letter). *Cleft Palate-Craniofacial Journal, 36,* 542–544.

Elliott, C., & Elliott, B. (1991). From the patient's point of view: Medical ethics and the moral imagination. *Journal of Medical Ethics, 17,* 173–178.

Evans, M. L., Oberg, K. C., Kirsch, W., Zhu, Y. H., & Hardesty, R. A. (1995). Intrauterine repair of cleft lip-like defects in lambs with a novel microclip. *Journal of Craniofacial Surgery, 6,* 126–131.

Fost, N. (1998). Ethical dilemmas in medical innovation and research: Distinguishing experimentation from practice. *Seminars in Perinatology, 22,* 223–232.

Harrison, M. R. (1996). Fetal surgery. *American Journal of Obstetrics and Gynecology, 174,* 1255–1264.

Helft, P. R., Siegler, M., & Lantos, J. (2000). The rise and fall of the futility movement. *New England Journal of Medicine, 343,* 293–296.

Holder, A. R. (1983). Parents, courts, and refusal of treatment. *Pediatrics, 103,* 515–521.

Iserson, K. V., & Chiasson, P. M. (2002). The ethics of applying new medical technologies. *Seminars in Laparoscopic Surgery, 9,* 222–229.

Johnson, N., & Sandy, J. R. (2003). Prenatal diagnosis of cleft lip and palate. *Cleft Palate-Craniofacial Journal, 40,* 186–189.

Jones, K. L. (1997). *Smith's recognizable patterns of human malformation* (5th ed.). Philadelphia: Saunders.

Jones, M. C. (1999). Prenatal diagnosis of cleft lip and palate: Experiences in Southern California. *Cleft Palate-Craniofacial Journal, 36,* 107–109.

Jones, M. C. (2002). Prenatal diagnosis of cleft lip and palate: Detection rates, accuracy of ultrasonography, associated anomalies, and strategies for counseling. *Cleft Palate-Craniofacial Journal, 39,* 169–173.

Jonsen, A. R., Siegler, M., & Winslade, W. J. (2006). *Clinical ethics: A practical approach to ethical decisions in clinical medicine* (6th ed.). New York: McGraw-Hill.

Lo, B. (2000). *Resolving ethical dilemmas: A guide for clinicians* (2nd ed.). Philadelphia: Lippincott, Williams & Wilkins.

Lowe, J. I., & Herranen, M. (1981). Understanding teamwork: Another look at the concepts. *Social Work Health Care, 7*(2), 1–11.

Mansfield, C., Hopfer, S., & Marteau, T. M. (1999). Termination rates after prenatal diagnosis of Down syndrome, spina bifida, anencephaly, and Turner and Klinefelter syndromes: A systematic literature review. European Concerted Action: DADA (decision-making after the diagnosis of a fetal abnormality). *Prenatal Diagnosis, 19,* 808–812.

Mast, B. A., Diegelmann, R. F., Krummel, T. M., & Cohen, I. K. (1992). Scarless wound healing in the mammalian fetus. *Surgery, Gynecology & Obstetrics, 174,* 441–451.

Matthews, M. S. (2002). Beyond easy answers: The plastic surgeon and prenatal diagnosis. *Cleft Palate-Craniofacial Journal, 39,* 179–182.

Matthews, M. S., Cohen, M., Viglione, M., & Brown, A. S. (1998). Prenatal counseling for cleft lip and palate. *Plastic and Reconstructive Surgery, 101,* 1–5.

McDermott, J. (2000). *Babyface: A story of heart and bones.* Bethesda, MD: Woodbine House.

McKneally, M. F. (1999). Ethical problems in surgery: Innovation leading to unforeseen complications. *World Journal of Surgery, 23,* 786–788.

McKneally, M. F., & Daar, A. S. (2003). Introducing new technologies: Protecting subjects of surgical innovation and research. *World Journal of Surgery, 27,* 930–935.

Parens, E., & Asch, A. (1999). The disability rights critique of prenatal testing: Reflections and recommendations. *Hastings Center Report, 29*(5), S1–S22.

Pearlman, R. A., & Uhlmann, R. F. (1988). Quality of life in chronic diseases: Perceptions of elderly patients. *Journal of Gerontology, 43,* M25–M30.

Ross, L. F. (1998). *Children, families, and health care decision making.* New York: Oxford University Press.

Saal, H. M. (2002). Prenatal diagnosis: When the clinician disagrees with the patient's decision. *Cleft Palate-Craniofacial Journal, 39,* 174–178.

Shaw, W. C., Mandall, N. A., & Mattick, C. R. (2002). Ethical and scientific decision making in distraction osteogenesis. *Cleft Palate-Craniofacial Journal, 39,* 641–645.

Slevin, M. L., Stubbs, L., Plant, H. J., Wilson, P., Gregory, W. M., Armes, P. J., et al. (1990). Attitudes toward chemotherapy: Comparing views of patients with cancer with those of doctors, nurses, and general public. *British Medical Journal, 300,* 1458–1460.

Spielman, B. J. (1993). Conflict in medical ethics cases: Seeking patterns of resolution. *Journal of Clinical Ethics, 4,* 212–218.

Strauss, R. P. (2002). Beyond easy answers: Prenatal diagnosis and counseling during pregnancy. *Cleft Palate-Craniofacial Journal, 39,* 164–168.

Strauss, R. P., & American Cleft Palate-Craniofacial Association Team Standards Committee. (1998). Cleft palate and craniofacial teams in the United States and Canada: A national survey of team organization and standards of care. *Cleft Palate-Craniofacial Journal, 35,* 473–480.

Wagner, W., & Harrison, M. R. (2002). Fetal operations in the head and neck area: Current state. *Head & Neck, 24,* 482–490.

Walker, B. (with Cooper, C.). (2004). Bree Walker interviewed by Chet Cooper. *Ability Magazine* [Online version]. Retrieved February 28, 2004, from www.abilitymagazine.com/walker_interview.html

Weir, R. F., & Peters, C. (1997). Affirming the decisions adolescents make about life and death. *Hastings Center Report, 27*(6), 29–40.

# CHAPTER 4

# Transcultural Care of Patients with Cleft Palate and Craniofacial Anomalies

*Virginia A. Hinton*

*Ask not what kind of disease a person has, but what kind of person has the disease.*

—Sir William Osler, 1849–1919

Providing complex interdisciplinary health care that is both culturally sensitive and effective requires the thorough commitment of all team professionals, as well as respect for and acceptance of the belief systems and traditions valued by patients and families from diverse cultures. A variety of specialized learning experiences and resources may assist the process, including in-service opportunities, relationships with community consultants and representatives, and partnerships with well-trained interpreters. The transition from an ethnocentric health care model to a system that communicates information with cultural proficiency also requires periodic review and self-assessment. In this chapter, Hinton describes the knowledge, considerations, and procedures that can help teams to develop the transcultural expertise necessary to improve service delivery to patients with cleft palate and craniofacial anomalies.

1. What are the changing U.S. demographics that compel the need for cultural proficiency in a health care team?
2. What are the risks to patient and family care created by a team that is restricted by its ethnocentric philosophies and procedures?
3. What are some of the critical influences of culture, religion, and socioeconomic backgrounds on attitudes and beliefs about health care? What impact might these biases have on the success of interdisciplinary team care for patients with cleft palate or craniofacial anomalies?

4. What are the six levels of cultural sensitivity that could characterize interdisciplinary team operation? Describe these levels and use a practical example of cleft palate and craniofacial team procedures or performance to illustrate.
5. What specific steps can be taken to reduce cultural bias in health care delivery? Propose a strategy that might enhance an interdisciplinary team's cultural proficiency in each of the five steps described.
6. What are specific suggestions that will improve communicative interactions using an interpreter? Discuss these recommendations for increasing the efficiency, sensitivity, and accuracy of interpreted messages.

With a current population of more than 281 million people, the United States is the most culturally, ethnically, and racially diverse country in the world. For the past four centuries, people from all parts of the planet have relocated to the United States through forced migration (i.e., slavery), through free immigration, and as refugees from violence and poverty. This influx of people from around the world has not resulted in the development of one homogeneous "American" culture, but rather a complex society that consists of many distinct and diverse cultural and ethnic communities that retain a high level of social identity (Taylor, 1986). Currently, more than 215 different ethnic groups reside in the United States. Data from the U.S. Bureau of the Census (2000) indicate that the population is becoming more diverse and that the traditional "minority groups" will continue to become larger percentages of the population (see Table 4.1). Hispanics represent the fastest growing minority group and will soon surpass African Americans in terms of percentage of the total population. Indeed, additional projection data from the U.S. Bureau of the Census (2000) suggest that by the end of the 21st century, people of Hispanic and Asian/Pacific Island heritage will make up a larger percentage of the U.S. population than individuals from Anglo and Western European backgrounds.

The changing demographics of the United States have increased the need for health care providers to incorporate knowledge of the cultural and ethnic characteristics of their patients into assessment and treatment plans. This chapter provides a framework (albeit limited) for members

**Table 4.1**
**Current and Projected Population Statistics (in Percentages) for the United States**

| Group | 2000 | 2010 | 2020 |
|---|---|---|---|
| African descent | 12.2 | 12.5 | 12.8 |
| Asian/Pacific Islander descent | 4.0 | 4.7 | 5.7 |
| Hispanic | 11.8 | 14.6 | 17.0 |
| Native American | 0.7 | 0.8 | 0.8 |
| White | 71.3 | 67.3 | 63.8 |

*Note.* Compiled by the Population Estimates Program, Population Division, U.S. Bureau of the Census, Department of Commerce (2000).

of cleft and craniofacial teams to use in developing an understanding of the many issues related to providing optimal clinical care to patients with diverse cultural and ethnic backgrounds.

## Definitions

Health care providers would benefit from understanding the terms that are commonly used when discussing diverse populations. Although there is not complete agreement on the definitions of these terms, the following represents common usage of the terms in the health care and social sciences literature.

> *Acculturation*—the degree to which an individual has given up the beliefs and social patterns of his or her original culture and adopted the traits of the predominant culture in which he or she currently resides (Huff & Kline, 1998).
>
> *Assimilation*—the social, economic, and political integration of an individual into the dominant society (Casas & Casas, 1994). For assimilation to occur, there must be some degree of personal integration into the mainstream society with respect to language, values, laws, and customs (Huff & Kline, 1998).

*Cultural competence or cultural proficiency*—the viewing of cultural differences as strengths, not deficits. In addition, cultural competence assumes that an individual has the ability to recognize the inherent merits and strengths of cultural groups other than one's own and to utilize knowledge about other groups to facilitate interactions that are satisfactory to all individuals (Campinha-Bacote, 1994).

*Culture*—common beliefs, ideas, experiences, knowledge, attitudes, and behaviors that are shared by a particular group of individuals. Further, a culture consists of the shared rules, values, and beliefs that underlie overt behavior and are learned as a consequence of being a member of a specific group or community. Members of a cultural group also share the same language or languages, through which the other aspects of the culture are transmitted (Slonim, 1991).

*Ethnicity*—the specifically identifiable characteristics of a culture, such as racial or national origin, dress, customs, and food (Taylor, 1986). In addition, ethnicity includes ancestral tradition, a shared sense of peoplehood, and the influence of the group on the lives of its members.

*Ethnocentricity*—the belief that one's own culture and its values are the standard against which the merits of all other groups are measured (Krajewski-Jaime, Brown, & Zeifert, 1996).

*Ethnorelativism*—the ability to accept and respect cultural differences and the ability to shift to another cultural world view (Krajewski-Jaime et al., 1996).

*Minority*—a group of individuals who are not members of the most populous group in a specific environment. For example, an individual may represent a minority population in his or her work environment but not in his or her neighborhood. In some contexts, this term may be associated with powerlessness and subordination (Clark, 1993).

*Multicultural/cultural pluralism*—any society that consists of many cultures with varying values, beliefs, languages, religions, customs, and traditions.

*Race*—the anatomic, physiologic, and biologic characteristics of an individual, including skin color and facial features. *Culture* and *race* are in no way synonymous terms. For example, a person with heavily pigmented skin may be a member of any number of African or Hispanic cultural groups.

*Transcultural*—adopting a set of beliefs or values that extend across cultural boundaries. Further, the term *transcultural* incorporates a functional knowledge of other cultures and the ability to use this knowledge constructively.

## Impact of Cultural Diversity on Health Care

The wide variety of cultural belief systems regarding health and illness poses a challenge to U.S. health care providers. To provide optimum care, professionals cannot remain indifferent to diverse cultural perspectives on health and wellness. Rather, they must understand that religious underpinnings and cultural values determine the beliefs and practices associated with illness and medical supervision (Page, 2005). It has been well established that Anglo Americans and people of Western European descent have a fundamentally different view of the world than most other cultures (Clark, 1993; Lynch & Hanson, 1992; Nilchaikovit, Hill, & Holland, 1993; Pachter, 1994; Taylor & Clarke, 1994). For example, members of many Asian, Native American, and Hispanic cultural groups ascribe states of wellness or illness to their relationship to God or nature, rather than to microbial disease processes or genetic defects (Gomez, Ruiz, & Rumbaut, 1985; Mattson, 1988; Nilchaikovit et al., 1993; Pachter, 1994; Spector, 2000). Clearly, these beliefs differ substantially from the predominant view of health and illness held by Western cultures. However, because Anglo Americans constitute the majority population of the country and of U.S. health care providers, an ethnocentric view of medical care frequently occurs. That is, many health care providers (e.g., physicians, nurses, speech-language pathologists) in the United States may assume that the Western, biomedical perspective on illness and disability is the only viable approach to diagnosis and treatment. Unfortunately, this attitude often leads to ineffective health care and the belief that some patients of diverse cultural backgrounds are "noncompliant." Therefore, the differences in culturally based perceptions of health care must be acknowledged, understood, and integrated into treatment plans for all patients before effective management of clefting or any other disorder can occur (Krajewski-Jaime et al., 1996; Nilchaikovit et al., 1993).

The relationship between cultural values and health-related beliefs and behaviors is very complex (Pachter, 1994). Each patient is a unique individual whose health-related attitudes arise not only from the beliefs and values of his or her cultural group, but also from personal experiences, length of residence in the United States, education, socioeconomic status, and degree of assimilation into the predominant culture. Further, to assume that all members of a given cultural group hold the same views regarding health-related issues is a form of stereotyping that may be as dangerous as ethnocentricity. Therefore, patients from any culture must be viewed as individuals from vastly different personal backgrounds who may subscribe to their culture in varying degrees and in varying situations, or perhaps not at all (Lassiter, 1995). To ascertain an individual patient's views on health-related issues, it is necessary to obtain a great deal of information that extends well beyond a complete medical history. Appendix 4A contains an example of such a questionnaire that explores cultural beliefs and attitudes relative to health care practices. Although obtaining information in such detail will be time-consuming, it is time well spent if the activity promotes enhanced communication between the health care provider and the patient and, therefore, results in maximally effective care.

In addition to differences in culturally based perceptions of health care, linguistic and physical barriers also exist. Physical barriers include financial constraints, lack of knowledge of the location of appropriate facilities, distance of available services, and inadequate transportation or lack of knowledge regarding transportation options (Bliatout, 1988). In addition, if clinic hours are incompatible with work schedules, patients or their parents may lose work time and wages. Although these physical barriers can present major problems for many patients, they are more easily corrected than other barriers to health care. Many social service or community agencies can provide transportation and information regarding the location of appropriate services. Professionals may accommodate patients' work schedules by extending clinic hours or by opening "satellite clinics" in outlying communities.

Language differences present one of the most substantial barriers to optimum health care in the United States. The U.S. Bureau of the Census (2000) estimates that approximately 30 languages other than English are spoken in the homes of more than 40 million U.S. residents. These data include only the major forms of a given language and not the various dialects that are spoken by members of a specific language community. Because Anglo Americans are rarely fluent in languages other than English, direct communication between the care provider and the patient may be difficult or impossible. If a patient is not proficient in English but is forced to use that language, he or she becomes immediately subordinate to the health care provider (Gomez et al., 1985). In addition, the communication barrier may preclude the possibility of obtaining an accurate medical history and may prevent the patient from understanding a health care provider's explanations of the problem and strategies for care. Clearly, the use of an interpreter is a reasonable solution to the linguistic barrier experienced by many patients of non-English speaking cultural groups. However, the health care provider must be aware that the use of an interpreter may interfere with adequate communication, if the interpreter is not familiar with medical terminology or treatment procedures, does not report all information, or inserts his or her own ideas. Suggestions for optimum communication with non-English speaking patients are located in Appendix 4B.

## Specific Cultural and Ethnic Variations That Influence Optimal Health Care

It is beyond the scope of this chapter to describe the myriad health care beliefs of members of various cultural and ethnic groups residing in the United States. To attempt to do so would be an excellent example of cultural stereotyping. Listing a set of general health care beliefs for Asian Americans would assume that the core values of an individual from a rural Hmong village would be the same as those of an individual from Beijing or Tokyo. Similarly, to assume that the beliefs of all Hispanic Americans, whether from Mexico or Haiti, are the same may lead to an ineffective health care relationship with an individual patient. Therefore, each cleft palate and craniofacial team must seek out information specific to the various populations that it serves. A list of initial references for information pertaining to the cultural beliefs of the major nondominant populations living in the United States is located in Appendix 4C.

## Poverty as a Cultural Barrier to Adequate Health Care

Regardless of cultural heritage or race, individuals living in poverty are faced with substantial barriers to appropriate care of any medical problem, including facial clefting. In many cases, poverty is the primary demographic barrier to adequate medical treatment (Spector, 2000). According to the U.S Bureau of the Census (2000), in 1999 approximately 12.7% of U.S. residents (32.3 million people) and 16.9% of all U.S. children lived at or below the poverty level. Children under 6 years of age are more likely to be poor than any other member of the population (Fitzgerald, Lester, & Zuckerman, 1995), and as many as 30% of all children are not covered by health insurance (Tingsley, Wang, Kwasmain, & Green, 1997). Although the overall poverty rate is the lowest since 1979, there are still substantial differences in the poverty rates for non-White versus White members of the population; Table 4.2 provides specific poverty rates for specific groups as reported by the U.S. Bureau of the Census (2000). Poverty levels also vary by geographic region. In 1999, according to the U.S. Census, 10.9% of residents in the Northeast, 12.6% of those living in the West, 9.8% in the Midwest, and 13.1% in the South lived at or below the poverty level.

Based on these data, it is reasonable to assume that all cleft palate and craniofacial teams will assess and treat many patients who live in poverty. Unfortunately, socioeconomic status and the culture of poverty may pre-

**Table 4.2**
**Estimates of Poverty Rates for the United States**

| Group | Total poverty rates in percentage of total population | Percentage of each cultural group living in poverty | Percentage of children living below poverty level |
|---|---|---|---|
| African descent | 7.7 | 25.9 | 30.0 |
| Asian/Pacific Islander descent | 12.5 | 10.3 | 11.5 |
| Hispanic | 23.6 | 46.1 | 30.0 |
| Native American | 22.8 | 3.6 | 19.7 |
| White | 25.9 | 23.1 | 9.4 |

*Note.* Compiled by the Population Estimates Program, Population Division, U.S. Bureau of the Census, Department of Commerce (2000).

vent these individuals from obtaining or benefiting from medical care. The most obvious poverty-related barriers to adequate care for patients include location and availability of health care services, inadequate transportation, hours missed from work, and lack of child care (Rodriguez, 1993). These factors may prevent clients from keeping scheduled appointments and from obtaining follow-up care away from the team. However, other, less obvious factors related to living in poverty may also have a negative impact on the overall development of and, therefore, long-term outcome for patients with facial clefts. These include lack of the following: parental education, appropriate nutrition, parental time spent with children, adequate local educational services, and sanitary living conditions. All of these factors may have a negative impact on the overall health status of the patient, the ability to comply with postoperative care instructions, and the ability to provide appropriate developmental activities for a child.

The presence of these poverty-related barriers indicates that what may be viewed by professionals as noncompliant behavior in very poor patients actually represents cultural differences from the mainstream health care community. Therefore, it is essential that health care providers determine the exact nature and source of the cultural barriers related to poverty and develop strategies that allow the patients to obtain the most appropriate services available. For example, changing parental beliefs about health-related issues is more realistic than increasing their income or changing their social class (Rodriguez, 1993; Tingsley et al., 1997). This can be accomplished primarily through education and identification of appropriate community agencies (e.g., state departments of health) that are accessible to the patient's family. Educational materials of appropriate literacy levels and the names of local facilities should be provided to all patients. If the patients or their parents have inadequate reading skills, then it may be necessary to present information orally to the families and to contact local health care providers to assist the families in obtaining appropriate follow-up care.

## Building a Culturally Proficient Team

Providing adequate care to all patients with facial clefts involves continuing education for the care providers. Therefore, all members of the cleft palate and craniofacial team must become culturally proficient. It is easy to say that teams should "treat all patients equally." However, this attitude does not allow for the most appropriate treatment for members of culturally and ethnically distinct groups. When discordant views of health care exist between the patient and the provider, it is incumbent upon the health care provider to adopt strategies and interaction styles that will allow the patient to obtain maximum benefit from the services that are available.

## Level of Cultural Sensitivity

To establish a culturally proficient cleft palate and craniofacial team, it is necessary to determine the attitudes of the team members toward non-dominant cultural groups. The following continuum (Randall-David, 1994) is appropriate for both assessing a team's current status and evaluating change over time.

1. *Cultural destructiveness*—attitudes, policies, and practices that are intentionally destructive to other cultures
2. *Cultural incapacity*—biased, paternalistic systems that lack the capacity to facilitate optimum health care in culturally diverse groups
3. *Cultural blindness*—the belief that culture, ethnicity, or race makes no difference in how services are provided
4. *Cultural precompetence*
   - awareness of the particular sets of attitudes, beliefs, and values associated with cultural groups other than one's own
   - awareness of the impact of culture on interactions, perceptions, and so forth
   - desire and attempts to provide services that are respectful of cultural diversity
   - engagement in workshops, training, and hiring of diversity staff
5. *Cultural competence*
   - acceptance of and respect for cultural differences
   - self-assessment regarding cultural competence
   - responsiveness to the unique needs of diverse groups
   - adaptation of service models
   - functional relationship between policy and practice
6. *Cultural proficiency*
   - attempts to add to the knowledge base of culturally competent practice

- development of culturally competent therapeutic approaches
- hiring of staff with specialization in cultural competence

## Steps to Achieving Cultural Proficiency

A great deal of information is available in written form and through workshops regarding the relationship between culture and health care. However, the development of a culturally proficient cleft palate and craniofacial team requires more than simply acknowledging the differences in the diverse populations served by the team. Information can be presented in many ways, but the health care providers must develop awareness, sensitivity, and appropriate skills. Listed below are steps that may facilitate the development of a culturally proficient team. However, each team member must make the decision to become a fully active participant in the process if successful changes are going to occur and culturally diverse patients are going to receive the most appropriate care.

**1.** Determine the current level of cultural bias and knowledge, using one of the many questionnaires available for this purpose. An example can be found in Appendix 4D (see Randall-David, 1994, and Goode, 2006, for other examples).

**2.** Obtain information about the culturally diverse groups whose members are current or future patients served by the team. Many types of information must be accumulated to begin to understand the perceptions of patients who are members of nondominant cultural groups. For example, this information should include lines of authority, family structure, sense of "community," the perceived value of education, verbal and nonverbal communication strategies, dietary needs and restrictions, beliefs pertaining to states of health and illness (including birth defects), interactions based on age and gender, and the use of biomedical treatment versus traditional healing (Mattson, 1988). In addition to continuing-education experiences, it is important for professionals to establish a functional and communicative relationship with nondominant cultural groups that are served by the team. One way to accomplish this goal is through the use of "cultural consultants." These individuals are typically prominent members of a specific cultural group, such as a local religious leader or community representative. In addition, the cultural consultant must have a detailed understanding of the group's current health-related attitudes and beliefs and must be willing to share this information with team members. The cultural consultant can provide specific examples of strategies and treatment approaches that will be most successful with members of a particular cultural group.

**3.** Develop culturally appropriate assessment and treatment procedures for members of *each* cultural group. It is crucial to identify materials and strategies that are appropriate for the culture of each individual being assessed. There are many resources available to speech-language pathologists for work with patients of diverse backgrounds (e.g., Battle, 1997; Goldstein, 2000). However, unless appropriate interaction strategies are employed with these materials, an optimal evaluation will not occur. Because physicians and dental specialists use fewer materials (i.e., written tests), their focus must be on developing and using culturally appropriate interactions. These may include asking permission to touch a patient, directing comments and recommendations to the appropriate person of authority, or refraining from making direct eye contact with members of the opposite sex. It is also crucial to identify models of treatment that are acceptable to patients of various cultural groups. For example, women of Asian or Middle Eastern descent should only be examined by other women.

In some cases, developing appropriate assessment and treatment procedures for members of nondominant cultural groups may involve negotiation with the patients or their families. Members of the cleft palate and craniofacial team need to learn to work collaboratively with patients so that appropriate care can occur. Specifically, the health care providers need to negotiate with the patient and family to eliminate potentially harmful folk medicine practices while not demeaning these practices. In addition, it may be useful to encourage or support the use of nonharmful traditional healing practices, such as the use of prayer or harmless herbal remedies. This will allow the health care provider and the patients to develop a more cooperative, respectful relationship.

**4.** Identify and train appropriate interpreters who can provide regular service to the cleft palate and craniofacial team. A list of suggestions for working effectively with interpreters in clinical examination and treatment is contained in Appendix 4B. Overall, it is important to verify that the individual who interprets is a qualified professional who can interpret knowledgeably and without bias. For example, information should be made available in advance to verify that the interpreter understands what he or she is being asked to interpret and has the appropriate medical terminology and vocabulary to communicate accurately. Whenever possible, it is useful for the cleft palate and craniofacial team to establish a recurring relationship with interpreters who may then become familiar with the terms, procedures, and other vocabulary associated with the clinical exchange. The clinician and interpreter must work together as a cohesive team to provide meaningful "chunks" of information that are not too short (i.e., "choppy") or too lengthy. Ultimately, the clinician has the responsibility to monitor the patient and family to ensure that the information is communicated successfully, by providing follow-up questions and opportunity for patient and family feedback that clarifies any potential misunderstandings (Purnell, 1998).

**5.** Evaluate the team's assessment and intervention procedures to determine potential areas of cultural bias or limits. Each team should develop procedures and standards for assessing the quality of team approaches to cultural proficiency. As with any good assessment, these procedures and standards should include gathering data from multiple sources. For example, questionnaires may be sent to patients following treatment sessions or hospitalizations. The questionnaire should focus on the patient's satisfaction with the treatment as it relates to the patient's personal beliefs about health and wellness. In addition, the team should interact with the cultural consultants consistently and should obtain written or oral evaluations from these individuals. The data collected from patients and cultural consultants should be shared with all members of the team. Based on these outcome data, the team can develop strategies to further enhance cultural proficiency.

## Summary

Providing optimal health care for patients with clefts and other craniofacial anomalies can be challenging under the most ideal circumstances. When patients and caregivers differ in their perspectives on health, wellness, illness, and medical care, the challenges facing cleft palate and craniofacial team members may increase substantially. Therefore, it is imperative that all team members actively seek to educate themselves regarding the diverse cultural beliefs of their patients. However, knowledge is not enough. Incorporating an informed, respectful understanding of cultural differences into daily practice will reduce frustration for the health care providers as well as for the patients and their families, thus ensuring that optimum treatment compliance and outcomes are achieved.

# APPENDIX 4A

# Cultural Beliefs and Attitudes Assessment

The following are questions to consider in caring for patients with cultural backgrounds that differ from the dominant health care culture.

1. How long has the patient been in the country?
2. Where and when was the patient born?
3. What is the patient's ethnic and/or cultural affiliation?
4. Why is the patient currently residing in the local area?
5. Who constitutes the patient's major support group?
6. What are the patient's primary and secondary languages and his or her reading and writing abilities?
7. What is the patient's preferred language?
8. How would you characterize the patient's nonverbal communication style?
9. What is the patient's religion, its importance in the patient's daily life and current practices, and its implications for medical care?
10. Have you determined the type of religious support that the patient needs for optimum health/medical care and/or hospitalization?
11. What are the patient's food prohibitions and preferences?
12. Are the patient's financial resources adequate to meet recommendations and follow-up care?
13. What are the patient's beliefs regarding health, illness, disability, and medical care?
14. Do you understand what the patient believes has caused or is causing the problem?
15. Are you aware of the patient's priorities for medical care?
16. Have you encouraged the patient to tell you about any issues, needs, or problems associated with health/medical care and/or hospitalization?

17. Have you determined the level of family and/or community involvement that the patient prefers or expects?
18. How have you determined the patient's level of understanding of the diagnosis, recommended treatments, follow-up procedures, and long-term outcomes?
19. Have you determined whether or not the patient is using alternative medical treatments?
20. Have you determined whether or not the patient has any unanswered questions?
21. Do you feel that the team's members and the patient have a shared understanding of the problem and the plan of action?
22. Do you know whether or not the patient agrees with the recommended plan of action?

## APPENDIX 4B

# Guidelines for Using Interpreters to Communicate with Non-English Speaking Patients

1. Use interpreters rather than translators. *Interpreters* decode the words and provide the meaning behind the words, whereas *translators* "convert" words from one language to another. Use a translator only if an interpreter is not available. In this case, realize that the information obtained may not be accurate or complete.
   - Use dialect-specific interpreters when possible.
   - Use interpreters trained in medical terminology when possible.
2. Provide adequate time for interpretation. Using an interpreter may take twice as long as a regular verbal interchange.
3. Consider both the patient's and the interpreter's gender, ethnicity, age, and language. For example, it may be inappropriate to use a male interpreter with a female patient or a Serbian interpreter with a Bosnian patient.
4. Be aware that class or social differences between the patient and the interpreter may result in incomplete reporting of information, if the interpreter views the content as unimportant, irrelevant, or superstitious.
5. Do not use relatives as interpreters. They may not report all relevant information if it is viewed as shameful, or they may provide their own opinion or interpretation rather than that of the patient.
6. Do not use children as interpreters, especially when discussing sensitive topics. In many cultures, it is inappropriate for children to converse with unfamiliar adults or to be more skillful at a particular task than an adult.

7. Meet with the interpreter before the session to discuss the purpose and goals of the session. Also, discuss the need for the interpreter *not* to add his or her own ideas or assessments and to include all information that the patient provides, whether or not the interpreter thinks that something is relevant or important.
8. Provide time for the interpreter and the patient to be alone. This allows the patient to become more comfortable with the interpreter and may produce more complete information.
9. Use appropriate language forms
    - Speak in short units of speech, without using long sentences or paragraphs.
    - Avoid technical terms and professional jargon to the extent possible.
    - Avoid use of idioms, abstractions, metaphors, colloquialisms, and slang.
10. Check the patient's understanding and the accuracy of the interpretation by asking the patient to repeat the message and/or instructions, facilitated by the interpreter.
11. Listen to the patient and notice nonverbal communications that indicate emotion and degree of understanding related to the topic.
12. Maintain eye contact with the patient if appropriate to the patient's culture.
13. Determine the legal implications pertaining to providing interpreters. In some cases, the facility may be legally liable if you do not provide appropriate interpreters. Always make a note in the chart indicating the name of the interpreter, how the interpreter was obtained, and any other pertinent information.

# APPENDIX 4C

# References for Information Related to Specific Cultural Groups

## African American and Sub-Saharan African Descent

African Americans are an extremely heterogeneous group. The majority of African Americans are the descendants of slaves from many regions of sub-Saharan Africa who were brought forcibly to the United States at approximately the same time as Europeans established permanent settlements. Although initially they represented many diverse cultures and spoke a wide variety of languages, the experience of slavery in America caused many African Americans to develop similar cultural values (Huff & Kline, 1998). More recent members of the group broadly defined as African American are refugees from poverty and war or civil unrest in countries as diverse as Haiti, the Sudan, and Zimbabwe. In addition, a wide variety of religious beliefs are practiced by African Americans, ranging from mainstream Catholic and Protestant to more traditional practices including voodoo. The specific relationship of these belief patterns to health care must be determined. The religious and health care practices of the Black Muslims in the United States may more closely resemble those of people from Middle Eastern countries than those of sub-Saharan African countries. The following references pertain to the cultural beliefs and health care characteristics of many of these groups.

Airhihenbuwa, C. O., & Harrison, I. E. (1993). Traditional medicine in Africa: Past, present and future. In P. Conrad & E. Gallagher (Eds.), *Healing and health care in developing countries.* Philadelphia: Temple University Press.

Congress, E. P., & Lyons, B. P. (1992). Cultural differences in health beliefs: Implications for social work practice in health care settings. *Social Work in Health Care, 17*(3), 81–96.

Herring, P., & Montgomery, S. (1996). Health beliefs and prevention, health promotion activities of Black and White women: A comparative study. *Journal of Wellness Perspectives, 12*, 188–197.

Iglesias, A., & Anderson, B. (1993). Dialectal variations. In J. E. Bernthal & N. Bankson (Eds.), *Articulation and phonological disorders* (3rd ed.). Englewood Cliffs, NJ: Prentice Hall.

Payne-Johnson, J. C. (1992). Communications and aging: A case for understanding African-Americans who are elderly. *Asha, 34*, 41–44.

Terrell, S. L., Battle, D. E., & Grantham, R. B. (1998). African-American cultures. In D. E. Battle (Ed.), *Communication disorders in multicultural populations* (2nd ed.). Boston: Butterworth-Heinemann.

Williams, D. R. (1996). The health of the African American population. In S. Petrosa & R. Rhomboid (Eds.), *Origins and destinies: Immigration, race and ethnicity in America*. Belmont, CA: Wadsworth.

Wolfram, W. (1994). The phonology of a sociocultural society: The case of African American vernacular English. In J. E. Bernthal & N. Bankson (Eds.), *Child phonology: Characteristics, assessment and intervention with special populations*. New York: Thieme.

## Asian and Pacific Islanders

The groups of people identified as Asian American and Pacific Islanders are arguably the most culturally diverse population residing in the United States. Asians may come from any of 30 different nations, while Pacific Islanders may come from any of 25 nations (www.census.gov). Each of these nations constitutes a very distinct ethnic cultural group with many subgroups. Although there are some commonalities among these groups in terms of health care practices, there just as many differences. The specific ethnic background of each patient must be explored and his or her personal health care practices identified. The following references offer a starting point for this process.

Asian and Pacific Islander American Health Forum, www.apiahf.org

Association of Asian Pacific Community Health Organization, www.aapcho.org

Chen, M. A. (1996). Demographics of Asian and Pacific Islander Americans: Health implications. *Asian American and Pacific Islander Journal of Health, 4*(1–3), 40–49.

Frye, B. A. (1995). Use of cultural themes in promoting health care among Southeast Asian refugees. *American Journal of Health Promotion, 9*, 269–280.

Hawks, B. L. (1996). Barriers to improvement for Asian Americans. *Asian American and Pacific Islander Journal of Health, 4*(1–3), 50–54.

Hughes, C. K., & Aluli, N. E. (1991). A culturally sensitive approach to health education for Native Hawaiians. *Journal of Health Education, 22,* 387–390.

McLaughlin, L., & Braun, K. (1998). Asian and Pacific Islander cultural values: Considerations for health-care decision making. *Health and Social Work, 23,* 116–126.

Mokuau, N. (1996). Health and well-being for Pacific Islanders: Status, barriers and resolutions. *Asian American and Pacific Islander Journal of Health, 4*(1–3), 55–67.

Uba, L. (1992). Cultural barriers to health care for Southeast Asian refugees. *Public Health Reports, 197,* 544–548.

van Breda, A. (1989). Health issues facing Native American children. *Pediatric Nursing, 15,* 575–577.

Yoon, E., & Chien, E. (1996). Asian American and Pacific Islander health: A paradigm for minority health. *Journal of the American Medical Association, 275,* 736–737.

## Hispanic/Latino Descent

Like African Americans, members of the group of Americans designated as Hispanic or Latino come from many different countries (e.g., Spain, Puerto Rico, Mexico, Central and South America) and have a wide variety of health care beliefs. Although demographic and medical literature generally refers to all individuals from these countries as Hispanic or Latino, individuals' culture, social structure, and medical practices can vary widely based on the country of origin and place of residence within a country (urban vs. rural). Religious practices (predominantly Roman Catholic) are an extremely important aspect of life for most Hispanics and have a substantial impact on health care beliefs. However, the type of Catholicism practiced in many Central and South American countries differs in form from that in the United States, and health care providers should explore the relationship between religion and health for each patient. In addition, heath care providers should determine if their patients also seek help from traditional healers, as well as priests and physicians. The following references provide some relevant information.

Carrasquillo, A. (1991). *Hispanic children and youth in the United States.* New York: Garland.

Erzinger, S. (1991). Communication between Spanish-speaking patients and their doctors in medical encounters. *Culture, Medicine and Psychiatry, 15*(1), 91–110.

Kayser, H. (1998). Hispanic cultures and language. In D. E. Battle (Ed.), *Communication disorders in multicultural populations* (2nd ed.). Boston: Butterworth-Heinemann.

Langdon, H. W., & Cheng, L. L. (1992). *Hispanic children and adults with communication disorders: Assessment and intervention.* Gaithersburg, MD: Aspen.

Mardiros, M. (1989). Conception of childhood disability among Mexican-American parents. *Medical Anthropology, 12*(1), 55–68.

Marin, G., & Marin, B. (1991). *Research with Hispanic populations.* Thousand Oaks, CA: Sage.

National Alliance for Hispanic Health, www.hispanichealth.org

National Hispanic Medical Association, www.nhmamd.org

## Native American

The native peoples in Canada and the United States do not form a unified ethnic group, but are members of many distinct cultural groups with separate languages, customs, religions, and beliefs relating to wellness and health care. Characterizing all native people as American Indians or First Americans ignores the fundamental differences in the distinct ethnic groups and may lead to generalizations in the manner in which all native patients are treated in a Western medical setting (Huff & Kline, 1998). Since it would be overwhelming to attempt to describe each separate native group, most demographic and medical research divides the native people of North America into the following groups: Northeastern Indians, Southeastern Indians, Southwestern Indians, Northern Plains Indians, Northwest Coast Indians, Alaska Natives, Oklahoma Indians, California Indians, and Indians of the Plateau, Great Basin, and Rocky Mountains. Although each group has differing beliefs regarding health, wellness, and illness, some general references are listed below.

American Academy of Pediatrics Committee on Native American Child Health & Committee on Community Health Services. (2004). Ethical considerations in research with socially identifiable populations. *Pediatrics, 113*(1), 148–151.

Association of American Indian Physicians, www.aaip.com

Beck, V., Walters, A., & Francisco, N. (1992). *The sacred.* Tsaile, AZ: Navajo Community Press.

Katz, J. R. (2004). Addressing the health care needs of American Indians and Alaska Natives. *American Journal of Public Health, 94*(1), 13–14

Lamarine, R. (1989). The dilemma of Native American health. *Health Education, 20*(5), 15–18.

Lowe, J., & Struthers, R. (2001). A conceptual framework of nursing in Native American culture. *Journal of Nursing Scholarship, 33,* 279–283.

Lyons, W. S. (1996). *Encyclopedia of Native American healing.* New York: Norton Press.

National Indian Child Welfare Association, www.nicwa.org

National Library of Medicine, www.nlm.nih.gov/medlineplus/nativeamericanshealth.html

Natural Health Notebook, www.naturalhealthnotebook.com

Perssini, S., Leake, J. L., Mayhall, J. T., Maar, M., & Trudeau, R. (2004). Prevalence of early childhood caries among First Nations children, District of Manitoulin, Ontario. *International Journal of Paediatric Dentistry, 14,* 101–110.

The Indian Health Service, www.ihs.gov

Wittig, D. R. (2004). Knowledge, skills and attitudes of nursing students regarding culturally congruent care of Native Americans. *Journal of Transcultural Nursing, 154*(1), 54–61.

## General Information References

American Public Health Association, www.apha.org

Chan, S. (1990). Early intervention of culturally diverse families of infants and toddlers with disabilities. *Infants and Young Children: An Interdisciplinary Journal of Special Care Practices, 3*(2), 78–87.

Cheng, L. L., & Hammer, C. S. (1992). *Cultural perceptions of disabilities.* San Diego, CA: Los Amigos Research Associates.

Hanline, M. F., & Daley, S. E. (1992). Family coping strategies and strengths in Hispanic, African American, and Caucasian families of young children. *Topics in Early Childhood Special Education, 12,* 351–366.

Huff, R. M., & Kline, M. V. (1998). *Promoting health care in multicultural populations: A handbook for practitioners.* Thousand Oaks, CA: Sage.

Julia, M. C. (1996). *Multicultural awareness in the health care professions.* Boston: Allyn & Bacon.

Lynch, E. W., & Hanson, J. (1992). *Developing cross-cultural competence: A guide for working with young children and their families.* Baltimore: Brookes.

National Center for Complementary and Alternative Medicine, http://nccam.nih.gov

Paniagua, F. A. (1994). *Assessing and treating culturally diverse clients: A practical guide.* Thousand Oaks, CA: Sage.

Resources for Cross Cultural Health Care, www.diversityRx.org

Roseberry-McKibbin, C. (1995). *Multicultural students with special language needs.* Oceanside, CA: Academic Associates.

Spector, R. E. (2004). *Cultural diversity in health and illness.* Upper Saddle River, NJ: Prentice Hall Health.

State of Queensland Health, www.health.qld.gov.au/multicultural/default.asp

Terrell, S. L., & Hale, J. (1992). Serving a multicultural population: Different learning styles. *American Journal of Speech-Language Pathology, 1,* 5–8.

U.S. Department of Health and Human Services. *Health Resources and Services Administration (HRSA) study on measuring cultural competence in health care delivery settings.* www.hrsa.gov/culturalcompetence/measures

# APPENDIX 4D

# Assessment of Personal Cultural Competence

| Yes | No | Competence |
|---|---|---|
| ☐ | ☐ | I have intentionally and aggressively sought to educate myself on the beliefs, attitudes, and values of cultural groups other than my own. |
| ☐ | ☐ | I have spent time reflecting on my upbringing/childhood and understand the source of my racial and cultural biases. |
| ☐ | ☐ | I have evaluated my use of language, particularly humor, and determined what might be insulting or degrading to members of other cultural groups. |
| ☐ | ☐ | I have openly disagreed with a culturally or racially biased joke. |
| ☐ | ☐ | I have grown aware of cultural and racial bias in broadcast and print media. |
| ☐ | ☐ | I have taken steps to increase my coworkers' knowledge of the beliefs, values, and attitudes of other cultural groups. |
| ☐ | ☐ | I have implemented strategies in my workplace that foster cultural proficiency. |
| ☐ | ☐ | I understand the relationship between (a) cultural and religious beliefs and (b) compliance with Western medical treatment. |
| ☐ | ☐ | I have accepted the premise that the behaviors associated with Western medical practice may not be the most appropriate for clients of other cultures. |
| ☐ | ☐ | I have taken steps to assess the cultural proficiency of my workplace and to improve areas that are culturally biased, culturally offensive, or paternalistic. |

# References

Battle, D. E. (1997). *Communication disorders in multicultural populations* (2nd ed.). Boston: Butterworth-Heinemann.

Bliatout, B. T. (1988, March 5). *Hmong refugees: Some barriers to some Western health care services.* Paper presented at the Conference on Southeast Asians in the United States, Tempe, AZ.

Campinha-Bacote, J. (1994). Cultural competence in psychiatric mental health nursing: A conceptual model. *Nursing Clinics of North America, 29*(1), 1–8.

Casas, J. M., & Casas, A. (1994). The acculturation process and implications for educational services. In A. C. Matiella (Ed.), *The multicultural challenge in health education.* Santa Cruz, NM: ETR Associates.

Clark, L. W. (1993). *Faculty and student challenges in facing cultural and linguistic diversity.* Springfield, IL: Thomas.

Fitzgerald, H. E., Lester, B. M., & Zuckerman, B. (1995). *Children of poverty.* New York: Garland.

Goldstein, B. (2000). *Cultural and linguistic diversity resource guide for speech-language pathologists.* San Diego, CA: Singular.

Gomez, R., Ruiz, P., & Rumbaut, R. (1985). Hispanic patients: A linguo-cultural minority. *Hispanic Journal of Behavioral Sciences, 7,* 177–186.

Goode, T. D. (2006). *Promoting cultural diversity and cultural competency: Self-assessment checklist for personnel providing services and supports to children with disabilities and special health needs and their families* (Rev. ed.). Washington, DC: Center for Child and Human Development, Georgetown University. Available online from www11.georgetown.edu/research/gucchd/nccc/documents/ChecklistBehavioralHealth.pdf

Huff, R. M., & Kline, M. V. (1998). *Promoting health care in multicultural populations: A handbook for practitioners.* Thousand Oaks, CA: Sage.

Krajewski-Jaime, E. R., Brown, K. S., & Ziefert, M. (1996). Utilizing international clinical practice to build inter-cultural sensitivity in social work students. *Journal of Multicultural Social Work, 4*(2), 15–29.

Lassiter, S. M. (1995). *Multicultural clients: A professional handbook for health care providers and social workers.* Westport, CT: Greenwood Press.

Lynch, E. W., & Hanson, M. J. (1992). *Developing cross-cultural competence: A guide for working with young children and their families.* Baltimore: Brookes.

Mattson, S. (1988). Health care delivery to Southeast Asian refugees. *Migration World, 17*(1), 30–35.

Nilchaikovit, T., Hill, J. M., & Holland, J. C. (1993). The effects of culture on illness behavior and medical care: Asian and American differences. *General Hospital Psychiatry, 15,* 41–50.

Pachter, L. M. (1994). Culture and clinical care: Folk illness beliefs and behaviors and their implications for health care delivery. *Journal of the American Medical Association, 271,* 690–694.

Page, J. B. (2005). The concept of culture: A core issue in health disparities. *Journal of Urban Health, 82*(Suppl. 3), 1135–1143.

Purnell, L. D. (1998). Purnell's model for cultural competence. In L. D. Purnell & B. J. Paulanka (Eds.), *Transcultural care: A culturally competent approach.* Philadelphia: Davis.

Randall-David, E. (1994). *Culturally competent HIV counseling and education.* Rockville, MD: National Hemophilia Program.

Rodriguez, R. (1993, May/June). Family violence and migrant women: Implications for practice. *Migrant Clinicians Network,* pp. 1–6.

Slonim, M. (1991). *Children, culture and ethnicity: Evaluating and understanding the impact.* New York: Garland.

Spector, R. E. (2000). *Cultural diversity in health and illness.* Upper Saddle River, NJ: Prentice Hall Health.

Taylor, O. (1986). *Nature of communication disorders in culturally and linguistically diverse populations.* San Diego: College-Hill Press.

Taylor, O. L., & Clarke, M. G. (1994). Cultural and communication disorders: A theoretical framework. *Seminars in Speech and Language, 15,* 103–113.

Tingsley, B. J., Wang, S. J., Kwasmain, A., & Green, D. (1997, April). *Between the cracks: Access to physical health care in children of the working poor.* Paper presented at the biennial meeting of the Society for Research in Child Development, Washington, DC.

U.S. Bureau of the Census. Retrieved December 12, 2007. http://www.census.gov/popest/national/asrh/NC-EST2006-asrh.html

# PART II

# Foundations of Cleft Lip and Palate and Craniofacial Anomalies

## CHAPTER 5

# Embryologic and Genetic Aspects of Clefting and Selected Craniofacial Anomalies

*Robert J. Gorlin and Adriane L. Baylis*

Gorlin and Baylis describe the clinical variability of cleft formation and the various types of clefts. How clefts develop embryologically from approximately the 5th through the 10th week and some possible mechanisms of cleft formation are presented. Multifactorial inheritance is discussed and presumed to be the cause for most examples of clefting. The genetics of clefting and the importance of genetic counseling for families with a child with clefting or a craniofacial anomaly are also discussed. In addition, the authors describe some common craniofacial anomalies and syndromes associated with clefting, including Robin sequence, Treacher Collins syndrome, Apert syndrome, Crouzon syndrome, oculo-auriculo-vertebral spectrum, and Stickler syndrome, and provide a more extensive section highlighting velocardiofacial syndrome because of the increased frequency with which clinicians might encounter this disorder.

1. What are the two basic types (entities, diagnoses) of clefting? How does incidence vary in males versus females and among racial groups?
2. Explain how the facial prominences form and merge from the 5th through the 10th week of embryological development. What can you conclude embryologically about a child born with a cleft uvula?
3. Why is so little known about specific mechanisms of cleft production?
4. Define *multifactorial inheritance*. What is the recurrence risk in first-degree relatives for multifactorial traits? Can you think of other multifactorial traits? What autosomal-dominant conditions frequently involve clefting?

5. What is meant by "nondirective genetic counseling"?
6. What are the most common craniofacial anomalies and syndromes associated with clefting? What are the major anomalies and speech-language features associated with each syndrome?
7. What is the role of the speech-language pathologist in the diagnosis and treatment of children with velocardiofacial syndrome?

## Types of Cleft Formations

Clinically, there is great variability in the degree of cleft formation. Relatively minor degrees of involvement include bifid uvula, linear lip indentations, so-called intrauterine-healed clefts, and submucous palatal clefts. Clefts may involve only a portion of the upper lip or may extend to the nostril and may be combined with defects of the hard and/or soft palates. Isolated palatal clefts may be limited to the uvula, or they may be more extensive, cleaving the soft palate or both soft and hard palates to just behind the incisor teeth (Gorlin, Cohen, & Hennekam, 2001).

### Cleft Lip and Cleft Palate

Orofacial clefting has been found to be the most prevalent birth defect in the United States, affecting approximately 6,800 infants annually, followed by Down syndrome (Centers for Disease Control and Prevention [CDC], 2006). A combination of cleft lip and cleft palate (CLP) is more common than cleft lip only or cleft palate only. The breakdown according to types seems to differ somewhat among several large surveys depending, in part, upon whether the data are gathered at birth or at the time of surgery. Data obtained from birth records are notoriously unreliable. Roughly, however, CLP represents about 50% of cases of clefting, and cleft lip only and cleft palate only each represent about 25% of cases, irrespective of race. By sorting clefts into three groups—isolated cleft lip, cleft lip and cleft palate, and isolated cleft palate—Fogh-Andersen (1942) was able to show that there are two separate entities: (1) cleft lip with or without cleft palate and (2) isolated cleft palate. From 1999 to 2001 in the United

States, cleft lip with or without cleft palate occurred in an average of 10.48 per 10,000 births, and cleft palate only occurred in 6.39 per 10,000 births (CDC, 2006). Cleft lip with or without cleft palate appears to occur in about 1 per 1,000 non-Hispanic Caucasian births (range 0.6–1.3 per 1,000). The prevalence is higher in Native American groups (over 3.6 per 1,000 live births) and in Japanese and Chinese populations (about 1.7 per 1,000 live births) but lower among African Americans (approximately 1 per 2,500 births) (Altemus, 1966; Bear, 1976; I. Emanuel, Huang, Gutman, Yu, & Lin, 1972; Lowry & Trimble, 1977; Natsume & Kawai, 1986; Robert, Käller, & Harris, 1996; Vanderas, 1987).

## Isolated Cleft Lip

Eighty percent of isolated clefts of the lip are unilateral (see Figure 5.1) and 20% are bilateral (see Figure 5.2). When unilateral, the cleft occurs on the left side about 70% of the time, although it is no more extensive than right clefts. About 85% of cases of bilateral cleft lip and 70% of cases of unilateral cleft lip are associated with cleft palate. Cleft lip with or without cleft palate is more common in males. Clefts of the lip do not always extend into the nostril, and in about 10% of the cases, there are bridges of skin (Simonart's bands) across the cleft (Semb & Shaw, 1991).

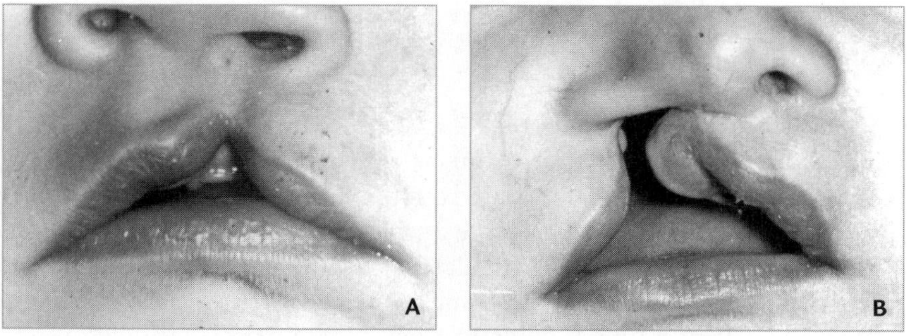


FIGURE 5.1. Unilateral cleft lip. Unilateral cleft lip may be incomplete (i.e., barely through the vermilion) as in view A, or complete (i.e., extending to the nostril) as in view B. *Note.* From "Lippen-, Kiefer-, Gaumenspalten," by W. Hoppe, 1965, *Archiv für Kinderheikunde, 171*(Suppl. 52:1), pp. 22, 27. Copyright 1965 by Springer Verlag. Reprinted with permission.

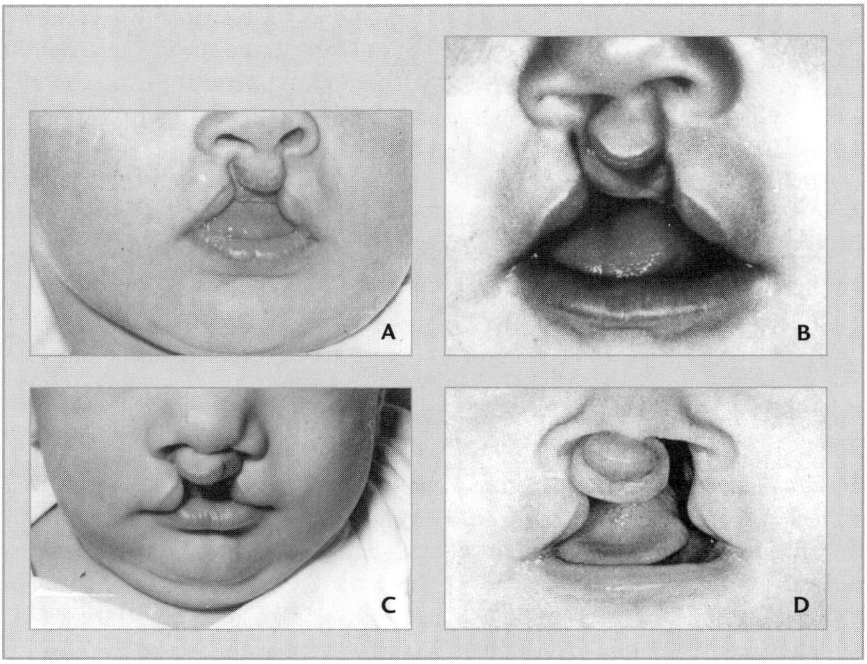


Figure 5.2. Bilateral cleft lip. Note the various degrees of clefting. In view D, the primary palate is attached only to the columella. *Note.* From "The Management of Bilateral Cleft of the Primary Palate," by T. Skoog, 1965, *Plastic and Reconstructive Surgery, 35,* p. 40. Copyright 1965 by Williams & Wilkins. Reprinted courtesy of the Estate of Tord Skoog.

## Isolated Cleft Palate

Isolated cleft palate (often referred to as "cleft palate only") (see Figure 5.3) appears to be an entity separate from cleft lip with or without cleft palate. Numerous investigators have pointed out that siblings of patients with cleft lip with or without cleft palate have an increased frequency of the same anomaly but not of isolated cleft palate, and vice versa. The frequency of isolated cleft palate among both Caucasians and African Americans appears to be between 1 per 2,000 and 1 per 2,500 births (Owens, Jones, & Harris, 1985). It may be slightly more common in the Japanese population (Natsume & Kawai, 1986). Cleft palate only occurs somewhat more often in females, who make up about 60% of the cases. However, studies of the extent of cleft palate clearly indicate that although there is a 2:1 female:

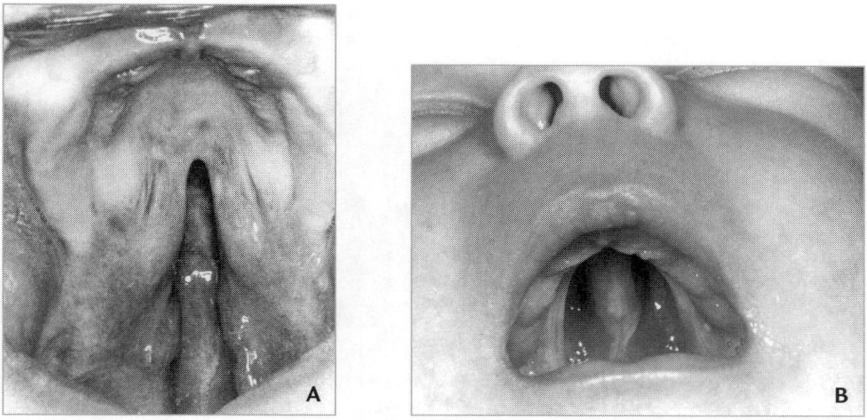


FIGURE 5.3. Cleft palate. Like cleft lip, cleft palate may be of variable extent. In the patient in panel A, note that cleft involves all of the soft palate and about one half of the hard palate.

male predilection for complete clefts of the hard and soft palate, the ratio approaches 1:1 for clefts of the soft palate only.

## Microforms

Minimal expressions (microforms) of cleft lip and/or cleft palate include cleft uvula, submucous palatal cleft, hairline indentation and lateral congenital sinus of the upper lip, and palatal defects demonstrated by laminographic examination (Heckler, Oesterle, & Jabaley, 1979). Minimal cleft lip has varied from defects in the orbicularis oris detected only by ultrasonagraphy to intrauterine-healed clefts of the lip (see Figures 5.4 and 5.5) and clefts extending through the vermillion (red portion of the lip) (Martin, Jones, & Benirschke, 1993). More extensive examination of patients with these microforms reveals an occasional nasal deformity, alveolar deformity, and anomalous tooth development on the affected side. Velopharyngeal inadequacy for speech may also occur in the absence of an overt cleft palate. This may be associated with bifid or absent uvula, short soft palate, or submucous cleft of the palate.

### Cleft Uvula

Cleft or bifid uvula varies in degree of completeness, with incomplete clefts being much more common. The incidence of cleft uvula (1 in 80

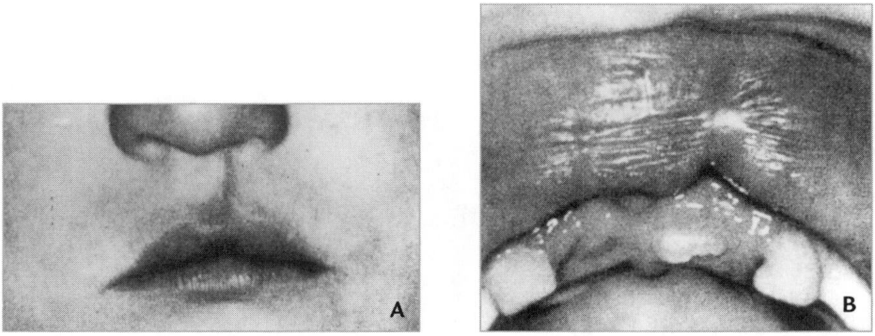


FIGURE 5.4. Intrauterine-healed unilateral cleft lip. Note the defect in the orbicularis oris. *Note.* From "Zur Histologie und Klinik der Lateralen Oberlippenfurchen," by G. Leutert and H. Heiner, 1962, *Archiv für Klinische Chirurgiae, 299,* p. 791. Copyright 1962 by Springer Verlag. Reprinted with permission.

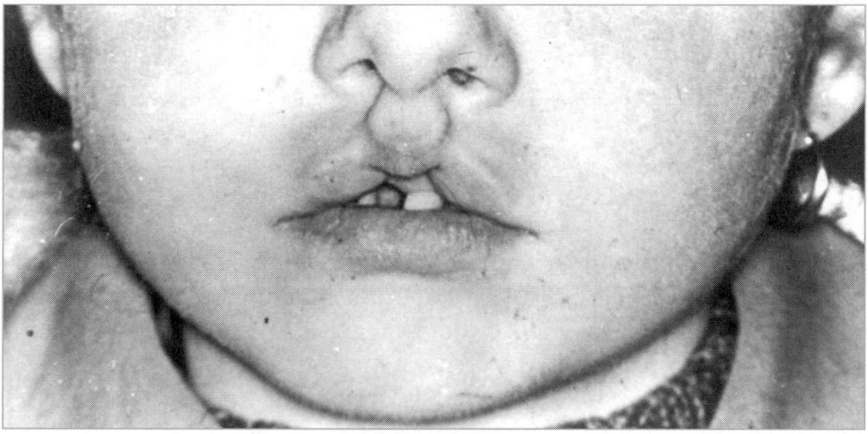

FIGURE 5.5. Intrauterine-healed bilateral cleft lip. *Note.* From "Zur Histologie und Klinik der Lateralen Oberlippenfurchen," by G. Leutert and H. Heiner, 1962, *Archiv für Klinische Chirurgiae, 299,* p. 792. Copyright 1962 by Springer Verlag. Reprinted with permission.

Caucasian individuals) is much higher than that for cleft palate. As with clefts of the soft palate, cleft uvula approaches a 1:1 sex ratio. The prevalence in parents and siblings of persons with clefts (probands) ranges from approximately 7% to 15% (Chosack & Eidelman, 1978; Lindemann, Riis, & Sewerin, 1977). The frequency of cleft uvula among Native American groups is quite high, ranging from 1 per 9 to 1 per 14 individuals, depending upon the tribal group. It is much less frequent in African Americans, with classic estimates ranging from 1 per 350 to 1 per 400 individuals (Cervenka & Shapiro, 1970; Jaffe & DeBlanc, 1972; Schaumann, Peagler, & Gorlin, 1970), although a more recent, smaller study suggested a frequency of 1 per 271 in a group of children from Jacksonville, Florida (Wharton & Mowrer, 1992). A cleft or bifid uvula is often a sign of an underlying submucous cleft palate, which may result in velopharyngeal inadequacy for speech in some individuals.

## Submucous Cleft Palate

Submucous cleft palate (SMCP) refers to imperfect muscle union across the soft palate underlying the mucous membrane (Heckler et al., 1979). The soft palate is typically short, and velopharyngeal closure may be inadequate for acceptable speech in some, but certainly not all, cases. Clinicians frequently describe the classic triad of symptoms for SMCP: (1) cleft uvula; (2) thin, bluish appearance of the midline of the soft palate ("zona pellucida"); and (3) median deficiency or bony notch in the posterior border of the hard palate (see Figure 5.6). This deficiency can usually be detected by palpation or by means of a light probe placed within the nose. Among those with SMCP, approximately 30% have cleft uvula and over 60% have a short soft palate, with poor mobility demonstrated in 20% of cases (Poswillo, 1974).

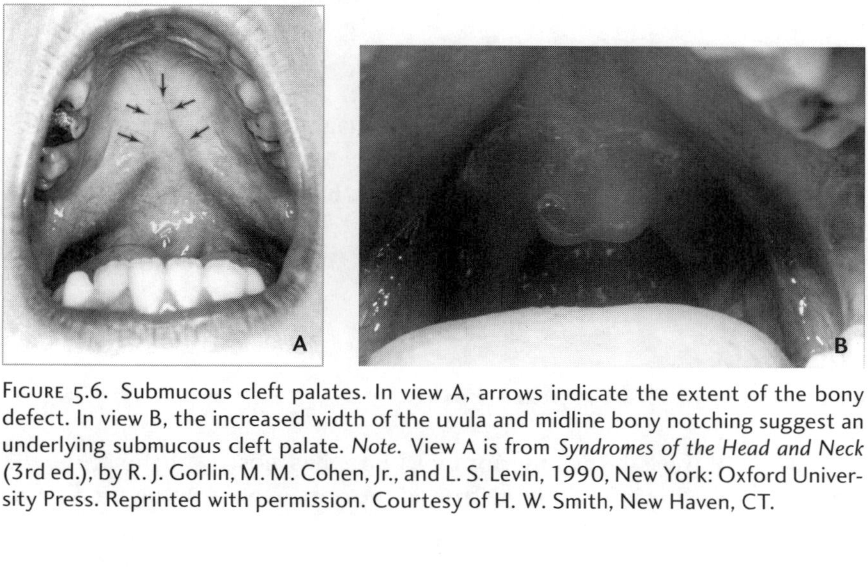


FIGURE 5.6. Submucous cleft palates. In view A, arrows indicate the extent of the bony defect. In view B, the increased width of the uvula and midline bony notching suggest an underlying submucous cleft palate. *Note.* View A is from *Syndromes of the Head and Neck* (3rd ed.), by R. J. Gorlin, M. M. Cohen, Jr., and L. S. Levin, 1990, New York: Oxford University Press. Reprinted with permission. Courtesy of H. W. Smith, New Haven, CT.

SMCP is relatively uncommon, occurring in 1 in 1,200 children, and there appears to be no sex predilection. Velocardiofacial syndrome (discussed later in this chapter) is the most common syndrome associated with SMCP. Thus, clinicians are urged to pursue comprehensive assessment in those patients presenting with SMCP to rule out the possibility of this diagnosis. In addition, some individuals may not have the "hallmark" signs of SMCP; however, upon flexible nasendoscopic examination, a furrowing in the nasal surface of the soft palate may be visible. This may be associated with a possible occult (hidden) submucous cleft palate (Peterson-Falzone, Hardin-Jones, & Karnell, 2001).

# Embryology of the Primary and Secondary Palates

The nature of this text does not permit us to "begin at the beginning." Many excellent treatises can guide the reader from the formation of the fertilized egg through development to the three embryonic germ cell layers. In this section, we discuss the period of embryonic development when the facial provinces form and merge, roughly the 5th to 10th week after conception. However, reference is made to earlier events that play a critical role (Gorlin & Slavkin, 1997; Johnston & Sulik, 1979).

## The Neural Crest

Neural crest cells play an integral part in facial morphology. At about the time when the neural folds fuse to form the neural tube, ectodermal cells adjacent to the neural plate migrate into the underlying regions. Those in the head and face form essentially all the skeletal and connective tissues of the face: bone, cartilage, fibrous connective tissue, and all dental tissues except enamel (Gorlin & Slavkin, 1997).

## Formation of the Primary Palate

By the end of week 4, the anterior neuropore has closed. At this time, the primitive face consists of a large frontal prominence overlying the first or mandibular arch. If one manually elevates the frontal prominence, one can see into the *primary mouth* or *stomodeum.* The primary mouth is separated from the foregut by the *buccopharyngeal membrane,* which undergoes selective cell death and ruptures about this time in development. On both sides of the frontal prominence, the *nasal placodes* are forming. These bilateral structures are located just above the primitive mouth and are represented by local thickening of the surface ectoderm. Rapid proliferation of tissue known as *nasal swelling* occurs both lateral and medial to the nasal placodes. By means of selective cell death and proliferation of tissues, *nasal* or *olfactory pits* (the primitive nostrils) are formed, which extend into the primitive mouth (see Figure 5.7).

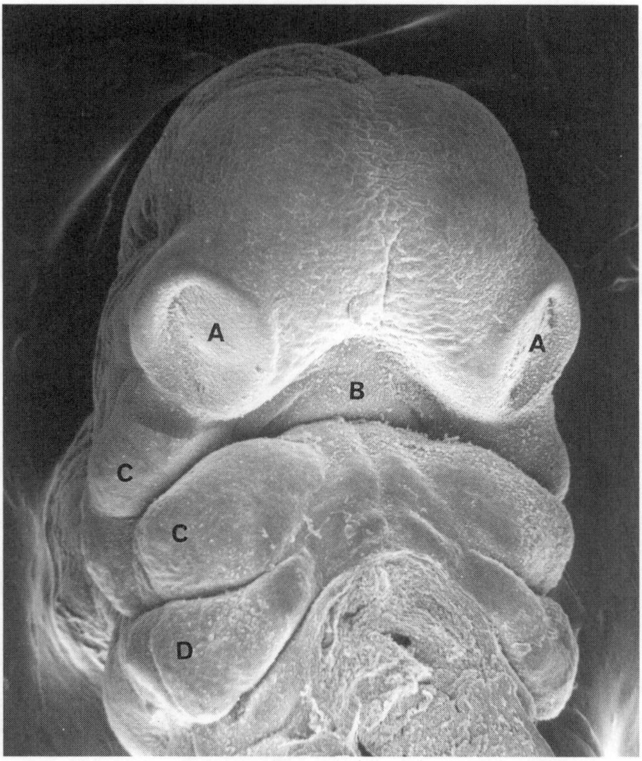


Figure 5.7. Scanning electron micrograph of 32-day-old embryo showing bilateral olfactory pits (A), buccopharyngeal membrane (B), mandibular arch (C), and hyoid arch (D). *Note.* From J. Jirasek and B. Shapiro, Minneapolis, MN. Courtesy of Burton Shapiro, Minneapolis, MN.

Extremely active growth occurs during the 5th and 6th weeks. The maxillary swellings, which represent the upper portion of the first pharyngeal arch, enlarge considerably and, by pushing the nasal swellings or prominences medially, cause them to approach one another in the midline. When the two prominences meet, merging takes place between the *median nasal prominences* and the maxillary swellings. Thus, the upper lip is formed laterally by the *maxillary prominences* and medially by the fused median nasal prominences (see Figure 5.8). This occurs around the 7th week. It should be emphasized that the *lateral nasal prominences* play no role in formation of the upper lip, but form the alae or wings of the nose.

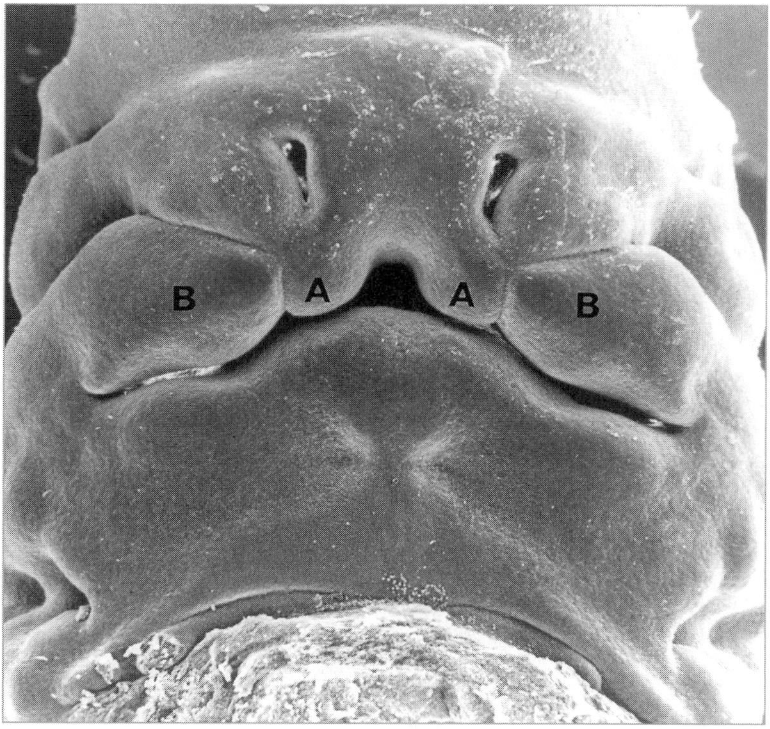


FIGURE 5.8. Scanning electron micrograph of 44-day-old embryo. Note that the upper lip will be formed from fusion of the median nasal prominence (A) and the maxillary part (B) of the mandibular arch bilaterally. *Note.* Courtesy of K. Sulik, Chapel Hill, NC.

The *primary palate* consists of the two merged nasal processes, which form the *intermaxillary segment.* This, in turn, consists of two portions: (1) a *labial component,* which forms the philtrum of the upper lip (i.e., the indented area flanked by roughly parallel ridges that run from the columella of the nose to the middle of the upper lip), and (2) the triangular *palatal component* of bone (also known as the *premaxilla*) that includes the four maxillary incisor teeth. The primary palate extends posteriorly to the incisive foramen or, clinically, to the incisive papilla.

## Formation of the Secondary Palate

The secondary palate makes up at least 90% of the hard and soft palate, or all except the anterior portion that houses the maxillary incisor teeth. Its development appears to be somewhat more complicated than originally thought. The palatal shelves originate as swellings or shelf-like burgeonings of the medial surfaces of the maxillary prominences. They appear in the 6th week and grow downward, lateral to and somewhat beneath the tongue. Elevation of the palatal processes to a horizontal plane is more "rigorous" anteriorly, that is, in the part closer to the primary palate. Elevation of the palatal processes begins during the 7th week.

What promotes this elevation has been called "intrinsic shelf force," which has a complex biochemical and physiochemical basis. The tongue appears to play little role in shelf elevation. This has been demonstrated in mouse embryos, where removal of the tongue prior to shelf elevation has been followed by partial elevation of the shelves to the horizontal plane.

In mammals, elevation of the shelves is associated with widening and forward growth of the mandible (see Figure 5.9A). This seems to be dependent upon growth of Meckel's cartilage, the evanescent stiffener of the first pharyngeal arch. Once the shelves are elevated to the horizontal plane, there is programmed cell death of the overlying epithelium. This has been demonstrated by noting the absence of certain cellular enzymes (cytochrome oxides) by histochemical study and by observing increased activity of other enzymes (e.g., cyclic adenosine monophosphate). When the shelf edges touch, the epithelium has thinned and is undergoing advanced stages of degeneration (see Figure 5.9B). This allows a flow of ectomesenchyme from each side to close the gap. Complete fusion takes place by the 10th week. In some infants, there is cystic degeneration of the epithelial remnants, which produces temporary midline palatal microcysts.

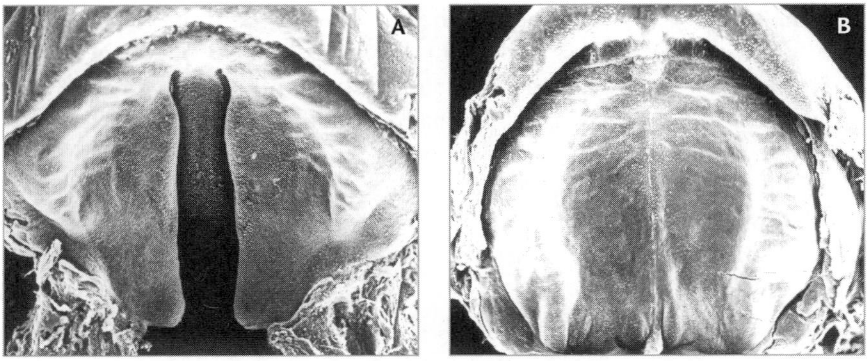


FIGURE 5.9. Scanning electron micrograph of a palate. In the 35-day-old embryo (A), fusion of primary palate only has occurred. At 59 days (B), there is complete fusion of secondary palate. *Note.* Courtesy of L. Russell, Chapel Hill, NC.

# Mechanisms of Cleft Production

By definition, cleft lip involves the failure of closure of the primary palate, whereas cleft palate involves the failure of closure of the secondary palate. Knowledge regarding mechanisms involved in regulation of embryonic growth is, at best, sparse. The blueprints for the rate at which facial prominences grow or burgeon, and in what direction they grow, is in part determined by the genetic template. The template is the deoxyribonucleic acid (DNA) code located in the nucleus of each cell. However, hereditary factors do not act alone. Growth patterns can be affected by environmental factors as well. For example, several mouse models exist for cleft lip and cleft palate. There are both susceptible and nonsusceptible strains. Furthermore, various teratogenic substances (corticosteroids, vitamin A, phenytoin, various folic acid antagonists, etc.) produce clefting in rodents. However, there is little evidence that any of these agents plays a role in cleft production in humans.

Cleft lip and cleft palate, for purposes of general discussion, are malformations evident at birth resulting from some failure in a normal embryologic event. For example, various genetic and/or environmental factors may inhibit the flow of neural crest cells or may affect their volume or mass so that contact between prominences is impossible or inadequate. The epithelium covering the ectomesenchyme may not undergo programmed cell death so that fusion cannot take place. Exact timing and exact positioning play critical roles. For example, Johnston and Sulik (1979) showed that if the bilaterally formed nasal placodes contact one another, the result is severe to complete suppression of development of median nasal prominences.

Altered positioning of the nasal placodes or abnormal direction of growth of the facial prominences may be responsible for clefting of the primary palate. This has been supported not only by animal models but by the clinical observation that parents of children with cleft lip exhibit some degree of reduction in overall midface size. Some parents of children with cleft lip have also been found to have subclinical clefting or discontinuity of the superior portion of the orbicularis oris muscle using ultrasound imaging.

Many mechanisms may lead to clefting of the secondary palate; however, some suggested mechanisms are doubtful causes. For example, it is extremely unlikely that a markedly large tongue could interfere with palatal closure. There is no known association with congenital hypothyroidism or macroglossia-omphalocele syndrome, although it may be argued that tongue enlargement in those disorders occurs late in gestation. Failure of growth of the mandible (micro- or retrognathia) may inhibit elevation of the palatal shelves since Robin sequence and mandibulofacial dysostosis (Treacher Collins syndrome) are associated with cleft palate (these will be discussed later in this chapter).

Clefts of both primary and secondary palates occur in association in about half of cases. Researchers have sought a common mechanism of production. One suggestion is that the tongue tip becomes wedged in the labial cleft produced by failure of fusion of the median nasal and maxillary prominences. This, it has been argued, would not allow the tongue to drop and, consequently, would interfere with midline contact and resultant closure. This explanation appears too simplistic, however. Reduction in size of both the labial maxillary prominence *and* the palatine process of the maxillary prominences seems to be a far more reasonable explanation (see Gorlin et al., 2001, for discussion).

Clefts of the secondary palate most likely result from either hypoplasia (underdevelopment) of the shelves or delay in timing of the shelf elevation. Experiments carried out on susceptible strains of mice have suggested that both mechanisms are operative, but at different times of gestation. For example, large doses of vitamin A given early in gestation inhibit palatal shelf growth, whereas cortisone given later in gestation inhibits palatal shelf elevation.

## Multifactorial Inheritance

Because most examples of cleft lip and/or cleft palate appear to have multifactorial inheritance, a short discussion of this type of hereditary transmission appears relevant. Multifactorial inheritance is far less familiar to most people than is single-gene inheritance, which is emphasized in high school biology courses. Study of multifactorial inheritance is usually reserved for college courses in genetics or human genetics, despite the major role that this form of inheritance plays in people's lives. Such diverse traits as height, hair color, and intelligence depend on the additive properties of many genes and environmental factors, as do schizophrenia, clubfoot, dislocated hips, most types of congenital heart disease, and most cases of cleft lip and/or cleft palate. Multifactorial disorders tend to cluster in families and follow different rules from those of single-gene inheritance.

A multifactorial disorder, by definition, is influenced by a combination of genetic and environmental factors. However, researchers do not know how many genes are involved, whether each gene has an equal influence (unlikely), or, in most cases, what environmental factors are operating. Multifactorial traits, such as stature, are unimodal. They generally follow a normal curve, if one ignores the tails of the distribution due to gigantism at one end and conditions such as achondroplasia (or other rare disorders of growth retardation) at the other. Development, in general, follows a continuous distribution. Failure in a developmental process, due to whatever cause, will interrupt the continuous distribution. If the failure in development after a certain point results in malformation, there are two classes, normal and abnormal, separated by a threshold. This is termed *quasi-continuous variation.*

Recurrence risks for multifactorial disorders are calculated from surveys of various populations. Analyses are then carried out on the frequencies of the disorder in assorted relatives: parents, children, uncles, aunts, nieces, nephews, grandparents, grandchildren, cousins, and so forth. From this data, empirical risk figures are calculated. An estimate that approximates the empirical risk in first-degree relatives may be easily calculated. This figure, known as the Edwards or Falconer approximation, equals the square root of the frequency of the specific disorders in the population. Thus, if a disorder has a population frequency of 1 in 2,500, the recurrence risk in first-degree relatives will be 1 in 50, or 2%. From this, it necessarily follows that the lower the population frequency, the greater the relative increased risk for affected siblings. For example, a disorder with a population frequency of 1 in 10,000 would have a recurrence risk of 1 in

100 (a 100-fold increase), whereas a disorder with a frequency of 1 in 900 would have a recurrence risk of 1 in 30 (a 30-fold increase).

Multifactorial disorders often occur more frequently in one sex. It follows that an affected individual of the less susceptible sex, who needs greater genetic and/or environmental factors to manifest the disorder, endows his or her offspring with a greater risk.

Multifactorial inheritance also differs from single-gene inheritance in that the recurrence risk increases as additional family members are affected. For single-gene traits, the risks stay the same regardless of the number of relatives affected. Risks for cleft lip and/or cleft palate are dealt with in great detail in the following sections. Another observation regarding multifactorial inheritance is that the more severe the malformation, the higher the risk of recurrence. The risk to subsequent siblings is also higher if there is parental consanguinity (i.e., marriage among relatives).

Twin studies are often employed for investigation of multifactorial traits to show the relative strengths of genetic and environmental factors. *Concordance* for a trait (i.e., when both twins are affected) is compared in both monozygotic (MZ) and dizygotic (DZ) twins. Concordance among MZ twins should be complete for single-gene disorders, but is rarely complete for multifactorial disorders. Thus, if the concordance rate is more than twice as great in MZ twins as in DZ twins, simple dominant inheritance can be excluded, whereas if concordance is more than four times as great, simple recessive inheritance can be excluded. A comparison between MZ and DZ twins will be made in the case of cleft lip and/or cleft palate in the following section.

## Genetics of Clefting

Following the belief in single-gene inheritance of clefting, as expressed during the early decades of the 20th century, it became evident that recurrence risks did not correspond to any simple pattern of inheritance. This was bolstered by twin studies, which indicate the relative roles played in cleft production by genetic and nongenetic influences. Table 5.1 reveals that among twins with cleft lip with or without cleft palate, concordance is far greater in monozygotic (36.2%) than in dizygotic twins (4.7%). In twins with cleft palate only, concordance is not quite as large between the two groups (monozygotic, 22.2%; dizygotic, 4.6%) (Blake & Wreakes,

**Table 5.1**
**Concordance in Facial Clefts in Twin Studies (1922–1988)**

| | Monozygotic twins | | Dizygotic twins | |
|---|---|---|---|---|
| | Cleft lip ± palate | Cleft palate | Cleft lip ± palate | Cleft palate |
| *N* studied | 84 | 27 | 191 | 44 |
| Concordance (*n*) | 34 | 6 | 9 | 2 |
| Percentage concordance | 36.2 | 22.2 | 4.7 | 4.6 |

*Note.* Adapted from *Syndromes of the Head and Neck* (3rd ed., p. 697), by R. J. Gorlin, M. M. Cohen, Jr., and L. S. Levin, 1990, New York: Oxford University Press.

1972; Gorlin et al., 2001; Shields, Bixler, & Fogh-Andersen, 1979; Wyszynski, Lewanda, & Beaty, 1996). These data suggest a stronger genetic basis for cleft lip with or without cleft palate than for isolated cleft palate. Microforms such as a submucous palatal cleft or bifid uvula could alter the data markedly. Although many investigators believe that cleft lip with or without cleft palate follows the rules of multifactorial threshold inheritance, others express skepticism that isolated cleft palate obeys the rules and have suggested that environmental factors play a major role. They have further suggested that cleft palate represents heterogeneity.

Both cleft lip with or without cleft palate and isolated cleft palate consist of three groups: sporadic (75%–80% occurrence rate), familial (10%–15%), and syndromal (1%–5%).

Clefting is heterogeneous, the variation and liability probably being determined by a number of major genes, minor genes, environmental insults, and a developmental threshold (Fraser, 1974; Reich, 1979). As indicated, cleft palate does not fit the multifactorial model very well. It is probably more heterogeneous than cleft lip with or without cleft palate (Chung, Bixler, Watanabe, Koguchi, & Fogh-Andersen, 1986; Melnick, Bixler, & Shields, 1980; Shields, Bixler, & Fogh-Andersen, 1981). Because one cannot, at this time, distinguish clearly among the multifactorial (polygenic) model, a major gene with reduced penetrance, and a mixture of sporadic cases, it seems foolish to argue for one or the other until more convincing evidence has been presented (Mitchell & Risch, 1992). Little error is made using empirical risk data or, in fact, mathematical model data, described below. The parents and relatives of an affected individual should also be examined carefully for such minor stigmata as cleft (bifid) uvula, submucous cleft palate, or velopharyngeal inadequacy for speech.

Within the past decade, much effort has been expended to discover major loci for nonsyndromic cleft lip with or without cleft palate. Several candidate regions have been investigated such as 2p13, 6p23, and 19q13. Although linkage and association have been found, no major gene related to cleft lip and palate has been defined with absolute certainty (Wong et al., 2000).

## Risk

In the random population, the risk for the occurrence of cleft lip and/or cleft palate ranges from 1 in 2,500 for cleft palate only, to essentially 1 in 2 for cleft lip with or without cleft palate or clefting of the secondary palate only, if in association with paramedian fistulas (pits) of the lower lip (known as Van der Woude syndrome). However, in the vast majority of cases, the cleft is either isolated or associated with a constellation of anomalies that do not form a recognizable syndrome. Although there may well be over 350 recognized cleft syndromes, they constitute a small number (2%–4%) of the total cases. However, efforts must be made to recognize a cleft syndrome, because the pattern of inheritance may be a simple one and the genetic risk for future affected children may then be made more precise. More specific reference is made to these syndromes later in this chapter (see "Selected Craniofacial Anomalies and Syndromes Associated with Clefting").

In the event of failure to recognize such a pattern, professionals must resort to empirical risk figures based on pooled data. These have been calculated by several investigators (Bonaiti et al., 1982; Bonaiti-Pellie & Smith, 1974; Mitchell & Christensen, 1996; Tolarová 1987a, 1987b). The reader is also referred to a mathematical model devised by Spence, Westlake, Lange, and Gold (1976) that yields results remarkably close to the empirical risk. In the use of tables, it should be borne in mind that the data apply only to risks for similar anomalies; for example, a parent with cleft palate only has no greater risk than anyone else of having a child with cleft lip with or without cleft palate, and vice versa.

As shown in Tables 5.2 and 5.3, in the case of uncomplicated clefts, the risk to a first-degree relative of an affected individual (proband) is on the order of 2%–4%. This is very close to the Falconer estimation of the square root of 1 in 900 (i.e., 1 in 30, or 3.3%). The risks increase as more individuals in the family are affected. For example, if a parent and child

Table 5.2
Facial Clefts—Empirical Recurrence Risks (%)

| Parents | Siblings | | Cleft lip ± palate | Cleft palate |
|---|---|---|---|---|
| | Affected | Normal | | |
| Normal parents | 1 | 0 | 4.0 | 3.5 |
| | 1 | 1 | 4.0 | 3.0 |
| | 2 | 0 | 14.0 | 13.0 |
| One parent affected | 0 | 0 | 4.0 | 3.5 |
| | 1 | 0 | 12.0 | 10.0 |
| | 1 | 1 | 10.0 | 9.0 |
| | 2 | 0 | 25.0 | 24.0 |
| Both parents affected | 0 | 0 | 35.0 | 25.0 |
| | 1 | 0 | 45.0 | 35.0 |
| | 1 | 1 | 40.0 | 35.0 |
| | 2 | 0 | 50.0 | 45.0 |

*Note.* Derived from "Empirical Recurrence Risk Figures for Genetic Counseling of Clefts," by M. Tolarová, 1972, *Acta Chirurgiae Plasticae* (Praha), *14,* p. 235. Copyright 1972 by Czechoslovak Medical Press. Adapted with permission.

have clefts, the risk for a future affected sibling increases to about 9%. These and other situations are presented in detail in Tables 5.2 and 5.3.

The severity of a facial cleft affects the recurrence risk. For example, if a parent has isolated unilateral cleft lip, the recurrence risk is about 2.5%. If there is unilateral cleft lip and cleft palate, the risk increases to 4%, whereas if there is bilateral cleft lip with cleft palate, the risk is over 5.5% (Gorlin et al., 2001).

## Genetic Counseling

Genetic counseling is sometimes sought by parents of a child with a craniofacial anomaly, such as cleft lip and/or palate, who want to know why it happened and whether it will happen to subsequent children. A counselee may be the individual with the disorder, or a close family member, or even someone who plans to marry into the family. The counselee may represent a social agency involved in adoption. Not uncommonly, a couple

**Table 5.3**
**Comparative Empirical Risks (%) for Cleft Lip ± Cleft Palate and for Cleft Palate**

| | Cleft Lip ± palate proband | | Cleft palate proband | |
|---|---|---|---|---|
| **Relative** | **Male** | **Female** | **Male** | **Female** |
| Brother | 6.7 | 6.8 | 1.8 | 2.8 |
| Sister | 2.8 | 4.4 | 3.7 | 1.7 |
| Father | 3.0 | 3.1 | 1.2 | 1.2 |
| Mother | 1.6 | 3.1 | 4.8 | 5.5 |
| Son | 6.7 | 2.4 | 11.5 | 6.0 |
| Daughter | 4.0 | 8.7 | 5.6 | 17.2 |

*Note.* Adapted from *The Etiology of Cleft Lip and Cleft Palate* (pp. 239 and 243), by M. Melnick, D. Bixler, and E. D. Shields (Eds.), 1980, *Progress in Clinical and Biological Research* (Vol. 46), New York: Alan R. Liss. Copyright 1980 by Alan R. Liss. Adapted with permission.

will seek genetic counseling prenatally or even during pregnancy. Some couples become concerned when they learn that they are distantly related to affected individuals.

The definition of genetic counseling has changed with time and is still in flux. One role of the genetic counselor is to help provide answers to individuals' questions. However, genetic counseling is much broader than merely communicating facts and probabilities regarding certain specific disorders. It also should help the person to cope with fear, anger, and guilt. The counselor also helps the counselee to understand the diagnosis or lack of diagnosis, the nature of the disorder, and the probable course of the condition if a diagnosis has been established. Counseling should also involve a discussion of management of the condition. The counselor should discuss various options, or courses of action, available to the counselee based on the risks in each case and the ethical, religious, and cultural views of each family. An inordinate number of concerns are of greater immediate importance in the counseling role than the presentation of a recurrence risk. These concerns often require the counselor to play a role in psychological support, trying to eliminate guilt if it exists or, if that fails, at least to distribute the guilt as much as possible, so that it becomes more easily vitiated.

The background of genetic counselors, until recently, has been quite variable. Some have had intensive training in human genetics. Others have developed an interest in counseling for only a single disorder or for a limited number of conditions. With the establishment of the American Board of Medical Genetics, it is reasonable to assume that all major health science centers will have certified genetic counselors and that requirements concerning training programs and qualifications will become more exacting.

Counselors' approaches to patients vary. In general, most genetic counseling is nondirective; that is, the genetic counselor attempts to stay removed from ultimate decision making, being careful not to transmit personal bias to the patient. Directive counselors, however, feel that some patients need to be led. They argue that the patient is asking for help and that it is the counselor's role to direct the patient in a positive manner toward reaching that goal. Many patients either consciously or unconsciously place the counselor in the position of making the decision for them by asking, "What would you do in my situation?" Most counselors respond by saying that they cannot be placed in such a position because they cannot know all the factors involved and that there are emotional aspects to the case that are not transferable. Most counselors try to be uninvolved and to avoid exhibiting preference for any single option. Nevertheless, subtle movements or facial expressions (or body language) often convey the counselor's bias to the counselee.

To counsel, one first needs the correct diagnosis. The counselor may or may not be the diagnostician. To blindly accept an unconfirmed diagnosis and to base one's discussion of the case on possibly spurious evidence is an untenable situation. Because of the desire to have a disorder labeled (which pleases both patient and diagnostician), individuals will be understandably discomfited if the original diagnosis is replaced with "disorder unknown." Even if the prognosis of the erroneously named disorder were grim, its replacement by an unknown prognosis produces fear. This fear and the attendant resentment, even though not articulated, may often inhibit the process of counseling. The counselor's use of clinical geneticists or other specialists, whether local, national, or international, to establish a diagnosis should be encouraged. The specialist should be supplied with a thorough medical and developmental history, laboratory findings, and high-quality color photographs and radiographs (if relevant). Computer-assisted diagnostic services are also available, but the answers obtained are only as good as the information supplied. A good clinician can often prevent countless dollars from being expended on a myriad of useless laboratory tests.

Once the diagnosis has been established, the counselor enters an informative role. A family pedigree should always be constructed, even in the "simplest" situations. It may not be possible to complete the pedigree in a single session; bits and pieces of information may be gathered over weeks or even months. Contacts may have to be made with various health professionals or agencies. Relatives who might provide useful information may be less than cooperative, resenting intrusion into matters they consider personal. In the process of data gathering, the skilled counselor may encounter information that could be detrimental were it to fall into the hands of unethical persons. Questions arise as to whether all information acquired regarding a patient or family should be made available to the person who seeks counsel, and whether other relatives are entitled to this information.

One cannot emphasize strongly enough the importance of keeping accurate records. They should be kept up to date and in good order, and should be easily accessible. Counseling sessions that are highly charged with emotion may be recorded and a transcript sent to the counselee. It is important that the counselee's nodding in agreement seldom be considered to reflect understanding. The psychological trauma of the birth of an infant with a craniofacial anomaly often works against parental comprehension of information. A reasonable test is to ask the counselee to repeat in his or her own words what the counselor has said. The revealed lack of understanding or fabricated misinformation is often shocking to the novice. In any event, a follow-up letter that summarizes the findings (both positive and negative), the diagnosis (if one has been determined), and the counseling information given (or nature of disorder) should be as explicit as possible. It is a good idea to have counselees sign a statement that they have received counseling and have understood the material presented (if they have, of course). A copy of this signed and witnessed statement should be kept in the patient's file.

Sometimes, especially in the case of an infant with an isolated malformation, a counselor cannot give the odds of recurrence (having another child with the same condition) because the underlying condition has not been identified. In those cases, should a counselor "bracket" the odds? For example, in the case of a male infant with severe developmental delays, a study of banded chromosomes reveals a normal karyotype. It would be inadequate to counsel a family and tell them that the chance for recurrence is somewhere between 0% and 25%. Although 25% would be the recurrence risk of a disorder with autosomal or X-linked recessive inheritance and 0% (or near that) would represent a new dominant mutation, the estimate would not cover the much higher chance of recurrence if a mother were still subject to the same unknown teratogen. Nor would it cover unaffected parents who have two or more children with a known dominant disorder due to segmental mutation in a testis or ovary. Although these are extremely rare examples, they are *real* examples. Obviously, one has to compromise, lest one scare parents from having future children.

Another aspect of counseling involves dealing with caveats reported by the sensationalist media. Most caveats are based on isolated case reports, rarely on prospective studies; however, retrospective data are always suspect. The associated feeling of guilt in having parented a child with a craniofacial anomaly may be transferred to something done or not done, or to some agent consumed or not consumed during pregnancy. It is important to remember that just because an agent is teratogenic in a mouse, does not mean that it is teratogenic in a rat, much less a human.

A marked increase in litigation has occurred regarding genetic malpractice. These cases have been largely concerned with "wrongful birth" (parents' claim) and/or "wrongful life" (child's claim). These cases have involved the failure of the health professional to meet a certain standard of care because of an error of omission or commission that injures or harms a patient, such as failing to advise the counselee (a) that the risk for recurrence is greater than normal or (b) to what degree the risk is enhanced. Thus, comprehensive and accurate clinical genetics evaluation, appropriate laboratory testing, and additional diagnostic evaluations needed to confirm a diagnosis are key components of care for families seeking genetic counseling.

## Selected Craniofacial Anomalies and Syndromes Associated with Clefting

Cleft lip and/or cleft palate most often occur as isolated craniofacial anomalies. In these cases, several thorough patient examinations conducted over several years have revealed no other *primary* physical abnormalities.(This statement excludes, for example, middle ear infections, which frequently occur *secondary* to cleft palate. In addition, although persons with cleft palate have been found to have an increased prevalence of language and learning disabilities, these conditions are also considered secondary to clefting because co-occurring speech or hearing disorders, such as velopharyngeal dysfunction, articulation disorders, and/or conductive hearing loss, may influence the development of language and reading skills.) Data secured at birth regarding congenital anomalies differ from data obtained at surgery, because those patients with more serious defects often succumb prior to surgery. When data are broken down according to subtype, there is general agreement that other congenital anomalies are far more often associated with cleft palate only (20%–50%) than with either cleft lip only (7%–13%) or cleft lip and palate (2%–11%). The frequency with which one or more malformations accompanied clefts of all types was almost 28% (I. Emanuel et al., 1972).

Additional physical malformations have been found more frequently in infants with bilateral cleft lip, with or without cleft palate, than in persons with unilateral clefting. Associated anomalies are more frequently noted in patients without a family history of clefting than in patients with affected relatives. Congenital velopharyngeal inadequacy for speech has been found to be frequently associated with other anomalies, such as cervical spine anomalies, and may suggest an underlying syndromic cause, such as velocardiofacial syndrome. Also, in general, birth weight decreases as the number of malformations increases.

Some of these associated findings form recognizable cleft syndromes. Perhaps as much as 5% of facial clefting is syndromal, and approximately 50% of cleft syndromes have single-gene inheritance (Shprintzen, Siegel-Sadowitz, Amato, & Goldberg, 1985). In 1971, Gorlin, Cervenka, and Pruzansky listed 72 such syndromes. This was increased to 133 such disorders by Cohen in 1978 and to over 204 cleft conditions by Lynch and Kimberling in 1981. The latter authors listed 47 autosomal-dominant, 55 autosomal-recessive, 6 X-linked, 32 chromosomal, and 64 disorders of unknown nature that are associated with facial clefting. A current estimate of the number of cleft syndromes is in excess of 350, with new ones described each year (Gorlin et al., 2001). Although there are currently hundreds of syndromes of which clefting is often a part, we have selected only a small number of these disorders to illustrate the points that we have raised earlier. These specific conditions are seen most often in our cleft palate and craniofacial clinic. We describe major anomalies and features of these syndromes associated with clefting, including speech-language, hearing, and cognitive features.

Readers may wonder at this point why a speech-language pathologist or audiologist should learn something about these relatively rare conditions. Although they might consider this information to be the province of the human geneticist or the pediatrician, it is actually the province of the *entire* interdisciplinary team. It is not at all unusual for parents to take a young child to a speech-language pathologist due to concerns about an unusual nasal speech quality or delayed sound production. In fact, this professional is often the first involved in cases of Stickler syndrome and velocardiofacial syndrome. The heart anomalies and distinctive personality of the latter syndrome may not be evident; thus, the phenotypic spectrum may not be recognized. The ability of the speech-language pathologist to recognize the phenotype and refer the child to a specialist or craniofacial team for definitive diagnosis (possibly followed by molecular genetic studies) will result in better patient care. For example, due to the high risk for early retinal detachment in Stickler syndrome, it is important that these patients be diagnosed as early as possible and then followed closely by an ophthalmologist to avoid debilitating visual impairment. Accurate diagnosis is important in aiding professionals in the assessment and treatment of the patient, helping parents make informed reproductive decisions, and helping the patient obtain earlier intervention and services as needed.

## Robin Sequence

Robin sequence (or Robin complex) is described as consisting of micrognathia, glossoptosis, and cleft palate, and was first reported in 1923 by Pierre Robin, a French physician (Cleft Palate Foundation, 1999; Cohen, 1999; Randall, Krogman, & Jahins, 1965). It should be recognized that this triad is not a specific disorder or diagnosis, but rather a malformation that can be seen in association with various conditions (Cohen, 1976, 1999). The facial features are often striking at birth (see Figure 5.10). The mandible is small and symmetrically receded. Congenital murmurs and/or heart disease have been observed in 15%–25% of those patients who die in early infancy, and necropsy has revealed a wide variety of congenital heart disorders (atrial septal defect, patent ductus arteriosus, ventricular septal defect, etc.) (Gorlin et al., 2001). Ocular findings are also common, especially esotropia and congenital glaucoma.

Pathogenesis is likely based on arrested development of the mandible, which then prevents the normal descent of the tongue between the palatal

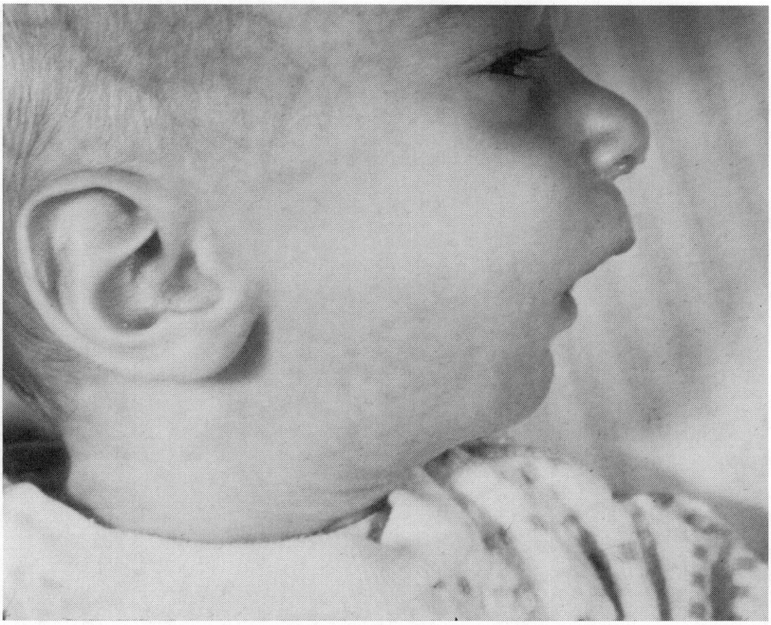

FIGURE 5.10. Severe micrognathia in an infant with Robin sequence.

shelves (hence the term *sequence*). Although many of the conditions with which the Robin sequence is associated are single-gene disorders, when it is not associated with any of these conditions, Robin sequence does not appear to have single-gene inheritance.

Although most individuals born with Robin sequence have normal intelligence, it has been established that about 20% of patients exhibit severe mental retardation, which may be primary or secondary to asphyxia (Hanson & Smith, 1975). The palatal defect may vary widely from cleft uvula to palatal clefting that involves two thirds of the hard palate and is often horseshoe- or U-shaped (see Figure 5.11). The majority of patients have a palatal defect of intermediate degree. In this disorder, cleft lip does not occur in combination with cleft palate. The small mandible may achieve catch-up growth by 4–6 years of age, although the angle is always somewhat abnormal (Vegter, Mulder, & Hage, 1997).

Infants with Robin sequence may have difficulty in the inspiratory phase of respiration, with periodic cyanotic attacks, labored breathing, and recession of the sternum and ribs, especially when the child is in the supine position. The respiratory difficulty is usually evident at birth,

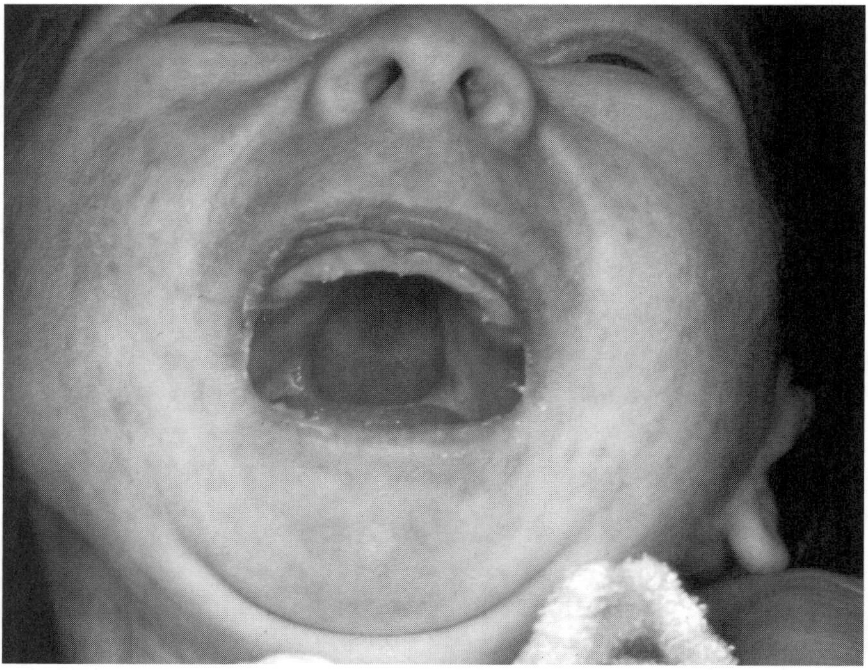

FIGURE 5.11. Complete cleft of the secondary palate in an infant with Robin sequence.

although it may not be severe until after the 1st week of life. The onset of respiratory problems is rarely delayed beyond the 1st month.

Airway obstruction in Robin sequence has been classified into four main types: (1) obstruction resulting from retroposition of the tongue, which contacts the posterior pharyngeal wall below the velum; (2) obstruction type 1 plus compression of the velum against the posterior pharyngeal wall when a cleft palate is present; (3) obstruction when the lateral pharyngeal walls move medially and obstruct the airway, but the tongue does not contact the posterior pharyngeal wall; and (4) obstruction due to excessive circular or sphincteric contraction of the pharynx, without the tongue contacting the posterior pharyngeal wall (Sadewitz & Shprintzen, 1986; Sher, 1992; Sher, Shprintzen, & Thorpy, 1986; Shprintzen, 1988).

Airway obstruction in this sequence has traditionally been treated using three main approaches. The most conservative includes prone positioning of the child at rest, having the child sit upright at feedings, and not placing the child on his or her back. Children with chronic airway obstruction may also require increased caloric intake due to increased caloric expenditure. Nasopharyngeal intubation (with "nasal trumpets" or respiratory support) and endotracheal intubation are slightly more aggressive treatment approaches to maintain airway integrity. Lastly, surgical approaches, including glossopexy (e.g., tongue-lip adhesion), tracheostomy, and mandibular distraction osteogenesis, are sometimes used in more severe cases of obstruction (Benjamin & Walker, 1991; Pashayan & Lewis, 1984; Sadewitz & Shprintzen, 1986; Sher, 1992; Sher et al., 1986; Shprintzen, 1988; Singer & Sidoti, 1992). In addition, all of these airway considerations must be taken into account when determining optimal timing and technique for cleft palate repair.

Not all children with Robin sequence experience such severe airway difficulties. In general, the feeding and swallowing difficulties of infants with Robin sequence are proportional to the severity of the airway impairment (Benjamin & Walker, 1991; Pashayan & Lewis, 1984; Sadewitz & Shprintzen, 1986; Sher, 1992; Sher et al., 1986; Shprintzen, 1988; Singer & Sidoti, 1992). These difficulties are usually similar to those encountered in children with cleft palate but magnified due to the respiratory obstruction, small jaw, and posterior tongue placement. The posterior tongue position further impedes sucking and bolus transit (Lehman, Fishman, & Neiman, 1995). To ensure adequate airway management, cleft palate repair may be delayed in children with Robin sequence, compared to those without it. In some children with Robin sequence, feeding and swallowing issues can be managed only with modified nipples during bottle feeding or palatal feeding obturators, whereas other children may require nasogastric or gastrostomy tube placement. The overall goal of feeding and swallowing management in these infants is to maintain airway patency and optimum nutrition while using a technique that is as natural as possible.

## Speech-Language Issues in Robin Sequence

Children born with Robin sequence that is not associated with other syndromes or anomalies generally have speech-language and cognitive expectations similar to those of children with isolated cleft palate, depending on the extent of early medical and respiratory complications, and the timing or duration of invasive treatment (Peterson-Falzone et al., 2001). In more severe cases, possible delays in palate repair could increase the child's risk for delayed speech-language skills and lead to the development of aberrant compensatory articulation patterns (Trost, 1981; Trost-Cardamone, 1987; Trost-Cardamone & Bernthal, 1993). In cases of severe micrognathia, tongue-backing articulation patterns may also be observed.

LeBlanc and Golding-Kushner (1992) examined the effect of glossopexy (for airway management) on speech sound production in children with Robin sequence. Their analysis suggested that glossopexy may delay the development of babbling and the initiation of first words; however, the delays were temporary. The only long-term effect was a tendency to produce tongue-tip sounds with the tongue blade, but production was perceptually normal.

About one third of cases of Robin sequence are associated with other anomalies that do not constitute a recognizable syndrome. The conditions most commonly associated with Robin sequence are Stickler syndrome and velocardiofacial syndrome, which may account for as many as 30% of the cases; however, Robin sequence can be seen with a wide variety of disorders (Gorlin et al., 2001). It is extremely important that an infant born with Robin sequence be evaluated by a geneticist to thoroughly investigate the possibility of an associated syndrome (Cleft Palate Foundation, 1999).

## Apert Syndrome (Acrocephalosyndactyly)

Apert syndrome is characterized by congenital craniosynostosis leading to turribrachycephaly (relatively pointed and shortened [front-to-back] appearance of the skull) (see Figure 5.12); syndactyly (webbing or joining together) of the hands and feet (see Figure 5.13); and various ankyloses and progressive synostoses (immobility and joint problems) of the hands, feet, and cervical spine (Buchanan, 1968; Gorlin et al., 2001; Schauerte & St. Aubin, 1966). Some patients with the disorder exhibit some degree of cognitive impairment, typically associated with central nervous system malformations, increased intracranial pressure, or postsurgical hydrocephalus complications.

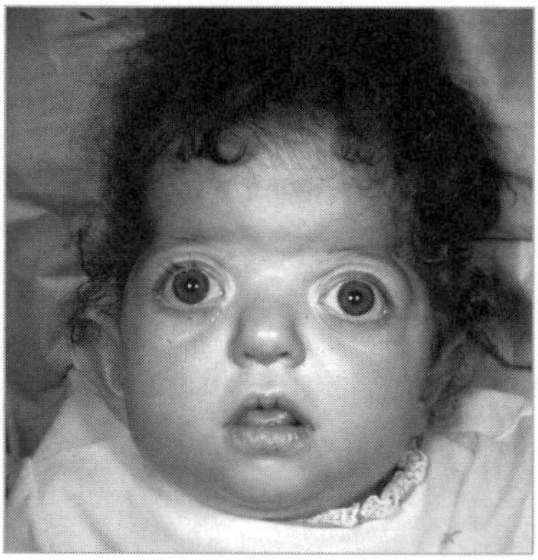

FIGURE 5.12. Craniosynostosis in infant with Apert syndrome.

This syndrome is due to mutations in fibroblast growth factor receptor 2 (FGFR2) on chromosome 10. There is autosomal dominant inheritance. Increased paternal age at the time of conception has been found. Although most cases are sporadic, there are sev-

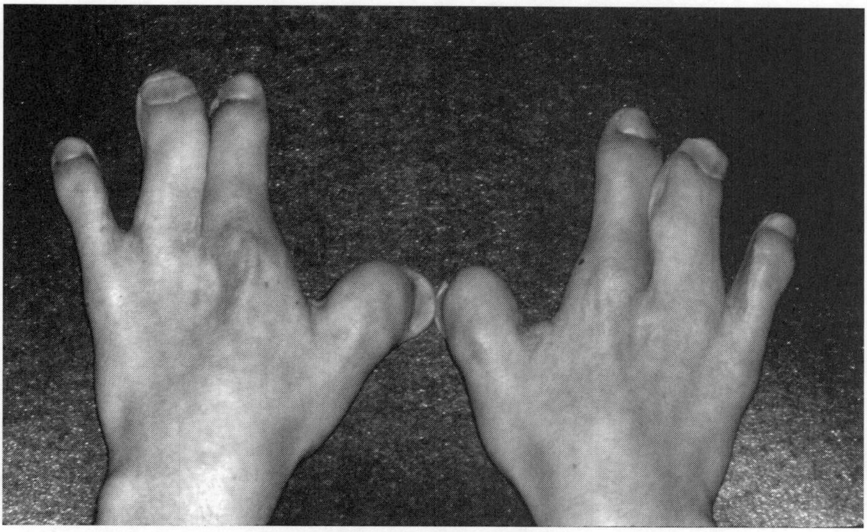

Figure 5.13. Syndactyly of the hands in Apert syndrome.

eral examples in which females with the disorder have given birth to an affected child. It is thought to occur in approximately 1 in 160,000 births; however, due to the high mortality rate in the neonatal period, there is approximately 1 case per 2 million in the general population.

In Apert syndrome, acne is commonly noted, with extension to the forearm. The eye orbits are quite hyperteloric (far apart). The midface is usually underdeveloped, lending prominent appearance to the mandible. The skull is malformed, with the frontal and occipital bones being flattened and the apex of the cranium located near or anterior to the bregma (junction of the coronal and sagittal sutures). Irregular early obliteration of the cranial sutures, especially the coronal suture, is common.

The hands and feet are symmetrically deformed (see Figure 5.13). A mid-digital hand with bony and soft-tissue syndactyly of digits two, three, and four is typical. Digits one and five are often incompletely attached to the mid-digital hand mass. In the feet, the hallux is frequently partially separated from the rest of the toes, which have complete soft tissue syndactyly and usually a common nail. Six metatarsals have been noted. The upper extremities may be shortened, and there may be ankylosis of joints, especially those of the elbow, shoulder, and hip. The bones of the hands, feet, and cervical spine become progressively synostosed.

The palatal vault of the maxilla is severely V-shaped ("byzantine" appearance), with ectopic eruption of teeth, severe Class III malocclusion, and open bite (Gorlin et al., 2001; Moller, 1994). (See Figure 5.14.) Malocclusion is common, due to midfacial hypoplasia. The palatal vault progressively accumulates soft tissue along the palatine shelves, which appears to be caused by an accumulation of acid mucopolysaccharides (Solomon, Medenica, Pruzansky, & Kreiborg, 1973). The palate is highly arched and constricted, and may have a median furrow. The palatal vault gradually changes in appearance with increasing age, from a deep narrow V shape to almost flat with a narrow slit or pseudocleft. The pharynx is reduced in height and depth. The velum is usually abnormally long and thick and may crowd or obstruct the nasopharyngeal airway (Peterson & Pruzansky, 1974; Peterson-Falzone, Pruzansky, Parris, & Laffer, 1981). Cleft of the soft palate has been observed in approximately 35% of cases (Gorlin et al., 2001).

In Apert syndrome, upper airway obstruction may be present secondary to bony or soft tissue abnormalities, choanal atresia, and a crowded nasopharyngeal space (Perkins, Sie, Milczuk, & Richardson, 1997; Peterson-Falzone et al., 2001). These pharyngeal anomalies can also contribute to inadequate aeration of the middle ear, chronic otitis media with effusion, and subsequent conductive hearing loss. Readers interested in a more detailed description of the physical anomalies associated with Apert syndrome are referred to Gorlin et al. (2001) and Cohen and Kreiborg (1996).

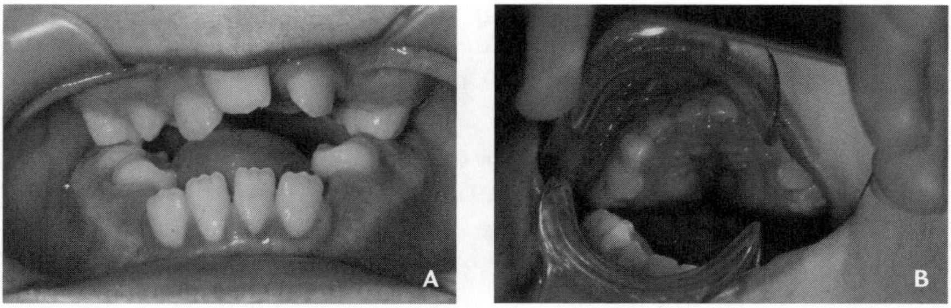


FIGURE 5.14. Anterior openbite and transverse crossbite (A) and V-shaped palatal vault (B) in Apert syndrome. *Note.* From "Apert Syndrome with Glucose-6-Phosphate Dehydrogenase Deficiency: A Case Report," by G. Tosun and Y. Sener, 2006, *International Journal of Paediatric Dentistry, 16,* pp. 218–221. Copyright 2006 by International Journal of Pediatric Dentistry. Reprinted with permission.

## Speech-Language and Hearing Issues in Apert Syndrome

In addition to oral and nasopharyngeal structural anomalies, persons with Apert syndrome are at risk for communicative impairments associated with possible cognitive deficits, hearing loss, reduced stimulation and interactions due to multiple hospitalizations, and negative psychosocial input because of their physical deformities (Solomon, Fretzin, & Pruzansky, 1970). Hyponasal resonance distortion is common, given altered nasopharyngeal dimensions, although mixed resonance may be observed if velopharyngeal inadequacy is also present.

Articulation errors are common and include obligatory distortions secondary to Class III malocclusion (anterior crossbite), developmental errors due to cognitive delays, and errors related to possible hearing loss or clefting. Class III malocclusion constitutes one of the most significant hazards to precise articulation because it interferes with tongue placement for sounds such as /s/, /ʃ/, and /tʃ/. Patients may find it easier to produce acceptable sibilants with a tongue tip down position. In addition, patients with Class III malocclusion may produce the /f/ and /v/ sounds with reversed labiodental approximation (Moller, 1994). Surgical midface and maxillary advancement is usually indicated and performed at a time when it will likely have a beneficial effect on occlusion, speech (resonance), and nasal airway patency.

Shipster, Hearst, Dockrell, Kilby, and Hayward (2002) explored speech, language, resonance/voice, attention, and cognitive skills in a group of 10 children with Apert syndrome. In all children for whom a BAS II–Early Years version Performance IQ was obtained ($n = 8$), abilities were reportedly within the average range and IQ scores were considerably higher than those reported in previous studies. Eight children had moderate or severe language difficulties, and expressive language difficulties were the most frequent. These language difficulties were not associated with a general cognitive deficit. All the children had problems with attention and speech, and 9 were considered to have abnormal voice quality. Multidisciplinary assessment is recommended to obtain a profile of each child's strengths and weaknesses to ensure that appropriate educational placements and early interventions are implemented.

# Crouzon Syndrome (Craniofacial Dysostosis)

First described by Crouzon in 1912, Crouzon syndrome is characterized by craniosynostosis, maxillary hypoplasia, shallow eye orbits, and ocular proptosis (Gorlin et al., 2001). (See Figure 5.15.) This syndrome has autosomal dominant transmission, with most cases being familial and about one third resulting from new mutations. Crouzon syndrome accounts for about 5% of all cases of craniosynostosis (Cohen & Kreiborg, 1992).

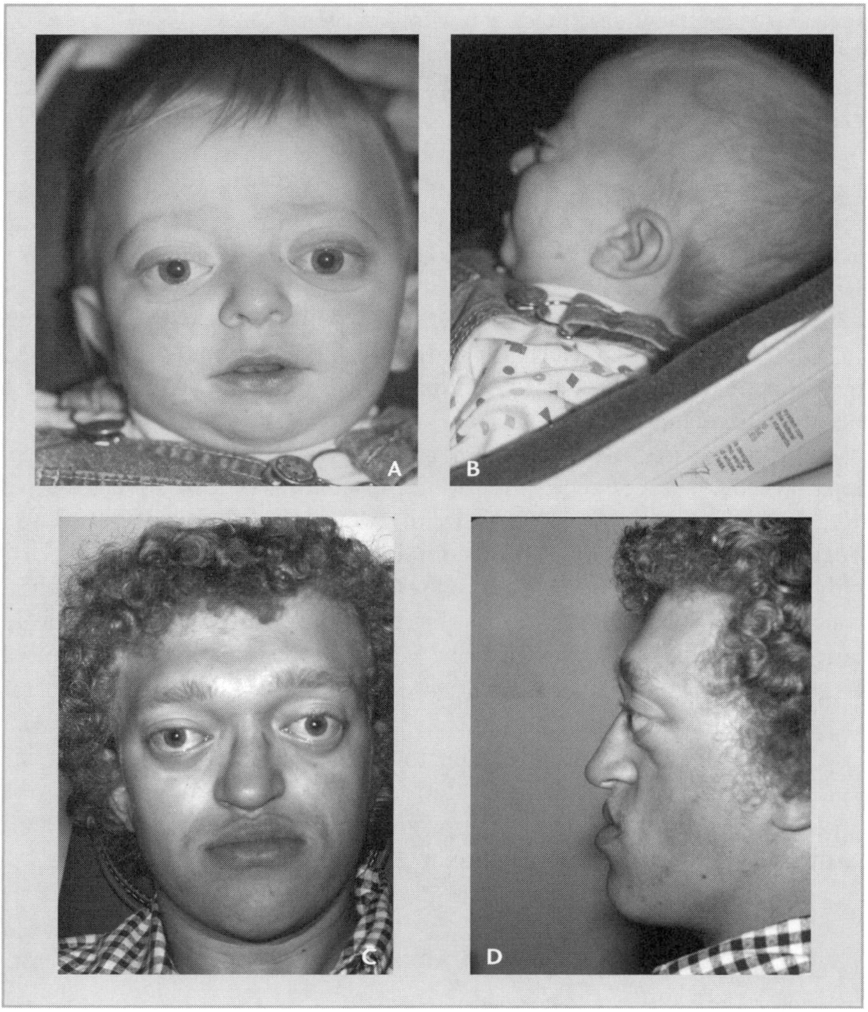


FIGURE 5.15. Craniosynostosis, maxillary hypoplasia, shallow eye orbits, and ocular proptosis in an infant (views A and B) and an adult (views C and D) with Crouzon syndrome.

Brachycephaly is most commonly observed, but scaphocephaly, triganocephaly, and cloverleaf skull also may be observed (Gorlin et al., 2001).

Maxillary hypoplasia results in a shortened maxillary dental arch and reduced arch width, which gives the appearance of a highly arched palate (although palatal height is normal by measurement) (Gorlin et al., 2001; Moller, 1994). Dental-occlusal anomalies are common. Ocular anomalies lead to increased risk for conjunctivitis, keratitis, and poor vision. Approximately 50% of individuals with Crouzon syndrome have visual impairments, with optic atrophy in 22% and blindness in 7% (Kreiborg, 1981). Hypertelorism is frequently observed. Progressive hydrocephalus and brain anomalies occur with significant frequency, as well as headaches, seizures, and cognitive impairment; however, a range of intelligence levels has been observed (Cinalli et al., 1995; Kreiborg, 1981; Martinez-Perez et al., 1996). Cervical spine anomalies are present in approximately 30% of cases (Kreiborg, Barr, & Cohen, 1992). Limb and hand anomalies are less common.

## Speech-Language and Hearing Issues in Crouzon Syndrome

Although clefting occurs with low frequency in Crouzon syndrome (Kreiborg, 1981), we believe it is important to briefly review the features of this condition because of (1) the often observed reduced nasopharyngeal dimensions (similar to Apert syndrome) that impact velopharyngeal function and resonance, (2) the dental-occlusal hazards to articulation, and (3) the presence of conductive hearing loss in over half of the patients with this syndrome (Gorlin et al., 2001; Kreiborg, 1981).

In Crouzon syndrome, maxillary hypoplasia is common, which results in reduced dimensions of the pharynx and velopharyngeal port and therefore contributes to frequent observations of hyponasality. Deviated septum has also been reported in one third of patients with Crouzon syndrome (Kreiborg, 1981).

The primary speech difficulties in persons with Crouzon syndrome are usually related to malocclusion. Speech-language delays may also be attributed to a history of hearing loss or other cognitive delays. Crowding of maxillary and mandibular teeth, anterior open bite, and Class III malocclusion are frequently observed (Gorlin et al., 2001) and may contribute to obligatory distortions of fricative or affricate sounds, or the use of compensatory placement for labiodental sounds, similar to persons with Apert syndrome (Moller, 1994). Tongue tip down placement for production of /s, z/ may be an appropriate speech therapy target, prior to orthognathic surgical procedures to improve the jaw relationship.

## Treacher Collins Syndrome (Mandibulofacial Dysostosis)

Treacher Collins syndrome was originally described by Franceschetti and Klein in 1949. Persons with this disorder have eye anomalies that include the following: antimongoloid obliquity (downward slant) of the palpebral fissures, coloboma (eye defect/notching) of the outer third of the lower lid, and a deficiency of cilia or lashes medial to the coloboma (Franceschetti & Klein, 1949; Gorlin et al., 2001). (See Figures 5.16 and 5.17.) The nose appears large due to lack of malar bone development, while the nares are often narrow and the alar cartilages hypoplastic. The nasofrontal angle is commonly severely reduced, and the bridge of the nose is raised. Choanal atresia has also been noted. Micrognathia is almost always present, and other oral manifestations include cleft palate (30%), high-arched palatal vault, dental malocclusion, and unilateral or, less often, bilateral macrostomia. The external ear is frequently deformed, crumpled forward, or misplaced. Some patients have an absence of the external auditory canal or ossicular defects associated with conductive hearing loss (see Figures 5.16B, 5.17B, and 5.17C). Anomalies of the ossicles include a fixed malleus, fusion of malformed malleus and incus, monopodal stapes, ab-

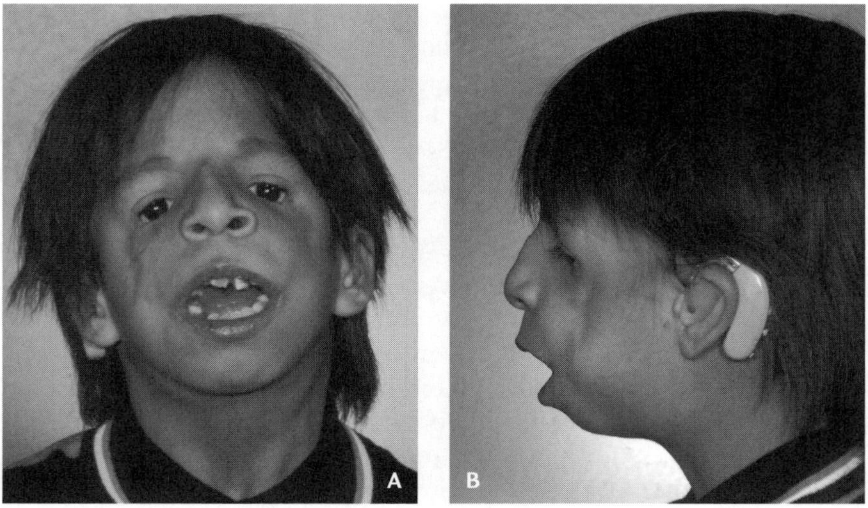


FIGURE 5.16. Hypoplastic malar bones, anterior openbite, mandibular hypoplasia, and conductive hearing loss in boy with Treacher Collins syndrome.

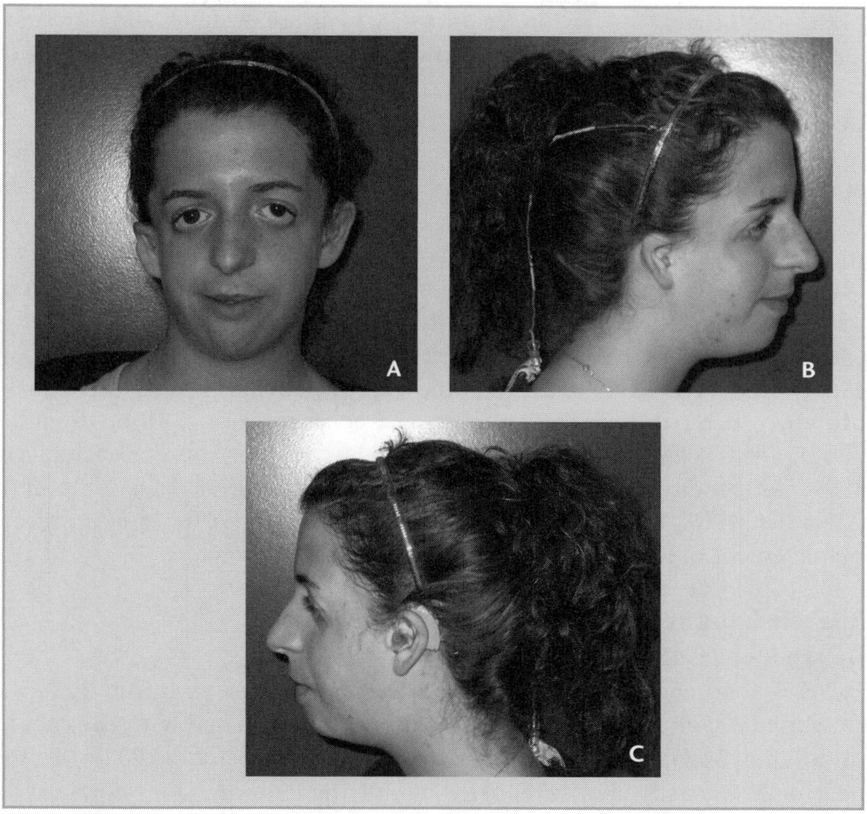


Figure 5.17. Downward slanting of the palpebral fissures, lack of malar bone development, bilateral external ear deformities, and conductive hearing loss in a teenager with Treacher Collins syndrome.

sence of stapes and oval window, and complete absence of the middle ear and epitympanic space. Extra ear tags and blind fistulas may be found anywhere between the tragus of the ear and angle of the mouth.

Treacher Collins syndrome has autosomal dominant inheritance. More than half the cases arise as new mutations, but before a patient is considered to represent a new mutation, careful examination of family members must be done, looking for minimal signs of the syndrome.

Radiographic studies of individuals with Treacher Collins syndrome may show a wide variety of findings involving the skull, such as poorly developed supraorbital ridges, hypoplastic malar bones with nonfusion of the zygomatic arches, sclerotic and nonpneumatized mastoids, sclerosis of the middle ear (and, rarely, the inner ear) with poor delineation of their structures, hypoplasia of the mandible, and flat or aplastic coronoid and condyloid processes. The undersurface of the body of the mandible is markedly concave.

Individuals with this syndrome have a pharynx that is small in diameter and often contributes to airway complications (Peterson-Falzone & Pruzansky, 1976; Shprintzen, Croft, Berkman, & Rakoff, 1979), in addition to mandibular and maxillary hypoplasia, posterior tongue positioning, retrognathia, and progressive "bending" of the cranial base which advances the position of the posterior pharyngeal wall into the airway (Figueroa, 1991; Kreiborg & Dahl, 1993; Peterson-Falzone & Figueroa, 1986). Infants with Treacher Collins experience significant respiratory difficulty at birth, with 23% requiring tracheostomies (Vallino-Napoli, 2002). Obstructive sleep apnea is often apparent (Arvystas & Shprintzen, 1991; Colmenero, Esteban, Albarino, & Colmenero, 1991; Fazen, Elmore, & Nadler, 1967) and must be taken into consideration for later surgical management of possible velopharyngeal issues for speech.

## Speech-Language and Hearing Issues in Treacher Collins Syndrome

Hearing loss, which is universal in Treacher Collins syndrome, is typically bilateral and conductive in nature, and is associated with ear canal, middle ear, and temporal bone deformities (Vallino-Napoli, 2002). Mixed hearing loss is occasionally reported. Following temporal bone computerized tomographic (CT) imaging of the course of the facial nerve (CN VII), consideration may be given to use of osseointegrated implants (e.g., bone anchored hearing aids [BAHAs]). Thomas (1996) found that associated abnormalities of jaw, teeth, and palate may amplify speech problems already affected by congenital hearing loss; however, spontaneous improvement in features such as voice pitch, quality, and intensity was observed in some patients following the fitting of a BAHA.

In addition to hearing limitations in Treacher Collins syndrome, cleft palate and velopharyngeal inadequacy can also contribute to speech delays and distortions. Vallino-Napoli (2002) reported palatal anomalies in 60% of individuals with Treacher Collins. In a series of 25 cases of Treacher Collins, Peterson-Falzone and Pruzansky (1976) found that 7 had cleft palate, 1 had complete unilateral cleft lip and palate, and 8 had "congenital palatopharyngeal incompetency" (CPI). The CPI appeared in four forms: (1) complete agenesis of the soft palate, (2) foreshortening of the soft palate associated with a submucous defect of the hard palate,

(3) submucous defect of the hard palate with adequate palatal length but inadequate elevation in speech, and (4) lack of adequate palatal elevation in the absence of a submucous defect or reduced length of the soft palate. Velopharyngeal inadequacy for speech may be masked by the presence of other speech problems in this syndrome, particularly by the "muffled" voice quality associated with an elevated and retracted tongue posture.

Hyponasality or muffled resonance is also frequently observed, secondary to the atypical size and shape of the oral and nasopharyngeal cavities, even in the presence of adequate velopharyngeal closure (Peterson-Falzone et al., 2001). In her study of 30 persons with Treacher Collins syndrome, Vallino-Napoli (2002) found that 77% had abnormal resonance, 63% had abnormal voice quality, and 100% demonstrated articulation errors. Although both prosthetic and surgical approaches are appropriate and viable treatment options for inadequate velopharyngeal function, both are more complicated in Treacher Collins because of the presence of other structural anomalies, including restricted oral opening and airway constriction (Peterson-Falzone & Pruzansky, 1976).

Articulation difficulties in Treacher Collins syndrome are typically related to malocclusion (e.g., open bite and overbite), velopharyngeal inadequacy, hearing loss, and/or other developmental causes of articulation or phonological delays. In some cases, the severe micrognathia causes persistent tongue backing with substitutions of posterior sounds for anterior sounds, abnormal tongue posturing, and dampened resonance. The mandibular deformity in Treacher Collins contributes in 60% of cases to a progressive open bite, which worsens over time (J. Goldberg, Enlow, Whitaker, Zins, & Kurihara, 1981; Roberts, Pruzansky, & Aduss, 1975; Vallino-Napoli, 2002). Anterior distortions secondary to open bite are common (see Figure 5.18) and may appear to worsen with age until appropriate orthodontic and surgical management is completed. The most common sounds negatively affected by the dental-occlusal hazards include the sibilants, apicoalveolar and bilabial stops (Vallino-Napoli, 2002). It is important for the speech-language pathologist to carefully determine which speech errors are obligatory (unchangeable due to structural differences) and which are amenable to articulation therapy.

Unlike some clefting syndromes, individuals with Treacher Collins typically have normal intelligence (Gorlin et al., 2001). For this reason, interdisciplinary team members, including the speech-language pathologist, must be alert to the need to refer these individuals for appropriate counseling and psychosocial support staff to help promote the development of self-confidence and healthy peer relationships.

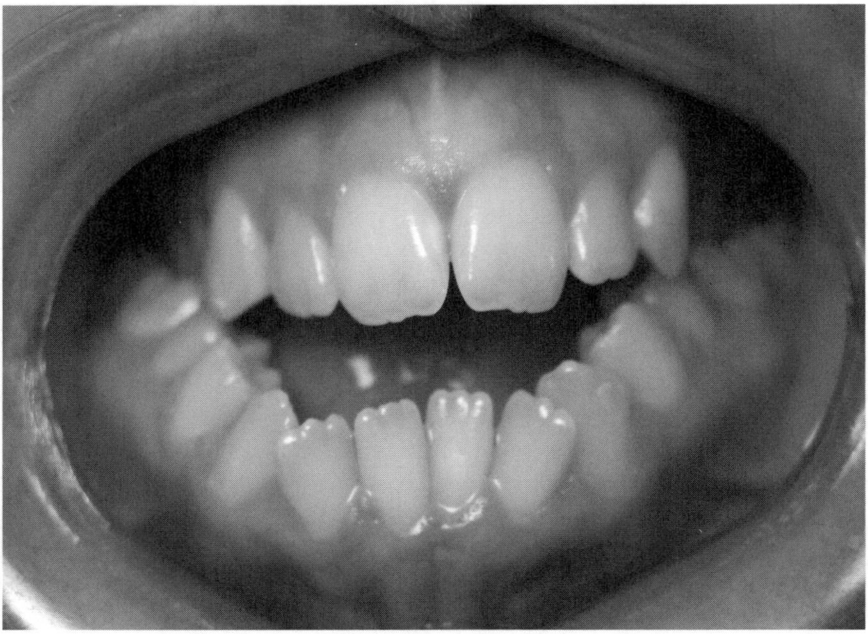

FIGURE 5.18. Open bite, which contributes to anterior distortions, in an individual with Treacher Collins syndrome.

## Oculo-Auriculo-Vertebral Spectrum (Goldenhar Syndrome, Hemifacial Microsomia)

In the 1960s, hemifacial microsomia, now known as oculo-auriculo-vertebral (OAV) spectrum, was defined as a condition affecting primarily aural, oral, and mandibular development (see Figure 5.19). This disorder varies from mild to severe, and involvement is typically more severe on the right side. Bilateral involvement has been found in approximately 10% of patients (Gorlin et al., 2001). Goldenhar syndrome is considered a variant of this disorder, characterized additionally by vertebral anomalies and epibulbar dermoids (benign tissue growth on the eye). Most cases of OAV are sporadic and of unknown etiology, but there is good evidence for genetic heterogeneity. Multifactorial transmission has been postulated by most authors. The frequency of the condition is about 1 in 3,000 live births. Recurrence risk in the isolated case is about 1%.

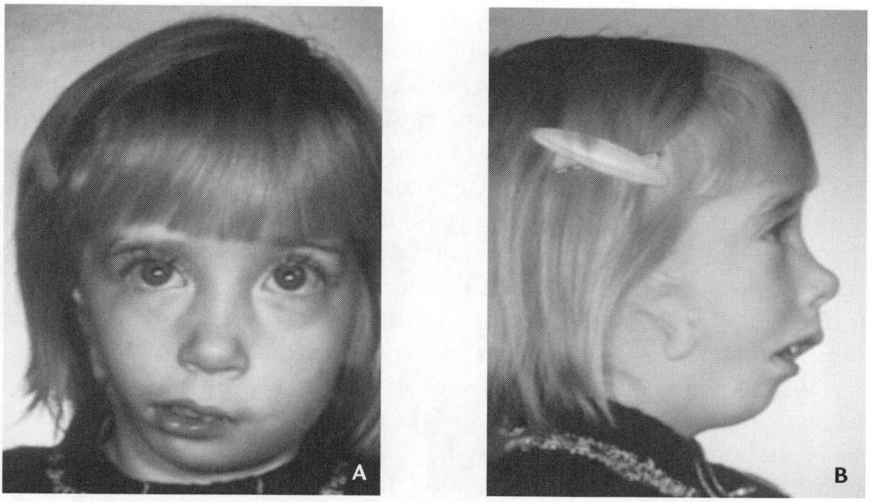


Figure 5.19. (A) Marked asymmetry and hypoplasia of the ear, mandible, and oral-facial structures in a female with oculo-auriculo-vertebral spectrum, primarily affecting the right side. (B) Ear malformations, including the lack of external ear structures and complete atresia of the auditory canal.

OAV spectrum is usually compatible with normal life span and intellect. Facial asymmetry is common but is remarkably variable. The maxillary, temporal, and malar bones on the involved side are reduced in size and flattened. The ipsilateral eye may be set lower than that on the opposite side. Malformation of the external ear may vary from complete aplasia to a crumpled, distorted pinna displaced anteriorly and inferiorly. Supernumerary ear tags may occur anywhere from the tragus to the angle of the mouth (see Figure 5.19B). There may be supratragal pits. When epibulbar dermoids are present, ear tags tend to be bilateral. Conductive hearing loss due to middle ear abnormalities and/or absence or deficiency of the external auditory meatus is found in approximately 40% of cases.

Eye anomalies including epibulbar dermoid and/or lipodermoid are variable findings. Dermoids are white to yellow in color, flattened, ellipsoidal, and solid. The dermoid is usually located at the limbus or corneal margin in the lower outer quadrant of the eye. Unilateral coloboma of the superior lid is common in those patients with epibulbar dermoids. Mental retardation is more common when unilateral microphthalmia (small eye) or anophthalmia (missing eye) is present.

Vertebral anomalies found in about half of patients with OAV include occipitalization of the atlas, cuneiform vertebra, complete or partial synostosis of two or more vertebrae, supernumerary vertebrae, hemivertebrae, and spina bifida. Anomalous ribs, talipes equinovarus (clubfoot), and other skeletal defects have been reported. Hypoplasia of muscles such as the masseter, temporalis, and pterygoideus, as well as muscles involved with facial expression on the involved side, has been observed. The palatal and tongue muscles may be asymmetrically hypoplastic and/or paralyzed, with intraoral examination revealing elevation deviating toward the unaffected side. Hypernasality and/or nasal air emission may also be found in those patients with OAV with asymmetrical palatal function.

Within the mouth there is decreased palatal width from the midline palatal raphe to the lingual surface of the teeth on the affected side. Agenesis of the mandibular ramus may be found in conjunction with macrostomia (i.e., lateral facial cleft of a mild degree). This is nearly always unilateral and on the side of the more affected ear. Dental malocclusion is common. Cleft lip with or without cleft palate is present in about 15% of individuals with OAV. Rare anomalies include occipital encephalocele, congenital heart disease, homolateral pulmonary agenesis or hypoplasia, various renal abnormalities (absent kidney, double ureter, anomalous blood supply to the kidney, etc.), and agenesis of the ipsilateral parotid gland (Gorlin et al., 2001).

## Speech-Language and Hearing Issues in OAV Spectrum

Normal cognitive functioning has been reported in the majority of OAV cases, even when speech and language delays are present. The most apparent hazards to the development of adequate communication skills include significant hearing loss and dental-occlusal hazards to articulation. The hearing impairment, typically conductive in nature, may be bilateral or unilateral regardless of the presence of a visible clinical deformity. The speech difficulties encountered in OAV typically depend on the severity of the physical deformity and the patient-specific capacity to adapt to or compensate for these structural differences. Thus, the more severe the facial and jaw asymmetry, the more severe the articulatory deviation. In the mildest cases, individuals may have only minor articulatory distortions.

The jaw deformity in OAV leads to an occlusal discrepancy that affects the individual's ability to produce precise speech and to maintain functional occlusion for eating. Hypotonia, paresis, or paralysis on the affected side(s) may lead to asymmetry of oral-facial muscle function (Caldarelli, Hutchinson, Pruzansky, & Valvassori, 1980; Sedee, 1973). This asymmetry of structure and function may also impact the velopharynx. Unilateral vocal fold paralysis is also possible (Shprintzen, 2000). Glossoptosis, ankylosis of the tongue, and retruded tongue positioning have also been reported (Peterson-Falzone et al., 2001; Shprintzen, 2000).

Approximately 50% of individuals with OAV have velopharyngeal inadequacy (VPI) and hypernasal speech, regardless of the presence of overt clefting (Shprintzen, Croft, Berkman, & Rakoff, 1980). VPI is often related to structural and physiological asymmetry of the pharynx. No relationship has been found between the severity of facial malformation and the presence of VPI. D'Antonio, Rice, and Fink (1998) described the occurrence and expression of pharyngeal and laryngeal anomalies in this population. This retrospective review reported a high occurrence of indicators of pharyngeal and laryngeal abnormalities, such as velopharyngeal inadequacy and airway obstruction. The presence and severity of pharyngeal and laryngeal abnormalities also were not correlated with the severity of expression of the spectrum based on mandibular morphology.

Van Lierde, Van Cauwenberge, Stevens, and Dhooge (2004) described the language, articulation, voice, and resonance characteristics in 4 children with OAV. All 4 had normal cognitive functioning but showed language delays. Articulation distortions were present along with some phonological processes in some of the children. Vocal roughness was seen in 2 of the children, and resonance distortion was present in only 1 child, who also had a cleft palate.

Mandibular distraction or advancement is a common dental-occlusal surgical treatment for persons affected by OAV. Guyette, Polley, Figueroa, Botts, and Smith (2001) examined the speech changes after unilateral mandibular distraction in 7 patients with this condition. Immediately after distraction, 28% (2 of 7) experienced temporary deterioration in articulation and 42% (3 of 7) experienced deterioration in nasal resonance. By the long-term follow-up evaluation (mean duration 14.1 months postsurgery), all had returned to their preoperative levels.

## Stickler Syndrome (Hereditary Arthroophthalmopathy)

Stickler syndrome manifestations are extremely variable and consist of flattened facial appearance, long philtrum, epicanthal folds, joint hypermobility, myopia, retinal detachment, cleft palate, micrognathia, and sensorineural hearing loss (Liberfarb, Hirose, & Holmes, 1981; Stickler & Pugh, 1967; Stickler et al., 1965). About 85% of the patients exhibit midfacial flattening, and the nasal bridge is depressed or saddle-shaped in about 65% (Gorlin et al., 2001) (see Figure 5.20). Cleft palate or submucous cleft palate is typically present in about 20% of the cases (Gorlin et al., 2001). In addition, up to 50% of persons with Stickler syndrome may have mitral valve prolapse (Liberfarb & Goldblatt, 1986).

Stickler syndrome has autosomal dominant inheritance but remarkably variable expressivity. There is genetic heterogeneity. The disorder is due to mutations in Type II collagen on chromosome 12, and in some cases, Type XI collagen on chromosome 6 (Gorlin et al., 2001).

Bony enlargement of the ankles, knees, and wrists may occur in the first few years of life. The joints at times are painful with use and become stiff at rest. The patient may experience difficulty walking if the capital femoral epiphyses are involved. Premature and progressive arthritis is common. Thoracic kyphosis or scoliosis is noted in about 25% of individuals with Stickler syndrome, with joint hypermobility in about 40% of cases (Lewkonia, 1992). Other less common skeletal anomalies may also be present, including pectus carinatum (protruding ribcage and sternum), genu valgum ("knock knees"), and pes planus (flat feet).

Congenital progressive myopia (as great as 20 diopters) with vitreous degeneration has been noted in about 75%–80% of individuals with Stickler syndrome (Blair, Albert, Liberfarb, & Hirose, 1979; Gorlin et al., 2001; Knobloch & Layer, 1972). Before the 10th year of life, broad zones of retinal detachment are experienced in about 20% of these individuals. By age 30 years, 75% have detachment. Retinal degeneration occurs in 80%–90% of cases (Maumenee, 1979). Cataracts (40%) and glaucoma (15%) complicate the clinical picture. Patients with this syndrome warrant close and consistent ophthalmologic follow-up through adulthood to minimize the potential for vision impairment.

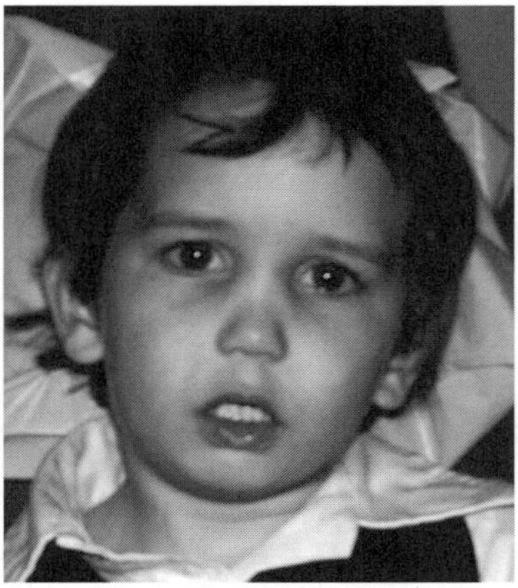

FIGURE 5.20. Midfacial flattening, elongated philtrum, and depressed nasal bridge are characteristics of Stickler syndrome.

Radiographically, about one third of patients exhibit multiple epiphyseal ossification disturbances and diminution in the width of the shafts of tubular bones (Gorlin et al., 2001). The overly thin diaphyses contrast with the normally broad metaphyses. The pelvic bones may be hypoplastic and the femoral neck poorly modeled and plump. There may be some coxa valga (hip deformity). Vertebral bodies tend to be flattened and irregular with a tendency to anterior wedging. The distal tibial epiphysis is usually wedge-shaped.

### Speech-Language and Hearing Issues in Stickler Syndrome

Individuals with Sticker syndrome are at risk for communicative disorders secondary to malocclusion, hearing loss, and possible overt or submucous cleft palate. Open bite and micrognathia with a hypoplastic maxilla can also pose hazards to precise articulation. For example, lingual protrusion may be observed along with distortions and other tongue-backing patterns if there is severe micrognathia. In the presence of clefting and/or velopharyngeal insufficiency, compensatory articulation patterns may also develop and require speech therapy services. Hypernasality may also be present, although mixed or hyponasal resonance distortion is common secondary to a small nasopharynx.

Close monitoring of hearing is critical, given the progressive nature of this disease. Progressive sensorineural hearing loss occurs in 60%–90% of individuals with Stickler syndrome (Gorlin et al., 2001), but they may be asymptomatic until middle age. Conductive hearing loss is less common, but may be secondary to a history of chronic otitis media. Persons with Stickler syndrome are also at risk for possible loss of vision later in life, so the preservation of adequate hearing and the development of functional speech skills are critical. Occasional learning difficulties are also encountered in Sticker syndrome, usually secondary to hearing loss, visual impairment, or communication disorders.

## Velocardiofacial Syndrome (22q11.2 Deletion Syndrome)

Velocardiofacial syndrome (VCFS) is a relatively common genetic disorder typically involving cardiac defects, cognitive-behavioral problems, speech-language disorders, palatal clefting, and a characteristic facial appearance (R. Goldberg, Motzkin, Marion, Scampler, & Shprintzen, 1993; Golding-Kushner, Weller, & Shprintzen, 1985; Gorlin et al., 2001; McDonald-McGinn et al., 1997; Shprintzen, Goldberg, Lewin, Sidoti, Berkman, Argamaso, & Young, 1978; Shprintzen, Goldberg, Young, & Wolford, 1981). (See Figure 5.21.) VCFS occurs in approximately 1 in

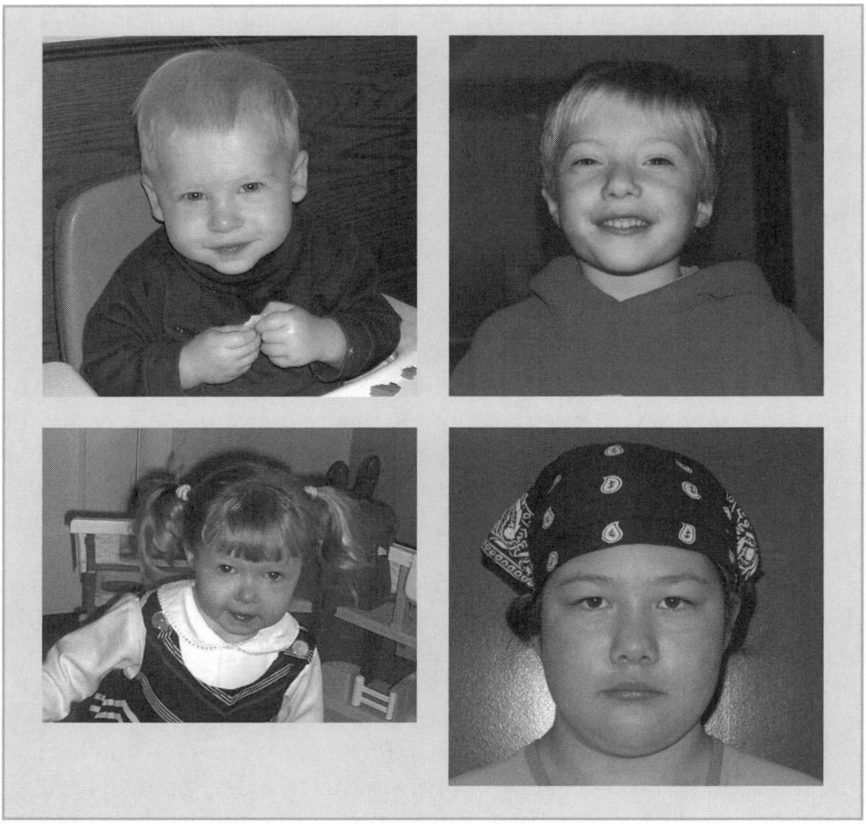

FIGURE 5.21. Four children with velocardiofacial syndrome (also known as DiGeorge syndrome). Note the characteristic, yet subtle, facial dysmorphology consisting of a bulbous nasal tip, broad nasal root, and "hooded" or narrow appearance of the eyelids.

4,000 births and is recognized as the most frequently occurring syndrome of clefting (Devriendt, Fryns, & Mortier, 1998; B. S. Emanuel, McDonald-McGinn, Saitta, & Zackai, 2001; Wilson et al., 1994).

In 1955, velofacial hypoplasia (Sedlackova syndrome) was first described by Sedlackova, a Czech phoniatrician, in a group of 26 children with congenital short soft palate, hypernasal speech, facial and ear dysmorphism, and muscle fiber differences (Sedlackova, 1955, 1967). (See Figure 5.22 for photos from one of the original cases diagnosed by Sedlackova.) In 1978, Shprintzen et al. reported a similar syndrome of typical facies, including a prominent nose and retruded mandible, cardiovascular

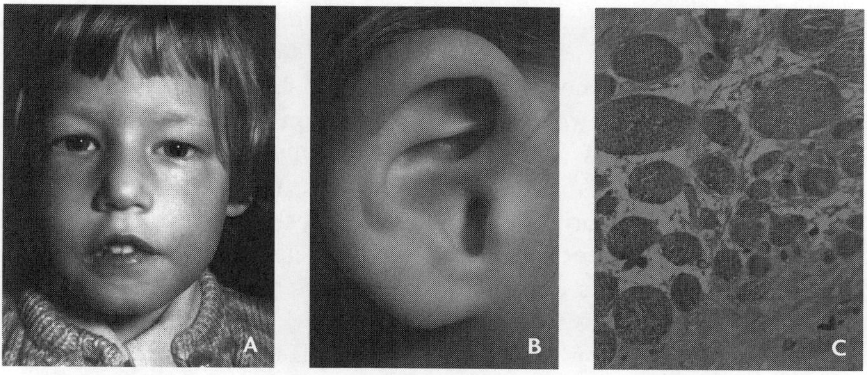


Figure 5.22. Photos from a female with velofacial hypoplasia, as described by Sedlackova in 1955, later found to overlap with the phenotype of velocardiofacial syndrome, as described by Shprintzen et al. in 1978. (A) Apparent facial hypotonia with reduced affect, narrow or "hooded" palpebral fissures, downturned upper lip, indistinct philtrum, and narrow nostrils with bulbous nasal tip. (B) Slight ear dysmorphism, including overfolded helix, simplistic ear architecture, and narrow external auditory canal. (C) Histologic slide of the levator veli palatine muscle, revealing marked variability in the diameter of the muscular fibers. *Note.* Courtesy of K. Vrticka, Zurich, Switzerland.

anomalies, cleft palate, and learning disabilities, later named "velocardiofacial syndrome." It now appears that both of these phenotypes share a common underlying genomic disorder. With advancements in genetic technology, researchers learned that approximately 85%–90% of cases of VCFS were caused by a genetic mutation on the long arm (the "q" arm) of chromosome 22; therefore, VCFS is also known as the 22q11.2 deletion syndrome (Driscoll et al., 1992; Scambler et al., 1992).

Currently, the diagnosis of VCFS is based on clinical and/or genetic presentation, since perhaps as many as 20% of cases do not have a detected deletion at 22q11.2 (Carlson et al., 1997; Gorlin et al., 2001). It is unknown whether these cases are also VCFS with deleted genetic material that has gone undetected (e.g., point mutations) or whether an entirely separate clinical entity exists (e.g., 10p deletion) (Gorlin et al., 2001; Lipson et al., 1991). In the past decade, the list of identified clinical features of individuals with VCFS has continued to grow. Thus, the extreme variability in expression of this syndrome is of key interest to researchers.

Inheritance of the 22q11.2 deletion is autosomal dominant with incomplete penetrance and variable expressivity (Devriendt et al., 1998; Gorlin et al., 2001; Shprintzen et al., 1981). In the majority of cases (approximately 85%), 22q11.2 deletions are de novo; therefore, only a small proportion of identified cases have been inherited through parental transmission (Carlson et al., 1997). Oskarsdottir, Persson, Eriksson, and Fasth (2005) reported on a cohort of 100 patients with 22q11.2 deletion presenting with a positively skewed, bimodal distribution of age at diagnosis. The median age at diagnosis was 6.5 years, with 26% diagnosed in infancy (92% of whom had a cardiac defect). However, of those diagnosed after 2 years of age, the majority presented with speech-language impairment (regardless of the presence of cleft palate), developmental delay, and recurrent infections, thus demonstrating the risk for diagnostic delay in some patients with this syndrome.

The 22q11.2 deletion is detected by specialized immunocytochemistry testing known as fluorescent in situ hybridization (FISH) analysis, in which the missing genetic material is highlighted for identification. It is widely recognized that there is both a phenotypic and genotypic overlap between VCFS and the DiGeorge anomalad, conotruncal anomaly face syndrome, and some cases of Opitz oculogenitolaryngeal syndrome or Opitz BBB/G Compound Syndrome (Gorlin et al., 2001; McDonald-McGinn et al., 1995). These genetic disorders have all been associated with the 22q11 deletion, but there is a predominant overlap of the hemizygous microdeletion shared with VCFS and the DiGeorge anomalad, which includes hypocalcemia, hypoparathyroidism, immune deficiency, and cardiac defects (DiGeorge, 1965; Driscoll et al., 1992; Gorlin et al., 2001; Taitz, Zarate-Salvador, & Schwartz, 1966). Many patients with 22q11.2 deletion are referred to as having DiGeorge syndrome when the phenotype may be virtually identical to those patients whom we refer to as having velocardiofacial syndrome; the initial diagnosis depends on the presenting features of the disorder when it is first suspected or diagnosed. For example, children identified through an immunology clinic or cardiology clinic may be more likely to be labeled as having DiGeorge syndrome, whereas those encountered in a cleft palate clinic or psychiatric clinic are more typically labeled as having velocardiofacial syndrome. Regardless, some have suggested the common use of the term *22q11.2 deletion syndrome* to avoid potential confusion and misnomers.

Currently, there are over 180 identified clinical features of VCFS (Shprintzen, 1997). Over 90% of cases present with speech and language disorders, velopharyngeal inadequacy (VPI) or cleft palate, learning disabilities, and/or mental retardation (Golding-Kushner et al., 1985; Gorlin et al., 2001; Niklasson, Rasmussen, Oskarsdottir, & Gillberg, 2001; Shprintzen et al., 1978; Solot et al., 2000; Swillen et al., 1997). Other frequent clinical findings include multiple cardiac defects and vascular anomalies in over 80% of cases, including ventricular septal defects (65%), Tetrology of Fallot (20%), right-sided or interrupted aortic arch (35%), and aberrant left subclavian (20%) and medial displacement and tortuosity of the internal carotid arteries (D'Antonio & Marsh, 1987; Hultman et al., 2000; Mackenzie-Stepner, Witzel, & Stringer, 1987; McDonald-McGinn, 2004; Mitnick, Bello, Golding-Kushner, Argamaso, & Shprintzen, 1996; Shprintzen, 2000; Tatum, Chang, Havkin, & Shprintzen, 2002; Young, 1980). Chiari malformation and cervical spine anomalies are also observed (Hultman et al., 2000). Upper respiratory illnesses in infancy are frequent, and about 25% of babies fail to thrive. Obstructive sleep apnea is noted in approximately 50%, and at least one third have short stature. About 15% of patients with Robin sequence have been found to have VCFS (Gorlin et al., 2001).

Typical craniofacial features of individuals with VCFS include microcephaly (40%), with long face and vertical maxillary excess, malar flatness, and mandibular retrusion. Prominent nose with a squared nasal root, bulbous nasal tip, and hypoplastic nasal alae are also consistent. Thirty-five percent have narrow palpebral fissures with "allergic shiners" (blue suborbital coloring) and tortuous retinal vessels. Also reported are long philtrum and thin upper lip, reduced facial affect, and frequent findings of minor ear anomalies, such as small pinnae (R. Goldberg et al., 1993; Gorlin et al., 2001; Shprintzen et al., 1978). The children depicted in Figures 5.21 and 5.22 demonstrate the consistent facial appearance in VCFS. For some patients, the facial features of VCFS become more noticeable with age (see Figure 5.23). Most studies report facial findings in Caucasian patients. McDonald-McGinn, Minugh-Purvis, et al. (2005) reported underrepresentation of African American patients in their large cohort with 22q11.2 deletion, possibly due to variations in facial features across different ethnic backgrounds. Craniosynostosis has also been found to be associated with 22q11.2 deletion (McDonald-McGinn, Gripp, et al., 2005).

Endocrine, immune, and renal abnormalities are also frequently identified in patients with 22q11.2 deletion (B. S. Emanuel et al., 2001; McDonald-McGinn, 2004; Shprintzen, 1997, 2000), as well as hypotonia (Solot et al., 2000; Swillen, Vogels, Devriendt, & Fryns, 2000; Wang, Woodin, Kreps-Falk, & Moss, 2000). Hypocalcemia of infancy and absent or small thymus (as part of the DiGeorge anomalad) have been found. The fingers appear slender and are often hyperextensible. Audiological findings include sensorineural hearing loss (15%) and conductive hearing impairment (45%), which is usually mild in severity and usually due

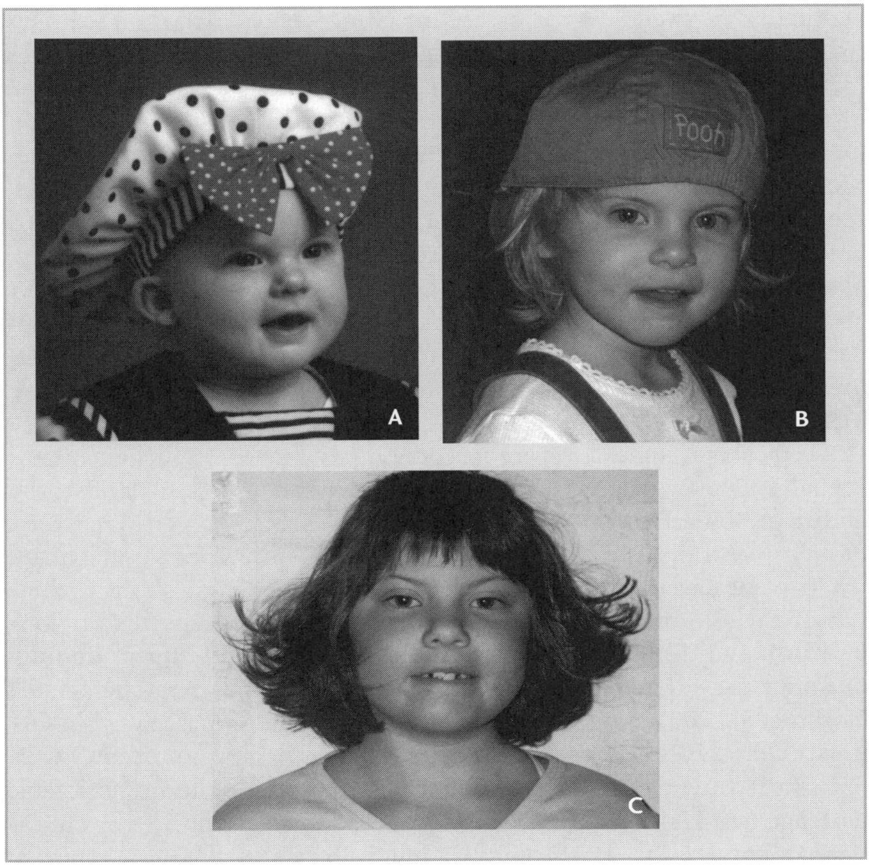


FIGURE 5.23. Photos of a female with 22q11.2 deletion (velocardiofacial syndrome) at ages (A) 1 year, (B) 2½ years, and (C) 8 years.

to frequent bouts of otitis, although significant inner ear anomalies have also been reported (Digilio et al., 1999).

Several studies of VCFS have emphasized the expanding psychiatric and behavioral phenotype, yielding frequent diagnoses of attention-deficit/hyperactivity disorder, obsessive-compulsive disorder, autism spectrum disorders, and even schizophrenia (Bearden et al., 2004; R. Goldberg et al., 1993; Niklasson et al., 2001; Papolos et al., 1996; Shprintzen, 2000; Swillen et al., 2000). Research continues to support previous studies that discovered that aside from having a monozygotic twin with schizophrenia, having the 22q11.2 deletion is the highest known risk factor for the development of the psychiatric illness, with approximately 25 times the risk of that of the general population (Van Amelsvoort et al., 2004). Children with VCFS are at risk for a variety of neurodevelopmental deficits and demonstrate considerable cognitive-behavioral overlap with other children at high risk for development of schizophrenia.

With advancements in functional and structural brain imaging capabilities, neurologic differences have also been identified. Eliez et al. (2001) and Simon et al. (2005) reported lower whole-brain total volume, including less gray and white matter, in children with VCFS compared with age- and gender-matched controls. The temporal lobe, parietal lobe, cerebellum, and hippocampus have all been found to be reduced in size in individuals with VCFS (Eliez et al., 2001; Eliez, Schmitt, White, & Reiss, 2001; Kates et al., 2001; Van Amelsvoort et al., 2004; Van Amelsvoort et al., 2001). Eliez et al. (2000) and Simon et al. (2005) also found that frontal lobe tissue tends to be enlarged relative to the overall reduction in brain volume. Children with 22q11.2 deletions have also been shown to have reduced size of the thalamus, as well as increased size of the caudate head of the basal ganglia (Bish, Nguyen, Ding, Ferrante, & Simon, 2004). Two studies investigating white matter differences using diffusion tensor imaging found reduced fractional anisotrophy in the frontal, parietal, and temporal regions and support for hypotheses regarding dysfunctional neural circuitry in VCFS (Barnea-Goraly et al., 2003; Simon et al., 2005). Finally, researchers are also beginning to investigate the syndrome-specific finding of a posteriorly displaced corpus callosum in persons with 22q11.2 deletion.

Learning disabilities and other language and cognitive impairments are among the most commonly identified characteristics of VCFS, with a prevalence rate as high as 99% (Glaser et al., 2002; R. Goldberg et al., 1993; Goorhuis-Brower, Dikkers, Robinson, & Kerstjens-Frederikse, 2003; Niklasson et al., 2001; Swillen et al., 1997). Studies have repeatedly found higher verbal than nonverbal IQ scores (McDonald-McGinn, 2004; Woodin et al., 2001); however, language impairment is also common (Glaser et al., 2002; Goorhuis-Brower et al., 2003; Solot et al., 2000). To some degree, verbal skills may be a relative strength of children with VCFS, with deficits more consistently shown in attention, visuospatial skills, and psychosocial functioning. There is more variability and disagreement regarding the cognitive-behavioral features of this syndrome than most of the other clinical characteristics. This has led to emerging research in this area, as well as increased debate as to how to counsel families regarding psychiatric risk and how to determine the type and timing of intervention approaches and educational services.

In addition to speech difficulties, many children present with feeding and swallowing problems before communicative impairments are identified. Dysphagia is typically due to pharyngeal hypotonia, upper airway obstruction, VPI, and esophageal dysmotility; however, serious gastrointestinal malformations have also been reported (Rommel et al., 1999; Shprintzen, 1997; Solot et al., 2000). Prolonged feedings, nasal regurgitation, and gastroesophageal reflux are reported as the most frequent problems, along with poor suck (difficulty creating positive intraoral pressure) and disorganized suck-swallow-breathe coordination (Eicher et al., 2000). However, few studies have examined these patterns in detail. Eicher et al. (2000) suggested that the degree and persistence of feeding dysfunction affecting these children exceeded that for other children with palatal or cardiac anomalies. Seventy percent demonstrated velopharyngeal inadequacy for swallowing with nasopharyngeal reflux observed.

VCFS may first be suspected and/or identified as part of an interdisciplinary evaluation by a cleft palate-craniofacial team, given the high incidence of cleft palate and velopharyngeal inadequacy. Studies cite a high incidence of cleft palate and submucous clefting, pharyngeal hypotonia, lymphoid (including adenoid) hypoplasia, and obtuse cranial base or deep retropharynx (termed "palatopharyngeal disproportion"), all of which can compromise velopharyngeal adequacy for speech (Arvystas & Shprintzen, 1984; R. Goldberg et al., 1993; Shprintzen, 1982; Solot et al., 2000). In addition to a short velum, palatal weakness, and reduced palatal and lateral pharyngeal wall movement, adenoidectomy surgery may also aggravate structural VPI in VCFS patients (Arvystas & Shprintzen, 1984; Croft, Shprintzen, Daniller, & Lewin, 1978; Finkelstein et al., 1993; Glander & Cisneros, 1992; Shprintzen et al., 1981; Witzel, Rich, Margar-Bacal, & Cox, 1986). Clefting in this population can include overt cleft palate, submucous cleft palate, and occult submucous cleft palate, while a few cases of cleft lip and palate have been identified (Gorlin et al., 2001; Lipson et al., 1991; Shprintzen et al., 1978). It is possible that more cases of VCFS with clefting of the primary palate exist but that a phenotypic bias has limited the identification of VCFS in this group. Unilateral palatal paresis has also been reported by Weik, Carneol, Marks, Denny, and Beste (1993) and by Hultman et al. (2000). Regardless of the identified (or unidentified) cause, VPI and hypernasal speech are among the most consistent findings in the speech of individuals with VCFS (Carneol, Marks, &

Weik, 1999; Goldberg et al., 1993; Gorlin et al., 2001; Persson, Lohmander, Jonsson, Oskarsdottir, & Soderpalm, 2003; Shprintzen et al., 1978).

## Speech-Language Issues in VCFS

Speech and language impairments are among the most commonly manifested symptoms of VCFS. The speech characteristics of children with VCFS were first described by Shprintzen et al. (1978), followed by a description of language impairments by Golding-Kushner et al. (1985). In addition to early signs of velopharyngeal inadequacy, generalized speech-language delays are commonly reported, with most children being nonverbal at age 2 years (Golding-Kushner, 2005; McDonald-McGinn et al., 1997; Scherer, D'Antonio, & Kalbfleisch, 1999; Shprintzen et al., 1978; Solot et al., 2000). Children may demonstrate hypernasality, articulation or phonological disorders, dysarthria and/or apraxia of speech, and high-pitched voice (Carneol et al., 1999; D'Antonio, Scherer, Miller, Kalbfleisch, & Bartley, 2001; Hultman et al., 2000; Persson et al., 2003; Scherer et al., 1999). Flat affect, reduced emotional expression, fast rate, and monotone speech are also observed in many children with VCFS, although no formal studies of voice or prosodic features have been done on children with VCFS at this point in time.

Several authors have found a high frequency of language impairment and delayed language development in children with VCFS (Carneol et al., 1999; Golding-Kushner et al., 1985; Scherer et al., 1999; Scherer, D'Antonio, & Rodger, 2001; Woodin et al., 2001). Similar to children with nonsyndromic cleft lip and/or palate, submucous cleft palate, and isolated velopharyngeal inadequacy, children with VCFS (regardless of the presence of clefting) have been found to exhibit delays in speech sound development. Younger children have been shown to exhibit glottal stop substitutions, which are the most common compensatory error in the speech of children with isolated cleft lip and palate or isolated cleft palate (D'Antonio, Scherer, et al., 2001; Golding-Kushner, 2005; Scherer et al., 1999; Trost-Cardamone, 1990); however, the articulation skills of children with VCFS have been shown to be poorer than those of children with nonsyndromic cleft palate or isolated velopharyngeal inadequacy (Baylis, Munson, & Moller, 2007; DeMarco, Moller, & Glaze, 2003) and of those children matched for cognitive deficits (Scherer et al., 2001).

Scherer et al. (1999) found that children with VCFS show limitations in speech sound inventory and early vocabulary development that are more severe than those of children with isolated cleft palate or cleft lip and palate. They also reported that the speech of children with VCFS contains an unusually high occurrence of glottal stop substitutions, compared to children with isolated clefting, regardless of the severity of VPI. This finding was confirmed by D'Antonio, Scherer, et al. (2001). Furthermore, Scherer et al. (1999) found that approximately 50% of the children with cleft lip and palate or isolated cleft palate demonstrated some mild to moderate symptoms of velopharyngeal inadequacy, whereas all the children in the VCFS group were perceived as having some hypernasality and/or nasal air emission. There was no apparent relationship between the age at palate repair and the number of consonant types, the PCC-R (*Percentage of Consonants Correct–Revised;* Shriberg, Aram, & Kwiatkowski, 1997) rating, or the percentage of glottal stop substitutions for the children in their sample. The authors also found no apparent relationship between the presence or severity of velopharyngeal inadequacy symptoms and the number of consonant types or PCC-R ratings. In a later study, Scherer et al. (2001) compared the speech and language skills of a small group of children with VCFS to language-matched peers with Down syndrome. Compared with the children with Down syndrome, the children with VCFS demonstrated poorer articulation and expressive language skills, disproportionately poorer than what their mental age predicted. Overall, structural factors related to velopharyngeal closure and severity of VPI alone do not explain why such differences in articulation and resonance characteristics exist between these groups of children. Baylis et al. (2006) found evidence that speech sound production deficits in VCFS are highly correlated with nonverbal intelligence skills, suggesting that a broader cognitive-linguistic deficit interacts with phonetic skills.

In addition to articulatory difficulties, hypernasal resonance distortion is a commonly reported speech finding in children with VCFS. Persons with VCFS tend to have hypernasal resonance of greater persistence, frequency, and severity than seen in other cleft and VPI populations (Baylis, Watson, & Moller, 2006; D'Antonio, Davio, Zoller, Punjabi, & Hardesty, 2001; D'Antonio, Scherer, et al., 2001; DeMarco et al., 2003; Kirschner et al., 2005; Persson et al., 2003). Rommel et al. (1999) and Nayak and Sell (1998) reported a frequency of hypernasality in the VCFS population ranging from 64% to 84%, depending on possible ascertainment biases related to each study. Persson et al. (2003) used an unselected, blinded consecutive series of 65 patients with a diagnosed 22q11.2 deletion for their study sample. They found that 32 of 65 patients had a "palatal anomaly," with 87% demonstrating "primary VPI" to some degree, and 55% with VPI warranting physical management.

In addition to these etiologic factors, differences in treatment history may also account for the difference in severity of velopharyngeal inadequacy in the VCFS population. The average age of diagnosis of VCFS (particularly when there are no cardiac anomalies identified) and subsequent diagnosis of velopharyngeal dysfunction is often years later than that of the diagnosis of VPI for children born with overt clefts. Hence, treatment could be considered "delayed" in the majority of the VCFS group compared to cleft populations, which may explain the increased severity of articulation disorders and VPI. It is possible that the delayed treatment in VCFS patients "misses" the critical period for motor learning and plasticity for velopharyngeal motor control during speech. It is unknown if earlier intervention would facilitate an improved prognosis for achieving adequate velopharyngeal closure for speech, and if it could eliminate the use of compensatory articulation productions in young VCFS patients. In addition, it is possible that earlier intervention directed at oral speech production may facilitate improved motor control and programming of velopharyngeal movements for speech.

Multiple obstacles to achieving adequate velopharyngeal closure for speech are encountered in this population, including a large velopharyngeal gap, hypoplastic muscles, hypotonia, and inadequate muscle movement during speech production. In a study by D'Antonio, Davio, et al. (2001), all patients with VCFS failed to achieve complete elimination of symptoms of VPI following a Furlow Z-plasty palatal lengthening procedure and required further secondary palatal management. However, there continues to be adamant disagreement among surgeons who advocate for a sphincter pharyngoplasty (Mehendale, Birch, Birkett, Sell, & Sommerlad, 2002; Witt, Cohen, Grames, & Marsh, 1999; Witt, Miller, Marsh, & Grames, 1997) versus a wide superiorly based pharyngeal flap (Kirschner et al., 2005; Tatum, 2002) in VCFS patients. (The reader is referred to Chapter 14 by Buckley and Landis for more detailed information about these procedures.) Overall, reports of surgical outcomes in this population point to a consistent failure to eliminate velopharyngeal inadequacy, which suggests that there is an underlying pathophysiology that differs from nonsyndromic or non-VCFS syndromic comparison groups (D'Antonio, Davio, et al., 2001).

Regardless of which surgical procedure is chosen, children with VCFS require preoperative magnetic resonance angiography to map out the course of the internal carotid arteries, which are sometimes medially displaced in this population and may heighten surgical risk (D'Antonio & Marsh, 1987; Hultman et al., 2000; Mackenzie-Stepner et al., 1987;

Mitnick et al., 1996; Tatum et al., 2002). Tatum (2002) and Kirschner et al. (2005) support the use of pharyngeal flaps in the VCFS population but also caution that, although speech will mostly likely improve postoperatively, VPI may still persist to some degree. Children with VCFS often have minimal movement of the lateral pharyngeal walls, which typically co-occurs with hypoplastic muscles, thus resulting in a hypodynamic or even adynamic velopharyngeal mechanism with a large velopharyngeal gap, complicated by an obtuse cranial base and atrophic adenoids.

Currently, there are no published reports regarding the use of speech prostheses for management of VPI in this population, although historically they are a viable and appropriate treatment option for selected patients. The less than ideal surgical outcomes for improved velopharyngeal closure in children with VCFS leave clinicians and surgeons with suspicion of neuromuscular abnormalities in this population. Surgical results (e.g., pharyngeal flap, sphincter pharyngoplasty) continue to be unacceptable when compared to nonsyndromic peers with cleft palate or VPI, and are more similar to the spectrum of populations with a history of muscle disorders (e.g., cerebral palsy, myotonic dystrophy) or neurologic insult (e.g., brain tumor, traumatic brain injury). VCFS patients are more likely to evidence VPI postsurgically and may have better treatment outcomes with a prosthetic approach or with novel behavioral speech treatment techniques in combination with surgical management.

Prosthetic options need to be explored in patients with VCFS, especially because of evidence of neuromuscular complications in this syndrome. It is possible that prosthetics will be effective as a temporary solution to improving velopharyngeal competence and enhancing therapy progress. In addition, if prostheses are used presurgically and can help to increase velopharyngeal movement, this may improve surgical outcomes. Lastly, for some patients whose medical complications are severe or placement of the internal carotid artery is anomalous and places them at great surgical risk, prostheses may be the only option and must be offered to families.

Researchers, clinicians, and surgeons continue to be puzzled by the following question: Why do children with VCFS have more pronounced and persistent velopharyngeal inadequacy and hypernasality than children with isolated clefts and VPI? In addition to structural defects, such as clefting, the following factors may contribute to the speech profile in VCFS: hypoplasia and hypotonia of the levator veli palatini and pharyngeal constrictor muscles, platybasia resulting in a deep pharynx, and pharyngeal asymmetry. Kuehn (2003) used magnetic resonance imaging

(MRI) to show that in patients with VCFS, the levator veli palatini muscle is in a more anterior position than in normal children. In addition to this evidence suggesting factors related to configuration and size of velopharyngeal structures, more recent evidence has begun to explore the possibility of neuromuscular problems in the velopharynx (Zim et al., 2003) and velopharyngeal closure timing differences (Baylis, Watson, & Moller, 2006).

After years of repeated claims of pharyngeal hypotonia, Zim et al. (2003) provided evidence for the existence of muscular abnormalities in the velopharynx in VCFS. In their MRI and histologic study of 26 patients with VCFS (ages 3–29 years), they found that the superior pharyngeal constrictor muscle is significantly less thick than in patients without VCFS. The superior pharyngeal constrictor muscle in VCFS contained a significantly greater proportion of Type 1 muscle fibers, smaller diameter of fibers, and increased endomesial space between fibers (suggesting that fibers were atrophied or more loosely packed). This evidence supported the claims of pharyngeal hypotonia that could be rooted either in an inherent muscle abnormality or in neurologic abnormalities that provided reduced neural input to these muscle fibers. Discerning the nature of the muscle abnormalities is important in leading professionals toward the design of improved speech treatment and surgical procedures for VPI in this population.

The brain differences previously discussed in this chapter lend support to a hypothesis of altered neural input to the muscular structures in individuals with VCFS. Cerebellar hypoplasia and atrophy, midline anomalies including agenesis of the corpus callosum, ventricular enlargement, and volumetric and morphologic changes in the thalamus, basal ganglia, and frontal and temporal parietal lobes may be related to the speech impairments seen in this syndrome (Bish et al., 2004; Eliez et al., 2001; Eliez et al., 2000; Simon et al., 2005; Swillen et al., 2000). Hultman et al. (2000) have also found significant evidence of neurologic deficits and cranial nerve abnormalities in VCFS. Given the mounting evidence of abnormal neural structures and subsequent neurologic functioning, there is a strong possibility that the speech disorders in VCFS are more neurologically based than purely determined by velopharyngeal structural hazards.

In conclusion, professionals are just beginning to understand the complex nature of the significant speech-language impairments in VCFS. All speech studies up to this point have been descriptive and cross-sectional in nature and often lack hypothesis-driven methods. Many studies lack control groups entirely. Those that do include a comparison group have matched for age and gender, and only one study has matched for language-comprehension age (Scherer et al., 2001). It is critical that future studies use control groups that are matched for IQ and socio-economic status, and possibly other family-related factors such as parent education level or language skills.

Speech-language pathologists and other interdisciplinary team members play a key role in the diagnosis and treatment of children with VCFS. Speech clinicians are often the first to encounter these children (particularly those without the cardiac defects) because speech-language delays are one of the earliest identified hallmarks of this syndrome. In addition, speech-language pathologists are involved in the treatment of the myriad communicative difficulties encountered by these children from infancy into adulthood. The profession's diagnostic sensitivity to VCFS has continued to grow, especially as speech-language pathologists learn more about the speech-language and neuropsychological characteristics of this disorder; however, treatment strategies continue to play catch-up with diagnostic skills. Clinical observations suggest some efficacy of behavioral speech therapy approaches that are typically used with other children with cleft palate or VPI but are modified as needed to take into account the hearing, attention, learning, and psychosocial difficulties present in the VCFS population.

## References

Altemus, L. A. (1966). The incidence of cleft lip and cleft palate among North American Negroes. *Cleft Palate Journal, 3,* 357–361.

Arvystas, M., & Shprintzen, R. J. (1984). Craniofacial morphology in the velocardiofacial syndrome. *Journal of Craniofacial Genetics and Developmental Biology, 4,* 39–45.

Arvystas, M., & Shprintzen, R. J. (1991). Craniofacial morphology in Treacher Collins syndrome. *Cleft Palate-Craniofacial Journal, 28,* 226–230.

Barnea-Goraly, N., Menon, V., Krasnow, B., Ko, A., Reiss, A., & Eliez, S. (2003). Investigation of white matter structure in velocardiofacial syndrome: A diffusion tensor imaging study. *American Journal of Psychiatry, 160,* 1863–1869.

Baylis, A. L., Munson, B., & Moller, K. T. (in press). Factors affecting articulation skills in children with velocardiofacial syndrome and children with cleft palate or velopharyngeal dysfunction: A preliminary report. *The Cleft Palate-Craniofacial Journal.*

Baylis, A. L., Watson, P. J., & Moller, K. T. (2006, April). *Aeromechanical and auditory-perceptual speech characteristics of children with 22q11.2 deletion and children with cleft palate.* Paper presentation at the annual meeting of the American Cleft Palate-Craniofacial Association, Vancouver, BC.

Bear, J. C. (1976). A genetic study of facial clefting in northern England. *Clinical Genetics, 9,* 277–284.

Bearden, C. E., Jawad, A. F., Lynch, D. R., Sokol, S., Kanes, S. J., McDonald-McGinn, D. M., et al. (2004). Effects of a functional COMT polymorphism on prefrontal cognitive function in patients with 22q11.2 deletion syndrome. *American Journal of Psychiatry 161,* 1700–1702.

Benjamin, B., & Walker, P. (1991). Management of airway obstruction in the Pierre Robin sequence. *International Journal of Pediatric Otorhinolaryngology, 22,* 29–37.

Bish, J. P., Nguyen, V., Ding, L., Ferrante, S., & Simon, T. J. (2004). Thalamic reductions in children with chromosome 22q11.2 deletion syndrome. *Developmental Neuroscience (Neuroreport), 15,* 1413–1415.

Blair, N. P., Albert, D. M., Liberfarb, R. M., & Hirose, T. (1979). Hereditary progressive arthro-ophthalmopathy of Stickler. *American Journal of Ophthalmology, 88,* 876–888.

Blake, G. B., & Wreakes, G. (1972). Clefts of the lip and palate in twins. *British Journal of Plastic Surgery, 25,* 155–164.

Bonaiti, C., Briard, M. L., Feingold, J., Pavy, B., Psaume, J., Migne-Tufferand, G., et al. (1982). An epidemiological and genetic study of facial clefting in France: I. Epidemiology and frequency in relatives. *Journal of Medical Genetics, 19,* 8–15.

Bonaiti-Pellie, C., & Smith, C. (1974). Risk tables for genetic counseling in some common congenital malformations. *Journal of Medical Genetics, 11,* 374–377.

Buchanan, R. C. (1968). Acrocephalosyndactyly or Apert's syndrome. *British Journal of Plastic Surgery, 21,* 406–418.

Caldarelli, D., Hutchinson, J., Pruzansky, S., & Valvassori, G. (1980). A comparison of microtia and temporal bone anomalies in hemifacial microsomia and mandibulofacial dysostosis. *Cleft Palate Journal, 17,* 103–110.

Carlson, C., Sirotkin, H., Pandita, R. K., et al. (1997). Molecular definition of 22q11 deletions in 151 velo-cardio-facial syndrome patients. *American Journal of Human Genetics, 61,* 620–629.

Carneol, S. O., Marks, S. M., & Weik, L. (1999). The speech-language pathologist: Key role in the diagnosis of velocardiofacial syndrome. *American Journal of Speech-Language Pathology, 8,* 23–32.

Centers for Disease Control and Prevention. (2006, January 6). Improved national prevalence estimates for 18 selected major birth defects: United States 1999–2001. *Morbidity and Mortality Weekly Report, 54*(51/52), 1301–1305.

Cervenka, J., & Shapiro, B. (1970). Cleft uvula in Chippewa Indians: Prevalence and genetics. *Human Biology, 42*(1), 47–52.

Chosack, A., & Eidelman, E. (1978). Cleft uvula: Prevalence and genetics. *Cleft Palate Journal, 15,* 63–67.

Chung, C. S., Bixler, D., Watanabe, T., Koguchi, H., & Fogh-Andersen, P. (1986). Segregation analysis of cleft lip with or without cleft palate: A comparison of Danish and Japanese data. *American Journal of Human Genetics, 39,* 603–611.

Cinalli, G. (1995). Chronic tonsillar herniation in Crouzon and Apert syndromes: The role of premature synostosis of the lambdoid suture. *Journal of Neurosurgery, 83,* 575–582.

Cleft Palate Foundation. (1999). *Factsheet: Information about Pierre Robin sequence/complex.* Chapel Hill, NC: Author.

Cohen, M. M., Jr. (1976). The Robin anomaly—Its nonspecificity in associated syndromes. *Journal of Oral Surgery, 34,* 587–593.

Cohen, M. M., Jr. (1978). Syndromes with cleft lip and palate. *Cleft Palate Journal, 15,* 306–328.

Cohen, M. M., Jr. (1999). Robin sequence and complexes. *American Journal of Medical Genetics, 84,* 311–315.

Cohen, M. M., Jr., & Kreiborg, S. (1992). Birth prevalence studies of the Crouzon syndrome: Comparison of direct and indirect methods. *Clinical Genetics, 41,* 12–15.

Cohen, M. M., Jr., & Kreiborg, S. (1996). A clinical study of the craniofacial features in Apert syndrome. *International Journal of Oral and Maxillofacial Surgery, 25,* 45–53.

Colmenero, C., Esteban, R., Albarino, A. R., & Colmenero, B. (1991). Sleep apnea syndrome associated with maxillofacial abnormalities. *Journal of Laryngology and Otology, 105,* 94–100.

Croft, C. B., Shprintzen, R. J., Daniller, A., & Lewin, M. L. (1978). The occult submucous cleft palate and the musculus uvulae. *Cleft Palate Journal, 15,* 150–154.

Crouzon, O. (1912). Dysostose cranio-faciale héréditaire. *Bulletin de la Société des Médecins des Hôpitaux de Paris, 33,* 545–555.

D'Antonio, L. L., Davio, M., Zoller, K., Punjabi, A., & Hardesty, R. A. (2001). Results of Furlow z-plasty in patients with velocardiofacial syndrome. *Plastic and Reconstructive Surgery, 107,* 1077–1079.

D'Antonio, L. L., & Marsh, J. L. (1987). Abnormal carotid arteries in the velocardiofacial syndrome. *Plastic and Reconstructive Surgery, 80,* 471–472.

D'Antonio, L. L., Rice, R. D., & Fink, S. C. (1998). Evaluation of pharyngeal and laryngeal structure and function in patients with oculo-auriculo-vertebral spectrum. *Cleft Palate-Craniofacial Journal, 35,* 333–341.

D'Antonio, L. L., Scherer, N. J., Miller, L. L., Kalbfleisch, J. H., & Bartley, J. A. (2001). Analysis of speech characteristics in children with CCFS and children with phenotypic overlap without VCFS. *Cleft Palate-Craniofacial Journal, 39,* 455–467.

DeMarco, A. L., Moller, K. T., & Glaze, L. E. (2003). *Speech production skills in children with velocardiofacial syndrome and children with isolated cleft palate and/or VPI.* Unpublished manuscript, University of Minnesota, Minneapolis.

Devriendt, K., Fryns, J. P., & Mortier, G. (1998). The annual incidence of DiGeorge/velocardiofacial syndrome. *Journal of Medical Genetics, 35,* 789–790.

DiGeorge, A. M. (1965). Discussion on a new concept of the cellular basis of immunology. *Journal of Pediatrics, 67,* 907.

Digilio, M. C., Pacifico, C., Tieri, L., Marino, B., Giannotti, A., & Dallapiccola, B. (1999). Audiological findings in patients with microdeletion 22q11.2 (diGeorge/velocardiofacial syndrome). *British Journal of Audiology, 33,* 329–334.

Driscoll, D. A., Spinner, N. B., Budarf, M. L., McDonald-McGinn, D. M., Zackai, E. H., Goldberg, R. B., et al. (1992). Deletions and microdeletions of 22q11.2 in velocardiofacial syndrome. *American Journal of Medical Genetics, 44,* 261–268.

Eicher, P. S., McDonald-McGinn, D. M., Fox, C. A., Driscoll, D. A., Emanuel, B. S., & Zackai, E. H. (2000). Dysphagia in children with a 22q11.2 deletion: Unusual pattern found on modified barium swallow. *Journal of Pediatrics, 137,* 158–164.

Eliez, S., Blasey, C. M., Schmitt, E. J., White, C. D., Hu, D., & Reiss, A. L. (2001). Velocardiofacial syndrome: Are structural changes in the temporal and mesial temporal regions related to schizophrenia? *American Journal of Psychiatry, 158,* 447–453.

Eliez, S., Schmitt, E., White, C., & Reiss, A. (2000). Children and adolescents with velocardiofacial syndrome: A volumetric MRI study. *American Journal of Psychiatry, 157,* 409–415.

Emanuel, B. S., McDonald-McGinn, D. M., Saitta, C., & Zackai, E. H. (2001). The 22q11.2 deletion syndrome. *Advances in Pediatrics, 48,* 39–73.

Emanuel, I., Huang, S-W., Gutman, L. T., Yu, F. C., & Lin, C. C. (1972). The incidence of congenital malformations in a Chinese population: The Taipei collaborative study. *Teratology, 5,* 159–170.

Fazen, L. E., Elmore, J., & Nadler, H. L. (1967). Mandibulofacial dysostosis. *American Journal of Diseases of Children, 113,* 405–410.

Figueroa, A. A. (1991). Commentary on craniofacial morphology in Treacher Collins syndrome. *Cleft Palate-Craniofacial Journal, 18,* 230–231.

Finkelstein, Y., Zohar, Y., Nachmani, A., Talmi, Y. P., Lerner, M., Hauben, D. J., et al. (1993). The otolaryngologist and the patient with velocardiofacial syndrome. *Archives of Otolaryngology-Head and Neck Surgery, 119,* 563–569.

Fogh-Andersen, P. (1942). *Inheritance of hairlip and cleft palate.* Copenhagen: A. Busck.

Franceschetti, A., & Klein, D. (1949). Mandibulo-facial dysostosis: A new hereditary syndrome. *Acta Ophthalmology, 24,* 143–224.

Fraser, F. C. (1974). Updating the genetics of cleft lip and palate. *Birth Defects, 10,* 107–111.

Glander, K., & Cisneros, G. J. (1992). Comparison of the craniofacial characteristics of two syndromes associated with Pierre Robin sequence. *Cleft Palate-Craniofacial Journal, 29,* 210–219.

Glaser, B., Mumme, D. L., Blasey, C., Morris, M. A., Dahoun, S. P., Antonarakis, S. E., et al. (2002). Language skills in children with velocardiofacial syndrome (22q11.2del). *Journal of Pediatrics, 140,* 753–758.

Goldberg, J., Enlow, D., Whitaker, L., Zins, J., & Kurihara, S. (1981). Some anatomical characteristics in several craniofacial syndromes. *Journal of Oral Surgery, 39,* 489–498.

Goldberg, R., Motzkin, B., Marion, R., Scampler, R. J., & Shprintzen, R. J. (1993). Velocardiofacial syndrome: A review of 120 patients. *American Journal of Medical Genetics, 45,* 313–319.

Golding-Kushner, K. J. (2005). Speech and language disorders in velocardiofacial syndrome. In K. C. Murphy & P. J. Scambler (Eds.), *Velocardiofacial syndrome: A model for understanding microdeletion disorders* (pp. 181–199). Cambridge, England: Cambridge University Press.

Golding-Kushner, K. J., Weller, G., & Shprintzen, R. J. (1985). Velo-cardio-facial syndrome: Language and psychological profiles. *Journal of Craniofacial Genetics and Developmental Biology, 5,* 259–266.

Goorhuis-Brower, S. M., Dikkers, F. G., Robinson, P. H., & Kerstjens-Frederikse, W. S. (2003). Specific language impairment in children with velocardiofacial syndrome: Four case studies. *Cleft Palate-Craniofacial Journal, 40,* 190–195.

Gorlin, R. J., Cervenka, J., & Pruzansky, S. (1971). Facial clefting and its syndromes. *Birth Defects, 7,* 3–49.

Gorlin, R. J., Cohen, M. M., Jr., & Hennekam, R. (2001). *Syndromes of the head and neck* (4th ed.). New York: Oxford University Press.

Gorlin, R. J., Cohen, M. M., Jr., & Levin, L. S. (1990). *Syndromes of the head and neck* (3rd ed.). New York: Oxford University Press.

Gorlin R. J., & Slavkin, H. C. (1997). Embryology of the face. In V. der Kaloustian & T. Tewfik (Eds.), *Congenital anomalies in otolaryngology.* New York: Oxford University Press.

Guyette, T. W., Polley, J. W., Figueroa, A., Botts, J., & Smith, B. E. (2001). Changes in speech following unilateral mandibular distraction osteogenesis in patients with hemifacial microsomia. *Cleft Palate-Craniofacial Journal, 38,* 179–184.

Hanson, J., & Smith, D. W. (1975). U-shaped palatal defect in the Robin anomaly: Developmental and clinical relevance. *Journal of Pediatrics, 87,* 30–33.

Heckler, R. R., Oesterle, L. G., & Jabaley, M. E. (1979). The minimal cleft revisited: Clinical and anatomic correlations. *Cleft Palate Journal, 16,* 240–247.

Hoppe, W. (1965). Lippen-, Kiefer-, Gaumenspalten. *Archiv für Kinderheikunde, 17*(Suppl. 52), 1–54.

Hultman, C. S., Riski, J. E., Cohen, S. R., Burnstein, F. D., Boydston, W. R., Hudgins, R. J., et al. (2000). Chiari malformation, cervical spine anomalies, and neurologic deficits in velocardiofacial syndrome. *Plastic and Reconstructive Surgery 106,* 16–24.

Jaffe, B. F., & DeBlanc, G. B. (1972, January). Cleft palate, cleft lip and cleft uvula in Navajo Indians. *Cleft Palate Journal, 7,* 301–305.

Johnston, M. C., & Sulik, K. K. (1979). Some abnormal patterns of development in the craniofacial region. *Birth Defects, 15,* 23–42.

Kates, W. R., Burnette, C. P., Jabs, E. W., Rutberg, J., Murphy, A. M., Grados, M., et al. (2001). Regional cortical white matter reductions in velocardiofacial syndrome: A volumetric MRI analysis. *Biological Psychiatry, 49,* 677–684.

Kirschner, R., Solot, C., Ruotolo, R., Catanzaro, J., McDonald-McGinn, D. M., Zackai, E., et al. (2005, April). *Speech outcome after surgical management of velopharyngeal dysfunction in 22q11.2 deletion syndrome.* Paper presented at the meeting of the American Cleft Palate-Craniofacial Association, Myrtle Beach, SC.

Knobloch, W. H., & Layer, J. M. (1972). Clefting syndrome associated with retinal detachment. *American Journal of Ophthalmology, 73,* 517–530.

Kreiborg, S. (1981). Crouzon syndrome. *Scandinavian Journal of Plastic and Reconstructive Surgery* (Suppl. 18), pp. 1–198.

Kreiborg, S., Barr, M., Jr., & Cohen, M. M., Jr. (1992). Cervical spine in the Apert syndrome. *American Journal of Medical Genetics, 43,* 704–708.

Kreiborg, S., & Dahl, E. (1993). Cranial base and face and mandibulofacial dysostosis. *American Journal of Medical Genetics, 47,* 753–760.

Kuehn, D. P. (2003). *MRI investigation of VCFS.* Paper presented at the meeting of the American Cleft Palate-Craniofacial Association, Greenville, SC.

LeBlanc, S. M., & Golding-Kushner, K. J. (1992). Effect of glossopexy on speech sound production in Robin sequence. *Cleft Palate-Craniofacial Journal, 29,* 239–245.

Lehman, J. A., Fishman, J. R., & Neiman, G. S. (1995). Treatment of cleft palate associated with Robin sequence: Appraisal of risk factors. *Cleft Palate-Craniofacial Journal, 32,* 25–29.

Leutert, G., & Heiner, H. (1962). Zur Histologie und Klinik der lateralen Oberlippenfurchen. *Archiv für Klinische Chirurgiae, 299,* 791–792.

Lewkonia, R. M. (1992). The arthropathy of hereditary arthroophthalmopathy (Stickler syndrome). *Journal of Rheumatology, 19,* 1271–1275.

Liberfarb, R. M., & Goldblatt, A. (1986). Prevalence of mitral valve prolapse in the Stickler syndrome. *American Journal of Medical Genetics, 24,* 387–392.

Liberfarb, R. M., Hirose, T., & Holmes, L. B. (1981). The Wagner-Stickler syndrome: A study of 22 families. *Journal of Pediatrics 99,* 394–399.

Lindemann, G., Riis, B., & Sewerin, I. (1977). Prevalence of cleft uvula among 2,732 Danes. *Cleft Palate Journal, 14,* 226–229.

Lipson, A. H., Yuille, D., Angel, M., Thompson, P. G., Vandervoord, J. G., & Beckenham, E. J. (1991). Velocardiofacial (Shprintzen) syndrome: An important syndrome for the dysmorphologist to recognize. *Journal of Medical Genetics, 28,* 596–604.

Lowry, R. B., & Trimble, B .K. (1977). Incidence rates for cleft lip and palate in British Columbia 1952–1971 for North American Indian, Japanese, Chinese and total populations: Secular trends over twenty years. *Teratology, 16,* 277–283.

Lynch, H. T., & Kimberling, W. J. (1981). Genetic counseling in cleft lip and palate. *Plastic and Reconstructive Surgery, 68,* 800–815.

Mackenzie-Stepner, K., Witzel, M. A., & Stringer, D. (1987). Abnormal carotid arteries in velocardiofacial syndrome: A report of three cases. *Plastic and Reconstructive Surgery, 80,* 347–351.

Martin, R. A., Jones, K. L., & Benirschke, K. (1993). Extension of the cleft lip phenotype: The subepithelial cleft. *American Journal of Medical Genetics, 47,* 744–747.

Martinez-Perez, D., Vander Woude, D. L., Barnes, P. D., Scott, R. M., & Mulliken, J. B. (1996). Case report: Jugular foraminal stenosis in Crouzon syndrome. *Pediatric Neurosurgery, 25,* 252–255.

Maumenee, I. H. (1979). Vitreoretinal degeneration as a sign of generalized connective tissue diseases. *American Journal of Ophthalmology, 88,* 432–449.

McDonald-McGinn, D. M. (2004, July). *Much ado about 22q: What's new with chromosome 22?* Paper presented at the 10th Annual International Meeting of the Velocardiofacial Educational Foundation and 4th International Congress for 22q11.2 Deletions, Atlanta, GA.

McDonald-McGinn, D. M., Driscoll, D. A., Bason, L., Christensen, K., Lynch, D., Sullivan, K., et al. (1995). Autosomal dominant "Opitz" GBBB syndrome due to a 22q11.2 deletion. *American Journal of Medical Genetics, 59,* 103–113.

McDonald-McGinn, D. M., Gripp, K. W., Kirschner, R. E., Maisenbacher, M. K., Hustead, V., Schauer, G. M., et al. (2005). Craniosynostosis: Another feature of the 22q11.2 deletion syndrome. *American Journal of Medical Genetics, 136A,* 358–362.

McDonald-McGinn, D. M., LaRossa, D., Goldmuntz, E., Sullivan, K., Eicher, P., Gerdes, M., et al. (1997). The 22q11.2 deletion: Screening, diagnostic workup, and outcome of results; report on 181 patients. *Genetic Testing, 1,* 99–108.

McDonald-McGinn, D. M., Minugh-Purvis, N., Kirschner, R. E., Jawad, A., Tonnesen, M. K., Catanzaro, J. R., et al. (2005). The 22q11.2 deletion in African-American patients: An underdiagnosed population? *American Journal of Medical Genetics, 134A,* 242–246.

Mehendale, F. V., Birch, M. J., Birkett, L., Sell, D., & Sommerlad, B. (2002). *Surgical management of velopharyngeal incompetence in VCFS.* Paper presented at the meeting of the Velocardiofacial Syndrome Educational Foundation, London, England.

Melnick, M., Bixler, D., & Shields, E. D. (Eds.). (1980). *The etiology of cleft lip and cleft palate.* In *Progress in clinical and biological research* (Vol. 46). New York: Alan R. Liss.

Mitchell, L. E., & Christensen, K. (1996). Analysis of the recurrence patterns for nonsyndromic cleft lip with or without cleft palate in the families of 3,073 Danish probands. *American Journal of Medical Genetics, 62,* 371.

Mitchell, L. E., & Risch, N. (1992). Mode of inheritance of nonsyndromic cleft lip with or without cleft palate: A reanalysis. *American Journal of Human Genetics, 5,* 323–332.

Mitnick, R. J., Bello, J. A., Golding-Kushner, K. J., Argamaso, R. V., & Shprintzen, R. J. (1996). The use of magnetic resonance angiography prior to pharyngeal flap surgery in patients with velocardiofacial syndrome. *Plastic and Reconstructive Surgery, 97,* 908–919.

Moller, K. T. (1994). Dental-occlusal and other oral conditions and speech. In J. E. Bernthal & N. W. Bankson (Eds.), *Child phonology: Characteristics, assessment, and intervention with special populations* (pp. 3–28). New York, Thieme Medical.

Natsume, N., & Kawai, T. (1986). Incidence of cleft lip and cleft palate in 39,696 Japanese babies born during 1983. *International Journal of Oral Surgery, 15,* 565–568.

Nayak, J., & Sell, D. (1998). *Communication disorders in velocardiofacial syndrome: A clinical audit.* Paper presented at the 4th Annual Meeting of the Velocardiofacial Educational Foundation, Boston.

Niklasson, L., Rasmussen, P., Oskarsdottir, S., & Gillberg, C. (2001). Neuropsychiatric disorders in the 22q11 deletion syndrome. *Genetics in Medicine, 3,* 79–84.

Oskarsdottir, S., Persson, C., Eriksson, B. O., & Fasth, A. (2005). Presenting phenotype in 100 children with the 22q11.2 deletion syndrome. *European Journal of Pediatrics, 164,* 146–153.

Owens, J. R., Jones, J. W., & Harris, F. (1985). Epidemiology of facial clefting. *Archives of Diseases in Childhood, 60,* 521–524.

Papolos, D. F., Faedda, G. L., Veit, S., Goldberg, R., Morrow, B., Kucherlapati, R., et al. (1996). Bipolar spectrum disorder in patients diagnosed with velocardiofacial syndrome: Does a hemizygous deletion of chromosome 22q11 result in bipolar affective disorder? *American Journal of Psychiatry, 153,* 1541–1547.

Pashayan, H. M., & Lewis, M. B. (1984). Clinical experience with the Robin sequence. *Cleft Palate Journal, 21,* 270–276.

Perkins, J. A., Sie, K. C., Milczuk, H., & Richardson, M. A. (1997). Airway management in children with craniofacial anomalies. *Cleft Palate-Craniofacial Journal, 34,* 135–140.

Persson, C., Lohmander, A., Jonsson, R., Oskarsdottir, S., & Soderpalm, E. (2003). A prospective cross-sectional study of speech in patients with the 22q11.2 deletion syndrome. *Journal of Communication Disorders, 36,* 13–47.

Peterson, S. J., & Pruzansky, S. (1974). Palatal anomalies in the syndromes of Apert and Crouzon. *Cleft Palate Journal, 11,* 394–403.

Peterson-Falzone, S. J., & Figueroa, A. A. (1986). Longitudinal changes in cranial base angulation in mandibulofacial dysostosis. *Cleft Palate Journal, 26,* 14–22.

Peterson-Falzone, S. J., Hardin-Jones, M. A., & Karnell, M. P. (2001). *Cleft palate speech* (3rd ed.). St. Louis, MO: Mosby.

Peterson-Falzone, S., & Pruzanksy, S. (1976). Cleft palate and congenital palatopharyngeal incompetency in mandibulofacial dysostosis: Frequency and problems in treatment. *Cleft Palate Journal, 13,* 354–360.

Peterson-Falzone, S. J., Pruzansky, S., Parris, P. J., & Laffer, J. L. (1981). Nasopharyngeal dysmorphology in the syndromes of Apert and Crouzon. *Cleft Palate Journal, 18,* 237–250.

Poswillo, D. (1974). The pathogenesis of submucous cleft palate. *Scandinavian Journal of Plastic and Reconstructive Surgery, 8,* 34–41.

Randall, P., Krogman, W., & Jahins, W. (1965, July). Pierre Robin and the syndrome that bears his name. *Cleft Palate Journal, 2,* 237–246.

Reich, T. (1979). The use of multiple thresholds and segregation analysis in analyzing the phenotypic heterogeneity of multifactorial traits. *Annals of Human Genetics, 42,* 371–390.

Robert, E., Käller, B., & Harris, J. (1996). The epidemiology of orofacial clefts: Some general epidemiological characteristics. *Journal of Craniofacial Genetics and Developmental Biology, 16,* 234–241.

Roberts, F., Pruzansky, S., & Aduss, H. (1975). An X-radiocephalometric study of mandibulofacial dysostosis in man. *Archives of Oral Biology, 20,* 265–281.

Rommel, N., Vantrappen, G., Swillen, A., Devriendt, K., Feenstra, L., & Fryns, J. P. (1999). Retrospective analysis of feeding and speech disorders in 50 patients with velo-cardio-facial syndrome. *Genetic Counseling, 10,* 71–78.

Sadewitz, V. L., & Shprintzen, R. J. (1986). *Pierre Robin: A new look at an old disorder* [Videotape]. White Plains, NY: March of Dimes Birth Defects Foundation.

Scambler, P. J., Kelly, D., Lindsay, E., Williamson, R., Goldberg, R. B., Shprintzen, R. J., et al. (1992). The velocardiofacial syndrome is associated with chromosome 22 deletions encompassing the DiGeorge locus. *Lancet, 333*(8802), 1138–1139.

Schauerte, E. W., & St. Aubin, P. M. (1966). Progressive synostosis in Apert's syndrome (acrocephalosyndactyly). *American Journal of Roentgenology, 97,* 67–73.

Schaumann, B. F., Peagler, F. D., & Gorlin, R. J. (1970). Minor craniofacial anomalies among a Negro population. *Oral Surgery, Oral Medicine and Oral Pathology, 29,* 566–575.

Scherer, N. J., D'Antonio, L. L., & Kalbfleisch, J. H. (1999). Early speech and language development in children with velocardiofacial syndrome. *American Journal of Medical Genetics (Neuropsychiatric Genetics), 88,* 714–723.

Scherer, N. J., D'Antonio, L. L., & Rodger, J. R. (2001). Profiles of communication disorders in children with velocardiofacial syndrome: Comparison to children with Down syndrome. *Genetics in Medicine, 3,* 72–78.

Sedee, G. (1973). Facial nerve and dysplasia of the temporal bone. *Journal of Otology, Rhinology, and Laryngology, 35,* 222–228.

Sedlackova, E. (1955). The syndrome of the congenital shortening of the soft palate (in Czech). *Cas Lek Ces, 94,* 1304–1307.

Sedlackova, E. (1967). The syndrome of the congenitally shortened velum—The dual innervation of the soft palate. *Folia Phoniatrica, 19,* 441–450.

Semb, G., & Shaw, W. C. (1991). Simonart's band and facial growth in unilateral clefts of the lip and palate. *Cleft Palate and Craniofacial Journal, 28,* 40–46.

Sher, A. (1992). Mechanisms of airway obstruction in Robin sequence: Implications for treatment. *Cleft Palate-Craniofacial Journal, 29,* 224–231.

Sher, A., Shprintzen, R. J., & Thorpy, M. J. (1986). Endoscopic observations of obstructive sleep apnea in children with anomalous upper airways: Predictive and therapeutic value. *International Journal of Pediatric Otorhinolaryngology, 11,* 135–146.

Shields, E. D., Bixler, D., & Fogh-Andersen, P. (1979). Facial clefts in Danish twins. *Cleft Palate Journal, 16,* 1–6.

Shields, E. D., Bixler, D., & Fogh-Andersen, P. (1981). Cleft palate: A genetic and epidemiologic investigation. *Clinical Genetics, 20,* 13–24.

Shipster, C., Hearst, D., Dockrell, J. E., Kilby, E., & Hayward, R. (2002). Speech and language skills and cognitive functioning in children with Apert syndrome: A pilot study. *International Journal of Language and Communication Disorders, 37,* 325–343.

Shprintzen, R. J. (1982). Palatal and pharyngeal anomalies in craniofacial syndromes. *Birth Defects, 18,* 53–78.

Shprintzen, R. J. (1988). Pierre Robin, micrognathia, and airway obstruction: The dependency of treatment on accurate diagnosis. *International Anesthesiology Clinics, 26,* 84–91.

Shprintzen, R. J. (1997). *Velo-cardio-facial syndrome specialist fact sheet.* Retrieved September 21, 2007, from www.vcfsef.org/articles/en/pdf/factsheet.pdf

Shprintzen, R. J. (2000). *Syndrome identification for speech-language pathology.* San Diego: Singular.

Shprintzen, R. J., Croft, C., Berkman, M. D., & Rakoff, S. (1979). Pharyngeal hypoplasia in Treacher Collins syndrome. *Archives of Otolaryngology, 105,* 127–131.

Shprintzen, R. J., Croft, C. B., Berkman, M. D., & Rakoff, S. J. (1980). Velopharyngeal insufficiency in the facio-auriculo-vertebral malformation complex. *Cleft Palate Journal, 17,* 132–137.

Shprintzen, R. J., Goldberg, R., Lewin, M. L., Sidoti, E. J., Berkman, M. D., Argamaso, R. V., et al. (1978). A new syndrome involving cleft palate, cardiac anomalies, typical facies, and learning disabilities: Velocardiofacial syndrome. *Cleft Palate Journal, 15,* 56–62.

Shprintzen, R. J., Goldberg, R., Young, D., & Wolford, L. (1981). The velocardiofacial syndrome: A clinical and genetic analysis. *Pediatrics, 67,* 167–172.

Shprintzen, R. J., Siegel-Sadowitz, V. L., Amato, J., & Goldberg, R. B. (1985). Anomalies associated with cleft lip, cleft palate, or both. *American Journal of Medical Genetics, 20,* 585–595.

Shriberg, L. D., Aram, D. M., & Kwiatkowski, J. (1997). Developmental apraxia of speech: II. Toward a diagnostic marker. *Journal of Speech, Language, and Hearing Research, 40,* 286–312.

Simon, T. J., Ding, L., Bish, J. P., McDonald-McGinn, D. M., Zackai, E. H., & Gee, J. (2005). Volumetric, connective, and morphologic changes in the brains of children with chromosome 22q11.2 deletion syndrome: An integrative study. *Neuroimage, 25,* 169–180.

Singer, L., & Sidoti, E. J. (1992). Pediatric management of Robin sequence. *Cleft Palate-Craniofacial Journal, 29,* 220–223.

Skoog, T. (1965). The management of bilateral cleft of the primary palate. *Plastic and Reconstructive Surgery, 35,* 40.

Solomon, L. M., Fretzin, D., & Pruzansky, S. (1970). Pilosebaceous abnormalities in Apert's syndrome. *Archives of Dermatology, 102,* 381–385.

Solomon, L. M., Medenica, M., Pruzansky, S., & Kreiborg, S. (1973). Apert syndrome and palatal mucopolysaccharides. *Teratology, 8,* 287–292.

Solot, C. B., Knightly, C., Handler, S. D., Gerdes, M., McDonald-McGinn, D. M., Moss, E., et al. (2000). Communication disorders in the 22q11.2 microdeletion syndrome. *Journal of Communication Disorders, 33,* 187–204.

Spence, M. A., Westlake, J., Lange, K., & Gold, D. P. (1976). Estimation of polygenic recurrence risk for cleft lip and palate. *Human Heredity, 26,* 327–336.

Stickler, G. B., Belau, P. G., Farrell, F. J., Jones, J. D., Pugh, D. G., Steinberg, A. G., et al. (1965). Hereditary progressive artho-ophthalmopathy. *Mayo Clinic Proceedings, 40,* 433–455.

Stickler, G. B., & Pugh, D. G. (1967). Hereditary progressive arthro-ophthalmopathy: II. Additional observations on vertebral anomalies, a hearing defect, and a report of a similar case. *Mayo Clinic Proceedings, 42,* 495–500.

Swillen, A., Devriendt, K., Legius, E., Eyskens, B., Dumoulin, M., Gewillig, M., et al. (1997). Intelligence and psychosocial adjustment in velocardiofacial syndrome: A study of 37 children and adolescents with VCFS. *Journal of Medical Genetics, 34,* 453–458.

Swillen, A., Vogels, A., Devriendt, K., & Fryns, J. P. (2000). Chromosome 22q11.2 deletion syndrome: Update and review of clinical features, cognitive-behavioral spectrum, and psychiatric complications. *American Journal of Medical Genetics (Seminar in Medical Genetics), 97,* 128–135.

Taitz, L. S., Zarate-Salvador, C., & Schwartz, E. (1966). Congenital absence of the parathyroid and thymus glands in an infant (III and IV pharyngeal pouch syndrome). *Pediatrics, 38,* 412–418.

Tatum, S. A. (2002). *Surgical management of velopharyngeal insufficiency in VCFS: Why is it so different?* Paper presented at the meeting of the Velocardiofacial Syndrome Educational Foundation, London, England.

Tatum, S. A., Chang, J., Havkin, N., & Shprintzen, R. J. (2002). Pharyngeal flap and the internal carotid in velocardiofacial syndrome. *Archives in Facial Plastic Surgery, 4*(2), 73–80.

Thomas, J. (1996). Speech and voice rehabilitation in selected patients fitted with a bone anchored hearing aid (BAHA). *Journal of Laryngology and Otology Supplement, 21,* 47–51.

Tolarová, M. (1972). Empirical recurrence risk figures for genetic counseling of clefts. *Acta Chirurgiae Plasticae (Praha), 14,* 234–235.

Tolarová, M. (1987a). Orofacial clefts in Czechoslovakia: Incidence, genetics and prevention of cleft lip and palate over a 19-year period. *Scandinavian Journal of Plastic and Reconstructive Surgery, 21,* 19–25.

Tolarová, M. (1987b). A study of the incidence, sex ratio, laterality and clinical severity in 3,660 probands with facial clefts in Czechoslovakia. *Acta Chirurgiae Plasticae (Praha), 29*(2), 77–87.

Tosun, G., & Sener, Y. (2006). Apert syndrome with glucose-6-phosphate dehydrogenase deficiency: A case report. *International Journal of Paediatric Dentistry, 16,* 218–221.

Trost, J. E. (1981). Articulatory additions to the classical description of the speech of persons with cleft palate. *Cleft Palate Journal, 18,* 193–203.

Trost-Cardamone, J. E. (1987). *Cleft palate misarticulations: A teaching tape* [Videotape]. Northridge: Instructional Media Center, California State University.

Trost-Cardamone, J. E. (1990). The development of speech: Assessing cleft palate misarticulations. In D. A. Kernahan & S. Rosenstein (Eds.), *Cleft lip and palate: A system of management.* Baltimore: Williams & Wilkins.

Trost-Cardamone, J. E., & Bernthal, J. E. (1993). *Articulation assessment and procedures and treatment decisions.* In K. T. Moller & C. D. Starr (Eds.), *Cleft palate: Interdisciplinary issues and treatment* (pp. 307–336). Austin, TX: PRO-ED.

Vallino-Napoli, L. D. (2002). A profile of the features and speech in patients with mandibulofacial dysostosis. *Cleft Palate-Craniofacial Journal, 39,* 623–634.

Van Amelsvoort, T., Daly, E., Henry, J., Robertson, D., Ng, V., Owen, M., et al. (2004). Brain anatomy in adults with velocardiofacial syndrome with and without schizophrenia: Preliminary results of a structural MRI study. *Archives of General Psychiatry, 61,* 1085–1096.

Van Amelsvoort, T., Daly, E., Robertson, D., Suckling, J., Ng, V., Critchley, H., et al. (2001). Structural brain abnormalities associated with deletion at chromosome 22q11: Quantitative neuroimaging study of adults with velo-cardio-facial syndrome. *British Journal of Psychiatry, 178,* 412–419.

Vanderas, A. P. (1987). Incidence of cleft lip, cleft palate, and cleft lip and palate among races: A review. *Cleft Palate Journal, 24,* 216–225.

Van Lierde, K. M., Van Cauwenberge, P., Stevens, I., & Dhooge, I. (2004). Language, articulation, voice, and resonance characteristics of 4 children with Goldenhar syndrome: A pilot study. *Folia Phoniatrica et Logopedica, 56,* 131–143.

Vegter, F., Mulder, J. W., & Hage, J. J. (1997). Major residual deformities in cleft patients: A new anthropometric approach. *Cleft Palate-Craniofacial Journal, 34,* 106–110.

Wang, P. P., Woodin, M. F., Kreps-Falk, R., & Moss, E. M. (2000). Research on behavioral phenotypes: Velocardiofacial syndrome (deletion 22q11.2). *Developmental Medicine and Child Neurology, 42,* 422–427.

Weik, L., Carneol, S. O., Marks, S. M., Denny, A. D., & Beste, D. (1993). *Velocardiofacial syndrome: Reassessment of the velo, cardio, and facial features.* Paper presented at the meeting of the American Cleft Palate Craniofacial Association, Pittsburgh, PA.

Wharton, P., & Mowrer, D. E. (1992). Prevalence of cleft uvula among school children in kindergarten through grade five. *Cleft Palate-Craniofacial Journal, 29,* 10–14.

Wilson, D., Cross, I., Wren, P., Scambler, P., Burn, J., & Goodship, J. (1994). Velopharyngeal insufficiency after adenoidectomy: An 8-year review. *American Journal of Human Genetics, 55,* 169.

Witt, P., Cohen, D., Grames, L. M., & Marsh, J. (1999). Sphincter pharyngoplasty for the surgical management of speech dysfunction associated with velocardiofacial syndrome. *British Journal of Plastic Surgery, 52,* 613–618.

Witt, P. D., Miller, D. C., Marsh, J. L., & Grames, L. M. (1997). Surgical management of speech dysfunction associated with velocardiofacial syndrome: Comparison of outcome characteristics following pharyngeal flap and sphincter pharyngoplasty. In *Transactions of the 8th International Congress on Cleft Palate and Related Craniofacial Anomalies* (pp. 355–360). Singapore: Stamford Press.

Witzel, M. A., Rich, R. H., Margar-Bacal, R., & Cox, C. (1986). Velopharyngeal insufficiency after adenoidectomy: An 8-year review. *International Journal of Pediatric Otolaryngology, 11,* 15–20.

Wong, F. K., Hagberg, C., Karsten, A., Larson, O., Gustavsson, J., Huggare, J., et al. (2000). Linkage analysis of candidate regions in Swedish nonsyndromic cleft lip with or without cleft palate families. *Cleft Palate-Craniofacial Journal, 37,* 357–362.

Woodin, M., Wang, P. P., Aleman, D., McDonald-McGinn, D., Zackai, E., & Moss, E. (2001). Neuropsychological profile of children and adolescents with the 22q11.2 microdeletion. *Genetics in Medicine, 3*(1), 34–39.

Wyszynski, D. F., Lewanda, A. F., & Beaty, T. H. (1996). Phenotypic discordance in a family with monozygotic twins and non-syndromic cleft lip and palate. *American Journal of Medical Genetics, 66,* 468–470.

Young, D. (1980). Cardiac malformations in the velocardiofacial syndrome. *American Journal of Cardiology, 46,* 643–648.

Zim, S., Schelper, R., Kellman, R., Tatum, S., Ploutz-Snyder, R., & Shprintzen, R. (2003). Thickness and histologic and histochemical properties of the superior pharyngeal constrictor muscle in velocardiofacial syndrome. *Archives in Facial Plastic Surgery, 5,* 503–510.

# CHAPTER 6

# Nursing Care, Feeding, and Nutrition in the First Year

*Mary L. Breen, Patricia D. Chibbaro, and Gerrilyn M. Hopper*

The nurse specialist on the interdisciplinary cleft palate team has a role that is both detailed and comprehensive. The nurse may provide direct care for the newborn and infant, teaching and counseling for the family, and interdisciplinary consultation for the team and the community. The nurse is often the most consistent provider before birth and throughout surgeries and recovery, until the family has adjusted satisfactorily to caring for a child with cleft lip or palate. In the child's 1st year, the family will learn about pre- and postoperative care, feeding options, nutritional requirements, and general markers of their child's healthy growth and development. Breen, Chibbaro, and Hopper explore the nurse's role in supporting the infant and family during this important early period.

1. The authors describe the specialized and multifaceted role of the nurse coordinator on the interdisciplinary cleft palate team. Describe the specific role of the nurse on the interdisciplinary cleft palate team.
2. What is the impact of prenatal diagnosis on parental responses to cleft lip and palate? What are the components of a prenatal consultation? What are the benefits of genetic testing and early diagnosis of clefting? Describe some of the common emotional challenges for parents facing an early diagnosis of clefting.
3. Describe the prefeeding assessment of a newborn with a cleft lip and palate. Explain the options for bottle feeding a baby with a cleft. When is direct breastfeeding indicated for babies with clefts? What techniques promote optimal feeding in these babies, and

what are signs of caution or concern for poor feeding or swallowing problems?

4. What measures and outcomes are available to assess adequacy of the infant's nutritional intake in the first year? What information and evidence can the nurse and coordinator elicit from families to verify that the infant is receiving sufficient nutrition? When can a baby with a cleft progress to solid foods?

From the moment an infant is born with a cleft lip or palate, a relationship between a family and a nursing professional is established. This professional relationship may begin even earlier if the condition is diagnosed prenatally. Throughout the early years, families will encounter and interact with many nursing professionals who have varied roles and responsibilities. The nurse in the delivery room may be the first professional to inform parents of their child's cleft. In the neonatal period, nurses in the newborn nursery and postpartum units focus on feeding interventions and provide emotional support for the family. Later, as the child undergoes surgical correction, operating room nurses are an integral part of the surgical experience. After surgery, inpatient hospital nurses provide direct care to the recovering child. However, the nurse that the family will encounter most often and rely on primarily throughout the habilitative process is the nurse on the interdisciplinary cleft team. The role of this nursing professional is to guide families through the maze of team care and the hospital system and to become a familiar face that families can seek as they meet and experience different specialists and different settings.

Nursing is defined as "the diagnosis and treatment of human responses to actual or potential health problems" (American Nurses' Association, 1995). In other words, the nurse assists the child and family in managing the impact of the cleft by providing education to increase the family's knowledge about cleft lip and palate. This education will include both specific information, such as how to feed the infant with a cleft lip or palate, and general support, such as how to monitor the child's growth and development.

Nursing education programs vary. Some are 3-year associate degree programs, and others are 4-year baccalaureate degree programs. Basic undergraduate nursing education prepares nurses for many areas of practice and covers a broad range of subjects. To achieve a license to practice nursing, candidates must pass a required exam administered by a state board of nurse examiners. Some nursing professionals will seek other advanced credentials. These advanced-practice nurses have completed supplemental graduate education to work as a clinical nurse specialist, as a nurse practitioner, or in a combined role. These credentials allow advanced-practice nurses to provide advanced-level case coordination or primary care.

The specialized pediatric nursing curriculum serves several important goals. First, nurses learn the technical knowledge and skills needed to care for pediatric patients. Second, they learn effective strategies to become family advocates, by being able to identify each family's goals and needs and plan effective interventions that best meet the family's problems. In addition, the pediatric nurse must be competent in health promotion and teaching, collaboration with other disciplines, and coordinating patient care (Wong, 1999). The nurse on the craniofacial team performs all of these functions. Often, the nurse is the team member with the most comprehensive knowledge of the child's and family's needs and is best suited to coordinate team care. A nurse's basic education, and in some cases graduate education, prepares the nurse for this case management role.

Thus, the multifaceted roles of the nurse on the craniofacial team include education, support, coordination, and consultation. Education and support of the child and family are ongoing processes, from the time of diagnosis through preoperative preparation and postoperative care. The nurse provides coordination and case management to communicate all of the treatment recommendations made by the different specialists to the family and to other health care providers. Additionally, the nurse verifies that the recommended interventions are implemented. As a consultant, the nurse provides outreach education to newborn nurseries, school nurses, and staff nurses on inpatient units. The nurse often serves as a resource and liaison to the primary care provider and other health providers in the community.

## Prenatal Diagnosis and Counseling of Cleft Lip and Palate

Although fetal ultrasound examination became available in the late 1950s, the first detection of a facial cleft by this technique was not reported until 1981 (Christ & Meininger, 1981; Johnson & Sandy, 2003). Since that time, the incidence of prenatal cleft diagnosis has increased greatly due to advances in high-resolution techniques (Bronshtein, Blumenfeld, & Blumenfeld, 1996; Chen, Chang, Yu, Cheng, & Chang, 2001; Chitty, Hunt, Moore, & Lobb, 1991; Jones, 2002; Robinson et al., 2001; Shaikh, Mercer, Sohan, Kyle, & Soothill, 2001). The literature reports detection rates ranging from 14% to 93% (Cash, Set, & Coleman, 2001; Jones, 2002; Shaikh et al., 2001; Smith, Estroff, Barnewolt, Mulliken, & Levine, 2004).

By gestational week 14, the fetal facial contour is almost complete (Bronshtein, Mashiah, & Blumenfeld, 1991). Clefts can be detected by transvaginal sonography as early as the 12th week (Blumenfeld, Blumenfeld, & Bronshtein, 1999). Transabdominal ultrasounds generally first identify clefts between week 16 and week 22, which corresponds to the timing of the first routine obstetrical sonogram (see Figure 6.1). Several studies have concluded that the optimal timing for ultrasound diagnosis of facial clefts is at 20–22 weeks gestation (Johnson & Sandy, 2003; Robinson et al., 2001; Shaikh et al., 2001).

The accuracy of a prenatal cleft diagnosis is quite variable (Robinson et al., 2001) and depends on the type and extent of the cleft, as well as the presence of associated anomalies (Smith et al., 2004). With the evolution of three-dimensional ultrasound, the precision of the diagnosis has increased (Chen et al., 2001; Chmait et al., 2002). However, it is still very unusual for an isolated cleft palate to be detected prenatally, as ultrasound remains limited in its ability to evaluate the structure of the secondary palate. Often, if a cleft palate is identified, it is actually the alveolus which is seen (Jones, 1999) (see Figure 6.1). Magnetic resonance imaging (MRI) is useful for evaluating fetal abnormalities that are difficult to identify on sonography, and it has been helpful in detecting some facial clefts (Smith et al., 2004). Incomplete cleft of the lip is not as easy to detect as complete bilateral and unilateral cleft lip or palate and may not be identified until the beginning of the third trimester (Benacerraf & Mulliken, 1993). This late finding can obviously be extremely overwhelming to a family who may previously have undergone sonograms that were reported as "normal."

Most facial clefts are isolated findings (Chmait et al., 2002), but they can be associated with other congenital defects, including over 350 syndromes (Chmait et al., 2002; Stoll, Alembik, Dott, & Roth, 2000). Studies report a wide range in associated birth incidence, from 4.3% to 63.4% (Croen, Shaw, Wasserman, & Tolarova, 1998; Jensen, Reiborg, Dahl, & Fogh-Andersen, 1988; Shprintzen, Siegel-Sadowitz, Amato, & Goldberg, 1985; Stoll et al., 2000). These associated malformations can be as mild as a preauricular skin tag or as severe as a potentially lethal deformity

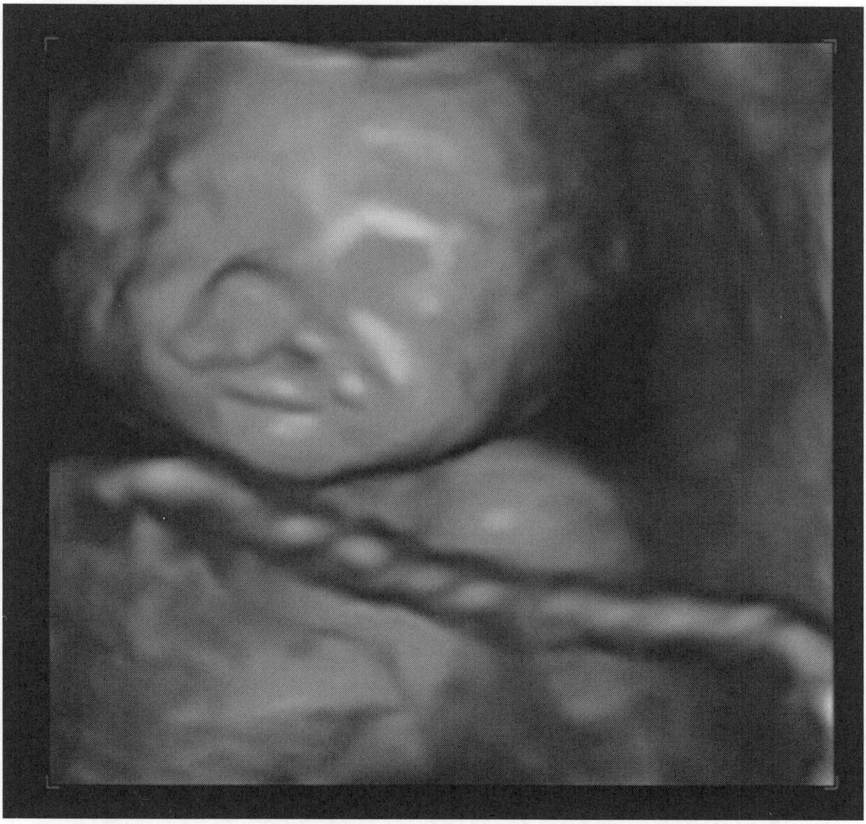

FIGURE 6.1. Prenatal three-dimensional ultrasound photo of a fetus with a cleft lip.

(e.g., Trisomy 13). The most common cleft-associated malformations are found in the central nervous and skeletal systems, followed by the urogenital and cardiovascular systems (Stoll et al., 2000). It is critical that the parents who receive a prenatal diagnosis of a fetal cleft be referred by their obstetrician to a genetics team for further evaluation and counseling. Ideally, this team should be associated with a cleft lip and palate center.

## The Issue of Pregnancy Termination

Genetics teams and cleft care professionals are often asked, "Do most parents decide to terminate the pregnancy after a cleft is identified?"

Matthews (2002) surveyed over 100 plastic surgeons who were members of the American Cleft Palate-Craniofacial Association. She concluded, "Most surgeons do not feel that they are being consulted about pregnancy termination. In fact, many indicated that the topic had never come up" (p. 181). Johnson and Sandy (2003), in reviewing several studies, found that the reported incidence of termination based solely on the diagnosis of an isolated facial cleft was very low (0%–27%), with one very clear outlier having a 92% termination rate. This outlier was reported in a study from Israel, and the high termination rate was thought to be the result of many factors. These include a very early date of diagnosis (12–16 weeks) by transvaginal ultrasound, an increased perception of burden by the cleft team, and a history of more prenatal counseling provided by nonprofessionals with personal life experience with clefts, rather than by the cleft team professionals (Blumenfeld et al., 1999; Davalbhakta & Hall, 2000; Johnson & Sandy, 2003; Jones, 1999; Saal, 2002). As discussed by Hinton in Chapter 4, each family's cultural influences, religious beliefs, and socioeconomic status must also be considered (Hager, 2002) when working with families who may consider terminating a pregnancy following a prenatal cleft diagnosis. A nonjudgmental, supportive approach is very important, although this approach can sometimes be difficult for the cleft team members, who have the overwhelming experience of seeing children with clefts grow up to lead very "normal" lives.

## The Pros and Cons of Prenatal Diagnosis of Cleft Lip and Palate

The benefits and limits of informing parents of their child's cleft diagnosis in the prenatal period have been well studied. Generally, parents and teams believe the practice is beneficial, but the issue is clearly complicated (Aspinall, 2002; Davalbhakta & Hall, 2000; Matthews, 2002; Matthews, Cohen, Viglione, & Brown, 1998; Strauss, 2002). Table 6.1 provides an overview of the perceived pros and cons of knowing a cleft diagnosis prenatally. One of the most important benefits is that the family is given the opportunity to learn more about cleft lip and palate, as well as to search for the appropriate cleft team for their baby. It is common for parents to visit three or four centers to obtain information, compare treatment options, and meet the team members. Parents who do not know the diagnosis prenatally often feel totally overwhelmed in the hospital and have no idea whom to consult or where to seek treatment.

**Table 6.1**
**Prenatal Diagnosis of Cleft Lip and Palate: The Pros and Cons**

**Pros**

- Opportunity to research information about clefts
- Ability to select and meet the cleft team prior to birth of infant
- Better prepared psychologically—increased sense of security
- Can optimize the delivery experience and decrease shock at time of birth
- Better prepared to feed baby—decrease in perinatal morbidity
- Ability to prepare family, siblings, and friends—increased support
- Decreased feelings of isolation
- Potential for fetal surgery (more research needed here)

**Cons**

- Increased anxiety for remainder of pregnancy
- Potential maternal complications secondary to anxiety (e.g., pre-eclampsia)
- Lack of specificity regarding extent of cleft and presence of other abnormalities
- Increased termination of pregnancy

Another advantage of knowing the diagnosis prenatally is that the family can prepare their own extended family, friends, and the hospital staff, to prevent a shocking, negative birth experience. Parents have the opportunity to make contact with as many people as possible at the birth hospital and to enlist their obstetrician and pediatrician in this effort. Many parents who did not know that their baby had a cleft have tearfully recalled that one could "hear a pin drop" in the delivery room and that the baby was often "whisked away" before the mother could even hold him or her. It is common for parents to remember hearing nurses and doctors "gasping" or seeing them "wince" at the sight of the baby. These are indelible and often very painful memories, which could be avoided (or at least minimized) if everyone knew what to expect.

In addition, prenatal diagnosis allows the parents an opportunity to communicate with families who have been down the road that they are about to travel and who can demonstrate the positive and joyous experience of parenting. Mothers who did not have an advance diagnosis often report feeling isolated on the postpartum unit, as well as on the playground or in mother and baby playgroups, as they were generally the only parent of an infant with a cleft. As with other illnesses, such as cancer or alcoholism, there is essential value in having the freedom to speak openly with and be immediately understood by another family that has an infant with a cleft. Family networking is an absolutely critical component of comprehensive care.

However, the difficult part of prenatal diagnosis is that, once known, many parents, especially mothers, report significant worry and anxiety about exactly what the child will look like and whether the child will have any other problems. It is common for the parents to have difficulty sleeping. Many talk about how preoccupied and distracted they are with the diagnosis, making attention to work or other children a significant challenge. For this reason, it is very important that prenatal diagnosis be followed by specialized counseling, to assist the family in adjusting to this new knowledge and dealing with the experience (Aspinall, 2002; Bender, 2000). Berk, Marazita, and Cooper (1999) found that parents of affected children have a strong desire for information, involvement in prenatal testing and counseling decisions and appear to value preparation in spite of acknowledging anxiety associated with prenatal information.

## Prenatal Counseling

Once a cleft is diagnosed prenatally, the parents are generally referred for a genetics evaluation and follow-up counseling, as well as a separate consultation with selected members of a cleft lip and palate team. This meeting usually involves the plastic surgeon and may include the nurse specialist, team coordinator, speech-language pathologist, social worker, and/or psychologist. The consultation can take several hours if the team members meet individually with the family and may be overwhelming emotionally. Each counseling session will have different components, depending on the team (see Table 6.2 for descriptions of some team members' duties), but there are many common elements (Rey-Bellet & Hohlfeld, 2004).

The genetics consultation will involve obtaining detailed pregnancy and family histories. If a three-dimensional ultrasound or an amniocentesis has not yet been performed, one or both may be recommended to contribute additional information about the extent of the cleft, as well as the presence of other structural abnormalities, a chromosomal disorder, or a syndrome. If other abnormalities are present, some of the possible associated syndromes are described to the parents.

**Table 6.2**
**Prenatal Consultation Checklist**

**Genetic Counselor**

- Obtain pregnancy and family history
- Review diagnostic studies and recommend additional studies
- Answer questions regarding cause of cleft, possible associated syndromes, and incidence of cleft in future pregnancies
- Clarify Internet information
- Offer follow-up appointment
- Provide written summary of consult

**Plastic Surgeon**

- Review ultrasound findings with parents
- Clarify information about cleft lip and palate
- Provide a roadmap of the treatment process
- Introduce and discuss the cleft team concept
- Review pre- and postoperative photographs of similarly affected infants

**Nurse Specialist/Team Coordinator (or other designated team member)**

- Clarify information from meetings with genetics counselor and surgeon
- Discuss and support parental feelings about the diagnosis
- Review pre- and postoperative photographs
- Offer advice on how to explain the diagnosis to family, friends, and siblings
- Network parents to others with cleft-affected babies
- Provide literature and American Cleft Palate-Craniofacial Association and Cleft Palate Foundation Web site information
- Discuss and demonstrate feeding options and provide sample of bottles
- Provide cleft team contact information for family and hospital staff to call after birth of infant

During this genetics consultation, the family is given ample time to ask questions such as, "Why did this happen?" "What could have been done to prevent this?" "What other problems could my baby have?" and "Will my baby be normal?" (Bender, 2000). This is also a good time to clarify and correct information parents have obtained from the Internet, where sources may be biased, inaccurate, or misleading. Genetics counseling sessions can be very emotional for the parents, who may have only recently received the sonogram result and who are still grappling with this unexpected diagnosis. In the case of a cleft-affected parent, feelings of guilt and anxiety associated with their own cleft are discussed in a sensitive, nonjudgmental, and informative manner. It is helpful for the genetics team to summarize in writing for the parents the information presented during the visit and to offer follow-up sessions as needed.

The plastic surgeon can reduce the parents' anxiety substantially by educating them about exactly what a cleft is and explaining the state of the art in cleft care. This approach involves as few surgeries as possible and will combine surgical intervention with pre- or postoperative orthodontic treatment to achieve an optimal outcome. Pre- and postoperative photographs of the surgeon's cleft patients are often available for the parents to view, if desired. A roadmap of expected treatment from birth through the end of adolescence can be presented in writing. This plan should include not only the range of possible surgical procedures, but also issues related to speech development, ear infections, hearing, dental and orthodontic treatment, and psychosocial concerns. The importance of comprehensive, long-term management by an experienced cleft team can be stressed at this time.

The nurse specialist (or other designated team member) can answer any questions the family has following the meetings with the genetic counselor and plastic surgeon. A very important part of the prenatal consultation is to assist the family in confronting their feelings about the discovery of the cleft. The family may want to meet with the team's social worker or psychologist as well. They are likely to experience a range of emotions, including shock, anger, fear, sadness, and depression (Aspinall, 2002). The family needs to be supported in their mourning of the loss of the "perfect infant." Many parents will blame themselves, especially parents who were born with a cleft and who may have negative, painful memories of their own surgery, hospitalization, and social development. In this case, it is important that they be informed of the major advancements in cleft treatment.

Parents should be given the option of reviewing pre- and postoperative photographs of infants with a range of clefts, in order to give them a sense of perspective and to help them better understand the impact of cleft (Matthews et al., 1998) (see Figure 6.2). We learned this helpful tip from a parent: Show photos in the opposite order (i.e., start with the "af-

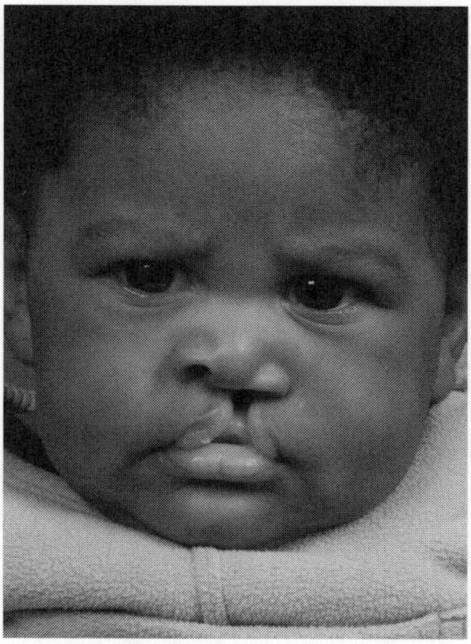
FIGURE 6.2. Preoperative photo of a child with cleft lip at age 2½ months.

ter" photos and then flip back to the "before" photos) to decrease the shock effect that some parents may feel. Parents should also be given suggestions on how to inform family, friends, and siblings about the baby's cleft. This is a very important time to extend a sense of hope and to give parents permission to believe that they will have a beautiful, smart, healthy child who has the potential to lead a relatively normal life, albeit with some challenges. For further support, parents can be networked by phone or email to other parents who had a prenatal cleft diagnosis. If a center has a parent and family support group, literature and contact information should be provided to parents. Many parents search the Internet for information, so it is helpful to warn them that some of the information on the Internet is simply not accurate and to provide them with the American Cleft Palate-Craniofacial Association (ACPA) and Cleft Palate Foundation address (www.cleftline.org). Finally, during this meeting, the nurse specialist can answer parents' questions and provide written materials to explain what to expect during surgery, hospitalization, and postoperative recovery following cleft lip and palate repairs.

Another important component of the prenatal visit is to help prepare the parents for how they will feed their infant. They need to understand that if the child has a cleft palate, the chance of breastfeeding directly and exclusively is very small. However, if the palate is intact, the mother should be encouraged to try breastfeeding. Another option is to express breast milk and feed the child with a special bottle for infants with clefts, which is an adapted form of breastfeeding. Even if the child has a cleft palate, the mother should feel free to put the baby to her breast to support the bonding process. The family should be given literature about feeding, both from the ACPA and from the individual cleft center. Centers should have available a variety of the special bottles for demonstration and give samples to the family to take with them to the birth hospital. It is also helpful for families to call the hospital's newborn nursery to inquire as to the availability of these bottles, as well as to connect with a lactation specialist.

A business card with the nurse specialist's pager number may be given to the family, so that they may call from the hospital after the baby is born. This contact can often be helpful if the hospital staff is not familiar with the care needed for a baby with a cleft. Many parents have called us with concerns that the staff is "overtreating" their baby. For example, occasionally a baby who has a cleft but who is otherwise healthy is placed in a neonatal intensive care unit, with placement of intravenous and nasogastric feeding tubes, apnea monitors, and so forth. The surgeon or nurse specialist may speak with the hospital's medical and nursing staff about appropriate treatment for the infant, especially in centers with less familiarity with cleft lip and palate. The birth nursery experience becomes a lifelong memory for most parents, so the cleft team can assist greatly in optimizing this very important encounter.

## Initial Management Needs: Newborn Period

When an infant is born with a cleft lip or palate that was not diagnosed prenatally, the family experiences a number of fears and concerns, such as "Why did this happen?" "Will the child ever look normal?" Will our child be able to talk?" "How will the child be able to feed?" Nursing interventions in the newborn period are aimed at answering these questions and guiding the family to acquire the skills and knowledge needed to handle their newborn competently and independently as quickly as possible.

The birth of an infant with a congenital anomaly is a crisis for the family. They must grieve for the loss of the anticipated healthy infant and often experience feelings of hurt, disappointment, and resentment (Caretto, 1984). Even those families who knew the cleft diagnosis prenatally may still experience some degree of shock and grief (Aspinall, 2002). It is important that parents see their infant as soon as possible after birth. Delay in seeing the baby may result in more anxiety and fantasizing that a defect is much worse than reality (Clifford & Crocker, 1971). A frequent comment from mothers who were delayed from seeing their infant for the first time is that the child's appearance was not as bad as they had imagined. Clifford and Crocker (1971) reported that although the parents' initial shock over the birth of an infant with a cleft is high, their anxiety seems to lessen quickly. The authors surmise this is because, in effect, "the worst has already happened" and parents have been told that surgery and treatment is available. This is in contrast to other conditions, such as mental retardation, where the future is uncertain.

When parents first see their infant, the nurse needs to create a supportive environment. Parents need to be allowed to express their feelings through crying, talking, or silence. The nurse may need to address questions that may not even be asked. Although parents frequently wonder why their child has a cleft and blame themselves, they may not always verbalize these feelings. It is important to reassure parents that they are not to blame. Once they are able to recover from the initial shock of seeing the cleft, they begin to need answers to their questions about the condition and its ramifications on the infant's well-being. In a study by Young, O'Riordan, Goldstein, and Robin (2001), parents of children with cleft lip or palate were asked to rank certain topics that they felt were important to discuss during the child's first day of life. Basic information such as feeding methods and home management were ranked high, whereas etiology, genetic basis, and the actual repair of cleft lip or palate were ranked lower.

Role modeling the acceptance and nurturing of the infant are important nursing interventions during the newborn period. Watching the nurse hold, cuddle, and care for the baby may lesson parents' anxiety (Wirt, Algren, & Arnold, 1992). Discussing other physical features of the infant can take the emphasis away from the cleft. Routine newborn care practices, such as bathing, signs of illness, and other day-to-day activities, are important topics to address and may provide opportunities for further education. For example, parents are sometimes reluctant to touch the cleft lip for fear that it hurts the child. They need to understand that it is no more sensitive than another infant's lip, and routine measures such as cleaning with a soft cloth and applying lubricant to the lip and gum area can be demonstrated.

As described previously, parents of newborns with clefts may benefit from seeing pictures of other infants before and after surgical correction to give them realistic optimism about the future. Contact with another parent or a support network is helpful for some families. During this emotional time for the parents, it is important for the nurse to remember that the mother is physically exhausted from the labor and delivery and may have physical discomforts from the birth process. Addressing the mother's physical needs can give her the energy needed to be able to care for the baby (Pate, 1987).

## Feeding

Feeding is perhaps the biggest challenge facing the parents of an infant with a cleft, as well as health care professionals. To successfully develop feeding interventions, one needs to understand the normal feeding process, which is comprised of sucking, swallowing, and breathing in a coordinated sequence (Glass & Wolf, 1999). Compressing the nipple results in positive pressure, which forces fluid into the mouth. Suction depends on negative pressure being generated in a sealed oral cavity to expel fluid into the mouth. Breathing must be coordinated with sucking and swallowing for effective feeding. With the presence of a cleft, it is difficult for the infant to form the seal necessary to create negative pressure. A cleft lip prevents the formation of an anterior seal on the nipple, and a cleft palate prevents formation of a seal in the oral cavity to create suction (Glass & Wolf, 1999). Even small clefts of the soft palate or submucous clefts can cause feeding problems (Curtin, 1990; Glass & Wolf, 1999). It is not unusual to hear health professionals or parents remark that it is just a "small cleft" and not understand the need to use special techniques. The result is often a poor feeder who fails to gain weight, resulting in increased anxiety and frustration for the parents.

### Breastfeeding

Infants with an isolated cleft lip may breastfeed successfully. However, for infants with cleft palate, direct breastfeeding is very difficult because they are not able to develop adequate suction to get milk from the breast. The benefits of breast milk are well known and include unique nutrients and antibody protection against development of otitis media. Therefore, it is important to encourage mothers who planned on breastfeeding to pump so they can feed their child expressed milk through a special bottle (Paradise, Elster, & Tam, 1994). An electric breast pump used at regular intervals is the best way to maintain an adequate milk supply. However, this can be very time-consuming and impractical for some mothers. They may have other small children to care for, work outside the home, or be too busy with medical appointments and routine infant care. The nurse should help the family strategize about the best way to provide adequate nutrition without inadvertently fostering the mother's feelings of guilt over being unable to breastfeed or supply breast milk.

## Bottle Feeding

A successful bottle-feeding method should provide adequate nutrition, use the infant's own suck and swallow mechanism, and be as normal appearing as possible. An infant with an isolated cleft lip may be a successful feeder by simply occluding the area of the cleft with the breast or nipple without any other modifications. There are several bottle options available for an infant with a cleft palate (see Figure 6.3). A soft squeeze bottle available from Mead Johnson allows the feeder to compress the bottle in rhythm with the infants' suck to deliver milk into the mouth easily. Different nipples can be used with the bottle. Parents should be instructed to squeeze at the beginning of the feeding and not wait until the infant is already fatigued. They should take cues from the infant as to how often to squeeze the bottle and how much pressure to apply.

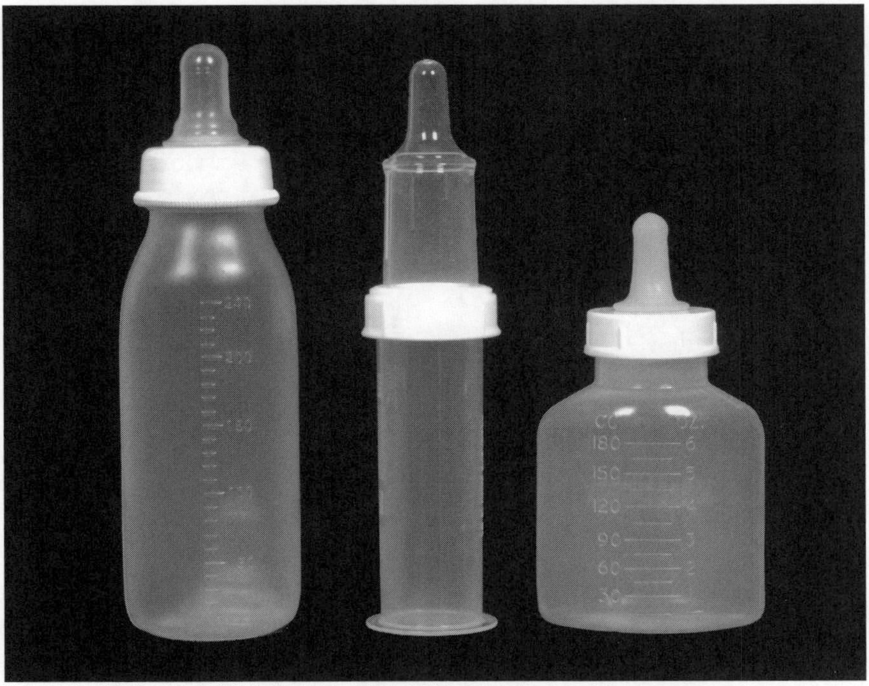

Figure 6.3. Bottles designed specifically for feeding babies with cleft lip and palate. Left to right: Pigeon Bottle, Haberman Feeder, Mead Johnson Cleft Lip/Palate Nurser.

The Haberman feeder by Medela has a one-way valve between bottle and nipple that allows compression of the nipple to substitute for suction. The feeder can control the rate of flow by rotating the slit opening relative to the infant's mouth (Glass & Wolf, 1999). Theoretically, this bottle enables the infant to have greater control over the flow and better coordination with breathing, but parents often have to squeeze the nipple to ensure adequate milk flow, and its use becomes similar to the other squeeze bottle techniques. The Pigeon Bottle, imported from Japan, has several features that make it a suitable option for babies with clefts. One side of the nipple is thinner than the other side so that milk flows with less effort. The thick side of the nipple is placed against the roof of the mouth. A one-way valve allows milk to flow when compressed by the infant's tongue. The flow can be regulated by tightening or loosening the collar.

It is critical that one bottle be chosen and used consistently by all feeders. Constantly changing equipment from one feeding to the next limits the success of the feeding. Whichever bottle is used, there are several additional techniques that should be used during feeding.

1. Hold the infant in an upright position (45–60 degrees) to decrease nasal regurgitation. Use a bulb syringe or cloth to clear the nose if regurgitation does occur.
2. Burp after every 30 ml if necessary due to air swallowing.
3. Limit feeding time to 30 minutes. Longer feeding sessions may tire the infant and increase caloric needs.
4. Focus attention on the infant and notice cues such as eye widening, choking, or milk leaking from the mouth, which could indicate too much flow.

Even with the use of a recommended bottle and technique, some infants may be unable to feed orally due to other factors such as cardiac, neurologic, or airway complications. Alternative methods such as a nasogastric or gastrostomy tube may be necessary for those babies.

## Going Home

Before discharge from the hospital, caretakers need to be confident in their ability to care for the infant, including both feeding and routine newborn care (see Appendix 6A for a hospital discharge checklist). An adequate supply of special bottles should be provided, as well as reordering information. Arrangements for a breast pump and supplies should be made for mothers who are planning to feed expressed breast milk. Parents are usually anxious about taking the new infant out in public and explaining the cleft to strangers or friends. A simple explanation about the condition and treatment is usually sufficient and serves as a way to educate others about clefting (About Face, 1992).

Ideally, the nurse on the cleft and craniofacial team should connect with the family in the newborn period either directly through a hospital visit or indirectly with a phone call to the family or nursery staff before discharge. Arrangements for follow-up with the interdisciplinary cleft team according to their particular protocol should be initiated. Additionally, the ACPA (2000) recommends that a team member, usually the nurse, provide the following services as needed:

1. Contact the family immediately after referral to provide assistance with feeding and to offer basic information, as needed, in conjunction with the primary care provider (e.g., the pediatrician or family physician).
2. Ensure weekly assessment of nutritional intake and weight gain during the first month of life.
3. Maintain support for the family through home visits, telephone calls, or a visiting nurse program.
4. Instruct caretakers of children with compromised airways in techniques of airway maintenance including positioning, nasogastric tube insertion, care of a tracheostomy, and apnea-bradycardia monitoring.
5. Recommend or arrange for hearing assessment of the child as soon as possible.

## Management Needs: Early Infancy

After the family's discharge from the birth hospital, the responsibility for managing the needs of the infant and family changes from the health professionals at the hospital to the specialists on the cleft team and the primary care provider (PCP). The collaboration between team and PCP is very important, and the PCP becomes, in effect, an extended member of the team (Mitchell & Wood, 2000). Their knowledge of normal growth and development, health maintenance practices including immunizations, and available community resources is the foundation of health care for the child (Nackashi, Dedlow, & Dixon-Wood, 1997).

## Feeding and Weight Gain

It is important to continue to monitor the baby's feeding and weight gain during the 1st month. Parents are usually happy to leave the birth hospital and settle into their own feeding routine at home; however, they need ongoing monitoring and re-evaluation of feeding techniques to ensure successful weight gain. Weekly weight checks should be done at the PCP's office or by the team nurse.

Birth weight and length in infants with clefts are usually considered identical to those of normal infants, when no other congenital malformations are present (Ranalli & Mazaheri, 1975). However, the growth rate after birth may be slower in patients with clefts due to feeding difficulties, chronic infections, syndrome-associated malformations, metabolic disorders, and repeated hospitalizations for surgery (Domet, 1986; Jensen, Dahl, & Kreiborg, 1983; Lee, Nunn, & Wright, 1997; Pandya & Boorman, 2001). Failure to achieve normal growth rates should be addressed through medical evaluation, including assessment of feeding and nutritional intake (Hall & Carroll, 2000). If intake continues to be inadequate, supplementation may be necessary and a referral to a registered dietitian for a more in-depth nutrition assessment may be warranted (Baer & Harris, 1997).

## Growth Assessment

Growth is one of the best indicators of an infant's nutritional status. Weight, length, and head circumference are important indicators of development and nutritional adequacy in infancy (Baer & Harris, 1997; Zlotkin, 1997). Careful measurements should be taken using appropriate and well-calibrated instruments. Recumbent length measurements should be used for infants younger than 2 years of age; the infant lies supine on a flat surface, and a length board is fitted against the soles of the feet and the crown of the head (Hall & Carroll, 2000). When taking measurements, the professional should take two readings and compute an average. Allowable differences in readings are 0.2 kg for weight, and 1.0 cm for recumbent length (Kleinman, 1998).

The measurements can be plotted on the four gender-specific growth charts: weight for age, length for age, head circumference for age, and weight for length. The values on each chart are compared by joining the dots to make a curve that provides a temporal depiction of an infant's progress. Revised pediatric growth charts from the Centers for Disease Control and Prevention (CDC) were published in 2000; these charts incorporate data from infants of diverse ethnic backgrounds, as well as from both formula-fed and breastfed infants (Roche & Guo, 2001). One concern of this diverse study group is that the charts may indicate falsely inflated rates of growth in breastfed infants up to 7 months of age (Roberts & Dallal, 2001). The WHO Multicentre Growth Reference Study (2006) presents new child-growth standards for height, weight, and age derived from a sample of healthy breastfed infants and young children worldwide.

The rate of growth is proportionately greater in early infancy; therefore, growth should be monitored at shorter intervals during this period. Short-term fluctuations in growth rates are common and cause little concern unless they are marked (Roche & Guo, 2001). With repeated measurements after birth, an individual growth trend can be established for each infant. Deviation from this established trend, such as a drift of more than 25 percentile points, can indicate problems with growth or nutritional intake. If this occurs, a global assessment of the infant is indicated to determine the source of the growth decline and to rule out a treatable problem (Tsang, Zlotkin, Nichols, & Hansen, 1997). A trend of persistent slow growth is important because it tends to be associated with disease, and, in the case of recumbent length and head circumference, it may have direct long-term health consequences (Roche & Guo, 2001). Absolute percentile value should only be taken as a starting point when evaluating an infant. Measurements outside of the 5th–95th percentile range may indicate developmental problems and should prompt further investigations (Kleinman, 1998).

## Nutritional and Energy Requirements

At present, there are no data to support the hypothesis that the nutritional requirements of an infant with cleft lip and palate differ from those of age-matched infants without clefts (Balluff, 1986). It is recognized, however, that feeding difficulties secondary to the abnormal anatomy of clefts and the associated surgical repairs can affect food intake, nutritional status, and growth (Balluff, 1986; Domet, 1986; Jensen et al., 1983; Lee et al., 1997; Pandya & Boorman, 2001). Until cleft-specific data are available to support specific nutritional recommendations, each infant with a cleft must first be assessed based on existing noncleft guidelines, which are then tailored to the individual based on clinical acumen, measurements, and observation.

There are no commonly accepted formulas to determine individualized energy requirements. A reasonable starting point is to compare the child's current estimated daily caloric intake with the appropriate Dietary Reference Intake (DRI) value for energy (see Table 6.3). The adequacy of energy intake can be monitored through close follow-up of weight gain and other growth pattern indicators, and then adjusted as required (Baer & Harris, 1997). Infants with syndromic clefts may have increased energy and nutrient needs due to comorbidities that result in breathing difficulties, metabolic dysfunction, cardiovascular malformations, or prematurity (Balluff, 1986; Domet, 1986; Pandya & Boorman, 2001). These infants should be assessed by a nutritionist and dietitian for more specialized nutritional assessment and treatment.

It is also important to make sure that infants meet the recommended daily intake of protein (see Table 6.4) and fluid (see Table 6.5). The fluid recommendations must be recognized as guidelines and taken into context with other nutritional parameters and volume of feed required.

**Table 6.3**
**Dietary Reference Intake Values for Energy**

| Age | Male (kcal/day) | Female (kcal/day) |
|---|---|---|
| Newborn–6 months | 570 | 520 (3 mo) |
| 7–12 months | 743 | 676 (9 mo) |

*Note.* From *Dietary Reference Intakes for Energy, Carbohydrate, Fiber, Fat, Fatty Acids, Cholesterol, Protein, and Amino Acids,* by Standing Committee on Scientific Evaluation of Dietary Reference Intakes, Food and Nutrition Board, Institute of Medicine, 2002, Washington, DC: National Academy Press. Copyright 2002 by National Academy Press.

**Table 6.4**
**Dietary Reference Intake Values for Protein**

| Age | Male (g/day) | Female (g/day) |
|---|---|---|
| Newborn–6 months | 9.1 (AI) | 9.1 (AI) |
| 7–12 months | 13.5 (RDA) | 13.5 (RDA) |

*Note.* AI = Adequate Intake; RDA = Recommended Dietary Allowance. From *Dietary Reference Intakes for Energy, Carbohydrate, Fiber, Fat, Fatty Acids, Cholesterol, Protein, and Amino Acids,* by Standing Committee on Scientific Evaluation of Dietary Reference Intakes, Food and Nutrition Board, Institute of Medicine, 2002, Washington, DC: National Academy Press. Copyright 2002 by National Academy Press.

**Table 6.5**
**Recommended Daily Fluid Requirements for Infants**

| Weight [kg (lbs)] | Fluid [mL/kg (oz/lb)] |
|---|---|
| 0.5–3 (1.1–6.6) | 120 (1.7) |
| 3–10 (6.6–22) | 100 (1.4) |
| 10–20 (22–44) | 1,000 mL (32 oz) + 50 mL/kg (0.7 oz/lb) for every kg (lb) above 10 kg (22 lb) |

*Note.* From "Infant Feeding," by R. T. Hall and R. E. Carroll, 2000, *Pediatrics in Review, 21,* pp. 191–199.

Table 6.6 lists the recommended daily intakes of iron, vitamin D, and fluoride for infants. Fluoride supplementation should not be provided during the first 6 months of life. From 6 months to 3 years of age, fluoride supplementation of 0.25 mg/d is needed only if the water supply contains less than 0.3 parts per million of fluoride (American Academy of Pediatrics, 2004; Gartner et al., 2005).

## Perioperative Considerations

Perioperative nutritional goals change based on the type of cleft, the age and weight of the infant, and the timing of repairs (Balluff, 1986; Pandya & Boorman, 2001). In general, prior to a surgery repair, extra calories and protein are required for anticipated wound healing (Escott-Stump, 1992) and adequate preoperative weight gain. If necessary, the delivery method

**Table 6.6**
**Dietary Reference Intake Values for Iron, Vitamin D, and Fluoride**

| Age | Iron (mg/day) | Vitamin D (μg/day) | Fluoride (mg/day) |
|---|---|---|---|
| Newborn–6 months | 0.27 (AI) | 5 (AI) | 0.01 (AI) |
| 7–12 months | 11 (RDA) | 5 (AI) | 0.5 (AI) |

*Note.* AI = Adequate Intake; RDA = Recommended Dietary Allowance. Adapted from *Dietary Reference Intakes for Vitamin A, Vitamin K, Arsenic, Boron, Chromium, Copper, Iodine, Iron, Manganese, Molybdenum, Nickel, Silicon, Vanadium, and Zinc,* by Standing Committee on Scientific Evaluation of Dietary Reference Intakes, Food and Nutrition Board, Institute of Medicine, 2001, Washington, DC: National Academy Press, and *Dietary Reference Intakes for Calcium, Phosphorus, Magnesium, Vitamin D, and Fluoride,* by Standing Committee on Scientific Evaluation of Dietary Reference Intakes, Food and Nutrition Board, Institute of Medicine, 1997, Washington, DC: National Academy Press.

of breast milk or formula can be altered to require less effort by the infant and decrease caloric output, thereby increasing the calories ingested to facilitate weight gain and growth (Redford-Badwal, Mabry, & Frassinelli, 2003). Postoperatively, some surgeons may prohibit breastfeeding or bottle feeding immediately after surgical repair; however, many surgeons support cautious reinstitution of normal feeding practices (Redford-Badwal et al., 2003). Also, in the days immediately after surgery, dietary intake can typically decrease, but nutritional requirements may temporarily increase. To compensate for this paradox, the caloric density, the frequency, or supplementation of the normal feeding may need to be increased (Balluff, 1986; Pandya & Boorman, 2001).

## Nutritional Assessment of Feeding

Analysis of an infant's dietary pattern can predict and prevent nutrient and energy deficiencies (Baer & Harris, 1997). A simple screening of dietary intake via a 24-hour recall should be done with a parent at every visit. If necessary, this review can be performed over the telephone. The following are examples of questions that could be asked:

- How many times a day did your child feed in the past 24 hours? Is this typical for your child?
- What was the average length of a feeding?

- Did your child spit up? If so, how often and how much?
- Did your child lose any food through the nose? If so, how often and how much?
- How many wet diapers did your child have in the past 24 hours?
- Did your child eat or drink anything other than breast milk or formula? If so, what were these foods and how much and how often did your child eat them?
- If the child takes formula: How many ounces did your child drink in the past 24 hours?
- What kind of formula do you use?
- How to do you prepare the formula?

Appendix 6B provides suggested nutritional assessment guidelines for infants with cleft lip or palate.

## Breastfeeding

To monitor nutrition in the infant with a cleft who is breastfed, the amount of breast milk consumed and the number and length of feedings should be noted. Breast milk contains approximately 680 kcal/L (20 kcal/oz) and approximately 10.5 g/L (0.3 g/oz) of protein (Hall & Carroll, 2000). The typical intake of breast milk is 46.9–62.5 mL (1.5–2 oz) every 2–3 hours, although this varies from child to child. The American Academy of Pediatrics guidelines for early breastfeeding recommend 8 to 12 feedings at the breast every 24 hours. Nondemanding infants should be aroused to feed if 4 hours have elapsed since the beginning of the last feeding (Gartner et al., 2005).

Any foods or supplementation given to the infant, such as vitamins, infant cereal, breast milk fortifiers, or supplementary bottle feedings of breast milk or infant formula, should also be noted when trying to calculate the day's intake. The American Academy of Pediatrics 2005 Policy Statement on Breastfeeding recommends that supplements (water, glucose water, formula, and other fluids) should not be given to breastfeeding newborn infants unless ordered by a health care provider when a medical condition exists (Gartner et al., 2005). The same policy recommends 200 IU of oral vitamin D drops daily for all exclusively breastfed infants within the first 2 months of life and continuing until the daily consumption of Vitamin D fortified formula or milk is 500 ml (Gartner et al., 2005). For infants under 6 months of age, routine iron supplements for term, healthy breastfed infants is not safe or necessary (Eglash, Kendall, & Fasher, 2005). For infants exclusively breastfed from 6 to 12 months of age, the American Academy of Pediatrics (2004) recommends iron from complementary foods and iron supplement of 1 mg/kg per day if intake from complementary foods is inadequate. The Academy also recommends that nonbreastfed infants under 12 months of age ingest iron-fortified formula (10–12 mg/L) until weaning at 12 months.

The number and quality of bowel movements and the amount and frequency of regurgitation are also important to take into consideration when trying to determine an infant's intake. For breastfed babies, at least four to six wet diapers each day (six to eight if cloth is used) can be a good indicator that the infant is consuming enough fluid. Yellowish crystals in a wet diaper can signal inadequate fluid intake or dehydration. It is difficult to assess breastfeeding intake accurately from historical information; therefore, accurate weights before and after breastfeeding may be required to determine the quantity consumed (Hall & Carroll, 2000).

The best overall indicator of breastfeeding progress is infant growth in the first 3 months of life. Healthy breastfed infants lose less than 10% of their birth weight initially and restore that weight by 2 weeks of age. From age 2 weeks to 3 months, they gain weight steadily at a minimum of 20 g per day. A thorough evaluation of the breastfeeding process by an infant feeding specialist may be needed if there is a strong deviation from this pattern (Powers, 2001).

## Infant Formula

If the infant with a cleft is being fed infant formula, the parent should provide details of the type of infant formula used, and the amount, length, and frequency of feedings, including night feedings. Only formula that the child actually ingested, not the amount prepared, should be recorded. If ready-prepared formula is not being used, it is also important to ask how caregivers are preparing the formula to determine whether they are using accurate measurements of powder or liquid concentrate for each feed. A useful verification is to ask how many cans of formula parents purchase at the store and how long these cans last. Standard infant formulas typically contain 676 kcal/L (20 kcal/oz) and approximately 14 g/L (0.4 g/oz) of protein. Some specialty formulas provide greater amounts of protein (Hall & Carroll, 2000). Formula intake generally ranges from 5 to 7 oz/kg (2.3 to 3.2 oz/lb) per day in the first 3 months of life, and then remains at 26–32 oz per day through 12 months of age. The American Academy of Pediatrics, Committee on Nutrition (2004), recommends iron-fortified formulas (10–12 mg/L)for all nonbreastfed infants. In general, an infant multivitamin and mineral supplement should be given if an infant is taking less than 16 oz of standard formula per day, and half a standard infant vitamin dose be given when an infant is taking between 16 and 32 oz per day.

In some infants with clefts, concurrent syndrome-related problems may prohibit the use of standard formula; therefore, enriched specialty formula may be required to meet their additional nutrient needs (Balluff, 1986). The previously stated recommendations for specific nutrient supplementation will change if an infant is consuming a formula that has higher levels of energy and nutrients per ounce. Failure to consider this formula difference can result in excess nutrient intake. Specialty formulas, such as soy protein formulas, lactose-free formulas, and protein hydrolysate formulas, are not routinely indicated for an infant with a cleft unless there is a dietary restriction or evidence of a specific medical condition to support their use. Examples of conditions that may support the use of these specialty products include certain enzyme deficiencies, cow's milk protein allergy, or some malabsorption syndromes (Balluff, 1986; Hall & Carroll, 2000). A registered dietitian and nutritionist should be consulted on the appropriateness of these specialty formulas for the individual infant, as many of these feeds are used inappropriately and sometimes unnecessarily.

## Solid Food

It is recommended that the introduction of solid foods be delayed until the infant is about 6 months of age (American Academy of Pediatrics, Work Group on Breastfeeding, 1997), although parents of infants with clefts may need to wait longer if there are concerns about the child's intake and oral-motor development. Before an infant is introduced to solid food, he or she should be able to sit upright and coordinate masticating and swallowing of nonliquid foods. Also, the infant's tongue-thrust reflex should have subsided. Infants typically show their readiness for solid foods by opening their mouths and leaning forward in a sitting position. They usually show satiety or lack of readiness by turning away (Hall & Carroll, 2000). Infants with clefts may aspirate food if they do not have the necessary oral-motor skills (Hall & Carroll, 2000); therefore, solid feeding in infants with clefts should be monitored carefully for excessive coughing, gagging, or other indicators of swallowing problems.

When solid foods are introduced, a small amount of food of smooth pureed consistency, which encourages slow swallowing, is recommended to prevent choking (Escott-Stump, 1992). In an infant with an open cleft, poorly swallowed food may enter the nasal cavity and come out the nose.

To avoid large losses of food through the nose, it is recommended that smaller bites be given more slowly until the child learns to direct the food more efficiently. Also, some foods, such as acidic and spicy foods, are irritating to the nasal passages, so they should be avoided until the child gains more control. Textured and lumpy foods can be introduced when indicated; however, some children with an open cleft handle lumps better by transitioning from strained foods to thickened foods, then from thickened foods to soft lumps in the thickened foods (Klein & Delaney, 1994).

When an infant with a cleft is started on solid foods, a 3-day record of typical dietary intake, including formula or breast milk, should be completed. Solid food intake should be assessed with reference to the basic food groups (Tsang et al., 1997). For example, is the child consuming a variety of different foods from the grains, fruit, vegetables, dairy, and meat groups? The caloric density of commercially prepared baby foods varies considerably, so labels should be consulted closely to determine a child's caloric intake. For example, an 8-oz jar of sweet potatoes contains 110 calories, whereas a similar jar of squash contains only 60 calories. The intake of solid food in infants 6 months of age should not decrease breast milk or formula intake to less than 32 oz per day (Escott-Stump, 1992) because these fluids still constitute the bulk of an infant's nutritional intake for the first 12 months of life. This is often not a concern in formula-fed infants; however, breastfed infants do tend to decrease their milk intake when introduced to solid foods (Hall & Carroll, 2000).

Particularly for breastfed infants, iron-fortified infant cereal should be one of the first solid foods introduced and should be a staple part of the diet until it is replaced by table foods at approximately 1 year of age (Aldous, 1999). The American Academy of Pediatrics recommends two servings of 4 tablespoons of dry cereal each day, which will provide 14 mg of iron per day (Kleinman, 1998). The cereal should be diluted with human milk or infant formula (Hall & Carroll, 2000). If iron-fortified cereal is delayed beyond 6 months of age, an iron supplement of 1 mg/kg per day is recommended (Kleinman, 1998).

Single-ingredient foods should be introduced first, with no more than one new food started each week to allow identification of intolerances (Baer & Harris, 1997). The introduction of pureed fruits, vegetables, and meats may be guided by individual taste and preference; however, they are usually most easily accepted in the order of vegetable, fruit, and meat (Escott-Stump, 1992). Juices are introduced around 7–9 months, or when the infant can drink from a cup, but they should not replace milk or formula or exceed 8 oz per day due to an increased risk of diarrhea and dental caries (Hall & Carroll, 2000). Fresh cow's milk, honey, and eggs should not be introduced until 12 months of age (Escott-Stump, 1992; Kleinman, 1998). Finely chopped foods may be introduced at 10–12 months of age, put parents must be watchful for potential aspiration of food particles. Nuts and seeds, hard pieces of raw fruit or vegetables, popcorn, hard candy, and hot dog wieners should not be fed to children younger than 2 years of age (Escott-Stump, 1992; Hall & Carroll, 2000). After surgical cleft repair, some foods are not well tolerated right away, especially if they are highly acidic or spicy (Escott-Stump, 1992).

## Otolaryngology and Audiology Considerations

As noted in Chapter 9 by Carlstrom and Nelson and Chapter 15 by Sidman, infants with cleft palate commonly have abnormal structure or function of the eustachian tube musculature, leading to impaired ventilatory function and subsequent otitis media (Paradise et al., 1994). Estimates of patients with cleft palate who have recurrent middle ear pathology range from 50% to 100% (Curtin, 1990; Mitchell & Wood, 2000). These middle ear problems increase the risk for hearing loss, which can adversely affect speech and language development. Consequently, infants with cleft palate need periodic audiology and otolaryngology evaluations to assess middle ear status. If they require ear procedures, often the surgery can be coordinated with lip or palate repair. Infants with isolated cleft lip or cleft lip and alveolus have the same risks of middle ear problems as the noncleft population and should also be monitored in case ear tubes are necessary. Cooperation between the infant's primary care provider and the team otolaryngologist is necessary. Monitoring and recognizing of middle ear disease by the primary care physician during routine well-child checks with subsequent referral to the team otolaryngologist are important. Parents should also be educated about the signs and symptoms of otitis media, such as irritability and fever, so they can seek help when needed.

## Dental Considerations

Children with clefts are at a greater risk for dental problems, including impacted teeth, supernumerary teeth, hypoplastic teeth, and congenitally missing teeth (Mitchell & Wood, 2000). Even in early infancy, caregivers should receive information regarding good oral hygiene and prevention of caries, especially nursing bottle caries.

As described previously, fluoride supplements should also be prescribed when appropriate (Chapple & Nunn, 2001). Detailed information about dental growth, development, and hazards in children with cleft palate is provided in Chapter 16 by Williams and Bevis and Chapter 17 by Swift.

## Primary Surgery: Nurse-Family Interactions

Perhaps the event that has the parents' primary focus during the child's first few months is the anticipated surgical repair. The nurse is involved in parent education from shortly after the child's birth, when parents begin asking questions about the timing of repairs, through consultations with the surgeon to discuss procedures. Because of the child's age, preoperative preparation for the first lip or palate surgery is aimed at the parents. The discussion should include the admission routines, anesthesia preparation, length of surgery, waiting room facilities, and recovery room and surgical pre- and postoperative routines. Child life specialists are available in most hospitals to provide preoperative hospital tours through the operating room area and nursing units. Networking with parents whose children have already had the same surgery can be helpful for practical advice and emotional support.

Postoperative routines vary, usually depending on the surgeon's preference, but are aimed at protecting the surgical site. Parents should understand the rationale for any postoperative restrictions so that they will be compliant. Typically, infants are hospitalized for 24 hours and receive intravenous fluids for hydration and pain medication until they can tolerate drinking liquids. Some surgeons allow immediate feeding by bottle or breast, whereas others prefer to use syringe or cup feeds for 1–3 weeks. Arm restraints may be used to prevent hands or other objects from reaching the surgical site. Positioning the infant on the side or back is preferable after lip repair, while prone positioning is encouraged after palate repair. Protocols for cleaning the sutures also vary, but usually involve cleansing with saline and applying antibiotic ointment, if prescribed. Again, it is important that parents are given information about these practices before surgery, so that they understand the rationale and are comfortable with their baby's care before being discharged home (see Figure 6.4).

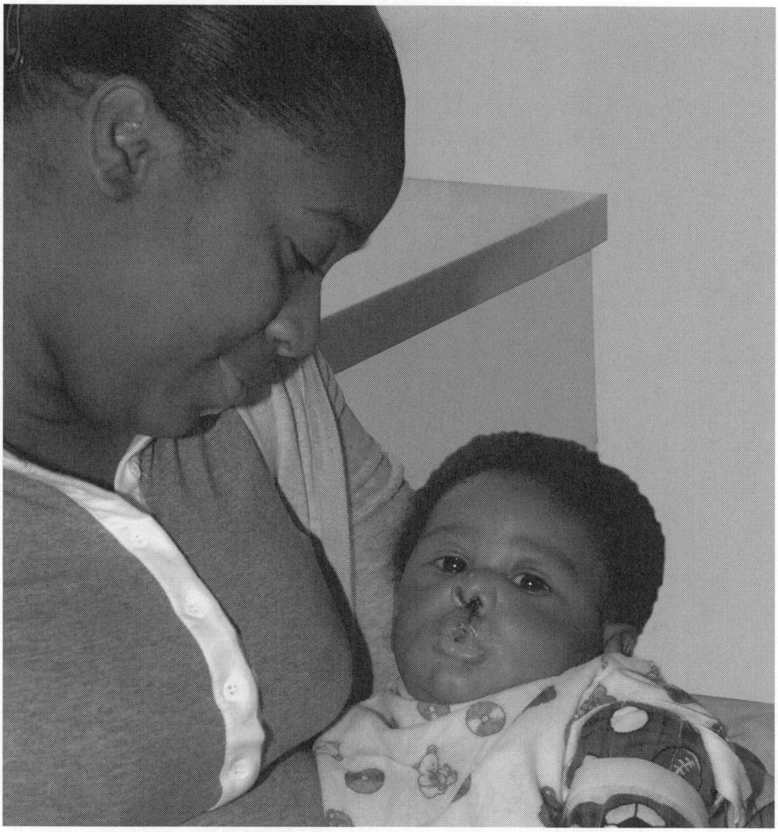

FIGURE 6.4. Mother and baby in early postoperative period.

## Summary

The first year of life for an infant born with a cleft is full of unique and sometimes challenging milestones, such as first successful feeding, first pound gained, and first surgery. They are all miraculous events yet can be frightening moments for the parents and family. The role of the nurse on the interdisciplinary cleft team is to be an educator, caregiver, service coordinator, and case manager. The nurse provides comprehensive assistance to help the child and family cope with and celebrate these "firsts" and achieve a successful outcome for the child's feeding, growth, and development.

## Authors' Note

We acknowledge with gratitude Wendy S. Looman, PhD, RN, CNP, for reviewing the nutrition section of this chapter.

## APPENDIX 6A

# Newborn Hospital Discharge Checklist

- Adequate feeding method has been established.
- Arrangements have been made for breast pump and bottle supplies.
- Parents have received routine infant care guidelines.
- Follow-up appointments have been made with cleft team specialists.
- An appointment has been made for a weight check by team or pediatrician 1 week after discharge.
- An appointment with the pediatrician has been scheduled for 2 weeks after discharge.
- The parents have received parent support group information.
- The parents have been advised about facing the public (dealing with friends and strangers).

# APPENDIX 6B

# Basic Nutritional Assessment Guidelines for Cleft Infants

## General Guidelines

1. Assess amount, length, frequency, and kind of feeding.
2. Assess appropriateness of feeding technique.
3. Assess number and quality of bowel movements.
4. Assess amount and frequency of regurgitation or loss of food through the nose.
5. Assess the appropriateness and the nutritional and caloric contribution of any food or beverage other than breast milk or formula to the overall diet.
6. Assess appropriateness of vitamin and mineral supplementation.
7. Assess growth parameters—that is, weight, length, and head circumference.

## Breastfeeding Guidelines

1. Infants should receive 8–12 feedings at the breast every 24 hours.
2. Infants should have at least four to six wet diapers each day, or six to eight if cloth is used.
3. Proper breastfeeding technique or breast milk bottle feeding technique should be assessed through continual observation in the first few weeks of life to determine if modifications are needed.
4. Infants should be weighed before and after breastfeeding for accurate assessment of intake when adequate intake is a concern.
5. Vitamin D supplementation in the form of a standard pediatric multivitamin should be provided to infants after 2 months of age.
6. Iron should be added to an infant's diet in the form of food or an iron supplement at approximately 6 months of age.

## Formula Feeding Guidelines

1. Infants should be fed iron-fortified formula—approximately 5–7 oz/kg (2.3–3.2 oz/lb) per day in the first 3 months of life and then 26–32 oz per day until 1 year old.

2. The actual amount of formula ingested and the accurateness of the preparation method (if applicable) should be assessed.
3. Proper bottle feeding technique should be assessed through continual observation in the first few weeks of life to determine if modifications are needed.
4. Supplementation with a standard pediatric multivitamin should be provided if the infant takes less than 16 oz (500 mL) of formula per day. Provide half a vitamin dose if formula intake is between 16 oz (500 mL) and 32 oz (1 L) per day.

## Solid Feeding Guidelines

1. Solid food should be introduced when the child is approximately 6 months of age. If the infant is not able to sit upright and coordinate masticating and swallowing of nonliquid foods, then solid foods should be delayed. An iron supplement is recommended for infants who are not receiving iron-fortified formula.
2. Infants should be monitored closely for excessive gagging, coughing, or other indicators of swallowing problems.
3. Infants who lose food through the nose should be given smaller bites each time and be fed more slowly until they learn to direct food more efficiently.
4. Infants should avoid foods that are acidic and spicy prior to and initially after surgical repair as these foods may be irritating to nasal passages and incision sites.
5. Small amounts of pureed food should be introduced slowly and one at a time. Iron-fortified cereal is usually recommended as the first food, then pureed vegetables, fruits, and meats as tolerated.
6. Juices should not be introduced until around age 7–9 months.
7. Cow's milk, honey, and eggs should not be introduced until age 12 months.
8. Finely chopped foods may be introduced at around 10–12 months of age if tolerated.
9. Nuts, seeds, hard pieces of fruit and vegetables, popcorn, hard candy, and hot dog wieners should not be fed to children younger than 2 years of age.

# References

About Face. (1992). *Making the difference.* Toronto, Ontario: Author.

Aldous, M. B. (1999). Nutritional issues for infants and toddlers. *Pediatric Annals, 28,* 101–105.

American Academy of Pediatrics, Committee on Fetus and Newborn, & American College of Obstetricians and Gynecologists. (1997). *Guidelines for perinatal care: Maternal and newborn nutrition.* Washington, DC: Authors.

American Academy of Pediatrics, Committee on Nutrition. (1989). Iron-fortified infant formulas. *Pediatrics, 84*(1, Pt. 1), 1114–1115.

American Academy of Pediatrics, Committee on Nutrition. (2004). *Pediatric nutrition handbook* (5th ed.). Elk Grove Village, IL.

American Academy of Pediatrics, Work Group on Breastfeeding. (1997). Breastfeeding and the use of human milk. *Pediatrics, 100,* 1035–1039.

American Cleft Palate-Craniofacial Association. (2000). *Parameters for evaluation and treatment of patients with cleft lip/palate or other craniofacial anomalies.* Retrieved September 19, 2007, from http://www.acpa-cpf.org/teamcare/Parameters00rev.pdf

American Nurses' Association. (1995). *Nursing's social policy statement.* Washington, DC: Author.

Aspinall, C. L. (2002). Dealing with the prenatal diagnosis of clefting: A parent's perspective. *Cleft Palate-Craniofacial Journal, 39,* 183–187.

Baer, M. T., & Harris, A. B. (1997). Pediatric nutrition assessment: Identifying children at risk. *Journal of the American Dietetic Association, 97*(10, Suppl. 2), S107–S115.

Balluff, M. A. (1986). Nutritional needs of an infant or child with a cleft lip or palate. *Ear, Nose and Throat Journal, 65,* 44–49.

Benacerraf, B. R., & Mulliken, J. B. (1993). Fetal cleft lip and palate: Sonographic diagnosis and postnatal outcome. *Plastic and Reconstructive Surgery, 92,* 1045–1051.

Bender, P. (2000). Genetics of cleft lip and palate. *Journal of Pediatric Nursing, 15,* 242–249.

Berk, N. W., Marazita, M. L., & Cooper, M. E. (1999). Medical genetics on the cleft palate-craniofacial team: Understanding parental preference. *Cleft Palate-Craniofacial Journal, 36,* 30–35.

Blumenfeld, Z., Blumenfeld, I., & Bronshtein, M. (1999, March). The early prenatal diagnosis of cleft lip and the decision-making process. *Cleft Palate-Craniofacial Journal, 36,* 105–107.

Bronshtein, M., Blumenfeld, I., & Blumenfeld, Z. (1996) Early prenatal diagnosis of cleft lip and its potential impact on the number of babies with cleft lip. *British Journal of Oral and Maxillofacial Surgery, 34,* 486–487.

Bronshtein, M., Mashiah, N., & Blumenfeld, Z. (1991). Pseudoprognathism—An auxillary sonographic sign for transvaginal sonographic diagnosis of cleft lip and palate in the early second trimester. *American Journal of Obstetrics and Gynecology, 165*(5, Pt. 1), 1314–1316.

Caretto, V. (1984). Maternal responses to an infant with cleft lip and palate: A review of the literature. *Maternal Child Nursing Journal, 10,* 197–205.

Cash, C., Set, P., & Coleman, N. (2001). The accuracy of antenatal ultrasound in the detection of facial clefts in a low-risk screening population. *Ultrasound in Obstetrics and Gynecology, 18,* 432–436.

Chapple, J. R., & Nunn, J. H. (2001). The oral health of children with clefts of the lip, palate, or both. *Cleft Palate-Craniofacial Journal, 38,* 525–528.

Chen, M. L., Chang, C. H., Yu, C. H., Cheng, Y. C., & Chang, F. M. (2001). Prenatal diagnosis of cleft palate by three-dimensional ultrasound. *Ultrasound in Medicine and Biology, 27,* 1017–1023.

Chitty, L. S., Hunt, G. H., Moore, J., & Lobb, M. (1991). Effectiveness of routine ultrasonography in detecting fetal structural abnormalities in low risk population. *British Medical Journal, 303*(6811), 1165–1169.

Chmait, R., Pretorius, D., Jones, M., Hull, A., James, G., Nelson, T., et al. (2002). Prenatal evaluation of facial clefts with two-dimensional and adjunctive three-dimensional ultrasonography: A prospective trial. *American Journal of Obstetrics and Gynecology, 187*(4), 946–949.

Christ, J. E., & Meininger, M. G. (1981). Ultrasound diagnosis of cleft lip and cleft palate before birth. *Journal of Plastic and Reconstructive Surgery, 68,* 854–859.

Clifford, E., & Crocker, E. C. (1971). Maternal responses: The birth of a normal child as compared to the birth of a child with a cleft. *Cleft Palate Journal, 8,* 289–304.

Croen, L. S., Shaw, G. M., Wasserman, C. R., & Tolarova, M. M. (1998). Racial and ethnic variations in the prevalence of orofacial clefts in California, 1983–1992. *American Journal of Medical Genetics, 79*(1), 42–47.

Curtin, G. (1990). The infant with cleft lip or palate: More than a surgical problem. *Journal of Perinatal and Neonatal Nursing, 3*(3), 80–89.

Davalbhakta, A., & Hall, P. N. (2000). The impact of antenatal diagnosis on the effectiveness and timing of counseling for cleft lip and palate. *British Journal of Plastic Surgery, 53,* 298–301.

Domet, M. J. (1986). The general pediatrician and the craniofacial defects team. *Ear, Nose and Throat Journal, 65*(7), 25–33.

Eglash, A., Kendall, S. K., & Fasher, J. (2005). What vitamins and minerals should be given to breastfed and bottle-fed infants? *Journal of Family Practice, 54,* 1089–1091.

Escott-Stump, S. (1992). *Nutrition and diagnosis-related care.* Philadelphia: Lea & Febiger.

Gartner, L. M., Greer, F. R., & Section on Breastfeeding and Committee on Nutrition. (2003). Prevention of rickets and vitamin D deficiency: New guidelines for vitamin D intake. *Pediatrics, 111*(4, Pt. 1), 908–910.

Gartner, L. M., Morton, J., Lawrence, R. A., Naylor, A. J., O'Hare, D., & Schanler, R. J. (2005). Breastfeeding and the use of human milk. *Pediatrics, 115,* 496–506.

Glass, R. P., & Wolf, L. S. (1999). Feeding management of infants with cleft lip and palate and micrognathia. *Infants and Young Children 12*(1), 70–81.

Hager, C. (2002). Termination of pregnancy with a prenatal diagnosis of cleft lip: Cultural differences and ethical analysis. *Plastic Surgical Nursing, 22*(1), 24–28.

Hall, R. T., & Carroll, R. E. (2000). Infant feeding. *Pediatrics in Review, 21,* 191–199.

Jensen, B. L., Dahl, E., & Kreiborg, S. (1983). Longitudinal study of body height, radius length and skeletal maturity in Danish boys with cleft lip and palate. *Scandinavian Journal of Dental Research, 91,* 473–481.

Jensen, B. L., Reiborg, S., Dahl, E., & Fogh-Andersen, P. (1988). Cleft lip and palate in Denmark, 1976–1981: Epidemiology, variability and early somatic development. *Cleft Palate Journal, 25,* 258–269.

Johnson, N., & Sandy, J. (2003). Prenatal diagnosis of cleft lip and palate. *Cleft Palate-Craniofacial Journal, 40,* 186–189.

Jones, M. C. (1999, March). Prenatal diagnosis of cleft lip and palate: Experiences in southern California. *Cleft Palate-Craniofacial Journal, 36,* 107–109.

Jones, M. C. (2002). Prenatal diagnosis of cleft lip and palate: Detection rates, accuracy of ultrasonography, associated anomalies and strategies for counseling. *Cleft Palate-Craniofacial Journal, 39,* 169–173.

Klein, M. D., & Delaney, T. A. (1994). *Feeding and nutrition for the child with special needs.* Austin, TX: PRO-ED.

Kleinman, R. E. (1998). *Pediatric nutrition handbook.* Elk Grove Village, IL: American Academy of Pediatrics.

Lee, J., Nunn, J., & Wright, C. (1997). Height and weight achievement in cleft lip and palate. *Archives of Disease in Childhood, 76*(1), 70–72.

Matthews, M. S. (2002). Beyond easy answers: The plastic surgeon and prenatal diagnosis. *Cleft Palate-Craniofacial Journal, 39,* 179–182.

Matthews, M. S., Cohen, M. B., Viglione, M., & Brown, A. S. (1998). Prenatal counseling for cleft lip and palate. *Plastic and Reconstructive Surgery, 101*(1), 1–5.

Mitchell, J. C., & Wood, R. J. (2000). Management of cleft lip and palate in primary care. *Journal of Pediatric Health Care, 14*(1), 13–19.

Nackashi, J. A., Dedlow, E. R., & Dixon-Wood, V. (1997). The craniofacial team: Health supervision and coordination. In K. R. Bzoch (Ed.), *Communicative disorders related to cleft lip and palate* (4th ed., pp. 169–190). Austin, TX: PRO-ED.

Pandya, A. N., & Boorman, J. G. (2001). Failure to thrive in babies with cleft lip and palate. *British Journal of Plastic Surgery, 54,* 471–475.

Paradise, J. L., Elster, B. A., & Tam, L. (1994). Evidence in infants with cleft palate that breast milk protects against otitis media. *Pediatrics, 94,* 853–860.

Pate, C. M. (1987). Care of the family following the birth of a child with a cleft lip and/or palate. *Neonatal Network, 5,* 30–37.

Powers, N. G. (2001). How to assess slow growth in the breastfed infant—Birth to 3 months. *Pediatric Clinics of North America, 48,* 345–363.

Ranalli, D. N., & Mazaheri, M. (1975). Height-weight growth of cleft children, birth to six years. *Cleft Palate Journal, 12,* 400–404.

Redford-Badwal, D. A., Mabry, K., & Frassinelli, J. D. (2003). Impact of cleft lip and/or palate on nutritional health and oral-motor development. *The Dental Clinics of North America, 47,* 305–317.

Rey-Bellet, C., & Hohlfeld, J. (2004). Prenatal diagnosis of facial clefts: Evaluation of a specialized counselling. *Swiss Medicine Weekly, 134,* 640–644.

Roberts, S. B., & Dallal, G. E. (2001). The new childhood growth charts. *Nutrition Reviews, 59*(2), 31–36.

Robinson, J. N., McElrath, T. F., Benson, C. B., Doubilet, P. M., Westgate, M. N., Holmes, L., et al. (2001). Prenatal ultrasonography and the diagnosis of fetal cleft lip. *Journal of Ultrasound Medicine, 20,* 1165–1170.

Roche, A. F., & Guo, S. (2001). The new growth charts. *Journal of Pediatric Nutrition and Development, 94,* 2–13.

Saal, H. M. (2002). Prenatal diagnosis: When the clinician disagrees with the patient's decision. *Cleft Palate-Craniofacial Journal, 39,* 174–179.

Shaikh, D., Mercer, N. S., Sohan, K., Kyle, P., & Soothill, P. (2001). Prenatal diagnosis of cleft lip and palate. *British Journal of Plastic Surgery, 54,* 288–289.

Shprintzen, R. J., Siegel-Sadowitz, V. L., Amato, J., & Goldberg, R. B. (1985). Anomalies associated with cleft lip, cleft palate, or both. *American Journal of Medical Genetics, 20,* 585–595.

Smith, A. S., Estroff, J. A., Barnewolt, C. E., Mulliken, J. B., & Levine, D. (2004). Prenatal diagnosis of cleft lip and cleft palate using MRI. *American Journal of Roentgenology, 183,* 229–235.

Standing Committee on Scientific Evaluation of Dietary Reference Intakes, Food and Nutrition Board, Institute of Medicine. (1997). *Dietary reference intakes for calcium, phosphorus, magnesium, vitamin D, and fluoride.* Washington, DC: National Academy Press.

Standing Committee on Scientific Evaluation of Dietary Reference Intakes, Food and Nutrition Board, Institute of Medicine. (2001). *Dietary reference intakes for vitamin A, vitamin K, arsenic, boron, chromium, copper, iodine, iron, manganese, molybdenum, nickel, silicon, vanadium, and zinc.* Washington, DC: National Academy Press.

Standing Committee on Scientific Evaluation of Dietary Reference Intakes, Food and Nutrition Board, Institute of Medicine. (2002). *Dietary reference intakes for energy, carbohydrate, fiber, fat, fatty acids, cholesterol, protein, and amino acids.* Washington, DC: National Academy Press.

Stoll, C., Alembik, Y., Dott, B., & Roth, M. P. (2000). Associated malformations in cases with oral clefts. *Cleft Palate-Craniofacial Journal, 37,* 41–47.

Strauss, R. P. (2002). Beyond easy answers: Prenatal diagnosis and counseling during pregnancy. *Cleft Palate-Craniofacial Journal, 39,* 164–168.

Tsang, R. C., Zlotkin, S. H., Nichols, B. L., & Hansen, J. W. (1997). *Nutrition during infancy: Principles and practice: Clinical skills for nutritional evaluation.* Cincinnati, OH: Digital Educational Publishing.

WHO Multicentre Growth Reference Study Group. (2006). WHO child growth standards based on length/height, weight, and age. *Acta Paediatrica Supplement, 450,* 76–85.

Wirt, S. W., Algren, C. L., & Arnold, S. L. (1992). Cleft lips and palates: A multidisciplinary approach. *Plastic Surgical Nursing, 12*(4), 140–147.

Wong, D. (1999). *Whaley and Wong's nursing care of infant and children* (6th ed.). St. Louis, MO: Mosby.

Young, J. L., O'Riordan, M., Goldstein, J. A., & Robin, N. H. (2001). What information do parents of newborns with cleft lip, palate, or both want to know? *Cleft Palate-Craniofacial Journal, 38,* 55–58.

Zlotkin, S. H. (1997). Clinical skills for nutritional evaluation. In R. C. Tsang, S. H. Zlotkin, B. L. Nichols, & J. W. Hansen (Eds.), *Nutrition during infancy: Principles and practice* (2nd ed., pp. 1–19). Cincinnati, OH: Digital Educational Publishing.

# CHAPTER 7

# Anatomy and Physiology of the Normal and Cleft Palate Speech Mechanism

*David L. Jones and Earl J. Seaver*

Jones and Seaver provide the reader with a selective review of the normal anatomy of the facial bones and the effect of a cleft on the muscles and physiology involved in speech production. They focus on velopharyngeal anatomy and discuss basic concepts of velopharyngeal function for speech. They stress the potential for interaction of muscles to bring about velopharyngeal closure for speech in speakers with normal and cleft structure.

1. List which skeletal bones are directly affected by a complete unilateral cleft lip and palate. What do Jones and Seaver say about more indirect effects of the cleft on other bones and muscles?
2. What are the potential speech and nonspeech consequences of an oral-nasal fistula?
3. Jones and Seaver stress two basic concepts regarding velopharyngeal closure and disordered nasalization of speech. What are these, and why do they consider them to be important?
4. According to Jones and Seaver, which velopharyngeal muscles control velopharyngeal closure, and how do these muscles interact?
5. How might the structural-motor differences of a cleft palate velopharyngeal mechanism hinder effective velopharyngeal closure for speech?
6. The authors discuss four patterns of velopharyngeal closure. What are they, and how do the velopharyngeal structures contribute to each pattern?

The production of normal speech is dependent upon the interaction between the form and function of the facial, mandibular, and palatopharyngeal structures. This chapter is designed to provide an abbreviated review and highlight those anatomic structures that are pertinent to cleft lip and palate and other craniofacial anomalies, and to discuss the effects of these anatomic abnormalities on oropharyngeal function for speech. Therefore, focus will be on the midfacial, palatal, and pharyngeal structures. A more comprehensive review of oropharyngeal anatomy can be obtained from Seikel, King, and Drumright (2005) and Zemlin (1998).

## Skeletal Characteristics: Normal

The midface and palate are made up of a complex matrix of bones, each of which is an important component in the overall structure of the face and mouth. The bones of the midface and palate serve as the framework for the oral and nasal cavities, as well as attachments for the soft tissues of the oral and nasal cavities, face, and orofacial musculature. Any abnormalities in bone structure can translate to (a) noticeable differences in facial appearance, (b) inadequate structure for the purpose of producing acceptable speech, and/or (c) possible deficiencies in the function of the orofacial musculature.

Figure 7.1 shows two views of the midfacial bones that are most "external." The most obvious, the maxillary bone, constitutes most of the upper jaw and hard palate. It serves as the base of the nasal cavity as well as the foundation for the soft tissues of the nose. The nasal bones are the two small bones that make up the "bridge" of the nose. The zygomatic bones are somewhat small bones that serve to couple the lateral aspects of the skull (temporal bones) to the medial-anterior aspect (the maxillary bone), thus forming the zygomatic arch. This combined structure serves as the framework for the base of the orbital cavity, and constitutes what is commonly referred to as the "cheekbone."

The left and right nasal cavities are separated by a structure that is referred to as the nasal septum (partition). The nasal septum consists of three parts. The superoanterior aspect is made up of septal cartilage, the inferior aspect is made up of the vomer bone, and the superoposterior aspect is comprised of the bony perpendicular plate of the ethmoid bone (see Figures 7.1–7.3).

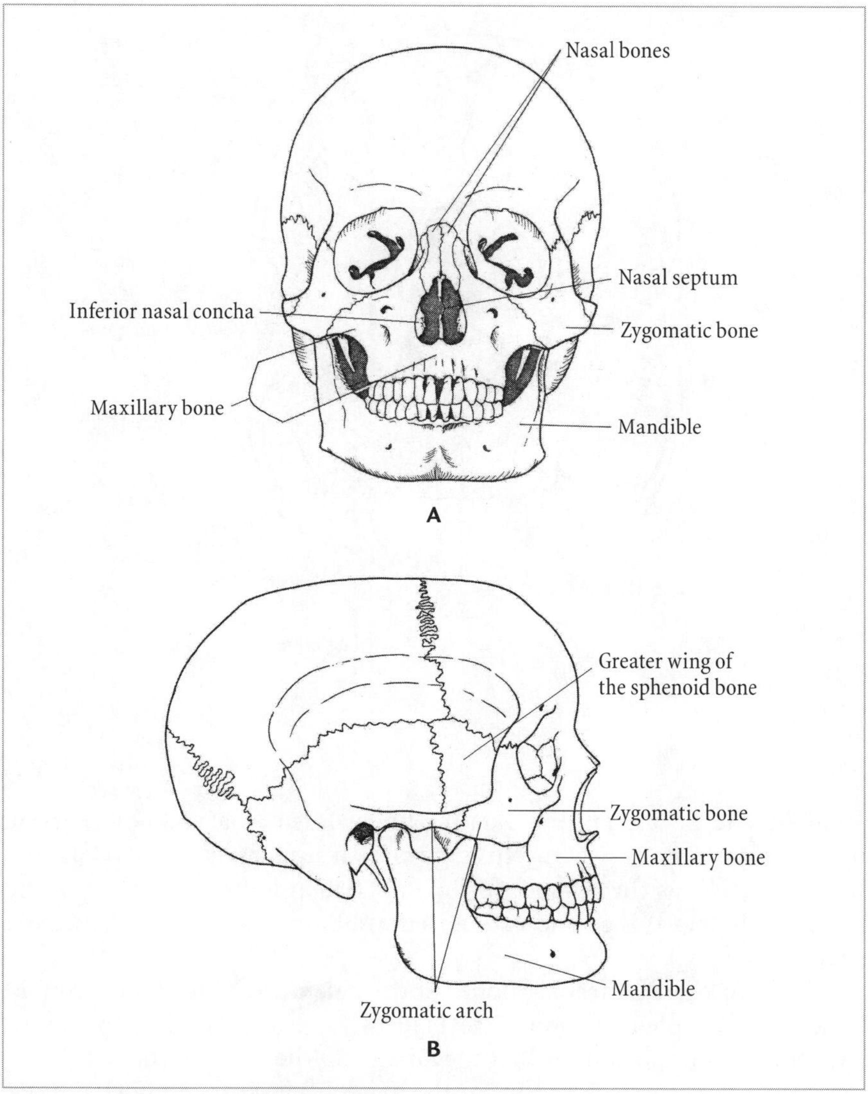


FIGURE 7.1. (A) Frontal view of skull. (B) Lateral view of skull.

Figure 7.2 shows a basal view of the normal palatal bone structure. The maxilla makes up the majority of the hard palate. The upper teeth erupt through the part of the maxilla that is called the alveolar process. Just posterior to the maxilla are the paired palatine bones. At their most

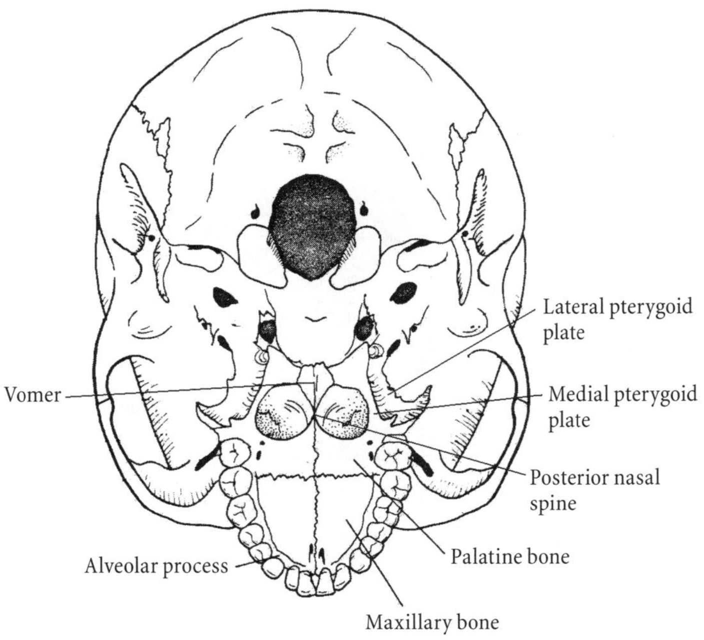


FIGURE 7.2. Basal view of skull.

medial-posterior aspect, the palatine bones form what is known as the posterior nasal spine (PNS). This landmark is important from a diagnostic perspective, as the absence of the PNS (when no overt clefting of the palate is observed) is an indication that a submucous cleft palate may be present.

The two most "internal" bones of the palatal structure, the ethmoid bone and the sphenoid bone (see Figures 7.2 and 7.3), are complex in structure and important in that they make up the walls of the nasal cavity and serve as the foundation for the base of the skull and posterior aspect of the midface. As noted previously, the perpendicular plate of the ethmoid is part of the nasal septum. On either side of the septum lie the middle and superior conchae (turbinates), which form most of the lateral walls of the nasal cavity. Among other structural roles, the sphenoid bone forms the pharyngeal cavity and the posterior part of the lateral walls of the nasal cavities. For the purpose of this discussion, perhaps the most

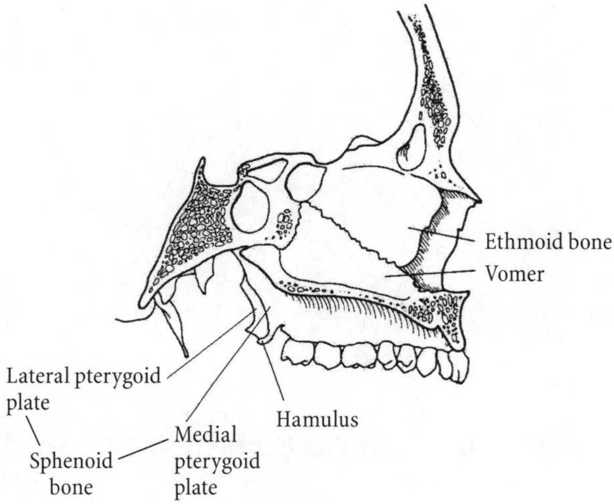


Figure 7.3. Medial view of left half of skull.

notable structures of the sphenoid are the medial pterygoid (winglike) plates. Each medial pterygoid plate descends inferiorly and terminates in a bony process called the hamulus. Although small in size, the hamulus serves an important role, as it is the point at which the tensor veli palatini muscle pivots as it courses from the palatal aponeurosis (inelastic broad, flat tissue connecting muscle to muscle or muscle to bone) to the auditory (eustachian) tube.

The mandible (Figure 7.4) is a relatively large bone that is critical for both mastication and speech. A number of muscles insert into or originate from various points along this bone. The structures to be highlighted include the ramus, which gives the mandible its height; the corpus (body), which comprises the anterolateral aspect and the alveolar process from which the lower teeth erupt; the coronoid process, to which the temporalis muscle attaches; and the condylar process, which articulates with the temporal bone to form the temporomandibular joint. During the production of speech, the mandible slides and rotates to change the positions of the tongue, lower lip, and vocal tract.

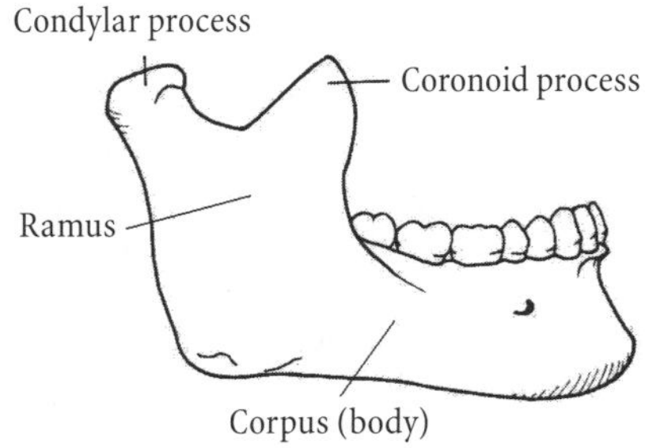


FIGURE 7.4. Lateral view of right side of mandible.

## Muscular Characteristics: Normal

As indicated earlier in this chapter, the production of normal speech is dependent on the interaction between the form and function of the facial, mandibular, and palatopharyngeal structures. The movements of the structures described previously for normal speech production are dependent on the control of the musculature of the oral-facial region.

The muscles of the lips are important for feeding, facial expressions, and the production of speech, along with providing forces that may contribute to dental alignment and development. During speech, the muscles of the lips are used for the production of the labial consonants (/p/, /b/, /f/, /v/) and for lip configuration (rounding and spread) for vowels (/u/ vs. /i/).

The orbicularis oris (Figure 7.5) muscle is typically viewed as the primary muscle of the lips. It is a complex muscle with fibers that are both intrinsic and extrinsic. The intrinsic fibers are contained within the structure of the lips and act as a sphincter upon contraction. This action results in a narrowing of the oral opening and a rounding (puckering) of the lips. There are a considerable number of extrinsic muscles that can affect the control of the lips. Two of the more prominent are the buccinator and risorius muscles (Figures 7.5 and 7.6). The buccinator muscles run from the corners of the upper and lower lips posteriorly and comprise the muscles of the cheeks. Contraction of these muscles pulls the edges of the lips to the side, resulting in a spreading as occurs in the production of the vowel /i/. The risorius muscles run parallel to those of the buccinator,

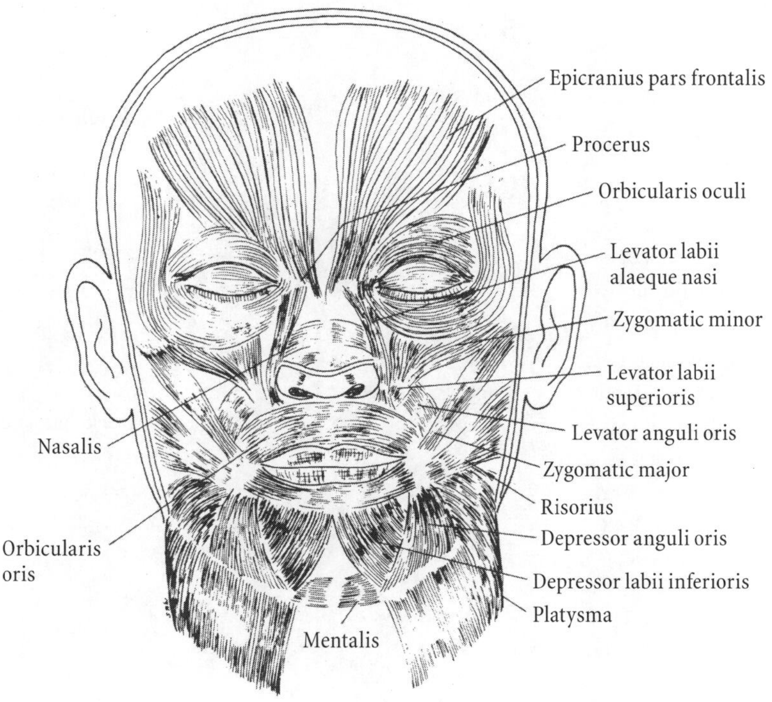


FIGURE 7.5. Frontal view of facial musculature. *Note.* From *Speech and Hearing Science: Anatomy and Physiology* (3rd ed., p. 230), by W. R. Zemlin, 1998, Boston: Allyn & Bacon. Copyright 1998 by Allyn & Bacon. Reprinted with permission.

also inserting into the corners of the lips, and their contraction results in a spread of the lips.

The muscles of the mandible function to change the positions of the tongue and lower lip and alter the shape of the vocal tract. All of these movements occur around the temporomandibular joint, which is formed by the condyle of the mandible and the temporal bone. For speech purposes, the muscles of the mandible can be divided into those that elevate the mandible (close the oral cavity) and those that depress the mandible (open the oral cavity). The muscles that function to elevate the mandible include the masseter, temporalis, and medial pterygoid (see Figures 7.7 and 7.8). The masseter muscle originates on the zygomatic arch (cheek bone) and inserts mostly into the ramus of the mandible. The temporalis

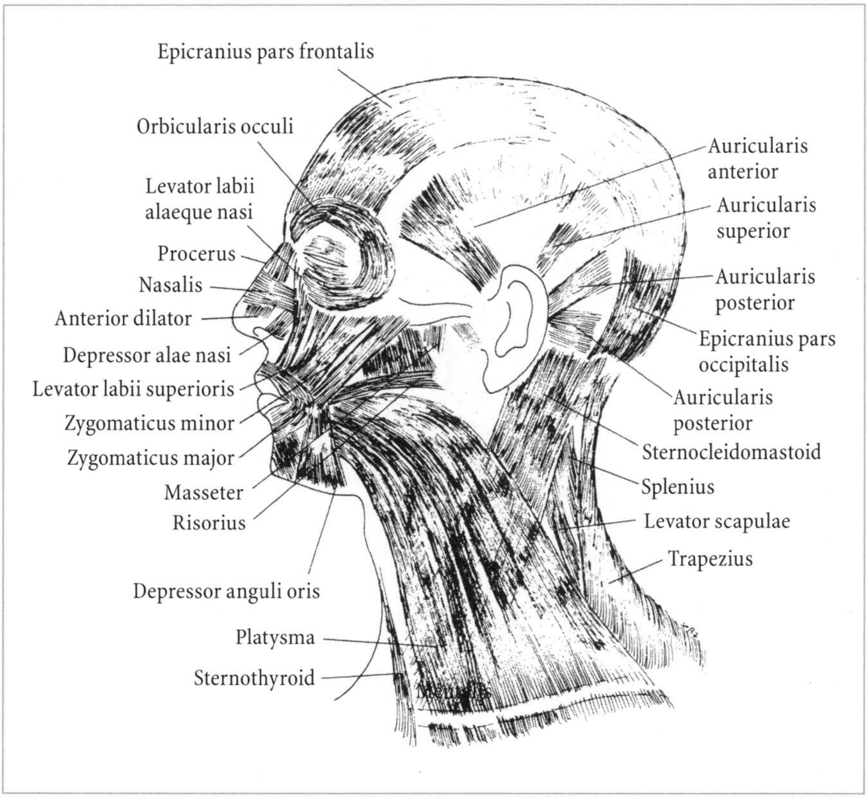


FIGURE 7.6. Lateral view of facial musculature and view of pterygomandibular ligament. *Note.* From *Speech and Hearing Science: Anatomy and Physiology* (3rd ed., p. 231), by W. R. Zemlin, 1998, Boston: Allyn & Bacon. Copyright 1998 by Allyn & Bacon. Reprinted with permission.

originates on the temporal and parietal surfaces of the skull and inserts into the ramus and coronoid process of the mandible. The muscle fibers of medial pterygoid run between the medial pterygoid plate of the sphenoid bone and the ramus of the mandible. All of the muscles that elevate serve to raise the mandible toward the more stable insertions of the muscles on the bones of the skull and face.

The muscles that serve to lower the mandible include the digastricus, mylohyoid, geniohyoid, and lateral pterygoid (see Figures 7.9 and 7.10). The two portions of the digastricus, anterior and posterior bellies, originate from the inner surface of the mandible and the mastoid process of

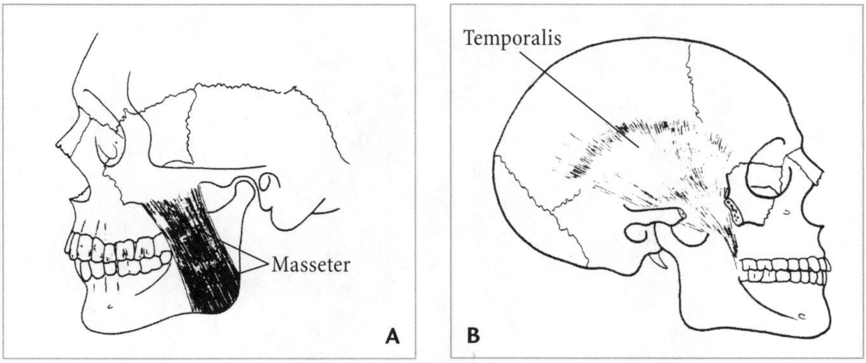


FIGURE 7.7. Masseter (A) and temporalis (B) muscles. *Note.* From *Anatomy and Physiology for Speech, Language, and Hearing: Instructor's Version* (2nd ed., p. 330), by J. A. Seikel, D. W. King, and D. G. Drumright, 2005, Clifton Park, NY: Thompson Learning. Copyright 2005 by Thompson Learning. Reprinted with permission.

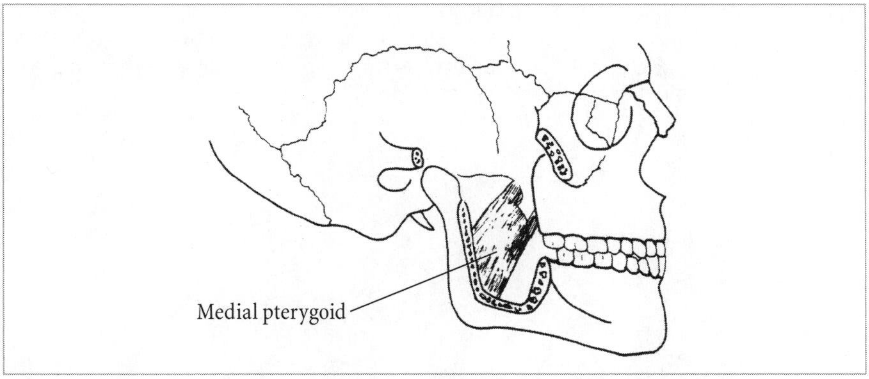


FIGURE 7.8. Pterygoid muscles. *Note.* From *Anatomy and Physiology for Speech, Language, and Hearing: Instructor's Version* (2nd ed., p. 331), by J. A. Seikel, D. W. King, and D. G. Drumright, 2005, Clifton Park, NY: Thompson Learning. Copyright 2005 by Thompson Learning. Reprinted with permission.

the sphenoid bone, respectively, and insert into the hyoid bone located just superior to the larynx. Both the mylohyoid and geniohyoid muscles run along the floor of the mouth from the mandible to the hyoid bone. The lateral pterygoid muscle originates from the sphenoid bone and inserts into the inner surface of the mandible on the condyle. Contraction of this muscle will cause the mandible to protrude as well as close the oral cavity.

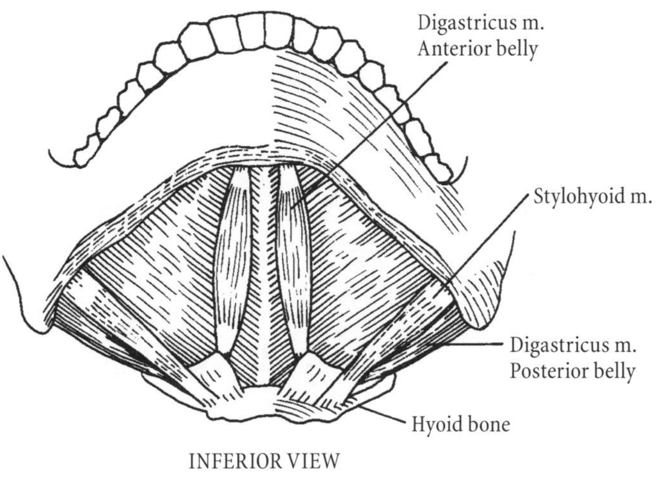


FIGURE 7.9. Inferior view of suprahyoid musculature. *Note.* From *Anatomy and Physiology for Speech, Language, and Hearing: Instructor's Version* (2nd ed., p. 204), by J. A. Seikel, D. W. King, and D. G. Drumright, 2005, Clifton Park, NY: Thompson Learning. Copyright 2005 by Thompson Learning. Reprinted with permission.

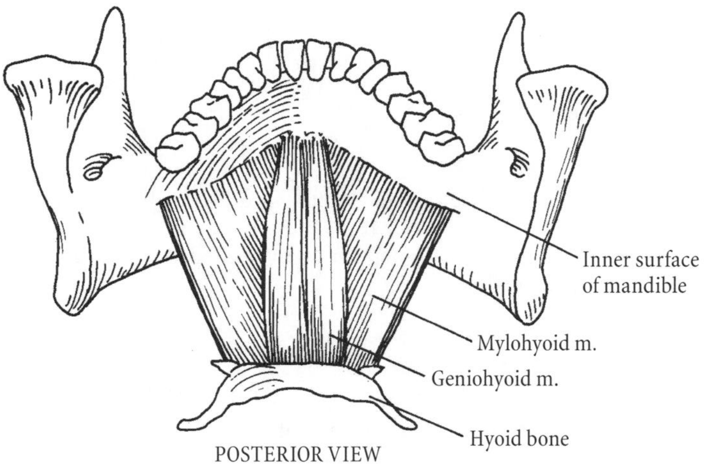


FIGURE 7.10. Posterior view of suprahyoid musculature. *Note.* From *Anatomy and Physiology for Speech, Language, and Hearing: Instructor's Version* (2nd ed., p. 205), by J. A. Seikel, D. W. King, and D. G. Drumright, 2005, Clifton Park, NY: Thompson Learning. Copyright 2005 by Thompson Learning. Reprinted with permission.

The tongue is a complex structure that is important for chewing, swallowing, and taste, along with providing forces that counter those provided by the lips and that contribute to dental alignment and development. The tongue is considered the single most important structure for the production of speech. The functioning of the tongue is controlled by a series of intrinsic and extrinsic muscles. A comprehensive description of these muscles can be found in the two speech anatomy texts listed at the end of this chapter. Two extrinsic muscles, the palatoglossus and palatopharyngeus, will be described later (see Figure 7.17) as to their relationship to velopharyngeal functioning. The lingual frenulum (Figure 7.11) is located under the tongue, running from the floor of the mouth to the tongue surface. On occasion the frenulum may be attached near the tip of the tongue, giving the impression of restricted tongue movement (i.e., tongue tied). In most cases, the individual is able to gain sufficient tongue elevation for the production of lingual consonants and does not require any intervention.

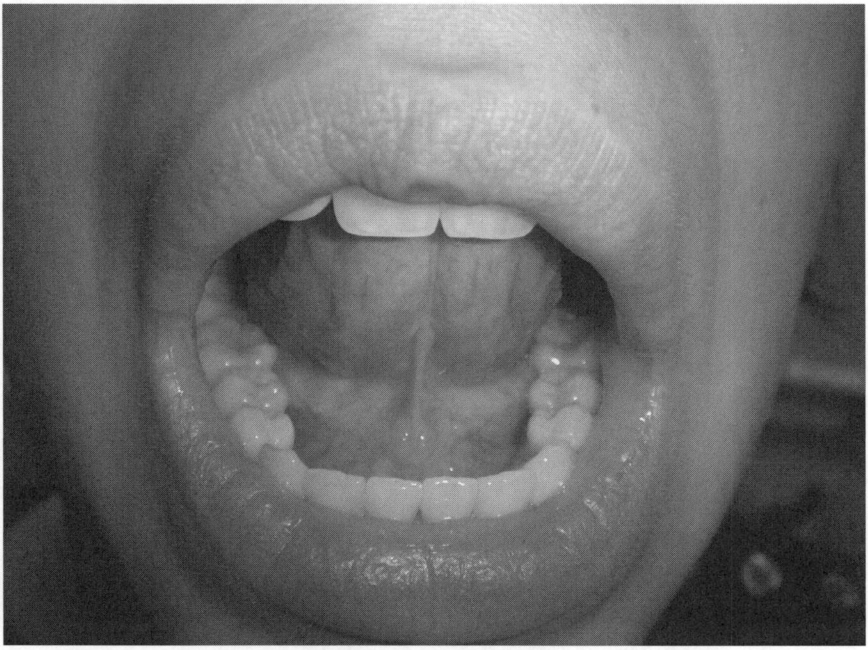

Figure 7.11. Oral view of lingual frenulum.

# Skeletal and Muscular Abnormalities: Cleft Palate

Most of the bony structures described earlier are directly or indirectly affected by the occurrence of a cleft palate (see, e.g., Figure 7.15, which shows the basic difference between a normal palate [view A] and a cleft palate at birth [view B]). Obviously, the maxillary and palatine bones are directly affected. Furthermore, because these bones are not positioned normally, the bones with which they articulate may not be positioned normally. For instance, because there is nothing with which to fuse at midline, the nasal septal cartilage, vomer, and perpendicular plate of the ethmoid may deviate to one side, resulting in a deviated nasal septum. Most importantly, the skeletal anomalies result in abnormal positioning of the musculature that is critical for normal velopharyngeal function.

## Functional Aspects: Skeletal Abnormalities in Cleft Palate

As stated previously, one consequence of the bony abnormality associated with cleft palate or other craniofacial anomalies is inadequate structure for the purpose of producing acceptable speech. The most significant structural problem involves the maxillary bone. Abnormalities include maxillary arch collapse, residual alveolar clefting, and oral-nasal fistulae following surgical repair. Each of these is easily identified during an oral peripheral examination. Maxillary arch collapse is characterized by a malpositioning of the anterior and/or lateral/posterior aspects of the dental arch in the lingual direction. In other words, the anterior and lateral/posterior maxillary teeth are posterior and medial, respectively, to the mandibular teeth, resulting in what is commonly referred to as an underbite, Class III malocclusion, or lingual crossbite (see Figure 7.12). When maxillary arch collapse is severe, lingual-alveolar articulation can be difficult because the reduced space within the oral cavity makes it difficult for the tongue to achieve precise alveolar placements. Labiodental articulation for /f/ and /v/ can also be more difficult, as the lower lip must be positioned posteriorly in order to approximate the retracted upper incisors. Fortunately, most patients demonstrate only a mild degree of maxillary arch collapse that can contribute to mild distortions of sibilants and affricates. Maxillary arch collapse can be treated with orthodontic

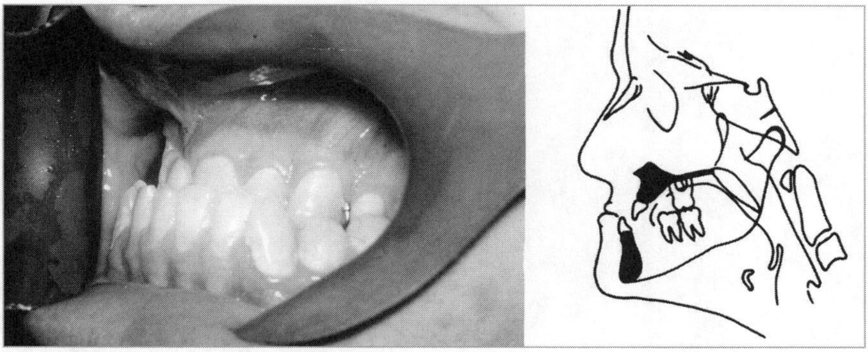

Figure 7.12. A Class III malocclusion.

intervention. For more severe upper to lower jaw discrepancies, orthognathic surgery may be required (see Chapter 16 by Williams and Bevis and Chapter 17 by Swift). Severe arch collapse is usually seen in cases where (a) the cleft palate was quite severe at birth and involved both sides, (b) the palate repair was not performed adequately, or (c) circumstances related to situation (a) or (b) were coupled with a lack of follow-up treatment by an orthodontist.

A residual alveolar cleft is shown in Figure 7.13. Surgical closure is usually performed when a child is 5–9 years of age. An alveolar cleft can occur unilaterally or bilaterally. The presence of an alveolar cleft translates to a lack of bony support and continuity for the maxillary dental arch, which can lead to maxillary arch collapse in the region of the defect. Also, teeth in the area of the cleft can be missing, malformed, and malpositioned. An alveolar cleft can have a negative effect on speech in one of two ways. First, when lingual-alveolar articulation is required, the tongue can protrude into the alveolar gap(s). Second, if the tongue cannot achieve a central constriction during the production of sibilants and affricates, airflow is likely to escape through the alveolar gap(s), resulting in a distortion of these consonants. Following surgical closure of the alveolar cleft and orthodontic alignment of teeth in the anterior maxillary area, articulation improvement is usually facilitated.

An oral-nasal fistula is an opening in the hard palate that communicates directly with the nasal cavity (see Figure 7.14A). It can also occur within the soft palate, but it is more commonly observed in the hard palate area. This fistula usually occurs as a result of a breakdown in the surgical repair of the palate. An oral-nasal fistula can vary in size and location

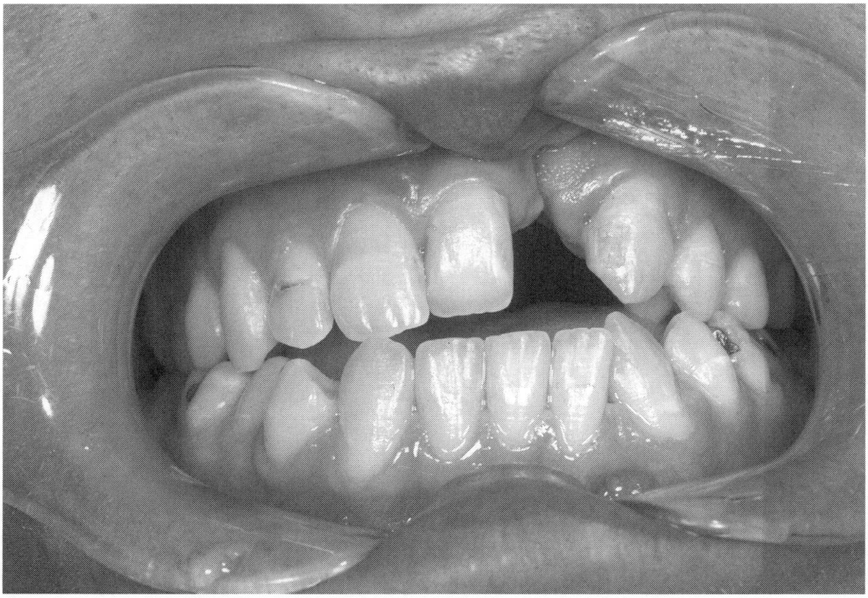

FIGURE 7.13. Alveolar cleft.

as well as its effect on speech. A nonspeech consequence of a fistula can be loss of food and/or liquids into the nose. It is not unusual for a fistula to be symptomatic for food and/or liquid loss, but not for speech. If a fistula affects speech, it will manifest itself as audible nasal emission of air or nasal turbulence during the production of pressure consonants that require an articulatory constriction anterior to the fistula. For example, in Figure 7.14B, audible nasal air emission would likely occur during production of anterior stops and fricatives, but not during production of the velar stops /k/ and /g/ because the articulatory constriction would occur posterior to the fistula. The perceptual effect of an oral-nasal fistula can be attributed erroneously to velopharyngeal inadequacy. However, when a fistula is sufficiently large, it can have a negative effect on velopharyngeal function (Isberg & Henningsson, 1987).

The mandible is not structurally abnormal in patients with cleft lip and palate; however, when a midfacial deficiency is present, it can result in a significant jaw discrepancy between the mandible and maxilla. Although it can appear that the mandible is too large (too far forward), it is generally the case that the maxilla is too small (retracted). In an attempt

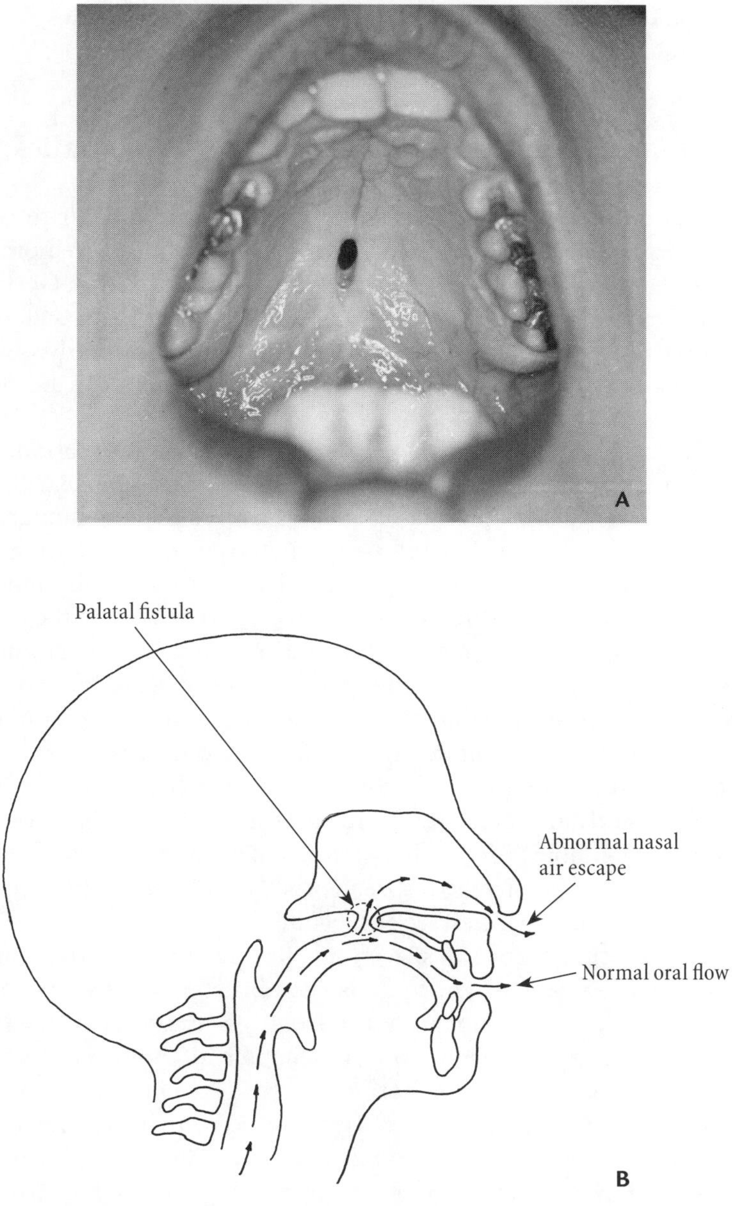


FIGURE 7.14. (A) Oral view of an oronasal fistula. (B) Aerodynamic consequence of an anterior oronasal fistula. When articulatory constriction is anterior to the fistula, air will escape through the fistula and nasal emission will result.

to compensate for the maxillary deficiency, mandibular movement patterns (e.g., during speech or chewing) may be altered, which can sometimes result in temporomandibular joint dysfunction.

## Skeletal Abnormalities: Other Craniofacial Anomalies

There are a number of craniofacial anomalies that can occur in the absence of cleft palate, but that involve deficiencies in the development of the midface and/or mandible. Conversely, and as discussed by Gorlin and Baylis in Chapter 5, there are perhaps over 350 syndromes in which clefting is a part. Only those conditions that are most commonly observed are discussed here, and photographs of these disorders can be seen in Chapter 5.

Unlike other conditions that will be mentioned in this section, Robin sequence (see Figures 5.10 and 5.11 in Chapter 5) is a craniofacial anomaly in which a cleft palate is present. The two features that set it apart from a "typical" cleft palate include glossoptosis (posterior positioning of the tongue into the pharyngeal airway) and micrognathia (small mandible). Because many of the attachments of the tongue are related to the position of the mandible, it is reasonable to conclude that posterior positioning of the tongue into the pharyngeal airway is due to the posterior position of the mandible. For an infant with Robin sequence, the tongue-mandible involvement can result in upper airway obstruction. In severe cases, surgical movement of the mandible forward or a tracheostomy may be required. Frequently, however, the discrepancy in size and/or position of the maxilla and mandible becomes less significant as the child grows. Thus, it does not introduce problems for speech production that are different from those of individuals with cleft lip and palate.

Oculo-auriculo-vertebral spectrum, also referred to as hemifacial microsomia or Goldenhar syndrome, is a condition in which one side of the craniofacial skeleton does not grow as normally as the other side, resulting in facial asymmetry (see Figure 5.19 in Chapter 5). However, the lack of normal development can be on both sides (see Chapter 5). Neuromuscular deficits are also evident on the affected side, which can affect movements of the tongue, soft palate, and mandible. The ear on the affected side usually shows some degree of malformation. Although clefting may also occur, it is not common. The craniofacial asymmetry can result in a significant dental malocclusion, which, when combined with hemiparesis of the tongue and/or soft palate, can result in marked distortions of consonants that require lingual articulation and/or velopharyngeal closure.

Craniofacial dysostosis, also called Crouzon syndrome (see Figure 5.15 in Chapter 5), is a disorder that consists of a bony deficiency in the midfacial region (also referred to as midfacial hypoplasia). The deficiency of bone is evident not only in the region of the maxilla but also in the orbital region, resulting in exophthalmos (the appearance of bulging eyes) and, in many cases, hypertelorism (eyes too far apart). It is common for the head to be abnormal in shape because some of the cranial sutures fuse prematurely during development. The hard palate is usually narrow and high arched; this, along with the typical severe underbite (Class III, anterior crossbite), can result in distortions of any consonants that require lingual articulation.

Mandibulofacial dysostosis, or Treacher Collins syndrome (see Figures 5.16–5.18 in Chapter 5), is one of the more severe craniofacial disorders with regard to its effect on speech production. The three most notable characteristics of this disorder are (a) significant micrognathia, (b) hypoplasia in the region of the zygomatic arch, and (c) malformations of the ears and hearing loss. In many cases, the mandibular hypoplasia is severe enough that a tracheostomy is required. Unlike in Pierre Robin sequence, the mandible in Treacher Collins does not "catch up" to the maxilla as the child grows, which results in significant problems with regard to speech production. Approximately 30% of patients with mandibulofacial dysostosis have a cleft palate (Jones, 1997; Peterson-Falzone & Pruzansky, 1976). The posterior positioning of the mandible and tongue, combined with velopharyngeal issues, results in a marked muffled-sounding resonance. In addition, lingual-alveolar articulation can be problematic because of the severe malocclusion (open bite) that usually accompanies this disorder.

## Velopharyngeal Anatomy

The velopharyngeal mechanism is made up of a complex system of muscles, tendons, and skeletal structures used to control the oral versus nasal distinction during speech. This section focuses on the muscles that can be used to control velopharyngeal closure during speech.

The levator veli palatini is considered to be the primary muscle of velar elevation and thereby is probably the most important muscle for velopharyngeal closure for oral speech production. This paired muscle originates from the petrous portion of the temporal bone and from the medial portion of the eustachian tube. The fibers on each side course in an inferior-anterior-medial direction to insert into the velum, blending with the fibers from the opposite side on the dorsal side of the velum, thereby forming a muscular sling (see Figures 7.15 and 7.16). Contraction of the levator veli palatini will result in the pulling of the velum toward the fixed attachment on the temporal bone, causing the velum to elevate toward the posterior wall of the pharynx (see Figure 7.16A).

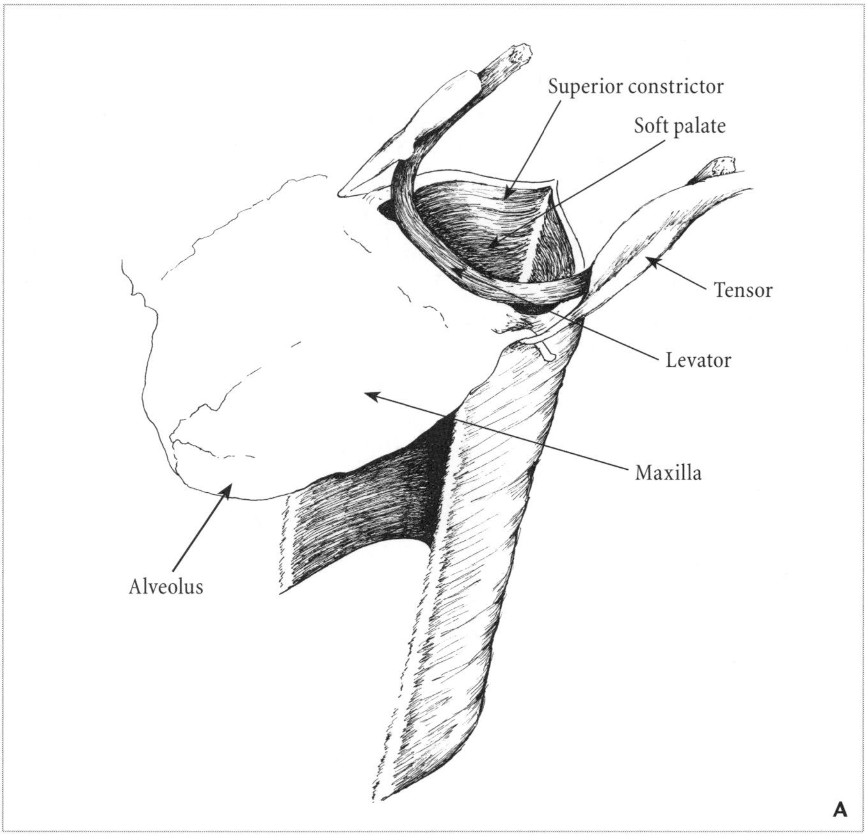


FIGURE 7.15. (A) Normal velopharyngeal musculature.

The tensor veli palatini, or tensor (see 7.15, 7.16A, and 7.16C), is a paired muscle that arises from the base of the skull at the medial pterygoid plates of the sphenoid and the lateral sides of the eustachian tubes. The fibers on each side form a tendon and wrap around the hamular processes of the sphenoid bones and broaden as they insert into the velum, forming the palatal aponeurosis. Fibers of the aponeurosis insert into the posterior portion of the hard palate. The aponeurosis forms a base for the attachment of other muscles, and it may serve as an anchor for muscles to work against. The tensor veli palatini serves no function during speech production. Contraction of this muscle serves to dilate the eustachian tube, resulting in pressure equalization in the middle ear cavity.

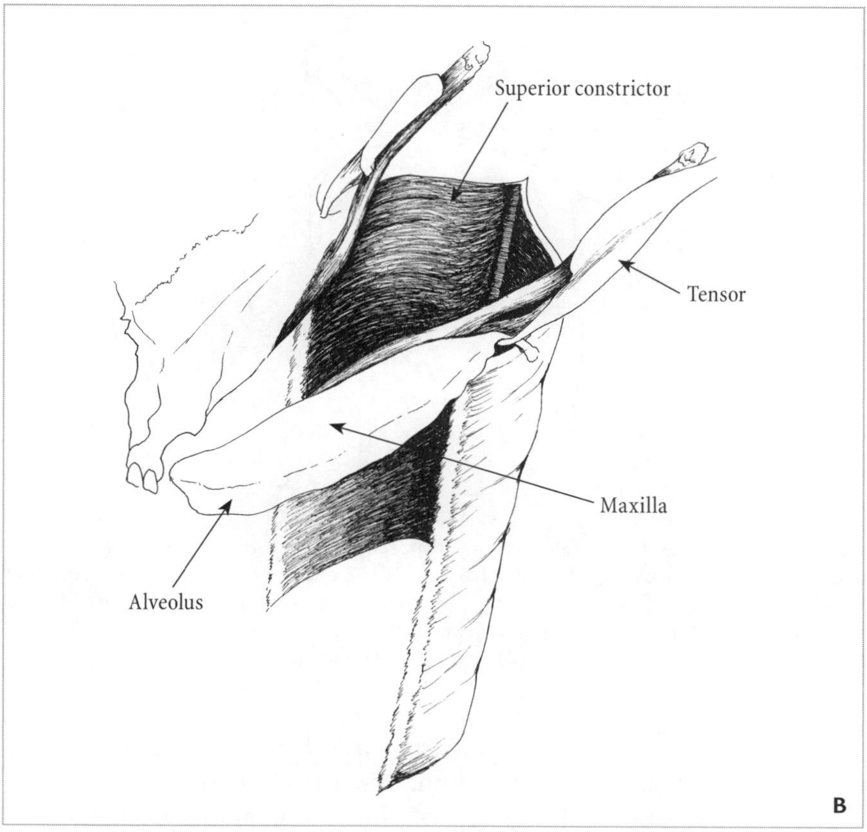


Figure 7.15. (B) Velopharyngeal musculature of the cleft palate.

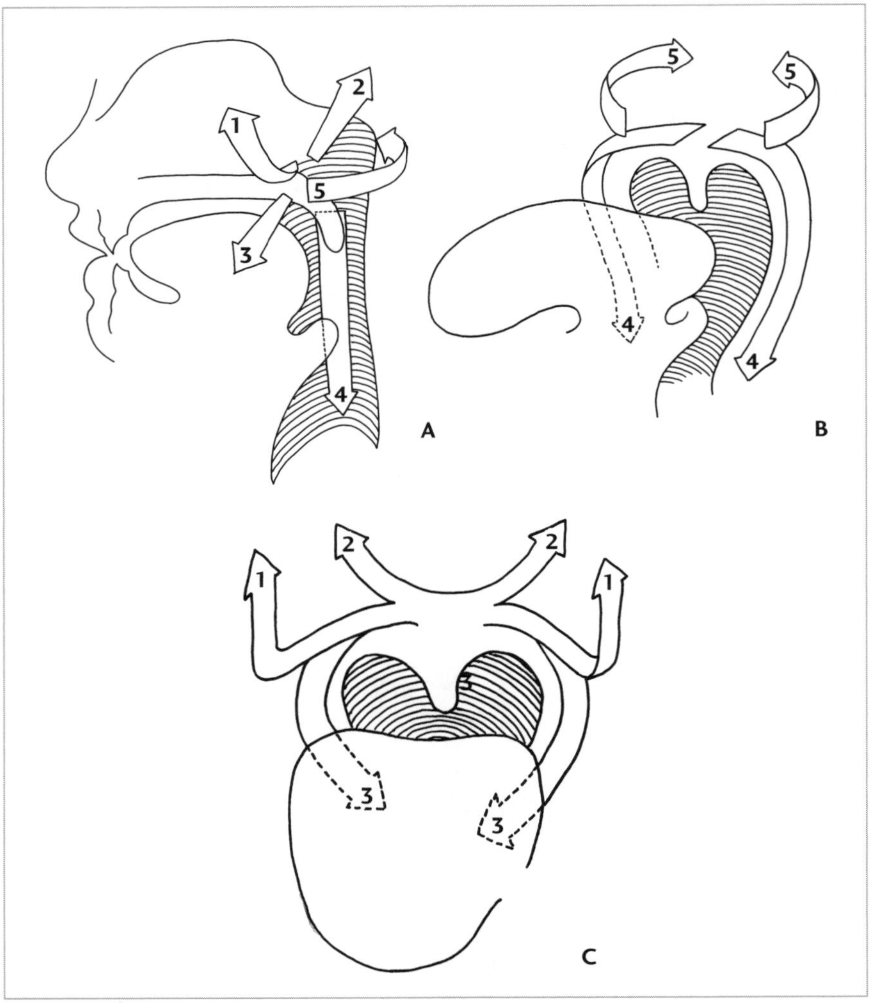


FIGURE 7.16. (A) Lateral view: Velopharyngeal muscle forces for tensor palatini (1); levator palatini (2); palatoglossus (3); palatopharyngeus (4); and superior pharyngeal constrictor (5). (B) Oblique view: Velopharyngeal muscle forces for palatopharyngeus (4) and superior pharyngeal constrictor (5). (C) Coronal view: Velopharyngeal muscle forces for tensor palatini (1); levator palatini (2); and palatoglossus (3).

The musculus uvulae is a paired muscle that forms the bulk of the superior (dorsal) surface of the velum. This muscle arises laterally to the posterior nasal spine of the hard palate in the region of the palatal aponeurosis and courses posteriorly to insert into the uvula. Contraction provides bulk to the superior surface of the velum, possibly assisting in achieving midline closure.

The palatoglossus muscles form the anterior faucial pillars (see Figures 7.16C and 7.17). The muscle fibers course superiorly from the longitudinal fibers of the tongue on each side and course to insert near the palatal aponeurosis on the inferior surface of the velum. The fibers from each side intermingle in the velum. Contraction of this muscle will produce a force (see Figure 7.16) that is in opposition to that provided by the

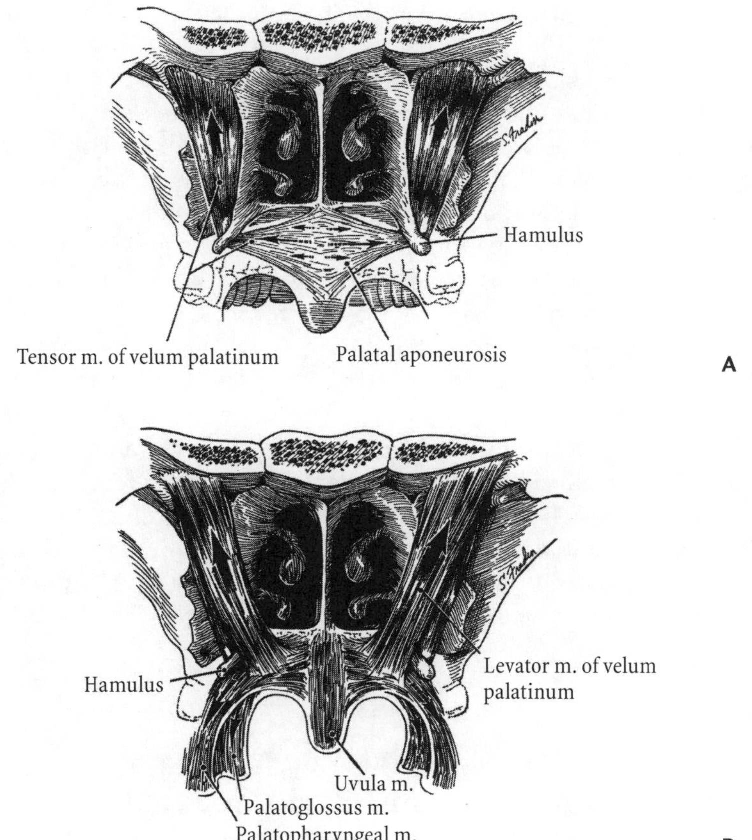


FIGURE 7.17. Posterior views of the soft palate. *Note.* From *Dental Prosthetics,* by R. J. Nagel and V. H. Sears, 1958, St Louis, MO: Mosby. Copyright 1958 by Mosby. Reprinted with permission.

levator veli palatini muscle (Moon, Smith, Folkins, Lemke, & Gartlan, 1994; Seaver & Kuehn, 1980).

The palatopharyngeus muscles are complex muscles, which may be thought of as consisting of two portions. Both portions comprise the posterior faucial pillars (see Figure 7.17B). The fibers, on both sides, arise from the velum laterally, while others arise from the walls of the pharynx. Both sets of fibers approximate in the midline of the velum and course down through the faucial pillars. One set of fibers continues to course inferiorly to insert into the thyroid cartilage. The positioning of the fibers of the palatopharyngeus would suggest that the muscle provides force (see Figure 7.16) in opposition to that provided by the levator muscle (Moon et al., 1994; Seaver & Kuehn, 1980). This muscle is probably important for swallowing.

Muscles of the pharynx also play an important role in controlling velopharyngeal opening. The superior constrictor muscle and the salpingopharyngeus muscle are likely the most significant in contributing to velopharyngeal activity. The superior constrictor muscle (see Figure 7.15) is a complex muscle of the pharynx consisting of different muscle bundles. Distinct portions of this muscle include the pterygopharyngeus, buccopharyngeus, mylopharyngeus, and glossopharyngeus muscles. Of these, the pterygopharyngeal portion, arising from the pterygoid plate and the hamular processes on both sides and inserting into the midline of the pharynx, is probably best situated to control the diameter of the pharynx in the area of the nasopharynx. This activity (see Figure 7.16) would reduce the size of the nasopharynx, assisting the velum in achieving velopharyngeal closure. In speakers believed to have inadequate velar tissue for closure, it is believed that the superior constrictor is responsible for the development of a localized anteriorly directed movement of the pharyngeal wall (Passavant's pad or ridge) as a form of compensation to narrow the velopharyngeal gap.

## The Velopharyngeal Speech Mechanism: Basic Concepts

When presented with a patient who demonstrates disordered nasalization, it is easy to draw conclusions regarding what the velopharyngeal mechanism may or may not be doing during speech. However, it is important to stress two basic concepts regarding velopharyngeal function and the perception of disordered nasalization. First, the preceding review of the velopharyngeal muscle anatomy should help to emphasize the fact that just as in other human motor activities, the closing and opening of the velopharyngeal port occur due to an interaction between a number of active and passive forces within the oropharynx. Second, when determining the cause of disordered nasalization, it is often necessary to consider the structural *and* functional aspects of the entire speech production system, not just the velopharyngeal mechanism.

### Velopharyngeal Gap Size and Nasality

There are two erroneous assumptions commonly made regarding velopharyngeal function and excessively nasal speech: (1) that the presence of hypernasality means there is a lack of velopharyngeal closure during speech, and (2) that the severity of hypernasality is directly related to the size of the velopharyngeal opening. Both of these clinical assumptions are based on the broader theoretical assumption that the perception of hypernasality is related solely to the presence and/or size of the velopharyngeal opening. *This is not the case.* Numerous studies have attempted to show the relationship between measures of velopharyngeal gap size and perceived nasality (Blackfield, Miller, Owsley, & Lawson, 1962a, 1962b; Carney & Morris, 1971; Dickson, 1969; Hagerty & Hoffmeister, 1954; Mazaheri, Millard, & Erickson, 1964; Subtelny, Koepp-Baker, & Subtelny, 1961). In general, these studies failed to show a strong correlation between the two measures. Acoustic studies of nasalization (Fant, 1960; House & Stevens, 1956) have demonstrated that nasality is related to the acoustic impedance of the nasal cavity relative to the acoustic impedance of the oral cavity. By moving the articulators, speakers manipulate the nasal-oral impedance relationship from moment to moment. This explains why phonetic context influences the degree of perceived nasality (Carney & Sherman, 1971; Moore & Sommers, 1973; Spriestersbach & Powers, 1959).

### Muscle Interaction

In a review of the anatomy and physiology of velopharyngeal movement, Fritzell (1969) presented the hypothetical actions of the velopharyngeal muscles, which are shown in Figure 7.16. While the action of the levator veli palatini is to pull the soft palate in a superoposterior direction (i.e., toward velopharyngeal closure), the palatoglossus and palatopharyngeus muscles act to pull down on the soft palate. Studies by Seaver and Kuehn (1980) and Kuehn, Folkins, and Cutting (1982) have shown that all three of these muscles are active during the act of velopharyngeal closure. Although it might appear that the palatoglossus and palatopharyngeal muscles are working against the levator muscle, this functional relationship appears to allow for better control of velar movement and position during speech. In other words, these muscle *interactions* are part of a normal process in the production of speech in individuals with normal structures.

Kuehn, Folkins, and Linville (1988) showed that the musculus uvulae is also active and in synchrony with the levator veli palatini during speech. They hypothesized that contraction of the musculus uvulae might serve two purposes. First, it might add bulk to the nasal surface of the soft palate, which results in more tissue available to close the velopharyngeal port. Second, given its position relative to the levator veli palatini, it may also function to increase velar stiffness so that the levator sling will have a stiffer surface to pull against, thereby maximizing the effect of levator muscle force and the control of velar movement. The reader is referred to Kuehn and Moller (2000) for a more detailed discussion of velopharyngeal anatomy and physiology.

## Velar Stretch

When the speech mechanism is viewed in the lateral plane via videofluoroscopy or lateral still X-ray, it appears that the soft palate increases in length as it moves toward the posterior pharyngeal wall. This phenomenon, known as velar stretch, is a common observation in speakers without cleft palate. Several studies have measured the degree of velar stretch in normal speakers. Simpson and Austin (1972) showed that the velum increased in length by an average of 20% in their adult subjects. Mourino and Weinberg (1975) found a lesser degree of stretch in 8- and 10-year-old children than in the adult subjects studied by Simpson and Austin. The 10-year-old children showed greater velar stretch than the 8-year-old children. The majority of the adolescent subjects studied by Simpson and Colton (1980) showed a degree of velar stretch that fell between the children and the adult subjects reported previously. An interesting finding in several studies (Mourino & Weinberg, 1975; Nieman & Simpson, 1975; Simpson & Austin, 1972; Simpson & Chin, 1981) has been that the degree of velar stretch correlates highly with the depth of the pharyngeal space. Thus, in the noncleft individual, velar stretch appears to be a common, albeit necessary, phenomenon that allows the soft palate to approximate the posterior pharyngeal wall during speech.

### Velar Movement and Position

It is oversimplistic to characterize the velopharyngeal mechanism as a "trap door" that maintains a closed position that is invariant across the production of nonnasal phonemes and a fully open position during the production of nasal phonemes. In fact, the control of velar movement—although somewhat predictable—is not that simple. The extent of velar displacement is dependent on phonetic context. Moll (1962) showed that velar height is greater for high vowels than low vowels, and that it is common for there to be a small gap (lack of complete velopharyngeal closure) during the production of low vowels. Vowels produced in nasal contexts result in lower velar height compared to vowels produced in nonnasal contexts.

### Patterns of Velopharyngeal Closure

Although the structural and functional aspects of the soft palate are considered critical to velopharyngeal function, it is also well understood that velopharyngeal closure does not necessarily occur due to palatal movement alone. For many speakers, the velopharyngeal mechanism functions in a sphincteric fashion. Several reports have documented that a number of velopharyngeal closure patterns exist within the population of normal speakers. Croft, Shprintzen, and Rakoff (1981) identified four patterns of velopharyngeal closure in 80 normal speakers and 500 patients with velopharyngeal inadequacy (VPI). A visual representation of these patterns is shown in Figure 7.18. It is interesting to note that the frequency with which the patterns were observed was somewhat similar in both groups. A coronal pattern was exhibited by 55% of the normal speakers and 45% of the speakers with VPI; a sagittal pattern was shown by 16% of the normal group and 11% of the VPI group; a circular pattern occurred in 10% of the normal group and 20% of the VPI group; and a circular with Passavant's ridge pattern was shown in 19% of the normal group and 24% of the VPI group. The authors emphasized that nearly 20% of the normal speakers exhibited a Passavant's ridge, a mechanism that previously had been considered to be exclusive to individuals with cleft palate and/or VPI.

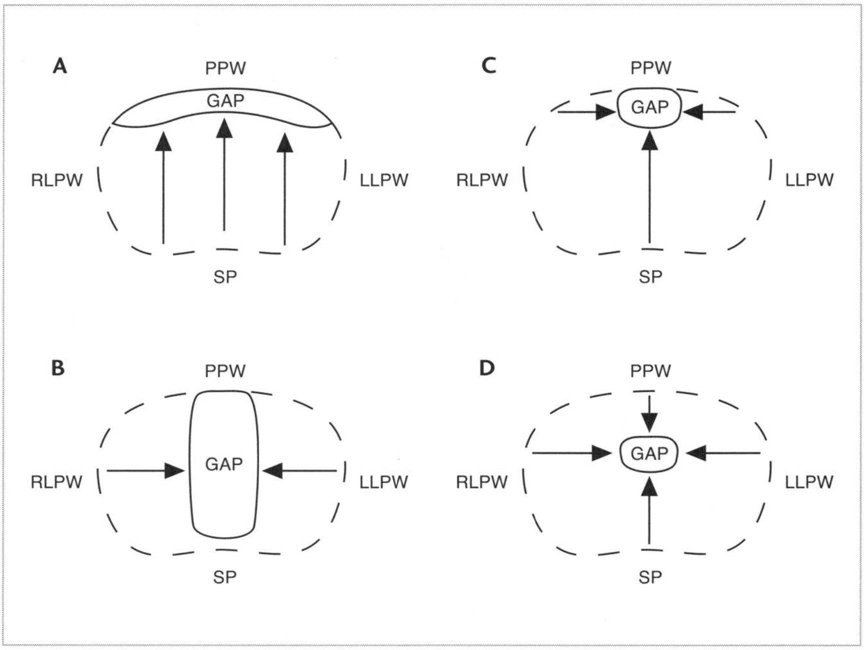


FIGURE 7.18. Patterns of velopharyngeal closure. (A) Coronal. (B) Sagittal. (C) Circular. (D) Circular with Passavant's ridge.

# Velopharyngeal Function: Cleft Palate

What is known about the function of the velopharyngeal muscles in individuals with repaired cleft palate? Although it has been demonstrated that a number of muscles are critical to velopharyngeal movement, the function of the levator veli palatini is of particular interest in the cleft palate population for several reasons. First, as Figure 7.15B shows, the muscle is not configured normally at birth. Second, even though it is now common for the surgeon to create the "sling" of the levator during the palatal repair (palatoplasty), the muscle is still not considered normal with regard to its position or bulk after the palate is repaired.

Two studies have demonstrated significant differences between levator muscle activity in individuals with cleft palate compared to those without cleft palate. Kuehn and Moon (1994) set out to characterize the relative degree of levator muscle activity that occurs during speech in noncleft speakers. To do this, they measured levator electromyographic activity during a series of speech tasks and compared this to the degree of muscle activity that was measured during a task that required maximum muscle activity (blowing with an intraoral air pressure of 60 cm $H_2O$). They found that "levator muscle activity for speech tended to occur in the lower region of its operating range" (p. 1269). In other words, for speakers without cleft palate, the degree of levator muscle activity required for palatal displacement that results in normal speech appears to be minimal relative to the magnitude of activity that the muscle can produce if needed.

Kuehn and Moon (1995) replicated this experimental paradigm with a group of speakers with repaired cleft palates. Whereas the previous study showed that noncleft speakers exhibit levator muscle activity in the lower end of its operating range during speech, the subjects with cleft palate demonstrated levator muscle activity in the middle to upper end of its operating range during speech. In other words, the speakers with repaired cleft palates were using the levator muscle at a level that was much closer to its maximum level of activity during speech. To explain why speakers with cleft palate might "expend relatively more physiologic effort" (p. 380) than speakers without cleft palate, the authors pointed to the anatomic deficiencies or differences that are inherent to the levator muscle in the repaired cleft palate and the possibility that more muscle activity is required to overcome stiffness within the soft palate that is secondary to scar tissue from the original palate repair.

Relating the palatal anatomy of the individual with cleft palate to the muscle function studies by Kuehn and Moon (1994, 1995), it is clear that a number of factors can prevent adequate palatal function even when the speaking environment is optimal. Each factor, along with its theoretical effect and probable consequence(s), is listed in Table 7.1. It is important to emphasize that although any individual factor may have a negative effect on palatal movement, it is more likely that these factors interact to affect the overall physiologic potential of the soft palate for speech. The challenge for clinicians and researchers alike is to determine the extent to which these structural and motor factors might interact in any individual with a repaired cleft palate. With this information, a treatment plan for a particular speaker with velopharyngeal issues should result in a speech outcome that is more optimal.

**Table 7.1**
**Structural and Motor Factors That Affect Velopharyngeal Function in the Cleft Palate Speech Mechanism**

| Factor | Possible effect | Possible consequence(s) |
|---|---|---|
| Lack of levator muscle bulk | Less muscle force | Less palatal displacement |
| Abnormal insertion of levator veli palatini muscle | Tethering of muscle to hard palate | Less palatal displacement<br>Greater levator muscle force required to move palate |
| Malpositioning of the repaired levator veli palatini muscle | Levator sling not positioned within same plane, resulting in less muscle force | Less palatal displacement<br>Greater levator muscle force required to move palate |
| Scar tissue within soft palate | Increased stiffness within the soft palate | Less palatal displacement<br>Less velar stretch<br>Greater levator muscle force required to move palate |
| Anterior/posterior faucial pillars | Passive force between tongue and mandibular position relative to soft palate | Greater levator muscle force required |
| Activity of palatoglossus and palatopharyngeus muscles | Active downward forces on soft palate | Greater levator muscle force required |

An example of the way in which these structural-motor factors may have a negative effect on speech comes from Zimmermann, Karnell, and Rettaliata (1984). In this study, 2 speakers with repaired cleft palates were compared. Both speakers were observed to achieve velopharyngeal closure; however, one speaker exhibited normal resonance and the other exhibited "inappropriate nasal resonance" (p. 299). The speaker with normal speech was shown to obtain maximum velopharyngeal constriction prior to voice onset, whereas the speaker with hypernasality achieved maximum velopharyngeal constriction after voice onset. For the hypernasal speaker, the mistiming of velopharyngeal closure to voice onset was considered to be related to movements of the tongue and mandible. Specifically, the authors suggested that the tongue and mandible placed mechanical constraints on the velum such that a delay occurred in achieving maximum velar displacement.

Although it is clear that structural-motor deficiencies are inherent in the surgically repaired cleft palate mechanism, it is also apparent that the vast majority of individuals with a repaired cleft palate exhibit velopharyngeal function that results in normal nasalization. This leads to two possibilities. First, it is possible that for many speakers, the structural-motor deficiencies are not great enough to prevent the speaker from using the velopharyngeal mechanism in the same way that speakers do without cleft palate. Second, it is possible that when a speaker with a repaired cleft palate achieves velopharyngeal closure that is adequate for perceptually acceptable speech, it may not be in a way that is similar to that of speakers without cleft palate. Karnell, Folkins, and Morris (1985) studied the speech movements of 4 adult speakers with repaired cleft palates relative to their perceived nasalization. Two subjects showed velar movements that were similar to normal speakers during the productions of consonant-vowel-consonant (CVC) utterances. That is, once maximum velopharyngeal constriction was obtained during production of the initial consonant, the velum moved downward slightly in association with production of the vowel prior to moving back upward for the final consonant. The other 2 subjects showed a "nonnormal" velar movement pattern. These subjects maintained a fixed velar position throughout the duration of the CVC utterance. The authors speculated that in order to produce more acceptable speech, some speakers with repaired cleft palate exploit their mechanism in ways that are different from the noncleft population.

The many advances in the surgical treatment of individuals with cleft palate-craniofacial disorders have resulted in minimizing the structural deficiencies that are inherent to the original anomaly. However, the fact that many individuals with these disorders continue to demonstrate speech disorders following surgery and behavioral treatment indicates that treatment is still not 100% successful. Furthermore, this suggests that the critical interactions that occur between structure and function are still not fully understood, and that continued basic science and clinical research are needed to facilitate improved treatment protocols and subsequent speech outcomes.

# Recommended Speech Anatomy Texts

Seikel, J. A., King, D. W., & Drumright, D. G. (2005). *Anatomy and physiology for speech, language, and hearing* (3rd ed.). Clifton Park, NY: Thomson Delmar Learning.

Zemlin, W. R. (1998). *Speech and hearing science: Anatomy and physiology* (4th ed.). Boston: Allyn & Bacon.

# References

Blackfield, H. M., Miller, E. R., Owsley, J. Q., Jr., & Lawson L. I. (1962a, October). Cinefluorographic evaluation of patients with velopharyngeal dysfunction in the absence of overt cleft palate. *Plastic and Reconstructive Surgery, 30,* 441–451.

Blackfield, H. M., Miller, E. R., Owsley, J. Q., Jr., & Lawson L. I. (1962b, February). Comparative evaluation of diagnostic techniques in patients with cleft-palate speech. *Plastic and Reconstructive Surgery, 29,* 153–158.

Carney, P. J., & Morris, H. L. (1971, July). Structural correlates of nasality. *Cleft Palate Journal, 8,* 307–321.

Carney, P. J., & Sherman, D. (1971). Severity of nasality in three selected speech tasks. *Journal of Speech and Hearing Research, 14,* 396–407.

Croft, C. B., Shprintzen, R. J., & Rakoff, S. J. (1981). Patterns of velopharyngeal valving in normal and cleft palate subjects: A multiview videofluoroscopy and nasendoscopic study. *Laryngoscope, 91,* 265–271.

Dickson, D. R. (1969, April). A radiographic study of nasality. *Cleft Palate Journal, 6,* 160–165.

Fant, G. (1960). *Acoustic theory of speech production.* The Hague, The Netherlands: Mouton.

Fritzell, B. (1969). The velopharyngeal muscles in speech. *Acta Otolaryngology, 250*(Suppl.), 1–81.

Hagerty, R., & Hoffmeister, F. S. (1954). Velopharyngeal closure: An index of speech. *Plastic and Reconstructive Surgery, 13,* 290–298.

House, A. S., & Stevens, K. N. (1956). Analog studies of the nasalization of vowels. *Journal of Speech and Hearing Disorders, 21,* 218–232.

Isberg, A., & Henningsson, G. (1987). Influence of open versus covered fistulas on velopharyngeal movements: A cineradiographic study. *Plastic and Reconstructive Surgery, 79,* 525–530.

Jones, K. L. (1997). *Smith's recognizable patterns of human malformation.* Philadelphia: Saunders.

Karnell, M. P., Folkins, J. W., & Morris, H. L. (1985). Relationship between perceived and kinematic aspects of speech production in cleft palate speakers. *Journal of Speech and Hearing Research, 28,* 63–72.

Kuehn, D. P., Folkins, J. W., & Cutting, C. B. (1982). Relationships between muscle activity and velar position. *Cleft Palate Journal, 19,* 25–35.

Kuehn, D. P., Folkins, J. W., & Linville, R. N. (1988). An electromyographic study of the musculus uvulae. *Cleft Palate Journal, 25,* 348–355.

Kuehn, D. P., & Moller, K. T. (2000). Speech and language issues in the cleft palate population: The state of the art. *Cleft Palate-Craniofacial Journal, 37,* 348-1–348-35.

Kuehn, D. P., & Moon, J. B. (1994). Levator veli palatini muscle activity in relation to intraoral air pressure variation. *Journal of Speech and Hearing Research, 37,* 1260–1270.

Kuehn, D. P., & Moon, J. B. (1995). Levator veli palatini muscle activity in relation to intraoral air pressure variation in cleft palate subjects. *Cleft Palate-Craniofacial Journal, 32,* 376–381.

Mazaheri, M., Millard, R. T., & Erickson, D. M. (1964, April). Cineradiographic comparison of normal to noncleft subjects with velopharyngeal inadequacy. *Cleft Palate Journal, 12,* 199–209.

Moll, K. L. (1962, March). Velopharyngeal closure on vowels. *Journal of Speech and Hearing Research, 5,* 30–37.

Moon, J. B., Smith, A. E., Folkins, J. W., Lemke, J. H., & Gartlan, M. (1994). Coordination of velopharyngeal muscle activity during positioning of the soft palate. *Cleft Palate–Craniofacial Journal, 31,* 45–55.

Moore, W. H., & Sommers, R. K. (1973, January). Phonetic contexts: Their effects on perceived nasality in cleft palate speakers. *Cleft Palate Journal, 10,* 72–83.

Mourino, A. P., & Weinberg, B. (1975, October). A cephalometric study of velar stretch in 8- and 10-year-old children. *Cleft Palate Journal, 12,* 417–435.

Nagel, R. J., & Sears, V. H. (1958). *Dental prosthetics.* St Louis, MO: Mosby.

Nieman, G. S., & Simpson, R. K. (1975, October). A roentgencephalometric investigation of the effect of adenoid removal upon selected measures of velopharyngeal function. *Cleft Palate Journal, 12,* 377–389.

Peterson-Falzone, S., & Pruzansky, S. (1976, October). Cleft palate and congenital palatopharyngeal incompetency in mandibulofacial dysostosis: Frequency and problems in treatment. *Cleft Palate Journal, 13,* 354–360.

Seaver, E. J., & Kuehn, D. P. (1980). A cineradiographic and electromyographic investigation of velar positioning in non-nasal speech. *Cleft Palate Journal, 17,* 216–226.

Seikel, J. A., King, D. W., & Drumright, D. G. (2005). *Anatomy and physiology for speech, language, and hearing: Instructor's version* (2nd ed.). Clifton Park, NY: Thompson Learning.

Simpson, R. K., & Austin, A. A. (1972, October). A cephalometric investigation of velar stretch. *Cleft Palate Journal, 9,* 341–351.

Simpson, R. K., & Chin, L. (1981). Velar stretch as a function of task. *Cleft Palate Journal, 18,* 1–9.

Simpson, R. K., & Colton, J. (1980). A cephalometric study of velar stretch in adolescent subjects. *Cleft Palate Journal, 17*(1), 40–47.

Spriestersbach, D. C., & Powers, G. R. (1959). Nasality in isolated vowels and connected speech of cleft palate speakers. *Journal of Speech and Hearing Research, 2*(1), 40–45.

Subtelny, J. D., Koepp-Baker, H., & Subtelny, J. D. (1961). Palatal function and cleft palate speech. *Journal of Speech and Hearing Disorders, 26,* 213–224.

Zemlin, W. R. (1998). *Speech and hearing science: Anatomy and physiology* (3rd ed.). Boston: Allyn & Bacon.

Zimmermann, G. N., Karnell, M. P., & Rettaliata, P. (1984). Articulatory coordination and the clinical profile of two cleft palate speakers. *Journal of Phonetics, 12,* 297–306.

# PART III

# Communication and Psychosocial Development

# CHAPTER 8

# Speech and Language of Children with Cleft Palate

## Interactions and Influences

*Kathy L. Chapman*

Chapman provides an overview of the speech and language characteristics of individuals with cleft palate. She also provides data on three children with cleft palate who show very different profiles of development in speech and language over time.

1. Children with cleft palate exhibit delays in early vocal development as well as delays in early lexical development. What contributes to the delays in both of these areas?
2. Why is it important to consider phonological and articulatory aspects of speech sound development of young children with cleft palate?
3. What are some of the factors that influence speech outcomes for children with cleft palate?
4. Inconsistencies exist across studies examining both speech and language development of children with cleft palate. What might account for these differences?

Learning to talk is one of the most significant accomplishments of early childhood. For many children, speech and language acquisition proceeds in a fairly predictable fashion. By 5 years of age, typical language learning children have mastered most of the sounds of their language, have an expressive vocabulary of over 2,000 words, and use a variety of grammatically correct simple and complex sentences as they assume the role of speaker and/or respondent during conversational interactions.

The process of speech and language learning may be more complicated for a child born with a cleft palate (with or without cleft lip).[1] Although various aspects of communication development may be delayed in this population, prior to palate repair, the most obvious concerns are difficulty with production of pressure consonants (i.e., stops, fricatives, and affricates) and hypernasal resonance due to oral-nasal coupling. Fortunately, primary palatal surgery is typically performed sometime during the first 18 months of life, with the goal of providing separation between the oral and nasal cavities and normal velopharyngeal function (Peterson-Falzone, Hardin-Jones, & Karnell, 2001). However, because communication development starts at birth, a baby born with cleft palate begins the task of speech and language learning with an impaired speech production mechanism.

The primary purpose of this chapter is to describe the speech and language development of individuals with cleft palate. A secondary purpose is to explore the interaction between oral structural deficits and learning and how both impact speech and language acquisition for babies and young children with cleft palate. The chapter includes (a) a brief overview of phonological theories, (b) a review of studies examining the speech and language development of individuals with cleft palate, and (c) case presentations of three children with cleft palate showing varying profiles of development (see Appendix 8A).

Although this chapter is meant to be an overview of what is "typically" seen in speech and language development of individuals with cleft palate, this population is extremely heterogeneous. Children with cleft palate vary in both type and extent of communication deficits, with some children showing no delays after a period of catch-up following palatal closure. Finally, it is important to remember that children with cleft palate may exhibit language and speech problems unrelated to clefting, just as any youngster may have difficulty learning various aspects of speech or language.

---

[1]This chapter focuses primarily on speech and language abilities of children with cleft palate with or without cleft lip. Although cleft lip alone may have some minor impact on articulation, most agree it is not an important risk factor for articulation problems (e.g., Kuehn & Moller, 2000; Peterson-Falzone, Hardin-Jones, & Karnell, 2001; Riski & DeLong, 1984).

## Phonological Theories

The acquisition of phonology entails learning about the sound system of the language. This includes not only articulation or motor learning (i.e., how to move and position the articulators for correct production of the sound), but also knowledge about the sound patterns of the language (e.g., the sound inventory of the language, permissible sound sequences, and variation in sound production related to context; Fey, 1992). Difficulties with perception and/or production of speech sounds will likely affect phonological learning (e.g., Fey, 1992; Schwartz, Mody, & Petinou, 1997). Further, because phonology "is the bridge to the expression and comprehension" of other aspects of language (i.e., semantics, syntax, morphology, pragmatics), a phonological deficit could potentially impact all language learning (Schwartz et al., 1997, p. 109). As already mentioned, children with cleft palate have limitations in structure and function that influence speech production. There is also some preliminary evidence to suggest that auditory perceptual deficits may be present in infants (Čeponienė et al., 2000; Cheour et al., 1999) and children with cleft palate (e.g., Čeponienė et al., 1999; Cheour et al., 1998; Whitehill, Francis, & Ching, 2003). It is not surprising then, that acquisition of speech and language may be difficult for this group of children.

Over the years, theories of phonology have provided important insights into the organization of the phonological system and the processes of phonological acquisition. Many of these theories have guided assessment and treatment of children with speech sound disorders. Although a detailed description of all of these theories is beyond the scope of this chapter, several that have significantly impacted the field of clinical speech-language pathology are described below. Additionally, there are a number of tutorials, books, and book chapters available for those interested in a more in depth review of the theories and implications for clinical practice (e.g., Ball & Kent, 1997; Barlow, 2001; Barlow & Gierut, 1999; Bernhardt & Stemberger, 1998; Bernhardt & Stoel-Gammon, 1994; Gierut & Morrisette, 2006; Schwartz, 1992).

*Generative phonology* (described by Chomsky & Halle, 1968, in their book *The Sound Pattern of English*) has contributed much to the understanding of phonological acquisition and phonological disorders in children (Ingram, 1997). This theory focuses not on phonemes but on phonological features. Phonemes are said to be represented (underlyingly) by a set of distinctive features, and sounds differ in terms of one or more of these features (e.g., /ᴛ/ and /δ/ vary with regard to the feature voicing). Generative theory also states that the phonology of the language can be described with an ordered "set of phonological rules that operate on *underlying representations*" to yield the "phonetic or *surface representation*" (Ingram, 1997, p. 9). *Rule ordering* can be seen in a child's production of [κε] for [ᴛεκ] (*take*) as the rule deleting word-final obstruents can only be applied after the rule that changes alveolars to velars when a velar occurs later in the word.

Although generative phonology appears to be waning in popularity, the major tenets of the theory are still relevant and have evolved into what is now referred to as *nonlinear phonology* (Ingram, 1997). Application of generative phonology to children with developmental phonological disorders can be found in the work of Gierut and colleagues (e.g., Elbert & Gierut, 1986; Gierut, Elbert, & Dinnsen, 1987).

*Natural phonology* (see Donegan & Stampe, 1979, and Stampe, 1979) has been applied very successfully to the clinical management of children with phonological disorders. A key aspect of this theory is the *phonological process*, which is described by Stampe as a "mental operation" that serves to simplify the process of speech production. This theory proposes that differences between the child's production and the adult target are due to these phonological processes (Stampe, 1979, p. vii). Because phonological processes are considered to be "responses to phonetic difficulties," they are applied across sounds that form "natural classes" and that are similar in level of difficulty (e.g., devoicing of final obstruents; Donegan & Stampe, 1979, p. 136). According to Stampe, processes are "innate" and with development they become suppressed until the child's productions are eventually adultlike (Stampe, 1979). Ingram (1976) is credited with application of *natural phonology* to management of children with phonological disorders, and numerous assessment instruments and intervention approaches have been developed based on this theory.

*Nonlinear phonologies* include a number of different "subtheories" (lexical, autosegmental, metrical, etc.) (for reviews, see, e.g., Bernhardt, 1992; Bernhardt & Stemberger, 1998; Bernhardt & Stoel-Gammon, 1994; Dinnsen, 1997; Schwartz, 1992). These theories differ from generative phonology because of their focus on "the hierarchical nature of relationships among phonological units" such as features, sounds, syllables, and words (Bernhardt & Stoel-Gammon, 1994, p. 123). As noted by Gierut and Morrisette (2006), the hierarchical structures "are arranged as nested tree structures," similar to syntactic tree diagrams (p. 268). Other important differences are related to (1) an emphasis on stress, (2) specification of features in the underlying representation, and (3) a reduction in the number of possible rules or operations (Bernhardt & Stoel-Gammon, 1994; Schwartz, 1992; Schwartz et al., 1997). Bernhardt and colleagues have provided guidelines for the clinical application of these theories to assessment and treatment of children with phonological disorders (e.g., Bernhardt, 1992, 1994; Bernhardt & Gilbert, 1992; Bernhardt & Stemberger, 2000; Bernhardt & Stoel-Gammon, 1994).

Finally, due to the efforts of a number of researchers, *optimality theory* (see McCarthy, 2002; McCarthy & Prince, 1994, 1995; Prince & Smolensky, 1997, 2004) is being applied to treatment of children with phonological disorders (e.g., Barlow, 2001; Barlow & Dinnsen, 1998; Barlow & Gierut, 1999; Bernhardt & Stemberger, 1998; Gierut & Morrisette, 2006; Goad, 1998). Principles of the theory as summarized by Barlow (2001) and Gierut and Morrisette (2006) are described below. In brief, *optimality theory* describes three distinct but coordinated mechanisms: the *Generator* (GEN), *Constraints* (CON), and *Evaluator* (EVAL). GEN produces all acceptable forms for any grammar. CON limits the number of potential forms by providing information about constraints. Finally, EVAL supplies language-specific information about constraint rankings, comparing the forms generated by GEN with the universal constraints of CON in order to choose the "optimal" output for an individual speaker. The "optimal" output is the "output candidate that violates the fewest number of high-ranked constraints in the grammar" (Gierut & Morrisette, 2006, p. 270). Constraints are central to this theory and can be likened to rules or processes in terms of explaining differences between the underlying representation and the surface form.[2] They are classified as either *faithfulness constraints* or *markedness constraints* and are universal across languages, although the rankings are language specific. With faithfulness constraints, the output (i.e., surface form) must be the same as the input (i.e., underlying representation). Violations occur when a segment or feature is changed or deleted. For example, deletion of the final /g/ in *dog* is a violation of the faithfulness constraint **Max** (no deletion). In contrast, "markedness constraints require outputs to be unmarked or simplified in structure" (Barlow, 2001, p. 243). Production of the final /g/ in *dog* is a violation of the markedness constraint **Coda** (no final consonants). Clearly, these constraints are in opposition to each other, and one or the other

[2]In optimality theory, the input and output representations are similar to underlying and surface forms in the other theories (see Barlow, 2001).

will be violated (lower ranked constraints are violated to maintain higher ranked constraints). So, the actual form chosen depends on the language-specific rankings, and phonological acquisition involves the child's learning how these constraints are rank ordered in his or her particular language (see Barlow, 2001; Barlow & Gierut, 1999; Bernhardt & Stemberger, 1998; and Gierut & Morrisette, 2006, for a more detailed review of this theory; for a case example of children with phonological disorders, including children with cleft palate, see Bernhardt & Stemberger, 1998).

Phonological theories have advanced the field's knowledge of phonological acquisition and improved professionals' management of children with phonological disorders. The theories are important for understanding how structure and learning interact to hinder or facilitate the speech sound acquisition of children with cleft palate. Because of limitations on speech production associated with palatal clefting, the acquisition of phonology cannot be expected to be the same as it is for children without clefts (called noncleft children in this chapter). Further, after surgery is performed, the patterns developed in response to these initial limitations do not disappear (Chapman, 1993; Fey, 1992; Schwartz, 1992). Therefore, considerations of phonological as well as articulatory processes are relevant to understanding the speech sound development of children with cleft palate.

## Vocal Development of Babies with Cleft Palate: Presurgery

Recent interest in studying the early vocal development of babies with cleft palate during the 1st year of life and prior to primary palatal surgery is likely related to (a) studies describing the prelinguistic development of typically developing babies and babies at risk for speech and language delays, (b) research documenting the relationship between prelinguistic and later speech and language outcomes in noncleft populations, and (c) research and writings attempting to delineate "the optimal age" of primary palatal surgery for children with cleft palate (Chapman, 2004b, p. 236). A review of that literature suggests that babies with cleft palate differ from their noncleft peers in many aspects of early vocal development. For example, differences have been reported in the cry behavior of babies with cleft palate and noncleft babies over the first 9 months of life (Wermke,

Hauser, Komposch, & Stellzig, 2002). Next, although babies with unrepaired clefts of the palate vocalized as frequently as their noncleft peers, they had smaller and less diverse consonant inventories (Chapman, Hardin-Jones, Schulte, & Halter, 2001). These inventories included fewer oral stops (e.g., Chapman, 1991; Chapman et al., 2001; Grunwell & Russell, 1987, 1988; Hutters, Bau, & Brøndsted, 2001; O'Gara & Logemann, 1988; Olson, 1965; Russell & Grunwell, 1993) but more nasals (Chapman, 1991; Chapman et al., 2001; Hutters et al., 2001; O'Gara & Logemann, 1988; O'Gara, Logemann, & Rademaker, 1994). Additionally, alveolars occurred less frequently (Chapman, 1991; Chapman et al., 2001; Hutters et al., 2001; O'Gara & Logemann, 1988; O'Gara et al., 1994; Olson, 1965) while glottals occurred more frequently (Chapman, 1991; Chapman et al., 2001; Hutters et al., 2001; O'Gara & Logemann, 1988; O'Gara et al., 1994; Olson, 1965). Finally, babies with cleft palate may be delayed in the onset of canonical babbling—that is, producing syllables containing a consonant (but not glottals) and a "fully resonant nucleus" (i.e., identifiable vowel) such as /bʌ/ (Oller & Eilers, 1988, p. 443)—with fewer canonical syllables noted in their spontaneous vocalizations overall. Chapman and colleagues (2001) found that only 57% of babies with cleft palate had reached the canonical babbling stage by 9 months of age compared to 93% of their age-matched peers.

Studies of the prespeech characteristics of the babies with cleft palate described above included participants with unrepaired clefts of the hard and soft palate. Data have also been reported on the prespeech vocalizations of babies with cleft palate receiving two-stage palatal surgery (e.g., Lohmander-Agerskov, Söderpalm, Friede, Persson, & Lilja, 1994; Willadsen & Albrechtsen, 2006; Willadsen & Enemark, 2000). In these cases, either the hard or the soft palate had been repaired at the time of testing. Willadsen and Enemark (2000) found that, in general, babies who had undergone primary veloplasty (i.e., repair of the soft palate) at 6–8 months performed as well as or better than babies with a repaired hard palate (surgery at 3 months) and an unrepaired soft palate on measures of consonant production at 13 months of age. Compared to noncleft babies of the same age, babies with cleft palate receiving early soft palate but delayed hard palate repair were similar for canonical babbling and number of consonants produced at 11 months of age (Willadsen & Albrechtsen, 2006); however, like babies with an unrepaired cleft of the hard and soft palate (see above), these babies produced fewer stops and alveolars, but more nasals, velars, and glottals than noncleft babies (Willadsen & Albrechtsen, 2006).

Delays in early vocal development have been reported regardless of cleft type (Hardin-Jones, Chapman, & Schulte, 2003) and regardless of whether the palate was obturated (Hardin-Jones et al., 2002; Konst, Weersink-Braks, Rietveld, & Peters, 1999[3]; Lohmander, Lillvik, & Friede, 2004). These latter results are interesting as several researchers have proposed that obturation of the hard palate might result in better consonant development, especially for sounds with an anterior place of production, for babies and young children with cleft palate (e.g., Dorf, Reisberg, & Gold, 1985; Hardin-Jones et al., 2002; Konst, 2002; Konst et al., 1999; Lohmander-Agerskov, 1998).

It is not surprising that babies with unrepaired cleft palate differ from their noncleft peers in many aspects of development. Avoidance of pressure consonants is obviously related to the fact that prior to surgery, babies with cleft palate are unable to impound intraoral air pressure required for production of these sounds. At the same time, the explanation for delays in canonical babbling is not as obvious. Because of constraints on production of oral consonants, the repertoire of sounds available for construction of canonical syllables is reduced. However, most babies with cleft palate produce nasals as well as glides during the prelinguistic stage, suggesting they have sounds within their repertoire that can be combined with vowels to form canonical syllables. So, why don't they use these sounds to produce canonical syllables at the same rate as their noncleft peers? Perhaps the "auditory experiences" of young infants with cleft palate may provide an explanation (e.g., Chapman et al., 2001; Kemp-Fincham, Kuehn, & Trost-Cardamone, 1990; Trost-Cardamone & Bernthal, 1993). It is often hypothesized that speech and language delays in babies and young children with cleft palate are due to otitis media. The occurrence of otitis media in babies with cleft palate has been well documented (see Chapter 15 by Sidman and Chapter 9 by Carlstrom and Nelson for discussion of otitis media and hearing problems in children with cleft palate). While the impact of otitis media and its accompanying hearing loss on communication development of noncleft children continues to be debated (e.g., see Casby, 2001; Paradise et al., 2000; Shriberg et al., 2000; Shriberg, Friel-Patti, Flipsen, & Brown, 2000), it has been shown that noncleft babies with early histories of otitis media produce

---

[3]Although Konst et al. (1999) found a statistically significant difference in the percentage of alveolar productions in their obturated and non-obturated groups at 12 months, the percent occurrence was small for each (3.7 and 0.6 for the obturated group and non-obturated group, respectively). Further, this finding did not hold up when the babies were evaluated at 18 months of age.

fewer canonical syllables in their early babbling (Rvachew, Slawinski, Williams, & Green, 1996, 1999). In contrast, a preliminary investigation of otitis media and babbling in 9-month-old babies with cleft palate found similarities in the early vocal development of babies with and without histories of otitis media. However, because of the small number of participants and lack of documentation of hearing thresholds, further research in this area is warranted (Chapman, Hardin-Jones, Cook, & Panelli, 2002).

It is also important to remember that, prior to palatal closure, nasal resonance is present in the vocalizations of babies with cleft palate, which may "reduce the acoustic contrasts between CV [consonant-vowel] syllables," making them less distinguishable (Kemp-Fincham et al., 1990, p. 740). Further, these nasalized productions may not match exactly with caregivers' speech, perhaps making them less salient to the baby (Chapman et al., 2001).

Additionally, studies have reported differences in the auditory discrimination abilities of infants with cleft palate and noncleft infants (Čeponienė et al., 2000; Cheour et al., 1999). For some tasks, differences in cleft type were also noted, as infants with cleft lip and palate exhibited better performance than infants with cleft palate only (Čeponienė et al., 2000).

In summary, clefting has the most obvious effect on the developing sound system of babies with cleft palate prior to palatal surgery. Additionally, the conductive hearing loss accompanying otitis media, distortion of babies' early speech attempts due to hypernasality, and possible deficits in auditory discrimination may impair their ability to (a) perceive important sound contrasts produced by caregivers, (b) obtain feedback from their own productions, and (c) reproduce and/or recognize similarities between their own babbled productions and the productions of their caregivers. All these are important for phonological and language learning (Chapman et al., 2001).

## Relationship Between Early Speech and Later Speech-Language Development

### Noncleft Children

In the previous section, research was cited documenting early delays in the prelinguistic-presurgery productions of children with cleft palate. Studies of typically developing and at-risk babies and young children have provided evidence for a relationship between prelinguistic vocalizations and later speech and language development. Researchers have documented consistencies in syllable (Vihman, 1992) and consonant characteristics (Stoel-Gammon & Cooper, 1984) across young children's prelinguistic and word productions (e.g., Oller, Weiman, Doyle, & Ross, 1976; Vihman, Ferguson, & Elbert, 1986; Vihman, Macken, Miller, Simmons, & Miller, 1985). There also appears to be a relationship between the quantity and complexity of babbling and later speech and/or language proficiency. For example, true consonant production early on was associated with more advanced speech sound development at 3 years of age for the babies studied by Vihman and colleagues (Vihman, 1986; Vihman & Greenlee, 1987). Menyuk, Liebergott, and Schultz (1986) found that use of syllables in babbling was related to accuracy of production of final consonants at 29 months. With regard to language, vocalization frequency (Camp, Burgess, Morgan, & Zerbe, 1987; McCathren, Yoder, & Warren, 1999), percentage of vocalizations with consonants, and vocalizations used interactively (McCathren et al., 1999) were related to later language performance (Camp et al., 1987; McCathren et al., 1999). Additionally, less complex babbling has been linked to slowed onset (Stoel-Gammon, 1989) and rate of lexical acquisition (Stoel-Gammon, 1989; Whitehurst, Smith, Fischel, Arnold, & Lonigan, 1991), as well as lower language performance at 6 years of age (Jensen, Boggild-Andersen, Schmidt, Ankerhus, & Hansen, 1988).

According to Stoel-Gammon (1992, 1998a, 1998b), the relationship between babbling and later speech and language development can be explained, in part, by practice and feedback. Practice is believed to increase both the "control and precision with which a movement is performed" (Stoel-Gammon, 1992, p. 451). Therefore, repetition of the same sound patterns over and over serves to stabilize them, making them more automatic and easily retrieved for word production (Stoel-Gammon, 1992, 1998a, 1998b). Fry (1966) described the role that feedback plays in speech-language acquisition. He believed that with repeated practice of speech sounds, a connection develops between the auditory and tactile-kinesthetic input the child receives. Stoel-Gammon (1992) proposed that "awareness of the links between one's own oral-motor movements and the acoustic signal that results is a prerequisite to auditory-vocal matching that underlies word production" (pp. 451–452). Further, this knowledge makes adult productions that match these babbled utterances especially salient to the child (e.g., Stoel-Gammon, 1992, 1998a; Vihman, 1993a,

1993b). Over time, the babbled productions (e.g., /dædæ/) that "match" words heard in the adult input (e.g., "daddy") are modified and strengthened, becoming likely candidates for early words (Stoel-Gammon, 1998a, 1998b; Vihman, 1993a, 1993b). As summarized previously in this chapter, there are a number of factors that might disrupt these processes for babies born with cleft palate. The consequence may be that these babies have a smaller repertoire of "practiced syllables" (Vihman, 1992) that have been reinforced and modified to resemble words, and thus their lexical development is delayed (Chapman et al., 2001; Kemp-Fincham et al., 1990; Stoel-Gammon, 1998b).

## Children with Cleft Palate

Chapman and colleagues (Chapman, 2004b; Chapman, Hardin-Jones, & Halter, 2003) studied the relationship between early speech production skills and later speech and language performance for children with cleft palate. The first of these studies (Chapman et al., 2003) examined the association (a) between speech production presurgery (age 9 months) and speech and language outcomes at age 21 months and (b) between speech production immediately postsurgery (age 13 months) and speech and language outcomes at age 21 months. A number of positive and significant correlations were noted, suggesting that babies who produced more true stops prior to surgery had better speech at 21 months, and those who produced more true stops immediately postsurgery had better speech and lexical development at 21 months. Finally, size of true consonant inventory postsurgery (age 13 months) was also related to general speech and lexical outcome measures at 21 months.

In a follow-up study, Chapman (2004b) was interested in determining if the relationships noted by Chapman et al. (2003) would still be evident at 39 months of age. In this study, correlations were performed on (a) speech measures presurgery (age 9 months) and speech and language outcome measures at 39 months and (b) speech measures postsurgery (age 13 months) and speech and language outcome measures at age 39 months. Results indicated two significant positive correlations: between true stop production postsurgery and mean length of utterance (MLU) at 39 months, and between true stop production postsurgery and number of different words (NDW) at 39 months. Unexpectedly, significant negative correlations were also noted for (a) true canonical babbling ratio (TCBR) presurgery and MLU at 39 months, (b) size of true consonant inventory presurgery and MLU at 39 months, and (c) size of true consonant inventory presurgery and NDW at 39 months. While it appears that babies who were good "babblers" presurgery had poorer language performance at 39 months, a more likely explanation is that a number of other factors in the 2nd and 3rd years of life, such as success of primary palatal surgery or early intervention, also influenced communication outcomes for these children. In some ways, these results were encouraging as they suggested that in spite of early deficits in prelinguistic-presurgery development for babies with cleft palate, significant improvements in speech and language development were possible. At the same time, if velopharyngeal inadequacy (VPI) or other problems were present, even those babies who were performing well presurgery showed poor speech and language outcomes later on (Chapman, 2004b).

Konst (2002) also described the results of a study examining the relationship between prelinguistic and later speech and language outcomes for children who received two-stage surgery (soft palate repair at age 12 months and hard palate repair at age 9 years). No correlations were noted between prespeech performance (measured at age 12 months, prior to repair of the soft palate) and speech and language outcomes at 30 months of age. However, moderate positive correlations were noted between prespeech measures at age 18 months, after repair of the soft palate, and speech and language outcomes at age 30 months. Children who produced more alveolars at age 18 months had fewer errors related to backing, palatalization, or lateralization at age 30 months. Similarly, children with more oral stops at 18 months were more intelligible and had higher MLUs at 30 months of age.

Although stop production has frequently been linked to better speech outcomes for children with cleft palate, these are the first studies suggesting that the ability to produce stops prior to initial palatal surgery is associated with better language skills in the early preschool years.

## Speech Sound Development of Children with Cleft Palate: Postsurgery

Most of the research on speech development of children with cleft palate has focused on the postsurgery period. Although increases in oral stop production have been reported at approximately 3 weeks postsurgery

(Grunwell & Russell, 1987), acquisition of age-appropriate speech is not achieved immediately or quickly for many children with cleft palate.

## The Early Postsurgery Period to Age 3

Only two investigations have examined longitudinal changes in speech abilities of children immediately following cleft palate surgery. Grunwell and Russell (1987) provided details on changes in development at four time points over the first few months following primary palate repair. Because of the small number of babies studied (i.e., $N = 3$) and the variability observed, it is difficult to make generalizations. However, all babies showed postsurgery increases in size of consonant inventories and use of multisyllabic productions by 3 to 7 weeks and 3 to 5 weeks, respectively.

More recently, Jones, Chapman, and Hardin-Jones (2003) studied the speech sound development of 14 children with cleft palate at approximately age 12 months (presurgery) and again at age 17 months (approximately 5 months postsurgery) to examine the impact of surgery on speech development. Comparisons were also made with 17-month-old noncleft toddlers to determine how their performance compared with that of their peers. Within-group comparisons suggested that while some improvements were noted 5 months postsurgery, not all aspects of speech production showed a similar change. For example, significant increases in canonical babbling ratio (CBR), size of consonant inventories, and production of the /b/ sound were noted postsurgery. In contrast, no significant changes were observed for TCBR, place and manner features, or production of other stops or nasals. The between-group comparisons suggested that toddlers with cleft palate were similar to their noncleft peers for CBR, TCBR, and production of fricatives, liquids, and all place features, with the exception of alveolars. Additionally, they were similar to their noncleft peers for accuracy of production of /p/, /t/, /g/, /m/, and /n/. At the same time, the children with cleft palate were lagging behind their peers in size of consonant inventories, overall frequency of stop production, and accuracy of production of /b/, /d/, and /k/. Finally, compared to the noncleft toddlers, those with repaired clefts produced more nasals and glides. Individual child comparisons revealed a great deal of variation across participants in their improvements in speech abilities postsurgery. For example, 5 of the 6 children who were not producing oral stops presurgery had added stops to their inventories by age 17 months. Additionally, new oral fricatives were also noted in the inventories of 6 toddlers postsurgery. Finally, at least 4 of the 14 toddlers with cleft palate appeared to be "catching up" to their peers as they had consonant inventories that were equal to or larger than their noncleft peers at age 17 months. At the same time, 3 of the toddlers showed little change in consonant production as a result of surgery (Jones et al., 2003).

Two additional studies, Chapman and Hardin (1992) and Chapman et al. (2003), also provided data on the speech development of children with cleft palate in the early postsurgery period. These two investigations differed from the Grunwell and Russell (1987) and the Jones et al. (2003) studies in that they were cross-sectional rather than longitudinal, and many of the analyses were performed on word productions rather than preword or unglossed words. Because intelligible words were analyzed, these investigators were able to examine accuracy of production rather than just frequency of occurrence for many of the variables under study. At the same time, these studies were different from each other in the types of analyses that were performed. Chapman and Hardin (1992) employed a phonological process framework to compare the speech production skills of 2-year-olds with cleft palate and their noncleft peers. In this study, more similarities than differences were noted. The two groups of toddlers were similar in size of consonant inventory and phonological process usage, with only a few exceptions. Backing and nasal assimilation, two processes that appear to be directly related to prior (or current) structural deficits, occurred more frequently in the speech of the toddlers with cleft palate. Also, cleft and noncleft toddlers differed in accuracy of production of nasals, liquids, and total consonants correct.

Chapman et al. (2003) found that 21-month-old toddlers with cleft palate were behind their peers in size of consonant inventories, emerging and stable consonant production, and production of true stops, liquids, labials, dentals, alveolars, and velars. Additionally, they were less accurate for production of words with initial /b/, /d/, /t/, and /k/. However, the cleft and noncleft toddlers were similar for production of fricatives, nasals, glides, glottals, and palatals, as well as word initial /p/ and /g/ sounds. Interestingly, the toddlers in the Chapman and Hardin (1992) study appeared to be doing better than the toddlers studied by Chapman et al. (2003) even though the former group of participants was selected because they had undergone late surgery. Differences between the two studies in the analysis procedures employed and the size of the comparison groups (only 5 typically developing toddlers participated in the Chapman and Hardin study) may explain the discrepancies.

Employing a somewhat different approach to studying the impact of clefting on early speech development, Estrem and Broen (1989) performed a detailed analysis of the phonological characteristics of the first 50 words acquired by 5 toddlers with cleft palate (4 of the 5 had undergone primary palate repair before the study began). Compared to noncleft peers matched for productive vocabulary and gender, the toddlers with cleft palate attempted fewer words beginning with oral stops, fricatives, and affricates and more words with initial nasals, glides, liquids, and vowels. Additionally, they continued to show a preference for labial, velar, and glottal sounds throughout the duration of the study. These results show how constraints on the speech sound system influence not only sound production but also lexical preferences of toddlers with cleft palate.

Clearly, young children with cleft palate show improvement in speech sound development as a result of surgical intervention. However, many deficits noted during the prelinguistic stage and prior to palatal closure are still apparent in the early postsurgery period. For example, the toddlers studied by Jones et al. (2003) and Chapman et al. (2003) were behind their noncleft peers in production of oral stops as well as other place and manner features in the 2nd year of life. At the same time, individual toddlers with cleft palate in the Jones et al. study were showing very good progress, and according to Chapman et al. (2003), fricatives, nasals, glides, palatals, and glottals, as well as word initial stops /p/ and /g/, were produced as accurately by the toddlers with cleft palate as by their noncleft peers at 21 months. Finally, although there does appear to be an association between presurgery and immediate postsurgery performance and later speech and language outcomes for young children with cleft palate, the relationship is strongest in the 2nd year of life. By 3 years of age, if VPI is present, even those children who were doing well early on are unable to maintain the same level of performance over time.

## The Later Preschool Years: Age 3 and Older

Children with cleft palate may also show delays in speech sound development into the preschool period. In fact, 5- and 6-year-olds with cleft palate did not perform as well as 3-year-old noncleft children when compared for number of speech sound errors (Bzoch, 1965; Philips & Harrison, 1969a) and intelligibility ratings (Philips & Harrison, 1969a). A more recent study of speech development of 5-year-olds with cleft palate from the United

Kingdom also documented "poor speech outcomes" for the children studied (Sell et al., 2001). Sell and colleagues found that 51% of the children in their study exhibited problems with speech intelligibility, 29% presented with hypernasal speech at some point in time, and 34% exhibited at least one speech sound error considered "serious" (e.g., backed patterns of articulation, nasal substitutions, deletion of pressure consonants). Finally, histories of VPI were present for 33% of the children.

The findings of the studies described above are in contrast to a report by Chapman (1993), who compared the occurrence of common phonological processes in the speech of 3-, 4-, and 5-year-olds with and without cleft palate. Results of this study indicated that the children with cleft palate employed more phonological processes than their noncleft peers at ages 3 and 4 years, but no differences between the groups were noted by 5 years. These findings led Chapman (1993) to conclude that children with cleft palate "catch up" to their noncleft peers, at least in terms of elimination of phonological processes, by 5 years of age. There are several possible explanations for the better outcome reported by Chapman (1993). Because the Bzoch and Philips and Harrison studies were undertaken 24 to 28 years earlier, perhaps the better performance by the 5-year-olds in the Chapman study can be attributed to improved management (including earlier and improved surgical techniques, earlier intervention, etc.) (Chapman, 1993). This explanation has some support in the literature, as better speech results have been reported for younger compared to older participants in several studies (e.g., Counihan, 1960; Riski, 1995; Van Demark, Morris, & Vandehaar, 1979). At the same time, this does not explain the poorer performance by the children in the Sell et al. (2001) study compared to the Chapman study. Although differences between these two studies might simply be related to differences in management of children with cleft palate in the United States versus the United Kingdom, another explanation should also be considered. Chapman (1993) performed a phonological process analysis on the speech of the children in her study, whereas Sell et al. (2001) and the other investigators conducted a traditional articulation analysis counting sound omissions, substitutions, and distortions to examine speech outcome. The process analysis employed by Chapman counted syllable structure, assimilatory, and substitution processes (i.e., omissions and substitutions), but not distortions, which may have underestimated the extent of the children's speech problems. A more detailed study of speech outcomes such as the one conducted in the United Kingdom would need to be carried out in the United States to reconcile the differences across studies. In the meantime, professionals can conclude that children with cleft palate perform at the level of their same-age peers by 5 years of age only if phonological process usage is considered. This does, however, bring up an important shortcoming of phonological process analyses and other assessment procedures that do not consider distortions when evaluating the speech sound systems of children with cleft palate.

Chapman and colleagues (Chapman, 1993; Chapman & Hardin, 1992) were not the first investigators to examine the speech of children with cleft palate using something other than a traditional articulation analysis. In fact, as early as 1983, Hodson, Chin, Redmond, and Simpson (1983) and Lynch, Fox, and Brookshire (1983) used "phonological" analysis procedures to describe the speech of a small number of children with cleft palate. In 1990, Powers, Erickson, and Dunn published a detailed phonetic and phonological analysis of 4 preschoolers with cleft palate. Although a comparison group was not included in the study, the authors described these children as more similar to "phonologically disordered children than normally developing children of the same chronological age" (Powers et al., 1990, p. 548). Interestingly, this report provided preliminary evidence for a relationship between the occurrence of phonological processes and lower overall language performance in children with cleft palate. Finally, two case studies of children with cleft palate who were not progressing in therapy employed detailed phonetic and phonological analyses of the children's speech sound system (Bernhardt, Doan, & Stoel-Gammon, 1995; Howard, 1993). Both articles highlighted the role that in-depth phonetic and phonological analyses play in management of children with cleft palate.

Some researchers and clinicians have questioned the contribution of phonological analyses to knowledge of speech development and/or management of children with cleft palate (see Golding-Kushner, 2001; Peterson-Falzone et al., 2001), and others have cautioned against ascribing "higher linguistic explanations to a child's use of phonological patterns or processes" (Trost-Cardamone & Bernthal, 1993, p. 309). I would argue that phonological-based analyses have provided and will continue to provide insights into the speech sound systems of children with cleft palate. The purpose of phonological analyses is to provide information about patterns of speech sound production and the systematic application of rules. The use of these procedures does not diminish the contribution of articulatory deficits to the sound patterns observed. Also, just as it may not be either appropriate or necessary to perform a detailed phonological analysis for all children with speech delays (e.g., those who exhibit sound distortions), the same is true for children with cleft palate. Additionally, it is important to remember that using phonological processes to describe or analyze children's sound systems is just one of several phonological approaches that might be employed to guide the assessment and intervention of children with speech sound disorders, and thus children with cleft palate (see earlier section on phonological theories). Finally, what should be clear is that structural deficits associated with clefting affect all aspects of phonological learning. As proposed by Russell and Grunwell (1993), youngsters with cleft palate "experience more difficulties with certain types of targets than would be expected from their increasingly more normal phonetic inventories" (p. 42). Several studies suggest that children with cleft palate may exhibit problems with speech production that are "phonological" in nature. For example, Whitehill et al. (2003) found that children with cleft palate who substituted /k/ for /t/ (i.e., backing) were unable to reliably identify synthetically generated /k/s and /t/s. However, this was not the case for a group of children with cleft palate without this sound substitution or for typically developing children. Next, Pamplona, Ysunza, and Espinosa (1999) found that phonological-based intervention was more effective than phonetic-based interventions in remediating compensatory articulation errors. Reportedly, less time was needed to change compensatory articulation errors when a phonological approach was employed. Finally, Chapman (2004a) used a nonlinear phonological analysis to describe the systematic use of pharyngeal fricatives by a preschooler with cleft palate.

## School Age to Adulthood

A literature review suggests that although speech proficiency improves with age, as a group, speakers with cleft palate may continue to exhibit speech problems into school age, adolescence, and beyond (e.g., Karnell & Van Demark, 1986; Lohmander-Agerskov et al., 1993; McWilliams, 1958; Pannbacker, 1971; Peterson-Falzone, 1995; Riski, 1995; Sell et al., 2001; Van Demark et al., 1979). The studies' findings were consistent in spite of varying methodologies and heterogeneous study populations (varying in age at time of testing, type and extent of clefting, integrity of the velopharyngeal mechanism, timing and types of management, etc.). Further, it appeared that although accuracy of production for most sound classes improved over time, fricatives (e.g., Albery & Grunwell, 1993; Grunwell et al., 2000; Lohmander-Agerskov et al., 1993; McWilliams, 1958; Pitzner & Morris, 1966; Van Demark et al., 1979) and affricates (Karnell & Van Demark, 1986; Van Demark et al., 1979) continued to pose problems for some speakers with cleft palate, and distortions replaced omissions and substitutions as the most common error type (e.g., Bardach et al., 1984; McWilliams, 1958).

As cautioned in the opening paragraphs of this chapter, these results represent group findings, and there are many children and adults with cleft palate who exhibit normal speech production from an early age (e.g., Chapman, 1993; Peterson-Falzone, 1995; Riski, 1995; Riski & DeLong, 1984). What, then, has the research on speech development of children with cleft palate indicated about variables mediating speech outcome across time? Presumably, a number of factors act singly or in combination to influence the child's acquisition of normal speech. These include but are not limited to the following:

1. Type and/or extent of initial clefting (e.g., Albery & Grunwell, 1993; Haapanen, 1994; Hardin-Jones & Jones, 2005; Karling, Larson, Leanderson, & Henningsson, 1993; Paliobei, Psifidis, & Anagnostopoulos, 2005; Riski, 1979; Riski & DeLong, 1984; Schönweiler et al., 1999; Van Demark & Hardin, 1985)
2. Otologic and/or hearing status (e.g., Hubbard, Paradise, McWilliams, Elster, & Taylor, 1985; Paliobei et al., 2005; Peterson-Falzone, 1995; Pitzner & Morris, 1966; Schönweiler et al., 1999; Van Demark et al., 1979)
3. Language functioning (Pamplona, Ysunza, Gonzáles, Ramírez, & Patiño, 2000)
4. Age (see Hardin-Jones & Jones, 2005; Peterson-Falzone et al., 2001; Rohrich, Love, Byrd, & Johns, 2000, for reviews), type (see LaRossa, 2000; Molsted, 1999; Peterson-Falzone et al., 2001, for reviews), and success of surgical interventions (e.g., Karnell & Van Demark, 1986; Peterson-Falzone, 1995)
5. Presence of VPI (e.g., Harding & Grunwell, 1993; Peterson-Falzone, 1995; Riski, 1979, 1995; Riski & DeLong, 1984; Van Demark, 1964, 1966; Van Demark et al., 1979)
6. Fistulae (e.g., Henningsson & Isberg, 1987, 1990; Karling, Larson, & Henningsson, 1993; Peterson-Falzone, 1995; Sell et al., 2001)

or dental/maxillary deviations (e.g., Albery & Grunwell, 1993; Bardach et al., 1984; Harding & Grunwell, 1993; Karnell & Van Demark, 1986; Pitzner & Morris, 1966; Riski, 1995; Van Demark et al., 1979)

7. Attendance at craniofacial team evaluations and follow-through with team recommendations (e.g., Peterson-Falzone, 1995)
8. Individual variation in the formation of the cleft (Molsted, 1999) and in learning strategies (e.g., Harding & Grunwell, 1993; Van Demark et al., 1979)
9. Access to intervention (e.g., Karling, Larson, Leanderson, & Henningsson, 1993; Riski & DeLong, 1984;) and type of intervention (Albery & Grunwell, 1993; Hardin-Jones & Chapman, 2005)

## Compensatory Articulations in the Speech of Children with Cleft Palate

A description of the speech development of children with cleft palate would not be complete without mention of their use of compensatory articulations. Compensatory articulations are typically backed patterns of articulation (e.g., a /ʔ/ is substituted for the /t/ in *two*) produced by the child to compensate for VPI, or they may occur as compensation for other structural problems such as malocclusions or fistulae (Peterson-Falzone et al., 2001). (See Chapter 11 for a more detailed discussion and description of compensatory articulations.)

Not all children with VPI produce compensatory sound substitutions. Instead, some children maintain the correct place of articulation but produce the sound with nasal emission of air. The reported occurrence of compensatory articulations varies across studies and centers, with the highest numbers being reported by Dorf and Curtin (1990). According to these authors, approximately 90% of children who had primary palate repair after age 12 months 15 days developed compensatory articulations compared to less than 5% of children who had surgery prior to that age. Their findings are somewhat difficult to evaluate as they did not provide important details such as information concerning the criteria employed to classify a child as a compensatory articulation user, the range of usage across children, and the age of children at time of testing.

Other investigators have reported a lower occurrence of compensatory misarticulations. According to Peterson-Falzone (1990) and Dalston

(1992), 22%–28% of children used these patterns. Chapman and Hardin (1992) found that although 90% of toddlers who had late surgery and were talking prior to surgery exhibited compensatory articulations, the overall occurrence for each child was very low. The child with the highest usage only had 14 instances of compensatory productions in a 100-word sample. More recent reports suggest that the percentage of children employing compensatory articulations has stayed fairly stable over time. Hardin-Jones and Jones (2005) and Chapman et al. (2007) found that 24% and 23% of the preschoolers they studied employed compensatory articulations.

There continues to be speculation about why some children develop compensatory misarticulations and others do not. According to Bzoch (1979), these patterns are produced and "reinforced" by listeners during the first few years of life. Another explanation attributes the development of these patterns to child preference for compensatory articulations over sounds produced with nasal emission (Morris, 1972). Although a few studies have attempted to test these two hypotheses, neither has been proven to date (Bradford & Culton, 1987; Paynter, 1987; Paynter & Kinard, 1979). At the same time, it does appear that words produced with compensatory articulations were considered to sound "better" by both parents (Bradford & Culton, 1987; Paynter, 1987) and children (Paynter, 1987; Paynter & Kinard, 1979[4]) than the same words produced with nasal emission of air.

Warren (1986) provided a physiologically based explanation for development of compensatory misarticulations. He suggested that the speech structures are responding like other regulating systems of the human body (e.g., respiration, temperature, cardiovascular) and using "control mechanisms" to preserve "steady state conditions" (Warren, 1986, p. 251). Following from this explanation, compensatory articulations were considered to be the result of a speaker's attempt to regulate oral pressure when pressure variations occurred as a result of VPI.

Dorf and Curtin (1982, 1990) suggested that use of compensatory articulations was tied to the child's "articulation age" at the time of surgery. That is, children who were more advanced with regard to "phonemic development" when palatal surgery was performed were more likely to

[4]This study found no difference in the children's preference for words produced with compensatory articulations or nasal emission if the children themselves produced compensatory articulations.

develop compensatory articulations. On the other hand, children who had later surgery and who demonstrated delays in "phonemic development" did not show evidence of these patterns.[5] According to the authors, this latter group did not develop compensatory patterns because, unlike the former group, they were not attempting productions beyond their speech production capabilities. Although these findings have received much attention in the literature, this study has not been replicated. In fact, both Peterson-Falzone (1990) and Dalston (1992) found a higher percentage of children with compensatory articulations in their early surgery groups (for a detailed discussion of these studies, see Peterson-Falzone et al., 2001). Although Chapman and Hardin (1992) did not compare two ages of surgery groups, all participants had received late surgery and all were producing words when surgery was performed. Yet, the median occurrence of compensatory articulations for any individual child was 6, which would hardly be considered significant.

More recently, Hardin-Jones and Jones (2005) found that age of surgery was not related to compensatory articulation usage in the preschoolers they studied. These authors speculated that lack of an association between age of surgery and compensatory articulation usage in their data was possibly related to the decrease in age of surgery and more aggressive management of VPI, providing "less opportunity for these patterns of articulation to stabilize in the developing phonology" (Hardin-Jones & Jones, 2005, p. 12).

Finally, Chapman et al. (2007) attempted to examine directly the impact of language level at time of surgery on speech outcome. This study included 40 children with cleft palate: 20 children who were less lexically advanced and younger and 20 children who were more lexically advanced and older when primary palatal surgery was performed. There was no

[5]Children studied by Dorf and Curtin (1990) were divided into groups based on age of surgery (i.e., before and after 12 months). For most children, it appeared that "articulation age" and chronological age were related. That is, most children in the early surgery group (i.e., surgery between 5 months 15 days and 12 months 15 days) also had less advanced speech development. However, it appeared that the children in the early surgery group who developed compensatory articulations had more advanced speech development. Conversely, the children in the late surgery group (i.e., surgery between 12 months 16 days and 27 months) who did not develop these patterns were reportedly delayed in speech development.

difference between the two groups in use of compensatory articulations at 3 years of age. As might be expected, however, compensatory articulation usage was related to VPI status in this study.

Investigators in Mexico have linked compensatory articulations to language deficits in children with cleft palate. Pamplona et al. (2000) found that children with VPI and compensatory articulations were more likely to exhibit delays in language than children with VPI but no compensatory articulations. The authors interpreted their findings as suggesting that a language deficit was related to the child's adoption of compensatory strategies. This proposal was also supported by studies showing that phonological intervention was successful in remediating compensatory articulations (Pamplona et al., 1999). The idea that compensatory articulation usage may be related to language status is an intriguing notion that needs additional study.

Although compensatory articulations are a much talked about characteristic of the speech of children with cleft palate, it is still not known why some children develop these patterns and others do not. However, the role of individual differences in acquisition of speech should be considered. For example, professionals know that some typically developing children without cleft palate may show preferences for and/or avoidance of words with certain sounds or syllable structures. According to Ferguson and Farwell (1975), these preferences are governed by children's production abilities. Further, different paths or approaches to phonological development have been identified. Some children take a more cautious approach initially and only attempt words that are within their phonetic and syllabic capabilities (e.g., Ferguson, 1979; Vihman & Greenlee, 1987). Others are more "exploratory" (Vihman & Greenlee, 1987, p. 519), producing words that are clearly beyond their production abilities (Ferguson, 1979; Vihman & Greenlee, 1987). Finally, the literature contains numerous examples of noncleft children who adopt unusual sound substitutions to compensate for some production constraint (see Ingram, 1997, for a description). Like their noncleft peers, children with cleft palate should be expected to adopt a variety of strategies, compensatory and otherwise, when acquiring the sound system of their language (Kuehn & Moller, 2000; Moller, 1990). Currently, most studies examining the speech development of children with cleft palate are group designs that describe average performance rather than focusing on individual patterns of development. Further, there has been no detailed analysis of the emergence, context of usage, or change over time in the child's production of compensatory articulations. Such data might provide additional insight into the development and maintenance of these patterns.

## Language Skills of Children with Cleft Palate

Just as vocal behaviors emerge during the 1st year of life, so do other aspects of language. In addition to reduplicated babbling, babies begin to show signs of linguistic comprehension and the ability to communicate nonverbally. Once the first words appear, vocabulary continues to grow. Single-word utterances are soon replaced by multiword constructions that reflect knowledge of syntax, morphology, pragmatics, and phonology. It is the interaction of all these complex linguistic systems that governs the overall communicative competence of children at different ages and stages of development.

Examination of the language functioning of children with cleft palate is not a new area of investigation. Like the study of speech sound development, this area received considerable attention in the 1950s through 1970s and experienced renewed interest in the 1990s. However, compared to the speech development literature, fewer studies have been performed, and there is less consistency of findings across studies. Regardless, most conclude that children with cleft palate are at risk for language delay.

### Status of Language Comprehension in Children with Cleft Palate

It is not easy to make a global statement about the language comprehension skills of young children with cleft palate as discrepancies exist across studies, and the cause of these differences is not clear. Some investigators have reported delays in the receptive language skills of children with cleft palate during the toddler and preschool years (Broen, Devers, Doyle, Prouty, & Moller, 1998; Chapman, Graham, Gooch, & Visconti, 1998; Fox, Lynch, & Brookshire, 1978; Jocelyn, Penko, & Rode, 1996; Morris, 1962; Nation, 1970; Philips & Harrison, 1969b), but others have not (Long & Dalston, 1983; Neiman & Savage, 1997; Scherer & D'Antonio, 1995; Spriestersbach, Darley, & Morris, 1958). It does appear, however, that school-age children with cleft palate are more likely to demonstrate age-appropriate comprehension (see Chapman et al., 1998). Interestingly, two of the studies showing delays in comprehension skills of young children with cleft palate found hearing status during the 1st year of life to be an important variable affecting comprehension performance (Broen et al., 1998; Jocelyn et al., 1996).

## Status of Language Production in Children with Cleft Palate

### Early Lexical and Later Semantic Development

Most researchers agree that young children with cleft palate are delayed in the acquisition of words (Broen et al., 1998; Chapman et al., 2003; Scherer & D'Antonio, 1995). The delay has been noted as early as 15 months (Broen et al., 1998) and may or may not continue into adolescence (Morris, 1962). Morris found differences, compared to normative data, for expressive vocabulary—number of different words produced in connected speech—in his youngest age group (3–8 years) but not his oldest group (9–16 years). Delays were also noted for 5- to 16-year-olds when they were asked to define words. A more recent study by Eliason and Richman (1990) showed no differences in defining words for 4-, 5-, and 6-year-old children with cleft palate. Again, the differences across these two studies may be related to improved management for children with cleft palate or differences across the studies in the age of children at testing.

Slower onset of babbling, lack of practice with supralaryngeal consonants, and difficulty in development of the feedback loop may be responsible for slowed vocabulary development in this population of children early on (Chapman et al., 2001). Or, as suggested by Broen et al. (1998), VPI and poor hearing may also be contributing factors. Whether VPI and poor hearing are contributing factors to language delays at later ages needs additional study.

### Standardized Measures of Language Production

Often, standardized measures have been administered to examine the language production abilities of children with cleft palate. A number of different measures have been used across studies, targeting various aspects of expressive language ranging from vocabulary to syntax to pragmatics. In some studies, the performance of the children with cleft palate was compared to the norms developed for the specific test employed (e.g.,

Neiman & Savage, 1997). Otherwise, investigators included a noncleft comparison group (e.g., Broen et al., 1998; Chapman et al., 1998; Fox et al., 1978; Jocelyn et al., 1996; Philips & Harrison, 1969b; Scherer & D'Antonio, 1995).

A majority of these studies suggested delays in expressive language for young children with cleft palate (Broen et al., 1998; Fox et al., 1978; Jocelyn et al., 1996; Neiman & Savage, 1997; Philips & Harrison, 1969b; Scherer & D'Antonio, 1995). However, at least one investigation found that children with cleft palate were similar to their peers on standardized tests of language production (Chapman et al., 1998).

## Spontaneous Speech Measures

A number of studies have attempted to examine the spontaneous language of young children with cleft palate in an attempt to gain more information about their linguistic abilities. Although Scherer and D'Antonio (1995) found differences between cleft and noncleft children in MLU, other studies carried out in the 1990s found children with cleft palate to be similar to their peers on this measure (Broen et al., 1998; Jocelyn et al., 1996). The landmark studies by Spriestersbach et al. (1958) and Morris (1962) showed mixed results. Both studies found delays in mean length of response; however, structural complexity was not found to be delayed except for the Morris participants at the youngest ages (Spriestersbach et al., 1958; Morris, 1962). In the Morris (1962) study, number of one-word responses (at all ages), number of different words, and mean length of five longest responses (for the youngest participants) were also significantly different from the normative samples. Finally, in a frequently cited study comparing adults with and without cleft palate, Pannbacker (1971) found differences for utterance length but not for structural complexity.

## Pragmatics

Pragmatics, or the use of language in social contexts, has been the least explored area of language for children with cleft palate. Early investigations suggested that if pragmatic deficits existed at all (see Long & Dalston, 1982a, 1982b[6]), they were no longer apparent by about 4 years of age (Shames, Rubin, & Kramer, 1966, as cited in Shames & Rubin, 1972). Next, a study

[6]No differences were noted in 12-month-olds' ability to express themselves with gestures alone; however, they differed from their peers in the ability to pair a vocalization with a gesture, suggesting that delays in other aspects of language may be a contributing factor (Long & Dalston, 1982a, 1982b).

by Warr-Leeper, Crone, Carruthers, and Leeper (1988) suggested just the opposite. They found that preschoolers with cleft palate scored within normal limits on the *Test of Pragmatic Skills* (Shulman, 1986), which required the child to respond to a variety of standardized situations using a specific communicative function (e.g., the child was asked to complete a task but was not given a pencil in an attempt to elicit an object request). However, the school-age children with cleft palate were delayed (based on the standardization sample, as a noncleft group was not included in the study design). The authors suggested that the poorer performance of the older children with cleft palate was not related to a problem in pragmatics per se, but rather to a tendency of children and adults with cleft palate to say less (i.e., produce shorter utterances) (Warr-Leeper et al., 1988).

In 1998, Chapman and colleagues attempted to study the pragmatic skills of preschool and school-age children with cleft palate by examining their performance on a standardized test of pragmatics (similar to Warr-Leeper et al., 1988) and during conversational interactions using the model of conversational participation described by Fey (1986). According to Fey, conversational participation varies on two parameters: (1) conversational assertiveness (i.e., "ability or willingness [or both] to take a conversational turn when none has been solicited by a partner") and (2) conversational responsiveness (i.e., how well the child responds to a partner's initiations) (Fey, 1986, p. 69). Children's conversational participation can be rated on both parameters, yielding four different conversational profiles (see Fey, 1986, for a complete description). The results of this investigation showed no statistically significant differences between either the preschool or school-age children with cleft palate on the standardized tests of pragmatics or the conversational measures. However, individual child comparisons indicated that 50% of the preschoolers and 20% of the school-age children showed a passive style of conversational interaction. That is, they were responsive to their partners' initiations but were less likely to initiate a conversational turn. The fact that so many of the preschool children exhibited a passive conversational style and that some of the comparisons were approaching significance suggested that the study may have been underpowered.

Frederickson, Chapman, and Hardin-Jones (2006) attempted to replicate and extend the findings of Chapman et al. (1998) by comparing the conversational skills of 17 preschool children with cleft palate and their noncleft peers using a similar study design. In addition to examining their conversational skills, these investigators were also interested in exploring the relationship between the children's performance in the area of pragmatics and other aspects of speech and language development. Results of this study suggested that 35% of preschoolers with cleft palate were either less assertive or less responsive than their noncleft peers. Additionally, the children with cleft palate were less assertive overall, as they produced fewer assertive conversational acts and maintained rather than extended the topic more frequently. They were also found to be less responsive to caregivers' comments. Finally, there was a positive relationship between level of conversational assertiveness and speech proficiency as children who were less assertive in conversation with their caregivers had poorer articulation skills. A number of explanations have been offered for why children with cleft palate might exhibit a more passive conversational style. First, they may have a pragmatic deficit that is interfering with their acquisition of conversational rules (Chapman et al., 1998). Second, they may know the rules for conversational interaction but appear passive because of an unwillingness to communicate secondary to problems with speech intelligibility (e.g., Faircloth & Faircloth, 1972; Pannbacker, 1971; Scherer & D'Antonio, 1995). Finally, the passive style may be a characteristic of a shy/withdrawn personality (Chapman et al., 1998). While the findings of the Frederickson et al. (2006) study cannot rule out explanations one and three, they do provide some support for explanation two because a relationship was found between conversational assertiveness and speech proficiency.

## Auditory Short-Term Memory Deficits and Language Skills of Children with Cleft Palate

Although there is debate about the role that auditory short-term memory deficits play in language impairment, several studies suggest that children with language impairment without cleft palate may show deficits in verbal working memory (see Montgomery, 2002, for a review). Investigators from Finland employed event-related potentials to examine short-term memory traces in children with cleft palate. Results of these studies suggested that school-age children with cleft palate exhibited deficits in auditory short-term memory that may be related to language and learning problems frequently reported in this population (Čeponienė et al., 1999). Interestingly, cleft type comparisons suggested that children with cleft lip only were similar to their noncleft peers, whereas those with cleft palate (with or without cleft lip) were significantly different from the noncleft group. Children with unilateral cleft lip and palate showed the largest differences on tasks measuring permanence of short-term memory traces. Clearly, more work is needed before a direct link can be made between deficits like those described here and poor language performance in children with cleft palate, but this work provides an exciting new direction for future study.

## Summary

The studies described in this chapter provide support for the proposal that children with cleft palate show early delays in speech that may continue into adolescence and beyond. Early constraints on production of supralaryngeal consonants are carried over into the period immediately following palatal surgery and may partially explain lexical delays in this population of children. Over time, however, the impact of the early structural deficits may be lessened as success of surgical and speech-language interventions begin to play a role in communication outcomes. Although children with cleft palate are at risk for language as well as speech delays, the language delays are not as easily tied to the structural deficits associated with clefting. However, it appears that children with poorer speech may be less assertive conversationalists. For example, children may shorten their utterances and/or be less willing to initiate conversational interactions due to past or present communication difficulties.

In Appendix 8A, descriptions are provided of three children with cleft palate. These children were chosen to represent the variability that is seen in this population. Additionally, each child will be compared with a noncleft peer who is matched for age, gender, and mother's educational level.

## Conclusion

Communication skills vary greatly in children with cleft palate. Early deficits related to palatal clefting may have obvious consequences for later speech and language development. Delays in one aspect of linguistic development (i.e., phonology) have implications for other aspects of language development (e.g., lexical development, conversational skills). In light of these apparent relationships, early surgery, aggressive treatment and monitoring of middle ear disease, and early and intensive speech and language intervention seem especially important to assure the best outcomes possible for these children.

## Acknowledgments

This work was supported by a research grant from the National Institute on Deafness and Other Communication Disorders (RO1 DC03193). I would like to thank the children described in Chapter 3 and their families for serving as research participants. I would also like to thank graduate students Trina DeHann, Rebecca Fenander, and Amy Krantz and the editors Karlind Moller and Leslie Glaze for helpful comments and careful editing of various drafts of this paper.

# APPENDIX 8A

# Speech and Language Profiles of Three Children with Cleft Palate

The children described in this appendix participated in a study of speech development of children with cleft palate ages 6 to 39 months. Data are presented showing changes in speech and language from 9 to 33 months of age, with the most detailed analyses being performed at 33 months. At the 33-month session, a 150-utterance spontaneous speech sample was analyzed for a number of indicators of speech and language functioning. These included overall accuracy of consonant production, accuracy of production for each manner category, percentage of intelligible utterances, mean length of utterance (MLU), number of different words (NDW), grammatical complexity (Scarborough's [1990] Index of Productive Syntax [IPSyn]), and conversational profile (Fey, 1986).

The first child, Child 1-CP, was a female with a unilateral cleft of the lip and palate. She underwent lip repair at 1;25 (months;days) and palate repair at 12;27. Based on parental report and observation of her spontaneous language sample at the presurgery session, it was determined that she produced approximately four words at the time of palatal surgery. Reportedly, Child 1-CP experienced only four episodes of otitis media prior to 33 months of age. She had pressure-equalization (PE) tubes inserted at the time of lip surgery and primary palatal surgery, and again at 24 months of age. Child 1-CP failed the tympanometry screening at one of the test sessions; however, results of audiological testing performed at her craniofacial team evaluations indicated hearing within normal limits. Unlike any of the other children to be described, Child 1-CP was not enrolled in therapy during this period nor was therapy recommended.

Table 8.1 provides information on size of consonant inventory for Child 1-CP and her noncleft peer (Child 1-NCP) from 9 to 33 months. Although Child 1-CP possessed a smaller consonant inventory at 9 months (i.e., presurgery) than Child 1-NCP, by 13 months the two babies produced a similar number of consonants. Further, the only difference noted for types of consonants present in their inventories was that Child 1-NCP produced two oral fricatives at 13 months and Child 1-CP did not produce oral fricatives until 17 months. However, from that point on, the makeup of their consonant inventories was very similar. Examination and comparison of their performance on the *MacArthur Communicative Development Inventories* (CDI; Fenson et al., 1993) and the *Preschool Language Scale–Third Edition* (PLS-3; Zimmerman, Steiner, & Evatt-Pond, 1992) suggested that Child 1-CP was performing as well as her noncleft peer, with a few exceptions (see Table 8.1). Examination of the data for both girls at 33 months also indicated very similar performance for production of stops, nasals, and glides (see Table 8.2). Child 1-CP was less accurate for production of fricatives, affricates, and liquids. Also, she was slightly less intelligible than Child 1-NCP (80% vs. 96%), and resonance was rated as mildly hypernasal. Examination of their spontaneous language samples suggested that the two girls were very similar for grammatical complexity, MLU, and NDW. Finally, both showed similar profiles with regard to assertiveness and responsiveness during conversational interactions with their mothers and were judged to be active conversationalists.

The second child, Child 2-CP, was a male born with a bilateral cleft of the lip and palate. This child was 2;23 at the time of lip repair and 12;14 at the time of primary palatal surgery. He was not producing any words at the time of palatal surgery. PE tubes were inserted at both lip and palatal surgeries. Audiological testing at all craniofacial team visits revealed normal hearing. He failed tympanometry screenings at three experimental sessions and reportedly had five episodes of otitis media from 6 until 33 months of age. Unlike Child 1-CP, Child 2-CP showed delayed speech development early on, and therapy was recommended. He was enrolled in early intervention from 20 months until 32 months of age, at which time he was dismissed as his speech and language development was judged to be within normal limits.

In contrast to both Child 1-CP and Child 2-NCP, Child 2-CP had a reduced consonant inventory through 27 months (see Table 8.1). In addition to quantitative differences in his consonant inventory, qualitative differences were also noted. For example, it was not until 21 months of age that oral stops and fricatives appeared in his inventory. With regard to lexical development (as measured by the CDI), it is clear that Child 2-CP was delayed until approximately 27 months, when he appeared not only to catch up but also to surpass his noncleft peer. Performance on the

(*text continues on p. 278*)

**Table 8.1**
Performance on Speech and Language Measures Over Time

| | Months | | | | | |
|---|---|---|---|---|---|---|
| **Child** | **9** | **13** | **17** | **21** | **27** | **33** |
| **Child 1-CP** | | | | | | |
| Size of inventory[a] | 5 | 9 | 18 | 23 | 22 | 23 |
| CDI[b] | 2 | 3 | 40 | 121 | 534 | — |
| PLS-3[c] | —[d] | — | 119(R) 124(E) | — | 115(R) 124(E) | — |
| **Child 1-NCP** | | | | | | |
| Size of inventory | 8 | 10 | 18 | 22 | 23 | 22 |
| CDI | 0 | 3 | 21 | 238 | 492 | — |
| PLS-3 | — | — | 132(R) 119(E) | — | 121(R) 119(E) | — |
| **Child 2-CP** | | | | | | |
| Size of inventory | 3 | 8 | 6 | 13 | 17 | 19 |
| CDI | 0 | 0 | 1 | 125 | 456 | — |
| PLS-3 | — | — | 123(R) 106(E) | — | 89(R) 96(E) | — |
| **Child 2-NCP** | | | | | | |
| Size of inventory | 10 | 14 | 13 | 17 | 23 | 19 |
| CDI | 0 | 3 | 8 | 220 | 283 | — |
| PLS-3 | — | — | 114(R) 100(E) | — | 105(R) 113(E) | — |

*(continues)*

**Table 8.1** *(continued)*

| Child | Months | | | | | |
|---|---|---|---|---|---|---|
| | 9 | 13 | 17 | 21 | 27 | 33 |
| **Child 3-CP** | | | | | | |
| Size of inventory | 8 | 7 | 8 | 15 | 19 | 20 |
| CDI | 0 | 12 | 28 | 105 | 482 | — |
| PLS-3 (R)(E) | — | — | 114(R) 112(E) | — | 97(R) 104(E) | — |
| **Child 3-NCP** | | | | | | |
| Size of inventory | 8 | 5 | 10 | 19 | 23 | 23 |
| CDI | 0 | 4 | 23 | 160 | 426 | — |
| PLS-3 (R)(E) | — | — | 132(R) 112(E) | — | 112(R) 100(E) | — |

[a]Number of consonants occurring at least two times in a spontaneous sampling session.

[b]Number of words reported on the *MacArthur Communicative Developmental Inventories* (CDI; Fenson et al., 1993).

[c]Standard scores for (R) receptive and (E) expressive subtests of the *Preschool Language Scale–Third Edition* (Zimmerman, Steiner, & Evatt-Pond, 1992).

[d]Dash indicates that assessment was not administered.

**Table 8.2**
**Performance of Children for Speech (% Accuracy for All Consonants and Different Manner Categories), Intelligibility, Resonance, and Language Measures at 33 Months**

| Measures | Child 1-CP | Child 1-NCP | Child 2-CP | Child 2-NCP | Child 3-CP | Child 3-NCP |
|---|---|---|---|---|---|---|
| All consonants | 71% | 86% | 78% | 62% | 40% | 82% |
| Stops | 83% | 85% | 84% | 64% | 20% | 75% |
| Nasals | 94% | 92% | 89% | 78% | 70% | 90% |
| Fricatives | 63% | 76% | 70% | 54% | 32% | 65% |
| Affricates | 46% | 95% | 0% | 7% | 0% | 75% |
| Liquids | 26% | 75% | 56% | 41% | 23% | 65% |
| Glides | 95% | 95% | 97% | 90% | 91% | 95% |
| Intelligible utterances | 80% | 96% | 90% | 79% | 69% | 88% |
| Resonance | Mild hypernasality | Normal | Normal | Normal | Mild hypernasality | Normal |
| IPSyn score | 84 | 84 | 77 | 82 | 76 | 79 |
| MLU | 2.74 | 3.02 | 2.74 | 2.62 | 2.03 | 3.06 |
| NDW | 156 | 142 | 145 | 136 | 92 | 162 |
| Conversational participation | Active conversationalist | Active conversationalist | Active conversationalist | Active conversationalist | Passive conversationalist | Active conversationalist |

*Note.* IPSyn = Index of Productive Syntax (Scarborough, 1990); MLU = mean length of utterance; NDW = number of different words.

PLS-3 appeared to be age appropriate and equal to or in advance of Child 2-NCP, except at 27 months. By 33 months of age, Child 2-CP not only had achieved normal speech and language functioning but also was outperforming Child 2-NCP on many measures (see Table 8.2). For example, he was more accurate for production of almost all sound classes, and his speech was more intelligible. Additionally, he performed somewhat better than his noncleft peer on all measures of language production with the exception of the IPSyn. Child 2-CP was similar to his noncleft peer in terms of conversational participation, and both were judged to be active conversationalists. Finally, his resonance was judged to be normal, and there was no concern regarding velopharyngeal function.

Child 3-CP was a female with a bilateral cleft of the lip and palate. Lip surgery was performed at 4;5. Initial primary palatal surgery was attempted at 11;26, but because the cleft was unusually wide, only the soft palate was repaired. The hard palate was repaired with a second surgery at 17;27. Child 3-CP had PE tubes inserted at lip surgery and again at 11 months of age. Results of audiological evaluations conducted at craniofacial team visits indicated hearing within normal limits. However, she failed three tympanometry screenings and reportedly experienced 11 episodes of otitis media from 6 until 33 months. Child 3-CP had an expressive lexicon of approximately 31 words when the hard palate was repaired at 17 months. She was enrolled in therapy at 22 months and was still receiving intervention at 33 months of age.

An examination of Table 8.1 shows that Child 3-CP did not differ from her noncleft peer in size of consonant inventory at 9 and 13 months, but seemed to fall behind over time. In fact, examination of Child 3-CP's consonant production at 33 months suggested that she was considerably behind Child 3-NCP in terms of speech development. As seen in Table 8.2, Child 3-CP was less accurate for production of all consonants except glides. Further, glottal stops were frequently occurring in her speech. Child 3-CP showed decreased intelligibility compared to her cleft and noncleft peers. Resonance was rated as mildly hypernasal, although it was difficult to judge because of her poor speech. In contrast, she appeared similar to her noncleft peer for lexical development (based on her mother's report of number of words produced on the CDI), performance on the PLS-3, and grammatical complexity as measured by the IPSyn. However, NDW and MLU at 33 months were lower than those seen for any of the other children described here (MLU was just outside the normal range for her age). Finally, on the measures of conversational assertiveness and responsiveness, compared to her noncleft peer, Child 3-CP produced fewer acts that were classified as assertive (19% vs. 40% for Child 3-CP and Child 3-NCP, respectively) or utterances that initiated or extended the topic. Instead, she produced more utterances that were classified as responsive and more topic-maintaining utterances, suggesting a more passive conversational style. Unlike her peers with cleft palate, Child 3-CP showed delays in speech development that were likely impacting her expressive language and conversational participation. For example, NDW may have been underestimated due to problems with speech intelligibility. Because of the late palatal repair, some of her error patterns were likely related to prior structural deficits.

## Summary

The three children with cleft palate described here followed different developmental paths. Child 1-CP evidenced steady progress beginning almost immediately following surgical repair of the palate. Although she was not quite as proficient as her noncleft peer in terms of overall speech intelligibility and production of fricatives, affricates, and liquids, she was functioning within normal limits for her age. A mild degree of hypernasality was present in her speech but was not of concern to her parents or the professionals overseeing her management. In contrast, Child 3-CP was behind her noncleft peer as well as her peers with cleft palate in speech intelligibility and accuracy of production of all sound classes except glides. It appeared that while she was performing within normal limits on standardized tests of language, she was behind in MLU, NDW, and conversational skills. Finally, Child 2-CP was a very interesting case because of the obvious delays in speech and lexical development early on. Apparently, surgical repair of the palate provided him with an appropriate mechanism; however, he did not experience the early progress that was seen for Child 1-CP. Eventually, he may have shown improvement on his own; with intervention, however, not only was he able to catch up but he performed slightly better than his noncleft peer by 33 months of age. Early intervention seemed to promote not only good speech, but overall communicative competence for this child.

Follow-up testing at 5 years of age revealed that Child 1-CP and Child 2-CP were continuing to do well in all areas of speech and language development. This was not the case for Child 3-CP, however. While she did not exhibit significant hypernasality, she was still receiving therapy for a speech sound disorder. Although her speech was intelligible, she continued to use compensatory substitutions. Recall that she was the child who received late hard palate repair and also had 11 reported episodes of otitis media, both of which may have contributed to her speech problems over the study period.

# References

Albery, E., & Grunwell, P. (1993). Consonant articulation in different types of cleft lip and palate. In P. Grunwell (Ed.), *Analysing cleft palate speech* (pp. 83–111). London: Whurr Publishers.

Ball, M. J., & Kent, R. D. (Eds.). (1997). *The new phonologies: Developments in clinical linguistics.* San Diego, CA: Singular.

Bardach, J., Morris, H. L., Olin, W., McDermott-Murray, J., Mooney, M., & Bardach, E. (1984). Late results of multidisciplinary management of unilateral cleft lip and palate. *Annals of Plastic Surgery, 12,* 235–242.

Barlow, J. A. (2001). Case study: Optimality theory and the assessment and treatment of phonological disorders. *Language, Speech, and Hearing Services in Schools, 32,* 242–256.

Barlow, J. A., & Dinnsen, D. A. (1998). Asymmetrical cluster development in a disordered system. *Language Acquisition, 7,* 1–49.

Barlow, J. A., & Gierut, J. A. (1999). Optimality theory in phonological acquisition. *Journal of Speech, Language, and Hearing Research, 42,* 1482–1498.

Bernhardt, B. H. (1992). The application of nonlinear phonological theory to intervention with one phonologically disordered child. *Clinical Linguistics and Phonetics, 6,* 283–316.

Bernhardt, B. H. (1994). Phonological intervention techniques for syllable and word structure development. *Clinics in Communication Disorders, 4,* 54–65.

Bernhardt, B. H., Doan, A., & Stoel-Gammon, C. (1995). Phonological and phonetic analysis of cleft palate speech. In K. Elenius & P. Branderud (Eds.), *Proceedings of the XIIth International Congress of Phonetic Sciences* (Vol. 4, pp. 108–115). Stockholm: KTH and Stockholm University Press.

Bernhardt, B. H., & Gilbert, J. (1992). Applying linguistic theory to speech-language pathology: The case for nonlinear phonology. *Clinical Linguistics and Phonetics, 6,* 123–145.

Bernhardt, B. H., & Stemberger, J. P. (1998). *Handbook of phonological development from the perspective of constraint-based nonlinear phonology.* San Diego, CA: Academic Press.

Bernhardt, B. H., & Stemberger, J. P. (2000). *Workbook in nonlinear phonology.* Austin, TX: PRO-ED.

Bernhardt, B. H., & Stoel-Gammon, C. (1994). Nonlinear phonology: Introduction and clinical application. *Journal of Speech and Hearing Research, 37,* 123–143.

Bradford, P. W., & Culton, G. L. (1987). Parents' perceptual preferences between compensatory articulation and nasal escape of air in children with cleft palate. *Cleft Palate Journal, 24,* 299–303.

Broen, P. A., Devers, M. C., Doyle, S. S., Prouty, J. M., & Moller, K. T. (1998). Acquisition of linguistic and cognitive skills by children with cleft palate. *Journal of Speech, Language, and Hearing Research, 41,* 676–687.

Bzoch, K. R. (1965). Articulation proficiency and error patterns of preschool cleft palate and normal children. *Cleft Palate Journal, 2*, 340–349.

Bzoch, K. R. (1979). Measurement and assessment of categorical aspects of cleft palate speech. In K. R. Bzoch (Ed.), *Communicative disorders related to cleft lip and palate* (pp. 161–191). Boston: Little, Brown.

Camp, B. W., Burgess, D., Morgan, L. J., & Zerbe, G. (1987). A longitudinal study of infant vocalization in the first year. *Journal of Pediatric Psychology, 12*, 321–331.

Casby, M. W. (2001). Otitis media and language development: A meta-analysis. *American Journal of Speech-Language Pathology, 10*, 65–80.

Čeponienė, R., Hukki, J., Cheour, M., Haapanen, M.-L., Koskinen, M., Alho, K., & Näätänen, R. (2000). Dysfunction of the auditory cortex persists in infants with certain cleft types. *Developmental Medicine and Child Neurology, 42*, 258–265.

Čeponienė, R., Hukki, J., Cheour, M., Haapanen, M.-L., Ranta, R., & Näätänen, R. (1999). Cortical auditory dysfunction in children with oral clefts: Relation with cleft type. *Clinical Neurophysiology, 110*, 1921–1926.

Chapman, K. L. (1991). Vocalizations of toddlers with cleft lip and palate. *Cleft Palate-Craniofacial Journal, 28*, 172–178.

Chapman, K. L. (1993). Phonologic processes in children with cleft palate. *Cleft Palate-Craniofacial Journal, 30*, 64–72.

Chapman, K. L. (2004a, November). *The interaction of phonological and articulation disorders in children with cleft palate.* Paper presented at the annual meeting of the American Speech-Language-Hearing Association, Philadelphia.

Chapman, K. L. (2004b). Is presurgery and early post surgery performance related to speech and language outcomes at 3 years of age for children with cleft palate? *Clinical Linguistics and Phonetics, 18*, 235–257.

Chapman, K. L., Graham, K. T., Gooch, J., & Visconti, C. (1998). Conversational skills of preschool and school-age children with cleft lip and palate. *Cleft Palate-Craniofacial Journal, 35*, 503–516.

Chapman, K. L., & Hardin, M. A. (1992). Phonetic and phonologic skills of 2-year-olds with cleft palate. *Cleft Palate-Craniofacial Journal, 29*, 435–443.

Chapman, K. L., Hardin-Jones, M., Cook, K., & Panelli, R. (2002, November). *The impact of otitis media on vocal development of babies with cleft palate.* Poster presented at the annual meeting of the American Speech-Language-Hearing Association, Atlanta.

Chapman, K. L., Hardin-Jones, M., Goldstein, J. A., Halter, K. A., Havlik, R. J., & Schulte, J. (2007, April). *The influence of linguistic level at the time of primary palatal surgery on speech outcome for children with cleft palate.* Poster presented at the annual meeting of the American Cleft Palate-Craniofacial Association, Broomfield, CO.

Chapman, K. L., Hardin-Jones, M., & Halter, K. A. (2003). The relationship between early speech and later speech and language performance for children with cleft palate. *Clinical Linguistics and Phonetics, 17*, 173–197.

Chapman, K. L., Hardin-Jones, M., Schulte, J., & Halter, K. (2001). Vocal development of 9-month-old babies with cleft palate. *Journal of Speech, Language, and Hearing Research, 44*, 1268–1283.

Cheour, M., Čeponienė, R., Hukki, J., Haapenen, M., Näätänen, R., & Alho, K. (1999). Brain dysfunction in neonates with cleft palate revealed by mismatch negativity. *Clinical Neurophysiology, 110*, 324–328.

Cheour, M., Haapenen, M., Čeponienė, R., Hukki, J., Ranta, R., & Näätänen, R. (1998). Mismatch negativity (MMN) as an index of auditory sensory memory deficit in cleft-palate and CATCH syndrome children. *NeuroReport*, 9, 2709–2712.

Chomsky, N., & Halle, M. (1968). *The sound pattern of English*. New York: Harper & Row.

Counihan, D. T. (1960). Articulation skills of adolescents and adults with cleft palate. *Journal of Speech and Hearing Disorders, 25*, 181–187.

Dalston, R. M. (1992). Timing of cleft palate repair: A speech pathologist's viewpoint. *Problems in Plastic and Reconstructive Surgery: Cleft Palate Surgery, 2*, 30–38.

Dinnsen, D. A. (1997). Nonsegmental phonologies. In M. J. Ball & R. D. Kent (Eds.), *The new phonologies: Developments in clinical linguistics* (pp. 77–126). San Diego, CA: Singular.

Donegan, P. J., & Stampe, D. (1979). The study of natural phonology. In D. A. Dinnsen (Ed.), *Current approaches to phonological theory* (pp. 126–173). Bloomington: Indiana University Press.

Dorf, D. S., & Curtin, J. W. (1982). Early cleft palate repair and speech outcome. *Plastic and Reconstructive Surgery, 70*, 74–79.

Dorf, D. S., & Curtin, J. W. (1990). Early cleft palate repair and speech outcome: A 10-year experience. In J. Bardach & H. L. Morris (Eds.), *Multidisciplinary management of cleft lip and palate* (pp. 341–348). Philadelphia: W. B. Saunders.

Dorf, D. S., Reisberg, D. J., & Gold, H. O. (1985). Early prosthetic management of cleft palate. Articulation development prosthesis: A preliminary report. *Journal of Prosthetic Dentistry, 53*, 222–226.

Elbert, M., & Gierut, J. (1986). *Handbook of clinical phonology*. London: Taylor & Francis.

Eliason, M. J., & Richman, L. C. (1990). Language development in preschoolers with cleft. *Developmental Neuropsychology, 6*, 173–182.

Estrem, T., & Broen, P. A. ( 1989). Early speech production of children with cleft palate. *Journal of Speech and Hearing Research, 32*, 12–23.

Faircloth, S. R., & Faircloth, M. A. (1972). Delayed language and linguistic variation. In K. R. Bzoch (Ed.), *Communicative disorders related to cleft lip and palate* (pp. 130–135). Boston: Little, Brown.

Fenson, L., Dale, P. S., Reznick, J. S., Thal, D., Bates, E., Hartung, J. P., Pethick, S., & Reilly, J. S. (1993). *MacArthur communicative development inventories*. San Diego, CA: Singular.

Ferguson, C. A. (1979). Phonology as an individual access system: Some data from language acquisition. In C. J. Fillmore, D. Kempler, & W. S.-Y. Wang (Eds.), *Individual differences in language ability and language behavior* (pp. 189–201). New York: Academic Press.

Ferguson, C. A., & Farwell, C. (1975). Words and sounds in early language acquisition. *Language, 51*, 419–439.

Fey, M. E. (1986). *Language intervention with young children.* San Diego, CA: College-Hill Press.

Fey, M. E. (1992). Clinical forum: Articulation and phonology treatment. Articulation and phonology: Inextricable constructs in speech pathology. *Language, Speech and Hearing Services in Schools, 23,* 225–232.

Fox, D., Lynch, J., & Brookshire, B. (1978). Selected developmental factors of cleft palate children between 2 and 33 months of age. *Cleft Palate Journal, 15,* 239–245.

Frederickson, M. S., Chapman, K. L., & Hardin-Jones, M. A. (2006). Conversational skills of children with cleft palate: A replication and extension, *Cleft Palate-Craniofacial Journal, 43,* 179–188.

Fry, D. B. (1966). The development of the phonological system in the normal and the deaf child. In F. Smith & G. A. Miller (Eds.), *The genesis of language: A psycholinguistic approach* (pp. 187–206). Cambridge, MA: MIT Press.

Gierut, J. A., Elbert, M., & Dinnsen, D. (1987). The functional analysis of phonological knowledge and generalization learning in misarticulating children. *Journal of Speech and Hearing Research, 30,* 462–479.

Gierut, J. A., & Morrisette, M. L. (2006). The clinical significance of optimality theory for phonological disorders. *Topics in Language Disorders, 25,* 266–280.

Goad, H. (1998). Consonant harmony in child language: An optimality-theoretic account. In S. J. Hannahs & M. Young-Scholten (Eds.), *Focus on phonological acquisition* (pp. 113–142). Amsterdam: Benjamins.

Golding-Kushner, K. J. (2001). *Therapy techniques for cleft palate speech and related disorders.* San Diego, CA: Singular.

Grunwell, P., Brøndsted, K., Henningsson, G., Jansonius, K., Karling, J., Meijer, M., Ording, U., Wyatt, R., Vermeij-Zieverink, E., & Sell, D. (2000). A six-center international study of the outcome of treatment in patients with clefts of the lip and palate: The results of a cross-linguistic investigation of cleft palate speech. *Scandinavian Journal of Plastic and Reconstructive Surgery and Hand Surgery, 34,* 219–229.

Grunwell, P., & Russell, J. (1987). Vocalisations before and after cleft palate surgery: A pilot study. *British Journal of Disorders of Communication, 22,* 1–17.

Grunwell, P., & Russell, J. (1988). Phonological development in children with cleft lip and palate. *Clinical Linguistics and Phonetics, 2,* 75–95.

Haapanen, M. L. (1994). Cleft type and speech proficiency. *Folia Phoniatrica Logopedics, 46,* 57–63.

Harding, A., & Grunwell, P. (1993). Relationship between speech and timing of hard palate repair. In P. Grunwell (Ed.), *Analysing cleft palate speech* (pp. 48–82). London: Whurr Publishers.

Hardin-Jones, M., & Chapman, K. L. (2005, March). *Early intervention: A retrospective look at outcomes.* Poster presented at the annual meeting of the American Cleft Palate-Craniofacial Association, Myrtle Beach, SC.

Hardin-Jones, M., Chapman, K. L., & Schulte, J. (2003). The impact of cleft type on early vocal development in babies with cleft palate. *Cleft Palate-Craniofacial Journal, 40,* 453–459.

Hardin-Jones, M. A., Chapman, K. L., Wright, J., Halter, K. A., Schulte, J., Dean, J. A., Havlik, R. J., & Goldstein, J. (2002). The impact of early palatal obturation on consonant development in babies with unrepaired cleft palate. *Cleft Palate-Craniofacial Journal, 39,* 157–163.

Hardin-Jones, M. A., & Jones, D. L. (2005). Speech production of preschoolers with cleft palate. *Cleft Palate-Craniofacial Journal, 42,* 7–13.

Henningsson, G., & Isberg, A. (1987). Influence of palatal fistulae on speech and resonance. *Folia Phoniatrica, 39,* 183–191.

Henningsson, G., & Isberg, A. (1990). Oronasal fistulas and speech production. In J. Bardach & H. L. Morris (Eds.), *Multidisciplinary management of cleft lip and palate* (pp. 787–792). Philadelphia: W. B. Saunders.

Hodson, B. W., Chin, L., Redmond, B., & Simpson, R. (1983). Phonological evaluation and remediation of speech deviations of a child with a repaired cleft palate: A case study. *Journal of Speech and Hearing Disorders, 48,* 93–98.

Howard, S. J. (1993). Articulatory constraints on a phonological system: A case study of cleft palate speech. *Clinical Linguistics and Phonetics, 7,* 299–317.

Hubbard, T. W., Paradise, J. L., McWilliams, B. J., Elster, B. A., & Taylor, F. H. (1985). Consequences of unremitting middle-ear disease in early life. *New England Journal of Medicine, 312,* 1529–1534.

Hutters, B., Bau, A., & Brøndsted, K. (2001). A longitudinal group study of speech development in Danish children born with and without cleft lip and palate. *International Journal of Language and Communication Disorders, 36,* 447–470.

Ingram, D. (1976). *Phonological disability in children.* New York: Elsevier.

Ingram, D. (1997). Generative phonology. In M. J. Ball & R. D. Kent (Eds.), *The new phonologies: Developments in clinical linguistics* (pp. 7–33). San Diego, CA: Singular.

Jensen, T. S., Boggild-Andersen, B., Schmidt, J., Ankerhus, J., & Hansen, E. (1988). Perinatal risk factors and first year vocalizations: Influence on preschool language and motor performance. *Developmental Medicine and Child Neurology, 30,* 153–161.

Jocelyn, L. J., Penko, M. A., & Rode, H. L. (1996). Cognition, communication, and hearing in young children with cleft lip and palate and in control children: A longitudinal study. *Pediatrics, 97,* 529–534.

Jones, C. E., Chapman, K. L., & Hardin-Jones, M. A. (2003). Speech development of children with cleft palate before and after palatal surgery. *Cleft Palate-Craniofacial Journal, 40,* 19–31.

Karling, J., Larson, O., & Henningsson, G. (1993). Oronasal fistulas in cleft palate patients and their influence on speech. *Scandinavian Journal of Plastic and Reconstructive Surgery and Hand Surgery, 27,* 193–201.

Karling, J., Larson, O., Leanderson, R., & Henningsson, G. (1993). Speech in unilateral and bilateral cleft palate patients from Stockholm. *Cleft Palate-Craniofacial Journal, 30,* 73–77.

Karnell, M. P., & Van Demark, D. R. (1986). Longitudinal speech performance in patients with cleft palate: Comparisons based on secondary management. *Cleft Palate Journal, 23,* 278–288.

Kemp-Fincham, S. I., Kuehn, D. P., & Trost-Cardamone, J. E. (1990). Speech development and the timing of primary palatoplasty. In J. Bardach & H. L. Morris (Eds.), *Multidisciplinary management of cleft lip and palate* (pp. 736–745). Philadelphia: W. B. Saunders.

Konst, E. M. (2002). *The effects of infant orthopaedics on speech and language development in children with unilateral cleft lip and palate.* Unpublished doctoral dissertation, University of Nijmegen.

Konst, E. M., Weersink-Braks, H., Rietveld, T., & Peters, H. (1999). Prelexical development of unilateral cleft lip and palate babies with reference to presurgical infant orthopaedics: A randomized prospective clinical trial. *Clinical Linguistics and Phonetics, 13,* 395–407.

Kuehn, D. P., & Moller, K. T. (2000). Speech and language issues in the cleft palate population: The state of the art. *Cleft Palate-Craniofacial Journal, 37,* 348-1–348-35. Retrieved January 15, 2001, from http://cpcj.allenpress.com/pdfserv/i1055-6656-037-04-0348.pdf

LaRossa, D. (2000). The state of the art in cleft palate surgery. *Cleft Palate-Craniofacial Journal, 37,* 225–228.

Lohmander, A., Lillvik, M., & Friede, H. (2004). The impact of early infant jaw-orthopaedics on early speech production in toddlers with unilateral cleft lip and palate. *Clinical Linguistics and Phonetics, 18,* 259–284.

Lohmander-Agerskov, A. (1998). Speech outcome after cleft palate surgery with the Goteborg regimen including delayed hard palate closure. *Scandinavian Journal of Plastic and Reconstructive Surgery and Hand Surgery, 32,* 63–80.

Lohmander-Agerskov, A., Havstam, C., Söderpalm, E., Elander, A. Lilja, J., Friede, H., & Persson, E. (1993). Assessment of speech in children after repair of isolated cleft palate. *Scandinavian Journal of Plastic Surgery and Reconstructive Surgery and Hand Surgery, 27,* 307–310.

Lohmander-Agerskov, A., Söderpalm, E., Friede, H., Persson, E., & Lilja, J. (1994). Prespeech in children with cleft lip and palate or cleft palate only: Phonetic analysis related to morphologic and functional factors. *Cleft Palate-Craniofacial Journal, 31,* 271–279.

Long, N. V., & Dalston, R. M. (1982a). Gestural communication in 12-month-old cleft lip and palate children. *Cleft Palate Journal, 19,* 57–61.

Long, N. V., & Dalston, R. M. (1982b). Paired gestural and vocal behavior in 1-year-old cleft lip and palate children. *Journal of Speech and Hearing Disorders, 47,* 403–406.

Long, N. V., & Dalston, R. M. (1983). Comprehension abilities of 1-year-old infants with cleft lip and palate. *Cleft Palate Journal, 20,* 303–306.

Lynch, J., Fox, D., & Brookshire, B. (1983). Phonological proficiency of two cleft palate toddlers with school-age follow-up. *Journal of Speech and Hearing Disorders, 48,* 274–285.

McCarthy, J. J. (2002). *A thematic guide to optimality theory.* Cambridge, UK: Cambridge University Press.

McCarthy, J. J., & Prince, A. (1994). The emergence of the unmarked: Optimality in prosodic morphology. *Northeastern Linguistic Society, 24,* 333–379.

McCarthy, J. J., & Prince, A. (1995). Faithfulness and reduplicative identity. In J. N. Beckman, L. W. Dickey, & S. Urbanczyk (Eds.), *University of Massachusetts occasional papers* (Vol. 18, pp. 249–384). Amherst: University of Massachusetts, Graduate Linguistic Student Association.

McCathren, R. B., Yoder, P. J., & Warren, S. F. (1999). The relationship between prelinguistic vocalization and later expressive vocabulary in young children with developmental delay. *Journal of Speech, Language, and Hearing Research, 42,* 915–924.

McWilliams, B. J. (1958). Articulation problems of a group of cleft palate adults. *Journal of Speech and Hearing Research, 1,* 68–74.

Menyuk, P., Liebergott, J., & Schultz, M. (1986). Predicting phonological development. In B. Lindblom & R. Zetterstrom (Eds.), *Precursors of early speech: Proceedings of an international symposium held at the Wenner-Gren Center* (pp. 79–94). New York: Stockton Press.

Moller, K. T. (1990). Early speech development: The interaction of learning and structure. In J. Bardach & H. L. Morris (Eds.), *Multidisciplinary management of cleft lip and palate* (pp. 726–731). Philadelphia: W. B. Saunders.

Molsted, K. (1999). Treatment outcome in cleft lip and palate: Issues and perspectives. *Critical Review Oral Biology and Medicine, 10,* 225–239.

Montgomery, J. W. (2002). Understanding the language difficulties of children with specific language impairments: Does verbal working memory matter? *American Journal of Speech-Language Pathology, 11,* 77–91.

Morris, H. L. (1962). Communication skills of children with cleft lips and palates. *Journal of Speech and Hearing Research, 5,* 79–90.

Morris, H. L. (1972). Cleft palate. In A. J. Weston (Ed.), *Communicative disorders: An appraisal.* Springfield, IL: CC Thomas.

Nation, J. (1970). Vocabulary comprehension and usage of preschool cleft palate and normal children. *Cleft Palate Journal, 7,* 639–644.

Neiman, G. S., & Savage, H. E. (1997). Development of infants and toddlers with clefts from birth to 3 years of age. *Cleft Palate-Craniofacial Journal, 34,* 218–225.

O'Gara, M. M., & Logemann, J. A. (1988). Phonetic analyses of the speech development of babies with cleft palate. *Cleft Palate Journal, 25,* 122–134.

O'Gara, M. M., Logemann, J. A., & Rademaker, A. W. (1994). Phonetic features by babies with unilateral cleft lip and palate. *Cleft Palate-Craniofacial Journal, 31,* 446–451.

Oller, D. K., & Eilers, R. E. (1988). The role of audition in infant babbling. *Child Development, 59,* 441–449.

Oller, D. K., Wieman, L. A., Doyle, W. J., & Ross, C. (1976). Infant babbling and speech. *Journal of Child Language, 3,* 1–11.

Olson, D. A. (1965). *A descriptive study of the speech development of a group of infants with cleft palate.* Unpublished doctoral dissertation, Northwestern University, Evanston, IL.

Paliobei, V., Psifidis, A., & Anagnostopoulos, D. (2005). Hearing and speech assessment of cleft palate patients after palatal closure: Long-term results. *International Journal of Pediatric Otorhinolaryngology, 69,* 1373–1381.

Pamplona, M. C., Ysunza, A., & Espinosa, J. (1999). A comparative trial of two modalities of speech intervention for compensatory articulation in cleft palate children: Phonologic approach versus articulatory approach. *International Journal of Pediatric Otorhinolaryngology, 49,* 21–26.

Pamplona, M. C., Ysunza, A., González, M., Ramírez, E., & Patiño, C. (2000). Linguistic development in cleft palate patients with and without compensatory articulation disorder. *International Journal of Pediatric Otorhinolaryngology, 54,* 81–91.

Pannbacker, M. (1971). Language skills of cleft palate children: A review. *British Journal of Disorders in Communication, 6,* 37–44.

Paradise, J. L., Dollahan, C. A., Campbell, T. F., Feldman, H. M., Bernard, B. S., Colborn, D. K., Rockett, H. E., Jankosky, J. E., Pitcairn, D. L., Sabo, D. L., Kurs-Lasky, & Smith, C. G. (2000). Language, speech sound production, and cognition in 3-year-old children in relation to otitis media in their first 3 years of life. *Pediatrics, 105,* 1119–1130.

Paynter, E. T. (1987). Parental and child preference for speech produced by children with velopharyngeal incompetence. *Cleft Palate Journal, 24,* 112–118.

Paynter, E. T., & Kinard, M. W. (1979). Perceptual preferences between compensatory articulation and nasal escape of air in children with velopharyngeal incompetence. *Cleft Palate Journal, 16,* 262–266.

Peterson-Falzone, S. J. (1990). A cross-sectional analysis of speech results following palatal surgery. In J. Bardach & H. L. Morris (Eds.), *Multidisciplinary management of cleft lip and palate* (pp. 750–757). Philadelphia: W. B. Saunders.

Peterson-Falzone, S. J. (1995). Speech outcomes in adolescents with cleft lip and palate. *Cleft Palate-Craniofacial Journal, 32,* 125–128.

Peterson-Falzone, S. J., Hardin-Jones, M. A., & Karnell, M. P. (2001). *Cleft palate speech* (3rd ed.). St. Louis, MO: Mosby.

Philips, B. J., & Harrison, R. J. (1969a). Articulation patterns of preschool cleft palate children. *Cleft Palate Journal, 6,* 245–253.

Philips, B. J., & Harrison, R. J. (1969b). Language skills of preschool cleft palate children. *Cleft Palate Journal, 6,* 108–119.

Pitzner, J. C., & Morris, H. L. (1966). Articulation skills and adequacy of breath pressure ratios of children with cleft palate. *Journal of Speech and Hearing Disorders, 31,* 26–40.

Powers, G. R., Erickson, C. B., & Dunn, C. (1990). Speech analyses of four children with repaired cleft palates. *Journal of Speech and Hearing Disorders, 55,* 542–549.

Prince, A., & Smolensky, P. (1997). Optimality: From neural networks to universal grammar. *Science, 273,* 1604–1610.

Prince, A., & Smolensky, P. (2004). *Optimality theory: Constraint interaction in generative grammar.* Malden, MA: Blackwell.

Riski, J. E. (1979). Articulation skills and oral-nasal resonance in children with pharyngeal flaps. *Cleft Palate Journal, 16,* 421–428.

Riski, J. E. (1995). Speech assessment of adolescents. *Cleft Palate-Craniofacial Journal, 32,* 109–113.

Riski, J. E., & DeLong, E. (1984). Articulation development in children with cleft lip/palate. *Cleft Palate Journal, 21,* 57–64.

Rohrich, R. J., Love, E. J., Byrd, H. S., & Johns, D. F. (2000). Optimal timing of cleft palate closure. *Plastic and Reconstructive Surgery, 106,* 413–421.

Russell, J., & Grunwell, P. (1993). Speech development in children with cleft lip and palate. In P. Grunwell (Ed.), *Analysing cleft palate speech* (pp. 19–47). London: Whurr Publishers.

Rvachew, S., Slawinski, E. B., Williams, M., & Green, C. L. (1996). The impact of early onset otitis media on prelinguistic speech development. *Journal of Speech-Language Pathology and Audiology, 20,* 247–255.

Rvachew, S., Slawinski, E. B., Williams, M., & Green, C. L. (1999). The impact of early onset otitis media on babbling and early language development. *Journal of the Acoustical Society of America, 105,* 467–475.

Scarborough, H. S. (1990). Index of productive syntax. *Applied Psycholinguistics, 11,* 1–22.

Scherer, N. J., & D'Antonio, L. L. (1995). Parent questionnaire for screening early language development in children with cleft palate. *Cleft Palate-Craniofacial Journal, 32,* 7–13.

Schönweiler, R., Lisson, J. A., Schönweiler, B., Eckardt, A., Ptok, M. Tränkmann, J., & Hausamen, J. (1999). A retrospective study of hearing, speech and language function in children with clefts following palatoplasty and veloplasty procedures at 18–24 months of age. *International Journal of Pediatric Otorhinolaryngology, 50,* 207–217.

Schwartz, R. G. (1992). Clinical forum: Phonological assessment and treatment—clinical application of recent advances in phonological theory. *Language, Speech, and Hearing Services in Schools, 23,* 269–276.

Schwartz, R. G., Mody, M., & Petinou, K. (1997). Phonological acquisition and otitis media: Speech perception and speech production. In J. E. Roberts, I. F. Wallace, & F. W. Henderson (Eds.), *Otitis media in young children: Medical, developmental, and educational considerations* (pp. 109–133). Baltimore: Brookes.

Sell, D., Grunwell, P., Mildinhall, S., Murphy, T., Cornish, T. A., Bearn, D., Shaw, W. C., Murray, J. J., Williams, A. C., & Sandy, J. R. (2001). Cleft lip and palate care in the United Kingdom: The clinical standards advisory group (CSAG) study. Part 3: Speech outcomes. *Cleft Palate-Craniofacial Journal, 38,* 30–37.

Shames, G., & Rubin, H. (1972). Psycholinguistic measures of language and speech. In K. R. Bzoch (Ed.), *Communicative disorders related to cleft lip and palate* (pp. 201–218). Boston: Little, Brown.

Shriberg, L. D., Flipsen, P., Thielke, H., Kwiatkowski, J., Kertoy, M. K., Katcher, M. L., Nellis, R. A., & Block, M. G. (2000). Risk for speech disorder associated with early recurrent otitis media with effusion: Two retrospective studies. *Journal of Speech, Language, and Hearing Research, 43,* 79–99.

Shriberg, L. D., Friel-Patti, S., Flipsen, P., & Brown, R. L. (2000). Otitis media, fluctuant hearing loss, and speech-language outcomes: A preliminary structural equation model. *Journal of Speech, Language, and Hearing Research, 43*, 100–120.

Shulman, B. B. (1986). *Test of pragmatic skills* (Rev. ed.). Tucson, AZ: Communication Skill Builders.

Spriestersbach, D. C., Darley, F. L., & Morris, H. L. (1958). Language skills in children with cleft palates. *Journal of Speech and Hearing Research, 1*, 279–285.

Stampe, D. (1979). *A dissertation on natural phonology.* Bloomington: Indiana University Linguistics Club.

Stoel-Gammon, C. (1989). Prespeech and early speech development of two late talkers. *First Language, 9*, 207–224.

Stoel-Gammon, C. (1992). Prelinguistic vocal development: Measurement and predictions. In C. A. Ferguson, L. Menn, & C. Stoel-Gammon (Eds.), *Phonological development: Models, research, implications* (pp. 439–456). Timonium, MD: York Press.

Stoel-Gammon, C. (1998a). Sounds and words in early language acquisition: The relationship between lexical and phonological development. In R. Paul (Ed.), *Exploring the speech-language connection* (pp. 25–52). Baltimore: Brookes.

Stoel-Gammon, C. (1998b). Role of babbling and phonology in early linguistic development. In A. M. Wetherby, S. F. Warren, & J. Reichle (Eds.), *Transitions in prelinguistic communication* (Vol. 7, pp. 87–110). Baltimore: Brookes.

Stoel-Gammon, C., & Cooper, J. A. (1984). Patterns of early lexical and phonological development. *Journal of Child Language, 11*, 247–271.

Trost-Cardamone, J. E., & Bernthal, J. E. (1993). Articulation assessment procedures and treatment decisions. In K. T. Moller & C. D. Starr (Eds.), *Cleft palate: Interdisciplinary issues and treatment* (5th ed., pp. 307–336). Austin, TX: PRO-ED.

Van Demark, D. R. (1964). Misarticulations and listener judgments of the speech of individuals with cleft palates. *Cleft Palate Journal, 1*, 232–245.

Van Demark, D. R. (1966). A factor analysis of the speech of children with cleft palate. *Cleft Palate Journal, 3*, 159–170.

Van Demark, D. R., & Hardin, M. A. (1985). Longitudinal evaluation of articulation and velopharyngeal competence of patients with pharyngeal flaps. *Cleft Palate Journal, 22*, 163–172.

Van Demark, D. R., Morris, H. L., & Vandehaar, C. (1979). Patterns of articulation abilities in speakers with cleft palate. *Cleft Palate Journal, 16*, 230–239.

Vihman, M. M. (1986). Individual differences in babbling and early speech: Predicting to age 3. In B. Lindblom & R. Zetterstrom (Eds.), *Precursors of Early Speech: Proceedings of an International Symposium Held at the Wenner-Gren Center* (pp. 95–109). New York: Stockton Press.

Vihman, M. M. (1992). Early syllables and the construction of phonology. In C. A. Ferguson, L. Menn, & C. Stoel-Gammon (Eds.), *Phonological development: Models, research, implications* (pp. 393–422). Timonium, MD: York Press.

Vihman, M. M. (1993a). Variable paths to early word production. *Journal of Phonetics, 21*, 61–82.

Vihman, M. M. (1993b). The construction of a phonological system. In B. de Boysson-Bardies, S. de Schonen, P. Jusczyk, P. McNeilage, & J. Morton (Eds.), *Developmental neurocognition: Speech and face processing in the first year of life* (pp. 411–449). Dordrecht: Kluwer.

Vihman, M. M., Ferguson, C. A., & Elbert, M. (1986). Phonological development from babbling to speech: Common tendencies and individual differences. *Applied Psycholinguistics, 7*, 3–40.

Vihman, M. M., & Greenlee, M. (1987). Individual differences in phonological development: Ages 1 and 3 years. *Journal of Speech and Hearing Research, 30*, 503–521.

Vihman, M. M., Macken, M. A., Miller, R., Simmons, H., & Miller, J. (1985). From babbling to speech: A re-assessment of the continuity issue. *Language, 61*, 397–444.

Warren, D. W. (1986). Compensatory speech behaviors in individuals with cleft palate: A regulation/control phenomenon? *Cleft Palate Journal, 23*, 251–260.

Warr-Leeper, G., Crone, L., Carruthers, A., & Leeper, H. (1988, April). *A comparison of the performance of preschool children with cleft lip and/or palate on the Test of Pragmatic Skills.* Paper presented at the annual meeting of the American Cleft Palate Association, Williamsburg, VA.

Wermke, K., Hauser, C., Komposch, G., & Stellzig, A. (2002). Spectral analysis of prespeech sounds (spontaneous cries) in infants with unilateral cleft lip and palate (UCLP): A pilot study. *Cleft Palate-Craniofacial Journal, 39*, 285–295.

Whitehill, T. L., Francis, A. L., & Ching, C. K-Y. (2003). Perception of place of articulation by children with cleft palate and posterior placement. *Journal of Speech, Language, and Hearing Research, 46*, 451–461.

Whitehurst, G. J., Smith, M., Fischel, J. E., Arnold, D. S., & Lonigan, C. J. (1991). The continuity of babble and speech in children with specific expressive language delay. *Journal of Speech and Hearing Research, 34*, 1121–1129.

Willadsen, E., & Albrechtsen, H. (2006). Phonetic descriptions of babbling in Danish toddlers born with and without unilateral cleft lip and palate. *Cleft Palate-Craniofacial Journal, 43*, 190–200.

Willadsen, E., & Enemark, H. (2000). A comparative study of prespeech vocalizations in two groups of toddlers with cleft palate and a noncleft group. *Cleft Palate-Craniofacial Journal, 37*, 172–178.

Zimmerman, I. L., Steiner, V. G., & Evatt-Pond, R. (1992). *Preschool language scale* (3rd ed.). San Diego, CA: Psychological Corp.

# CHAPTER 9

# Hearing Assessment and Management

*Jane E. Carlstrom and Peggy B. Nelson*

The audiologist has the primary responsibility for performing hearing assessment and follow-up to identify potential hearing loss in children born with cleft palate or craniofacial anomalies. Fortunately, audiologists have access to a variety of diagnostic techniques that provide very early and accurate information on a patient's hearing status. By performing newborn hearing screenings and, later, indirect and direct behavioral tests, the audiologist can achieve a thorough description of any hearing loss and describe its potential impact on learning and communication. In collaboration with the otolaryngologist, the audiologist helps to define and support healthy hearing in children with cleft palate or craniofacial anomalies. Carlstrom and Nelson describe the audiologist's role in identifying hearing loss, recommending amplification or other treatments, performing periodic reassessments and reviews, and educating the family, caregivers, and teachers on the critical association between adequate hearing and academic performance.

1. The authors describe the benefits of newborn hearing screenings. Explain how hearing can be tested in a newborn, and describe the follow-up that is required if a newborn does not pass a screening.
2. In the 1st year, there are a number of indirect measures that can serve as diagnostic tools to detect and define hearing thresholds in infants and toddlers. Name and describe the major applications of these early assessment tools.
3. What components are essential to perform visual reinforcement audiometry (VRA)? What are the advantages and limits to this behavioral diagnostic technique?
4. If hearing loss is detected, what amplification options are available to babies, infants, and toddlers in the early years? What support

will a family need to ensure that an amplification device is accepted and tolerated by the child?

5. What association exists between early hearing thresholds and learning speech and language? Academically, what evidence is available to support the need for adequate hearing in the classroom? How can this be achieved in larger, busier, and louder preschool and elementary settings?

The partnership between physicians, speech-language pathologists, and audiologists is more important than ever for diagnosing and treating hearing disorders in children with cleft palate. The incidence of hearing disorders among children with cleft palate remains high.

Children with cleft palate that is not part of a syndrome show an incidence of sensorineural hearing loss similar to that of children without a cleft palate. However, because of the anatomical differences caused by the cleft, children with cleft palates almost universally experience episodes of persistent otitis media that may lead to conductive hearing loss. Between 30% and 90% of children with cleft palate require placement of middle ear tubes to ventilate the middle ear space and improve hearing (e.g., Broen et al., 1996; Muntz, 1993; Zanzi, Cherpillod, & Hohlfeld, 2002). Following palatal repair the incidence of otitis media falls, but children with cleft palate continue to experience middle ear problems more frequently than their peers without clefts. The audiologist's role on the cleft palate team is to identify and describe the nature and degree of any hearing problems and to provide information about the effects of the hearing loss on communication and about options for follow-up and management. Fortunately, audiometric test techniques have been refined, new tools for early identification have been developed, and amplification options have expanded. We can and *should* assess auditory function in all children with cleft palate.

The impact of hearing loss on learning remains profound. Although most children with recurrent otitis media presumably catch up to their peers (e.g., Haggard, 1996; Paradise, 2007), some reports suggest that there are long-term language and learning effects of reduced hearing sensitivity due to otitis media (for a review, see Roberts, Rosenfeld, & Zeisel, 2004). Most children with permanent hearing loss show long-term language and educational delays due to impaired hearing (e.g., Ross, 1990). On average, children with mild hearing losses read more than a grade level below their peers.

Overwhelming evidence (Moeller, 2000; Yoshinaga-Itano & Gravel, 2001) suggests that the negative consequences of hearing loss can be minimized with early identification and remediation. Unfortunately, early identification of hearing loss is still not universal. The average age of identification of mild hearing loss is older than 2 years (Harrison, Roush, & Wallace, 2003). Hearing loss can be identified at birth and described in detail by the time a child reaches 3–6 months of age. Even before this age, there are reliable diagnostic and treatment strategies available to the otolaryngologist, audiologist, and speech-language pathologist team, including effective treatment for middle ear pathologies, use of appropriate hearing aid technology, and behavioral interventions to enhance language stimulation and development in early childhood. All of these approaches will play a role in preventing secondary learning difficulties (Carney & Moeller, 1998). The message must be promoted: Young children can be tested and treated for hearing disorders.

## Tools for Evaluating Auditory Function

For children of every developmental age, audiologists, speech-language pathologists, and physicians can work together to determine the following:

- When to screen for hearing loss and what techniques to use
- When and how to do diagnostic tests to confirm and describe hearing loss
- When and how to measure other auditory function
- How to conduct appropriate follow-up for medical management, amplification, family counseling, and/or speech-language and educational services

### Screening Tools

Newborn hearing screening has gained widespread acceptance. In 2007, approximately 95% of newborns in the United States participated in a hearing screening program (National Center for Hearing Assessment and

Management, 2007). Newborn hearing screening is important to identify congenital hearing loss, but children with cleft palate are at risk for later developing hearing loss in large part due to middle ear disorders. The importance of screening infants who are at risk for developing hearing loss cannot be overemphasized (Joint Committee on Infant Hearing, 2007). Table 9.1 outlines the hearing risk factors for newborns and older infants. These include factors often encountered at the cleft palate clinic, including craniofacial anomalies, conditions requiring a period of 5 or more days in the neonatal intensive care unit, syndromes associated with progressive hearing loss, and recurrent caregiver concerns. Clearly, all children with cleft palate should be screened regularly, due to their known risk for hearing loss caused by otitis media (Muntz, 1993). Currently, two screening tools are used for newborn hearing screening: transient-evoked otoacoustic emissions and auditory brainstem response.

*Transient-evoked otoacoustic emissions* (TEOAE) reflect the nonlinear echo response of normal cochlear outer hair cells to a click stimulus. A small probe with a soft tip is inserted into the ear canal, a series of clicks is presented, and a sensitive microphone picks up the cochlear emission. When outer hair cells from the cochlea are functioning normally, they generate a "cochlear echo" in response to stimulation. When the middle ear is normal, the cochlear echo response can be measured in the ear canal and displayed on a screen. A TEOAE screening provides a quick, reliable assessment of outer hair cell function over a broad frequency range using a soft probe in the infant's ear canal (Maxon, White, Behrens, & Vohr, 1995). Although TEOAE is adversely affected by infant and environmental noise, and by fluid in the newborn ear canal and/or middle ear space, they have been successfully measured in over 90% of neonatal ears.

*Auditory brainstem response* (ABR) screening measures the evoked response of the VIIIth cranial nerve and the brainstem to broadband click stimuli. ABR screening requires the placement of electrodes on the newborn's scalp, mastoid, and earlobe. As with the TEOAE test, a series of clicks is presented through a soft earpiece in the child's ear. The response to sound is seen as changes in electrical activity in the brainstem. ABR is considered a slightly more invasive procedure than TEOAE. ABR also requires more time (and therefore money) and disposable supplies. The two tools can be used in tandem, resulting in good test sensitivity and specificity.

The critical element of a successful screening program is follow-up. Those children referred for additional testing must be located and brought to an audiologic/otologic facility. If hearing loss is identified, then medi-

**Table 9.1**
**2007 Joint Committee on Infant Hearing Risk Indicators Associated with Permanent Congenital, Delayed-Onset, or Progressive Hearing Loss in Childhood**

1. Caregiver concern regarding hearing, speech, language, or developmental delay
2. Family history of permanent childhood hearing loss
3. Neonatal intensive care of >5 days, or any of the following regardless of length of stay: ECMO (Extra Corporeal Membrane Oxygenation), assisted ventilation, exposure to ototoxic medications (gentamycin and tobramycin) or loop diuretics (furosemide/lasix), and hyperbilirubinemia requiring exchange transfusion
4. In-utero infections, such as cytomegalovirus, herpes, rubella, syphilis, and toxoplasmosis
5. Craniofacial anomalies, including those involving the pinna, ear canal, ear tags, ear pits, and temporal bone anomalies
6. Physical findings, such as white forelock, associated with a syndrome known to include a sensorineural or permanent conductive hearing loss
7. Syndromes associated with hearing loss or progressive or late-onset hearing loss, such as neurofibromatosis, osteopetrosis, and Usher syndrome
8. Other frequently identified syndromes, including Waardenburg, Alport, Pendred, and Jervell and Lange Nielson
9. Neurodegenerative disorders, such as Hunter syndrome, or sensory motor neuropathies, such as Friedreich ataxia and Charcot-Marie-Tooth syndrome
10. Culture-positive postnatal infections associated with sensorineural hearing loss, including confirmed bacterial and viral (especially herpes viruses and varicella) meningitis
11. Head trauma, especially basal skull/temporal bone fracture requiring hospitalization
12. Chemotherapy

*Note.* From Joint Committee on Infant Hearing. (2007). Year 2007 position statement: Principles and guidelines for early hearing detection and intervention programs. *Pediatrics, 120,* 898–921.

cal, audiologic, and educational remediation services must be available without delays. The Joint Committee on Infant Hearing (2007) recommends that those who do not pass the newborn hearing screening receive diagnostic hearing evaluation before age 3 months and receive appropriate amplification and enroll in an early intervention program if necessary by age 6 months. These goals are rarely accomplished; typical delays between identification and intervention are reported to be 9 months to 1 year (Harrison & Roush, 1996), resulting in a loss of valuable time.

## Diagnostic Test Tools

Referral from screening must be followed by detailed diagnostic testing of the child's hearing sensitivity and auditory function. The only direct test of hearing is the assessment of *behavioral responses* to sound. Although the ability to do this behavioral testing is limited for very young infants (0–5 months of age), it is the "gold standard" for testing all children who are at or beyond the 5-month developmental level. Procedures for each age range are outlined below. Together with indirect measures of auditory function (outlined in a later section), audiologists and physicians can complete testing and implement treatment by the time the child is 6 months of age, as recommended by the National Institutes of Health consensus conference on early identification (1993).

### Direct Measures of Hearing

***0- to 6-Month-Olds.*** Limited behavioral information can be obtained about hearing function during a child's first 6 months of life. Behavioral testing is not usually feasible until a developmental age of 5–6 months, when the child can be conditioned to respond selectively to sound. Behavioral observation audiometry (BOA) involves the observation of changes in a child's behavior when sounds are presented. The observed behaviors may include eyeblinks, a startle response, arousal from sleep, or quieting. BOA is considered unreliable and is not recommended because unacceptably high numbers of false positive and false negative results have been reported. For example, children with hearing loss may show reflexive responses to nonauditory stimuli at the same time the sound is presented, and the observers may misinterpret the infant's behavior as a response to sound (a false negative result). Conversely, children with normal hearing may fail to respond as expected and thus may be misidentified as having hearing loss (Diefendorf & Gravel, 1996). Thus, physiological measures of auditory function are the only appropriate tests before a child is 5 months of age.

***6-Month- to 2-Year-Olds.*** Pediatric audiologists consider 6 months to 2 years the ideal age range for thorough behavioral evaluation of hearing and auditory function. Complete behavioral test results (ear-specific air- and bone-conduction thresholds) can be obtained by experienced pediatric audiologists, although multiple test sessions may be necessary. The clinic must be equipped to appeal to parents and young children. Behavioral testing is accomplished successfully by skilled personnel using *visual reinforcement audiometry* (VRA) equipment. VRA is based on the principles of operant conditioning and on the natural tendency of infants to turn toward an interesting or novel sound. Audiologists obtain good estimates of hearing threshold by appropriately distracting the child, conditioning the child to turn toward the sound, and reinforcing the child for an appropriate response. During conditioning trials, tones or speech are presented at levels that are presumed audible. When the child turns toward the sound, animated toys (that are otherwise invisible) are lit up to reinforce that behavior. Once the child is conditioned, the intensity of the signals is systematically decreased, and thresholds are obtained. Control trials (with no sound presented) ensure that the child is turning only in response to a sound. Multiple and interesting lighted toys are necessary to maintain conditioning over time to test a variety of signals, including speech. The audiologist assesses threshold for hearing the child's name, nonsense syllables, or familiar objects and body parts to confirm pure tone results.

Typically, two audiologists and a caregiver are involved in VRA testing. One audiologist is in the room with the child and caregiver, maintaining the child's attention between trials; the other audiologist is outside the booth, controlling the audiometer and reinforcers. Figure 9.1 shows a child (on her mother's lap) who has just heard the sound through the insert earphone and has turned toward the reinforcer. Remote-controlled systems are commercially available that allow a single audiologist to control the audiometer and reinforcers from inside the room with the child.

Some young children object to using earphones, and the audiologists may elect to begin testing in the sound field. In this case, asymmetric hearing losses cannot be identified because the child will respond using the better ear only. Thresholds of the poorer ear, then, cannot be measured when the stimuli are presented through loudspeakers rather than earphones. When possible, ear-specific information is obtained using insert earphones with young children. One earphone is inserted and taped into place while the child is distracted. Testing is initiated immediately, before the child can object to the earphone. After thresholds are obtained in one ear, the earphone is repositioned in the opposite ear for testing.

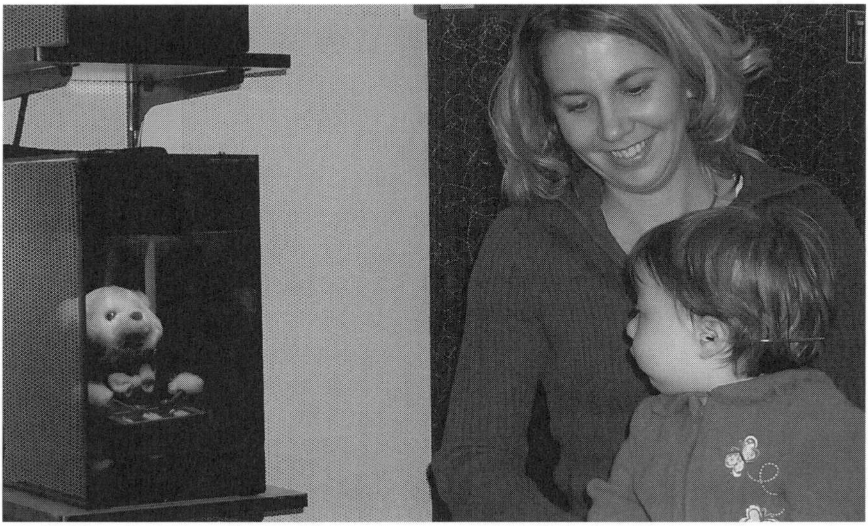

FIGURE 9.1. A 14-month-old child and her parent involved in visual reinforcement audiometry. After hearing the sound, the child turns toward the reinforcer to her right.

*2-Year-Olds.* Although experience with children leads us to conclude that each child is unique, it is apparent that many 2-year-olds are challenging to test. VRA techniques may be boring for these children, effective reinforcers may be difficult to find, and play audiometry (outlined below) may be inappropriate. Unfortunately, the decision to assess a child's hearing is often delayed by parents and physicians until the child's speech and language delay is significant. This delay may result in the recommendation for initial hearing testing around the child's 2nd birthday. Patience and flexibility are required of the audiologist to obtain the necessary behavioral test results from many 2-year-old children using the VRA techniques outlined above. Any conditioned response to sound is acceptable (banging on a table, pushing a button) and should be reinforced, as long as adequate controls ensure that the behavior is a response to sound. Young children are likely to respond to speech at lower levels than tones. Thresholds for hearing speech are used to confirm pure tone or warble tone test results. Speech awareness thresholds are tested in the same manner as pure tones. When the child has learned the names of objects or body parts, speech recognition thresholds can be measured by asking the child to point to objects such as the child's shoe or nose or a favorite toy, or to a picture of an object.

***Preschoolers.*** Play audiometry is a fun and effective tool for assessing hearing in preschool children who love to play games. Although play audiometry is also loosely based on operant conditioning procedures, the actual games incorporated into the test session are assumed to be rewarding and to reinforce appropriate behavior from the child. In play audiometry, the child is instructed to toss a block into a bucket, put a peg into a pegboard, or do a quiet game activity each time a sound is heard. The audiologist provides intermittent social reinforcement and enough control trials to ensure the validity of the child's responses. With adequate reinforcement and appropriate selection of games, the audiologist can obtain pure tone air- and bone-conducted threshold estimates for each ear in one session. When the child has learned the names of objects or body parts, speech recognition thresholds can be measured by asking the child to point to an object or a picture of the object. Speech recognition thresholds can be obtained using picture spondees or by asking the child to repeat words. Word recognition tests are presented at suprathreshold levels and give information about the child's ability to understand speech. Tests for preschool children may also make use of a picture-pointing response; these tests include the *Northwestern University Children's Perception of Speech* (NU Chips; Chermak, Pederson, & Bendel, 1984) and *Word Intelligibility by Picture Identification* (WIPI; Ross & Lerman, 1971).

## Indirect Measures of Hearing

Batteries of indirect measures of auditory function are useful for evaluating children of all ages. These measures often provide confirmation of findings from behavioral tests, additional information about middle ear pathologies, and, when behavioral tests are incomplete, sufficient information to begin intervention. Indirect measures of auditory function include (a) acoustic immittance testing for evaluation of middle ear function in children older than 2 months of age, (b) otoacoustic emissions testing for evaluation of cochlear outer hair cell function for all ages, and (c) auditory brainstem testing for the evaluation of VIIIth cranial nerve and brainstem auditory responses to sound for all ages.

*Acoustic immittance tympanometry* provides an indirect assessment of middle ear function by measuring the reflectance of acoustic energy from the eardrum as the pressure in the ear canal is changed systematically (see Figure 9.2). *Reflectance* is a measure of the fraction of sound reflected back into the ear canal from the eardrum relative to the fraction transmitted through the eardrum. A soft probe is placed in the ear, and a pressure seal is obtained. A constant probe tone is played while the pressure in the ear

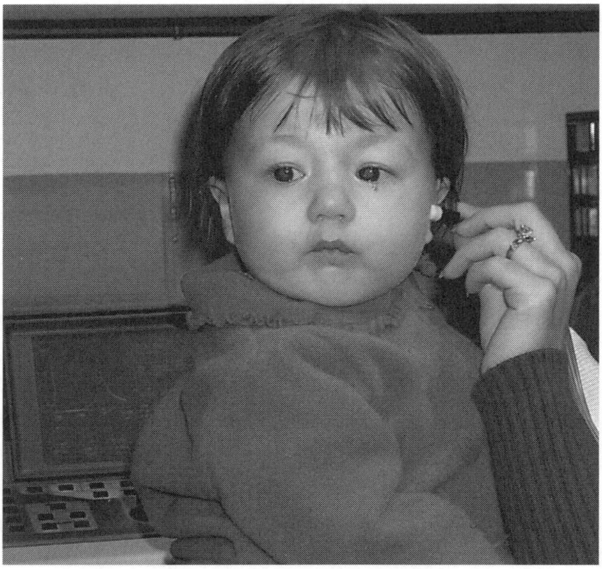

FIGURE 9.2. The child shown in Figure 9.1 having completed tympanometry. The tympanogram on the screen shows normal eardrum mobility, which is consistent with a normal middle ear system.

canal is changed. As the eardrum is pushed and pulled by the change in air pressure, the level of the reflected sound in the ear canal is measured automatically. This procedure is invaluable for the diagnosis and management of otitis media with effusion (OME) in young children. Fluid-filled middle ears cause increased mass and stiffness of the middle ear system, resulting in flat tympanograms with increased sound reflection at all ear canal pressures.

In Figure 9.3, panels A through D show a variety of tympanograms that are typical of children with occasional or chronic middle ear disorder. The child with the tympanogram in panel A (upper left) would pass the test. It is consistent with normal middle ear function, normal eardrum mobility, only slight negative pressure, and an intact tympanic membrane. Panel B (lower left) may reflect an ear with otitis media. The compliance or mobility of the eardrum is low (i.e., the middle ear system is stiff), the tympanogram curve is wide, and the ill-defined peak is seen at a significantly negative pressure. A child whose tympanogram resembled this one would be referred for medical management. Panels C (upper right) and D

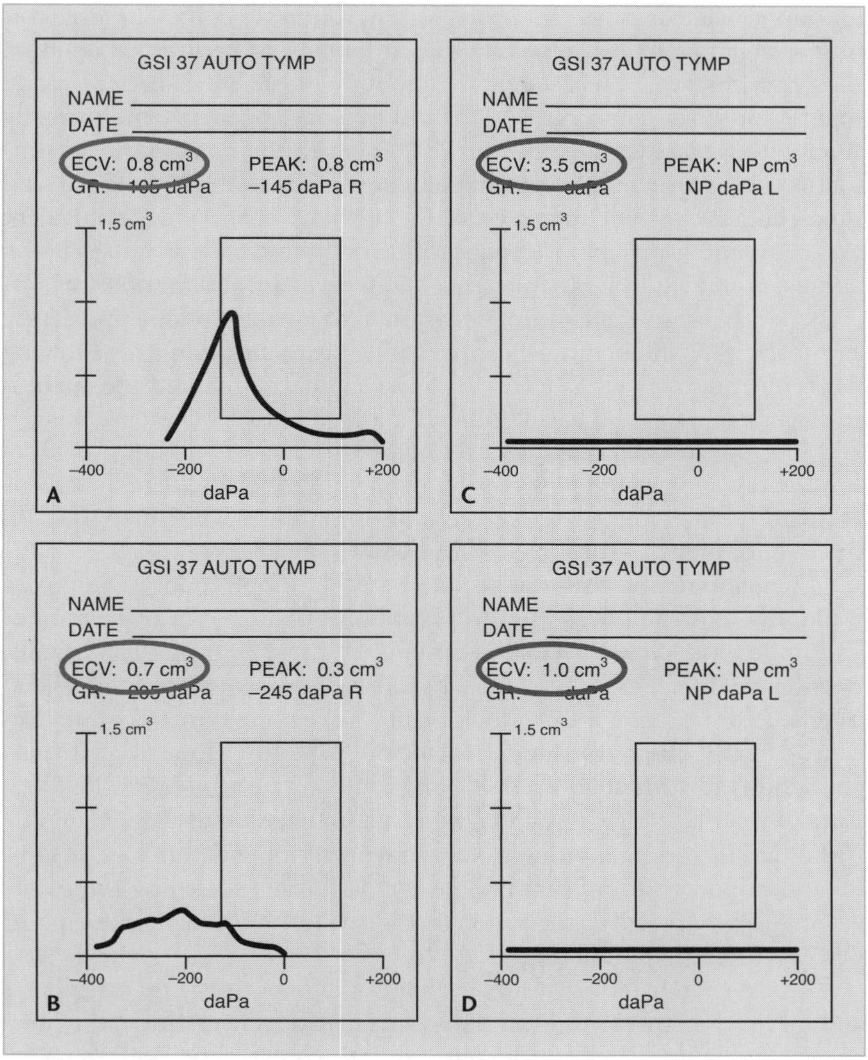


FIGURE 9.3. Four sample screening tympanograms. Panel A shows a normal Type A tympanogram, with classic bell shape, normal compliance, and only slightly negative pressure.

(lower right) show flat tympanograms with no definable peak. These two tympanograms represent cases where the eardrum is immobile regardless of the pressure introduced to the ear canal. Of interest is the ear canal volume (ECV), circled in each panel. Panel C shows a very large volume

(3.5 $cm^3$), whereas panel D shows a normal volume (1 $cm^3$). The large volume seen in panel C suggests that the eardrum has a perforation and that the tympanogram is measuring the mobility of the entire ear canal and middle ear space. This occurs when children have open, patent, normally functioning pressure equalization (PE) tubes in their eardrums for ventilation. This would be the desired outcome when testing a child with PE tubes, because it would indicate that the tubes are open. A high equivalent volume reading may be of concern if a ventilation tube is not in place, because it may indicate the presence of an eardrum perforation. In contrast, panel D shows a flat tympanogram with normal volume, indicating a probable fluid-filled middle ear with intact eardrum. Children showing flat tympanograms with normal volume should be referred for medical management. If a child has PE tubes, but that child's tympanogram is flat with normal volume, the tubes are apparently clogged and not providing ventilation. This would be a reason for medical referral. Regular screening with tympanometry can be useful for monitoring the function of PE tubes, once they have been placed in a child's ears.

Tympanometric test results obtained for infants under the age of 2 months must be interpreted with caution because of immature outer and middle ear systems (Holte, Margolis, & Cavanaugh, 1991; Margolis, Bass-Ringdahl, Hanks, Holte, & Zapala, 2003). Neonates with fluid-filled middle ears may have normal looking but misleading tympanograms because of early differences in ear canal wall mobility. However, flat tympanograms for infants do reflect abnormal eardrum mobility. Between 2 and 4 months of age, tympanograms begin to look like those of adults. Although diagnostic and multiple-frequency tympanograms are helpful for the diagnosis of unusual middle ear pathology, screening tympanograms give sufficient information for identification and monitoring of OME and ventilation tubes.

*Acoustic reflex testing* (ART) evaluates the integrity of the peripheral auditory system by monitoring change in acoustic reflectance in the presence of loud stimuli due to middle ear muscle contraction. With the tympanometry probe still in the ear canal and the pressure seal maintained, loud sounds are presented. When the entire auditory system is normal, the loud sound triggers middle ear muscle contractions, and the eardrum stiffens. This requires normal function of the middle ear, cochlea, VIIIth cranial nerve, brainstem, and VIIth cranial nerve. ART in children older than 3 months of age can help confirm conductive, cochlear, and retrocochlear pathology by evaluating the pattern of reflexes obtained from ipsilateral (same-ear) and contralateral (opposite-ear) stimulation. Practiced audiologists and good distracting toys are essential for obtaining the cooperation of young children and their parents for both tympanometry and acoustic reflex testing. Unfortunately, the acoustic reflex response may be obscured when the child moves, cries, or talks during the test.

## Testing Cochlear Outer Hair Cell Function

*Otoacoustic emissions* (OAE) test results complement behavioral and immittance results for all children. OAE tests can be performed in a very short time and only require the child to remain somewhat still for the measurement (see Figure 9.4). Emissions are especially informative when behavioral and tympanometric results are inconclusive or when a child is unable to participate in behavioral testing. One cannot, however, differentiate mild from more severe degrees of hearing loss, and emissions are absent with middle ear pathology commonly found in children with cleft palates.

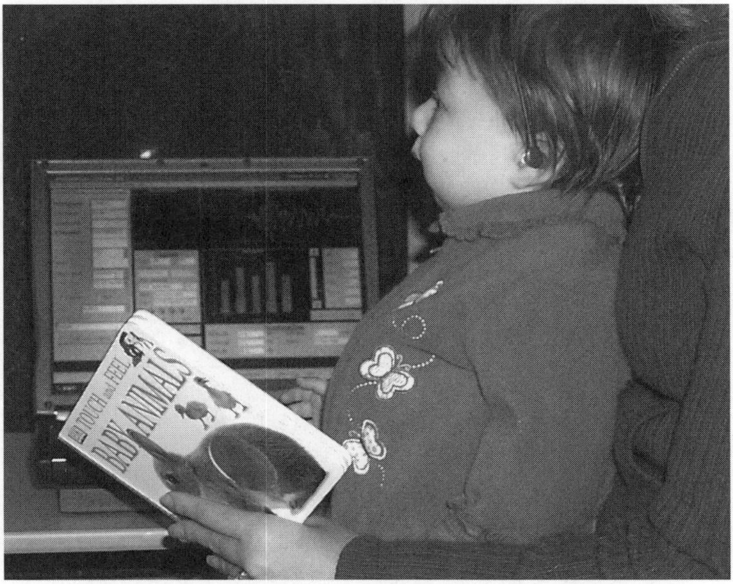


Figure 9.4. A child completing otoacoustic emission testing. The pattern of response on the computer screen is consistent with normal outer hair cell and middle ear function.

## Testing the Auditory Brainstem

*Diagnostic auditory brainstem response (ABR) testing* using pure-tone stimuli provides frequency-specific and ear-specific thresholds to sound that closely approximate behavioral hearing thresholds. Electrodes are placed on the child's head, a small eartip is placed in the ear canal, and a series of tone bursts are presented at varying frequencies. The electrical responses of the brainstem to the tones are recorded and averaged. Near-threshold ABR peaks occur later in young children than in adults (for norms, see Gorga, Kaminski, Beauchaine, Jesteadt, & Neely, 1989; Gorga, Reiland, Beauchaine, Worthington, & Jesteadt, 1987). ABR thresholds may be obtained in young children by depriving the child of sleep prior to testing and by encouraging a feeding and subsequent nap after the family arrives at the test center. If this strategy is unsuccessful, sedation may be necessary. Diagnostic ABR results can also be used in the diagnosis of brainstem tumors and central nervous system dysfunction.

Recent work on *auditory steady-state response* (ASSR) evoked potentials (Cone-Wesson, Dowell, Tomlin, Rance, & Ming, 2002) has shown them to be an effective alternative to ABR tests, especially for identifying conductive hearing losses in children. The ASSR uses a combination of sustained, modulated tones to monitor changes in central auditory activity. Electrodes are placed on the child's scalp, as in ABR testing. The eartip in the ear canal presents sustained modulated tones, and responses to the modulated tones are averaged and recorded. Conductive losses (in which bone-conducted sound is more easily detected than air-conducted sound) are most common in children with cleft palate. Proponents of ASSR suggest that using bone-conducted noise to mask the ASSR may distinguish between infants and children with conductive hearing losses and those with sensory losses. Their evidence suggests that when ASSR tests are used as part of the diagnostic evaluation for infants and children, the results can yield important information about the child's audiometric contour and residual hearing, which aids in treatment and habilitation decisions (Cone-Wesson, Rickards, et al., 2002).

# Follow-up and Referral

Once hearing loss is identified and described, the most critical element for minimizing communication problems is appropriate follow-up. Follow-up can include medical management of middle ear disorder, as well as amplification when chronic hearing loss may put the child at risk for speech and language delays. Cochlear implants offer options to children who do not benefit from traditional amplification, such as those with profound hearing loss. For those children with mild to severe hearing loss, hearing aid fitting strategies specially geared for young children are available to ensure appropriate gain without overamplification (American Academy of Audiology, 2003; American Speech-Language-Hearing Association Pediatric Working Group, 1996). Hearing aid fittings can be modified as the child is able to perform behavioral measures of hearing, around the age of 5–6 months. Most children with hearing loss adapt well to behind-the-ear hearing aids that fit appropriately, as long as they are met with patience, firmness, and cooperation from parents, audiologists, and physicians. Children with persistent conductive hearing loss, especially those with malformations of the pinna and ear canal, may be candidates for bone-conduction hearing aids. These hearing aids (see Figure 9.5) have microphones and amplifiers, along with oscillators held to the mastoid area that stimulate the bones of the skull. A traditional bone-conduction hearing aid is held in place by a metal or elastic headband. For children who are expected to need a bone-conduction hearing aid on a very long-term or permanent basis, a bone-anchored hearing aid (BAHA) system may be recommended. The BAHA uses a surgically placed titanium implant to couple the hearing aid to the mastoid bone. Children as young as 18 months have been fit with BAHA devices (Seemann, Liu, & DiToppa, 2004); however, the current recommendation is to wait until the child's skull is thick and strong.

For both bone-conduction and conventional hearing aids, special adaptations for young children should be considered, such as battery compartment covers to prevent battery ingestion, hearing aid retention devices to prevent hearing aid loss during strenuous activities, and direct audio input jacks to accommodate external microphones and receivers. Many children with hearing aids will test their parents' authority by threatening to throw the hearing aids away, plant them in the garden, or flush them down the toilet. These behaviors are common and are not necessarily indicators that the hearing aids are inappropriate. Hearing aid insurance policies, however, are essential for families.

Educating parents and teachers about the importance of the hearing aid to the child's learning is essential. Studies of children's hearing aids worn at school suggest that up to 50% of hearing aids are not functioning appropriately or are not being worn at any given time (Hawkins, 1990).

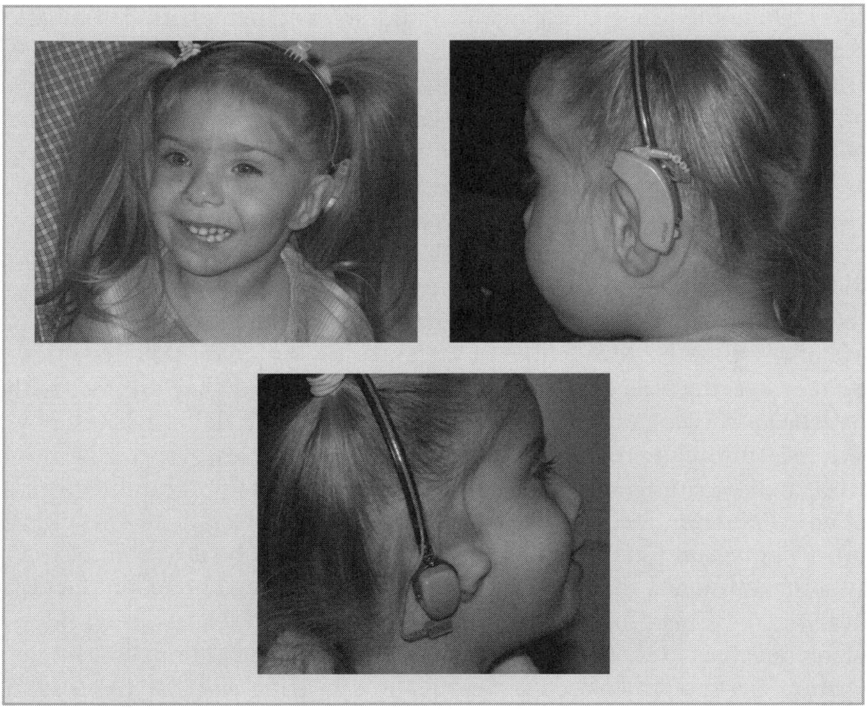

FIGURE 9.5. Bone-conduction hearing aids for chronic middle ear disorder.

Wearing a hearing aid that is turned off or is malfunctioning only adds to the degree of hearing loss experienced by the child. To avoid this problem, audiologists and speech-language pathologists need to collaborate and develop a manageable hearing aid monitoring program for each child. Someone at home or at school needs to perform a hearing aid listening check at least once each day. Additionally, the function and fit of the aids worn by preschool and elementary school children should be evaluated every 3–6 months by an audiologist. Older children need at least annual hearing and amplification review.

Children with fluctuating hearing loss who are attending school may be helped through the use of sound field amplification systems in their classrooms. With these amplification systems, a wireless microphone worn by the teacher transmits the teacher's voice throughout the classroom to loudspeakers. The amplified signal is broadcast throughout the room at a slightly higher level than normal. All children in the room can benefit from the system, but those children with slight hearing losses show significant benefit from such systems (Anderson & Goldstein, 2004).

Speech and language evaluation and services are almost always indicated for children with cleft palate and/or hearing loss. Partnership between the family, physician, audiologist, speech-language pathologist, and school officials is critical. Each team member can have a significant positive impact on the child's educational success by showing an interest in the child's progress, asking questions of the parents and the child, and writing reports that are useful to school personnel. Each child with a hearing loss and each family with a hard-of-hearing or deaf child bring to the professional a unique set of abilities and needs. Parents and professionals may need to review and discuss the child's current school placement annually. Changes may be recommended, depending on the child's academic success and overall happiness. Involvement and counsel by the team help to empower parents to make appropriate decisions for their child.

Many children with hearing loss are identified early and are successfully referred for appropriate intervention services. Early intervention enables these children to become well-adjusted and well-educated adults who achieve comprehensive social, academic, and professional goals. Some have become audiologists themselves. They are proof that the available tools can successfully minimize the secondary effects of reduced communication that were previously associated with childhood hearing loss.

## References

American Academy of Audiology. (2003). *Pediatric amplification protocol.* Retrieved March 14, 2007, from www.audiology.org

American Speech-Language-Hearing Association Pediatric Working Group. (1996). Amplification for infants and children with hearing loss. *American Journal of Audiology, 5,* 53–68.

Anderson, K. A., & Goldstein, H. (2004). Benefits of three FM devices to speech perception of children who are hard of hearing listening in a typical classroom. *Language, Speech and Hearing Services in Schools, 35,* 169–184.

Broen, P. A., Moller, K. T., Carlstrom, J., Doyle, S. S., Devers, M., & Keenan, K. M. (1996). Comparison of the hearing histories of children with and without cleft palate. *Cleft Palate-Craniofacial Journal, 33,* 127–133.

Carney, A. E., & Moeller, M. P. (1998). Treatment efficacy: Hearing loss in children. *Journal of Speech and Hearing Research, 41,* S61–S84.

Chermak, G. D., Pederson, C. M., & Bendel, R. B. (1984). Equivalent forms and split-half reliability of the NU-CHIPS administered in noise. *Journal of Speech and Hearing Disorders, 49,* 196–201.

Cone-Wesson, B., Dowell, R. C., Tomlin, D., Rance, G., & Ming, W. J. (2002). The auditory steady-state response: Comparisons with the auditory brainstem response. *Journal of the American Academy of Audiology, 13,* 173–187.

Cone-Wesson, B., Rickards, F., Poulis, C., Parker, J., Tan, L., & Pollard, J. (2002). The auditory steady-state response: Clinical observations and applications in infants and children. *Journal of the American Academy of Audiology, 13,* 270–282.

Diefendorf, A., & Gravel, J. (1996). Behavioral observation and visual reinforcement audiometry. In S. Gerber (Ed.), *The handbook of pediatric audiology* (pp. 55–83). Washington, DC: Gallaudet University Press.

Gorga, M. P., Kaminski, J. R., Beauchaine, K. L., Jesteadt, W., & Neely, S. T. (1989). Auditory brainstem responses from children three months to three years of age: Normal patterns of response. *Journal of Speech and Hearing Research, 32,* 281–288.

Gorga, M. P., Reiland, J. K., Beauchaine, K. L., Worthington, D. W., & Jesteadt, W. (1987). Auditory brainstem responses from graduates of an intensive care nursery: Normal patterns of response. *Journal of Speech and Hearing Research, 30,* 311–318.

Haggard, M. (1996). Optimizing an outcome battery for OME in 3–7 year olds. *Abstracts of the Nineteenth Midwinter Research Meeting, Association for Research in Otolaryngology, 69.*

*Hard of hearing pupils in the schools* (2nd ed.). Washington, DC: U.S. Department of Education, Office of Special Education and Rehabilitative Services, Office of Special Institutions.

Harrison, M., Roush, J., & Wallace, J. (1996). Trends in age of identification and intervention in infants with hearing loss. *Ear and Hearing, 24,* 89–95.

Holte, L., Margolis, R. H., & Cavanaugh, R. M., Jr. (1991). Developmental changes in multifrequency tympanograms. *Audiology, 30,* 1–24.

Joint Committee on Infant Hearing. (2007). Year 2007 position statement: Principles and guidelines for early hearing detection and intervention programs. *Pediatrics, 120,* 898–921.

Margolis, R. H., Bass-Ringdahl, S., Hanks, W. D., Holte, L., & Zapala, D. A. (2003). Tympanometry in newborn infants–1 kHz norms. *Journal of the American Academy of Audiology, 14,* 383–392.

Maxon, A. B., White, K., Behrens, T. R., & Vohr, B. R. (1995). Referral rates and cost efficiency in a universal newborn hearing screening program using transient evoked otoacoustic emissions. *Journal of the American Academy of Audiology, 6,* 271–277.

Moeller, M. P. (2000). Early intervention and language development in children who are deaf and hard of hearing. *Pediatrics, 106*(3), E43.

Muntz, H. R. (1993). An overview of middle ear disease in cleft palate children. *Facial Plastic Surgery, 9,* 177–180.

National Center for Hearing Assessment and Management. (2007). *State summary statistics: Universal newborn hearing screening.* Retrieved December 14, 2007, from www.infanthearing.org/status/unhsstate.html

National Institutes of Health. (1993, March 1–3). Early identification of hearing impairment in infants and young children. *NIH Consensus Statement, 11*(1), 1–24.

Paradise, J. L., Feldman, H. M., Campbell, T. F., Dollaghan, C. A., Rockette, H. E., Pitcairn, D. L., et al. (2007). Tympanostomy tubes and developmental outcomes at 9 to 11 years of age. *New England Journal of Medicine, 356*, 248–261.

Pediatric Working Group. (1996). *Recommended protocol for pediatric amplification.* Minneapolis: Minnesota Department of Health.

Roberts, J. E., Rosenfeld, R. M., & Zeisel, S. A. (2004). Otitis media and speech and language: A meta-analysis of prospective studies. *Pediatrics, 113*(3, Pt. 1), e238–e248.

Ross, M. (1990). Educational impact. In J. Davis (Ed.), *Our forgotten children: Hard of hearing pupils in the schools* (2nd ed.). Washington, DC: U.S. Department of Education, Office of Special Education and Rehabilitative Services, Office of Special Institutions.

Ross, M., & Lerman, J. (1971). *Word intelligibility by picture identification.* Pittsburgh, PA: Stanwix House.

Seemann, R., Liu, R., & DiToppa, J. (2004). Results of pediatric bone-anchored hearing aid implantation. *Journal of Otolaryngology, 33*, 71–74.

Yoshinaga-Itano, C., & Gravel, J. S. (2001). The evidence for universal newborn hearing screening. *American Journal of Audiology, 10*, 62–64.

Zanzi, M., Cherpillod, J., & Hohlfeld, J. (2002). Phonetic and otological results after early palate closure in 18 consecutive children presenting with cleft lip and palate. *International Journal of Pediatric Otorhinolaryngology, 66*, 131–137.

# CHAPTER 10

# Evaluation of Velopharyngeal Function

*Jerald B. Moon*

*This chapter is dedicated to the memory of Herbert A. Leeper, Jr., a friend, colleague, and mentor, who was taken from us far too soon.*

Any management plan for cleft palate or a speech resonance disorder relies on an accurate description of the structure and function of the velopharyngeal mechanism. This chapter provides a detailed description of the various instrumental and noninstrumental techniques that may be used to evaluate velopharyngeal function and assess its impact on speech production and communication. Because no single method serves all clinical needs, Moon outlines the procedures, special considerations, and clinical importance of a comprehensive array of evaluation approaches that help professionals understand the limits and capabilities of this complex articulator.

1. Velopharyngeal closure can be evaluated from three interactive perspectives: kinematic, acoustic, and aerodynamic. Describe the expectations for normal velopharyngeal closure in each of these domains. Then explain how velar movements, speech sound contexts, and pressure and flow may be disrupted or altered in disordered velopharyngeal articulation.
2. Moon distinguishes among various categories of evaluation techniques: direct versus indirect, and primary versus secondary. How are these categories defined? How may various categories be used in combination to strengthen the validity of interpreting velopharyngeal performance accurately? What limits are present in each category?
3. Describe the assets and limitations of the various imaging techniques used to evaluate velopharyngeal function. Besides allowing

a direct view of the physical structure, what are the other distinct advantages of each technique? What technical limits are present for each? Finally, what patient selection criteria might limit one's ability to use or interpret each approach?

4. How do indirect evaluation techniques support the difficult task of assessing the perceptual quality of speech resonance and articulation? For each approach, describe what is being measured (e.g., airflow magnitude, movement timing, acoustic output). Then explain how that measure relates to the perceptual judgment of velopharyngeal closure and speech resonance.

All speech clinicians involved with persons with cleft palate regularly face the challenge of evaluating a velopharyngeal (VP) mechanism to determine how it functions, or why it does not perform as it should. The results of VP evaluation are also important to surgical and dental colleagues serving on interdisciplinary teams because these specialists are frequently called upon to treat a VP mechanism that does not function appropriately for speech. In this chapter, some of the instruments that the diagnostician may use for VP evaluation are presented.

Before continuing, however, some discussion regarding terminology used to describe VP function is warranted. Terms such as *inadequacy*, *incompetence*, and *insufficiency* appear in literature references and clinic reports. According to Loney and Bloem (1987), application of these different terms in a redundant or contradictory manner hinders discussion of the problem, especially in the context of a multidisciplinary team. They suggested using *incompetence* to describe a deficit in neuromuscular functioning and *inadequacy* as a descriptor of imperfect VP closure caused by a deficit of tissue. They recommended that *insufficiency* be used to refer to any malformation resulting in imperfect closure. This term, therefore, would encompass the terms *incompetence* and *inadequacy*. Folkins (1988) correctly pointed out that use of the term *perfect*—and by extension, Loney and Bloem's "imperfect"—might cause some significant problems of interpretation. Is "perfect" closure a prerequisite to normally perceived speech? Although it may be true that VP disorders are rooted in anatomical (structural) and/or neuromuscular (movement) deficits, Folkins (1988) argued that professionals do not yet possess the quantitative ability, or the theoretical need, to separate speakers on the basis of neuromuscular versus structural deficits. *Incompetent* is defined in the dictionary as "lacking the qualities needed for effective action" and "inadequate to or unsuitable for a particular purpose" (*Merriam-Webster's Collegiate Dictionary,* 2003). This definition implies not causation, but simply that a particular result cannot be attained. The result in this case is speech that is perceived to be within normal limits. Therefore, the term *incompetent* is applied throughout this chapter to refer to abnormal function of the VP mechanism.

Evaluation of any mechanism must be based on knowledge of normal form and function; that is, the diagnostician must know the anatomy of the normal VP mechanism (form) and must understand the physiological events associated with normal VP movement (function). Moon and Kuehn (1997) and Cassell, Moon, and Elkadi (1990) provided comprehensive descriptions of VP anatomy. For purposes of orientation, a schematic diagram of the head showing the VP region in relation to other craniofacial structures and cavities (i.e., form) is presented in Figure 10.1. The physiological events associated with VP closing and opening gestures during speech (i.e., function) are complex. It is beyond the scope of this chapter to discuss the physiology of VP function in detail; however, because this discussion of instrumental analysis of the velopharynx is predicated on a basic understanding of the physiological events associated with normal VP movement, a brief review of those events is presented here. Other sources provide more detailed explanations of VP physiology (e.g., Cassell et al., 1990; Kummer, 2001; Moon & Kuehn, 1997; Peterson-Falzone, Hardin-Jones, & Karnell, 2001).

## Physiological Events Associated with Normal VP Movement

### Kinematics

Normal VP closure is thought to consist of a velar and a pharyngeal movement component (Skolnick, McCall, & Barnes, 1973). The velar component includes elevation and posterior elongation or stretching of the velum (Simpson & Chin, 1981). According to Skolnick et al. (1973), the pharyngeal component includes all movements of the nasopharyngeal walls. No distinction is made between lateral and posterior pharyngeal

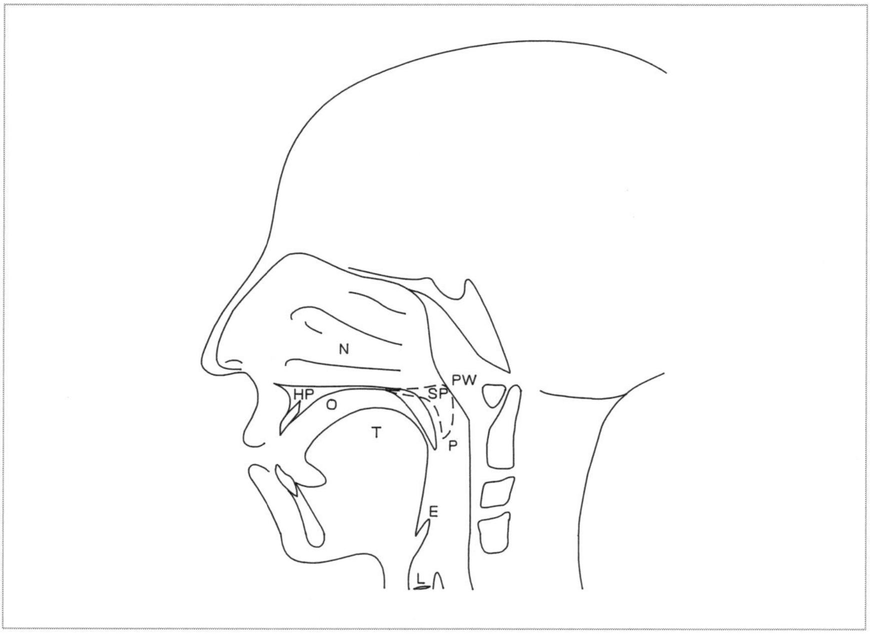


Figure 10.1. Sagittal schematic view of the head showing structures of the oral and pharyngeal region in relation to other craniofacial structures. Soft palate (SP) is shown at rest (solid line) and during /s/ production (dotted line). N = nasal cavity, O = oral cavity, P = oropharynx, HP = hard palate, PW = posterior pharyngeal wall, E = epiglottis, L = larynx, T = tongue.

wall movement, and the nasopharyngeal walls are thought to move as a single functional unit. It is generally accepted, however, that mesial movement of the lateral pharyngeal walls constitutes a most significant aspect of the "nasopharyngeal" component (Iglesias, Kuehn, & Morris, 1980). The relative contribution of the velum and lateral pharyngeal walls to closure has been studied by Croft, Shprintzen, and Rakoff (1981), Skolnick (1975), and Zwitman, Sonderman, and Ward (1974), who described a number of patterns, ranging from exclusive velar movement to exclusive lateral pharyngeal wall movement.

## Acoustics

Acoustic events associated with VP function involve the movement of vibrational energy through the vocal tract. During normal speech production, VP closure serves to impede the transmission of sound energy into and through the nasal cavity. The sound resonator, in this case, comprises the pharyngeal and oral cavity. Differing oral cavity shapes that result from articulator movements give rise to different acoustic filters. The passage of acoustic energy through these filters produces complex sounds with different spectral "shapes" that are perceived as different oral speech sounds (Daniloff, Schuckers, & Feth, 1980; Peterson & Barney, 1952). In some instances (e.g., nasal consonants /m/, /n/, /ŋ/), the VP mechanism offers minimal impedance to sound transmission relative to much greater oral impedance. Here, the nasal tract contributes to sound resonation and the oral cavity outlet is closed. Energy in the nasal airway is dissipated in two principal ways: While the primary output is an acoustic signal at the nares, some energy can also be expected to vibrate the nasal mucosa and overlying nasal bones. This vibration is easily demonstrated by placing a finger on the nasal bone while humming.

## Aerodynamics

Perhaps the most basic physiological event associated with normal speech production is the movement of a pressurized airstream through the vocal tract. The aerodynamics of speech production has been studied extensively (Stathopoulos & Weismer, 1985; Thompson & Hixon, 1979; Warren, 1979, 1982). Simply stated, normal oral articulation involves no (or at least very little) nasal airflow and a large pressure drop across the VP orifice. The result is an infinite (or at least very large) VP aerodynamic resistance and the ability to develop oral airflows and pressures of sufficient magnitude to produce appropriately resonated speech output. Conversely, normal nasal resonance involves airflow through the nasal cavity. Lowering of the velum to allow for the passage of air results in a much lower pressure drop across the VP port and much lower VP resistance. The magnitude of these parameters will depend, among other things, on the amount of VP opening present.

## Interactions Among Levels—Prerequisites for Normal Function

Simply described, the VP mechanism is a valve that must open and close during a variety of speech and nonspeech tasks. However, its role in the production of speech is anything but simple. The velopharyngeal mechanism is an articulator. It must function according to principles of neuromotor programming and coordination. It must be moved in concert with other articulators (upper lip, lower lip, jaw, tongue) and with other anatomical/physiological systems (laryngeal, respiratory) to appropriately valve the airstream and contribute to the production of an acoustic product perceived as normal. On a moment-to-moment basis, VP movements (and the movements of all these structures) are influenced by the phonetic and linguistic demands of the speaker.

In addition to considering coordination between the VP mechanism and the rest of the speech production system, one must also consider control of VP activity itself. Activation of the numerous muscles of the VP mechanism in response to neural commands must result in opening and closing gestures that couple and decouple the oral and nasal cavities. The timing and magnitude of muscle activations must be sufficient to close the aperture with a force or tightness sufficient to prevent inappropriate acoustic influence or unwanted air movement.

It is important to realize that normal speech production is the result of activity on a number of levels physiologically. Disordered speech can occur as a consequence of abnormal activity at any one or combination of those levels. Further, behavior observed at any level of the speech production system may be related to a combination of events at preceding levels. It is critical to bear this in mind while reading the discussion of instruments used to "tap into" the physiology of speech production in general and velopharyngeal function specifically.

## Instrumental Evaluation

The many approaches to instrumental evaluation of the VP mechanism vary from fairly simplistic in concept and design to highly sophisticated. VP evaluation is usually undertaken because someone perceives that an individual's speech deviates from normal. It is widely accepted that the ear is the first and primary clinical diagnostic tool:

> If the individual's speech is "normal" sounding during conversational speech, then there is no need to do any further testing—except for research purposes . . . The most valid measure of adequate functioning is

the sound produced while talking. When conversational speech deviates from normal, our task is to determine why. (Bensen, 1977, p. 46)

Ultimately, by simply listening, a speech clinician judges a person's speech to be within normal limits or suspects a potential VP problem that warrants, as termed by McWilliams, Morris, and Shelton (1984), a definitive assessment.

Given that a patient is suspected of speaking with a dysfunctional system, the clinician should evaluate the structure of the VP mechanism and its ability to move appropriately during speech. The structure of the mechanism is best evaluated by comparing it with normal. Study of the motion (kinematics) of the mechanism can be accomplished in a number of ways. One can simply watch the mechanism move, or one can evaluate the consequences of VP movement. For example, acoustic and aerodynamic events in the vocal tract are intimately related to movements of VP structures. In defining VP inadequacy, Schwartz (1975) referred to "an opening between the nasopharynx and the oropharynx during speech of sufficient magnitude to produce a condition of acoustic coupling between nose and mouth great enough for trained listeners to perceive a quality called hypernasality," and to "an opening between oral and nasopharynx great enough to allow an escape of air from the nose during the production of high intraoral air pressure consonants and to thereby create a condition known as nasal emission" (p. 305).

Lubker and Moll (1965) referred to those evaluative approaches that allow the diagnostician to make direct observations of the articulatory structures as "direct techniques," and those approaches that provide data that may be used to make inferences regarding VP movement as "indirect techniques." Evaluative techniques may be grouped further into primary measures (measures of structure and movement per se) and secondary measures (acoustics and aerodynamics); that is, primary measures are those that allow for evaluation of the structure and kinematics of the VP mechanism, whereas secondary measures are those that involve an evaluation of the consequences of VP function on other speech physiological parameters. In this chapter, I present the techniques in these groupings, as illustrated in Table 10.1. This categorization is not meant to suggest that primary measures are more important than secondary measures. The distinction is offered simply to differentiate between the types of data that might be collected that provide information about the VP mechanism and its function at some level physiologically. This information should

**Table 10.1**
**Evaluative Techniques Used to Assess Velopharyngeal Form and Function**

| Type of measures | Direct | Indirect |
|---|---|---|
| **Primary** | Unaided-eye visual oral exam | Phototransduction |
| | Lateral still radiography | Electromyography |
| | Motion picture radiography/ videofluoroscopy | Movement transduction |
| | Computed tomography (CT scan) | Velar closure force |
| | Magnetic resonance imaging (MRI) | |
| | Ultrasound | |
| | Endoscopy | |
| **Secondary** | | |
| Acoustics | | Listener judgment |
| | | Sound spectrography |
| | | Sound pressure (nasometry) |
| | | Accelerometry |
| | | Acoustic rhinometry |
| Aerodynamics | | Airflow detection |
| | | Air pressure detection |
| | | Orifice area estimation |

contribute to the clinical decision regarding what the speaker can and cannot do velopharyngeally to produce acceptable speech.

A further distinction would be to separate approaches commonly used in clinical practice from those typically used in experimental or laboratory-based situations. Such a differentiation, while perhaps meaningful at the time of this writing, could prove to be inaccurate in the future. That is, many currently accepted clinical approaches began as experimental techniques. As technology advances, new approaches to the study of speech production will emerge first in the laboratory, and then, if appropriate, gain acceptance in routine clinical practice. Similarly, some clinical diagnostic instrumentation commonly employed in the past has fallen by the wayside; therefore, some currently accepted diagnostic tools may fall out of practice in the future, replaced by newer approaches.

This chapter is written to provide an overview of both past and present instrumental approaches to the study of velopharyngeal function. Because one cannot predict which approaches now considered experimental will someday become routine, no such distinction will be made.

## Direct Primary Measures

Direct primary measures used to evaluate the structure and movement abilities of the VP mechanism include visual intraoral examination, a number of radiographic procedures, magnetic resonance imaging, ultrasound, and endoscopy.

### Visual Intraoral Examination

It seems intuitively obvious to begin an evaluation of the VP mechanism by looking in the mouth (Figure 10.2). In fact, 88% of the speech pathologists surveyed by Schneider and Shprintzen (1980) utilized intraoral examination in assessing VP function. Intraoral examination should be targeted toward an inspection of the lips, teeth, tongue position and function, tonsils, hard palate, soft palate, uvula, and pharyngeal walls (Kummer, 2001; McWilliams et al., 1984). Various questions should be considered: How do these structures function during speech? Are there any observable fistulae in the hard or soft palate? Is there notching of the uvula that would indicate a submucous cleft of the palate? Does the velum move on phonation? What is the extent of movement? Does it move symmetrically? Does the length of the velum appear normal? Is there pharyngeal wall movement on phonation?

Neither researchers nor clinicians uniformly agree on the utility of the unaided visual examination of the oral cavity. Yules and Chase (1971) suggested that one should view the mechanism in order to estimate

> length of soft palate, soft palate thickness, palate closure, quickness of motion, amplitude of motion, depth of nasopharynx, presence or absence of Passavant's ridge, presence or absence of an adenoidal mass, movement of posterior and lateral pharynx, characteristics of the hard palate . . . presence or absence of fistulas. (p. 454)

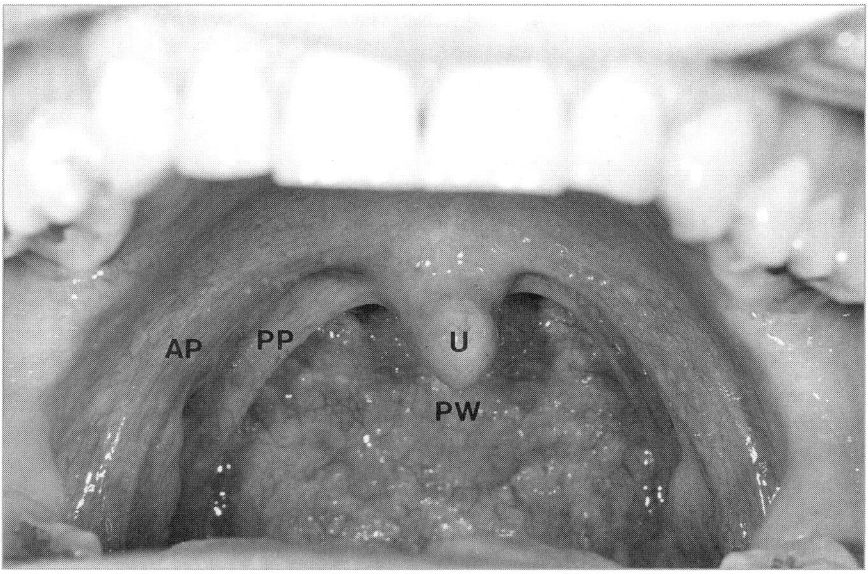


Figure 10.2. Intraoral view of the oral cavity and pharynx at rest. U = uvula; PW = posterior pharyngeal wall; AP = anterior faucial pillar; PP = posterior faucial pillar.

Others support the view that although the intraoral examination can provide some useful information and should not be ignored, it should be much more limited in scope. Evaluation of length and mobility of the soft palate from this perspective can be misleading (Pigott, 1980). The posterior pharyngeal wall cannot be visualized well from the front of the oral cavity. The soft palate may show considerable movement from this view but still not contact a recessed posterior pharyngeal wall. McWilliams et al. (1984) suggested a number of aspects of VP form and function that cannot be reliably assessed on visual exam. These include

> the adequacy of velar length, palatal elevation, movement of lateral and posterior pharyngeal walls, VP valving, occult submucous cleft palate wherein the levator muscles insert into the hard palate instead of forming a muscle sling for velar elevation . . . [and] malformation of the musculus uvulae. (p. 287)

Using lateral-view cinefluorography as the referent, Eisenbach and Williams (1984) evaluated the accuracy of statements made on the basis of unaided visual examination of the VP mechanism. Statements regarding velar length, depth of nasopharynx, VP closure, and velar mobility were compared with objective data obtained from cinefluorographic films. Rates of agreement ranged from 52% (velar mobility) to 71% (VP closure). The overall rate of agreement was only 60%. Not surprisingly, the data supported the view that more objective assessments of VP form and function should be utilized.

## Lateral Still Radiography

Lateral-view still or cephalometric radiography represents one of the oldest instrumental approaches to the evaluation and study of the VP mechanism. The technique of lateral-view still radiography involves positioning the patient between the X-ray tube and a sheet of X-ray film. The head is immobilized with rubber pads to ensure that the head is not tilted to one side. This also maintains each patient's head at a constant distance from the film, allowing for a constant magnification factor. Accurate measurements of the size of various structures can then be made from the exposed and developed film. High-speed electrons are emitted from the X-ray tube. They pass into the body part in their path and are selectively absorbed by the tissue. The amount of absorption depends on, among other things, the density of the tissue. Those electrons not absorbed pass through to the X-ray film, where the degree of exposure at any given point varies with the magnitude of electrons hitting it. The result is a radiograph or X-ray (see Figure 10.3).

Because this approach involves a picture taken at one instant in time, the speech tasks that may be employed are somewhat limited. Typically, radiographs have been taken at rest, during a sustained /s/, and perhaps during prolongation of a vowel. In some instances, a barium solution is injected either nasally or orally to coat the surfaces of the velum and pharyngeal walls. Because barium is a radiopaque material, it allows for better visualization of the margins of the velum and pharyngeal walls. Interpretation of lateral-view still radiographs may be subjective or objective. Van Demark, Kuehn, and Tharp (1975) developed a subjective X-ray rating scheme in an attempt to standardize interpretation of lateral radiograph images. They used the scale, in one instance, to predict the need for secondary management of the soft palate. On the basis of X-ray ratings alone, eventual outcome (i.e., pharyngeal flap required vs. not required) was correctly predicted in 92% of their patients.

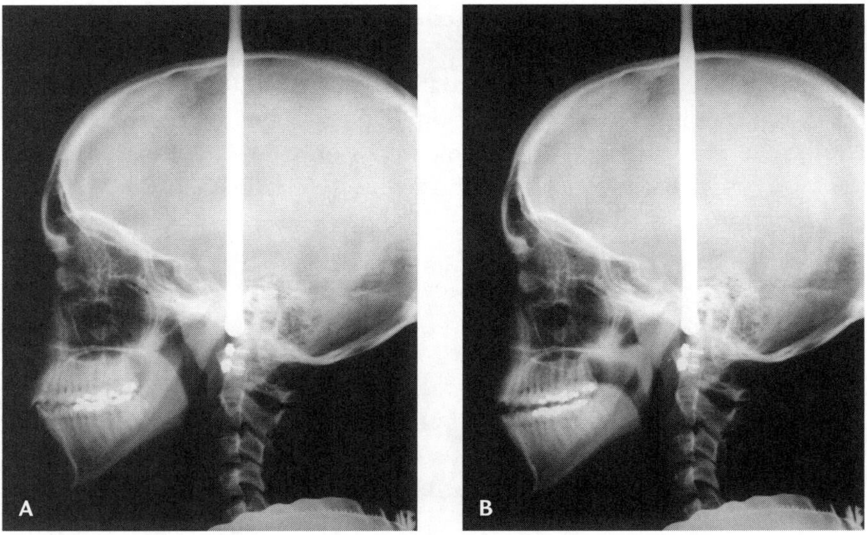


Figure 10.3. Lateral still radiographs taken at rest (A) and during production of /s/ (B). Vertical white bars are ear rods used for head immobilization. Elevation of soft palate to contact posterior pharyngeal wall may be seen during /s/ production.

The relationship between the presence of adenoid tissue and the ability to achieve VP closure in cleft palate is well documented. Subjective interpretation of lateral-view still radiographs was used by Mason and Warren (1980) to predict possible VP closure problems following adenoid size reduction. They suggested, however, that lateral-view still radiographs should not be used routinely for this purpose. Objective measures of structural features and relationships among VP structures have included hard palate length, velar length, velar thickness, pharyngeal depth, level of velopharyngeal contact with the posterior pharyngeal wall, and soft palate extension (e.g., Birch, Sommerlad, Fenn, & Butterworth, 1999; D'Antonio et al., 2000; Pae et al., 1994; Satoh, Wada, Tachimura, Sakoda, & Shiba, 1999; Witt, Marsh, McFarland, & Riski, 2000; Wu, Huang, Huang, & Noordhoff, 1996). These measures have been and continue to be made in attempts to assess the effects of growth and surgical alteration on the mechanism.

Lateral-view still X-rays were once a mainstay of the evaluation process at some centers. An obvious advantage of this approach is that it does allow for direct observation of the VP mechanism. The procedure is relatively simple to complete, is reliable, and provides quantifiable data. However, these positive aspects are outweighed by the liabilities of the approach. It is important to stress that the VP mechanism is a three-dimensional structure. Movements occur during opening and closing in both the sagittal (lateral) and frontal planes. By contrast, lateral X-rays are two-dimensional. Only structural features lying in the sagittal plane (anterior-posterior and superior-inferior) are represented. A second major disadvantage is that data collected is static in nature; that is, the radiograph depicts events occurring at one instant in time. The two common tasks (rest vs. prolonged /s/) yield information only on the extremes of movement. Events happening in between are not captured.

Proponents of the technique (e.g., Bzoch, 1968; Lubker & Morris, 1968) have argued that velar "activity" seen on lateral-view still X-ray is an accurate indicator of velar activity actually occurring during ongoing speech. However, Williams and Eisenbach (1981) compared decisions regarding the functional status of the VP mechanism made from lateral-view still radiographs with those made from motion picture radiographs (cinefluoroscopy). Inaccurate evaluation "of the competency or incompetency of the VP sphincter as viewed during the production of the sustained vowel /i/ would have occurred on 27% of the cases and 30% of the cases during the production of the CV [consonant-vowel] syllable /pi/" (p. 49). The point is further illustrated by Stringer and Witzell (1989), who found that for assessing adequacy of closure, the lateral view alone produced a large number of false positives. Finally, the exposure to ionizing radiation must also be considered a disadvantage of this approach and, in fact, all of the radiographic approaches to be discussed in this section.

Despite its disadvantages, lateral-view still radiography continues to be part of the diagnostic battery in some clinics and centers. For example, Wu et al. (1996) argued for the use of lateral-view still radiographs to screen the velopharyngeal area before evaluation with more sophisticated instrumentation.

## Cinefluoroscopy/Videofluoroscopy

In contrast to the lateral-view still technique, cineradiography allows for the visualization of VP structures in motion. The procedures involved in obtaining dynamic or moving radiographs are not significantly different from those discussed for still radiographs. The patient is seated between the X-ray tube and the film at right angles to the path of the X-ray beam with the head stabilized to prevent image blurring movements. Instead of a sheet of photographic film, an intensifying screen and motion picture or video camera are used. Electrons hitting the intensifying screen cause it to emit light, which is then filmed by the camera. The intensity of light emitted at any point on the screen is a function of the number of electrons hitting the screen, which in turn varies with the density of the body part being traversed. With this technique, the speech sample is not limited to prolonged vowels or sibilants, but can include syllables and sentences or connected speech.

Cineradiography (also referred to as cinefluoroscopy) has a rather extensive history of use in both clinical and research applications. Images have been rated with respect to extent of VP closure (McWilliams-Neely & Bradley, 1964) or measured to determine structural relationships in the pharyngeal cavity during speech (Moll, 1960, 1964). The technique has been employed in research studies to evaluate the mechanism of VP closure (Warren & Hofmann, 1961), articulatory movements (Wada, Yasumoto, Ikeoka, Fujiki, & Yoshinaga, 1970), results of pharyngeal flap surgery (Harrington, 1970), velar movement (Kuehn & Moll, 1976; Seaver & Kuehn, 1980; Shaw, Folkins, & Kuehn, 1980), and relationships between perceived nasality and VP movement (Karnell, Folkins, & Morris, 1985).

With advances in technology, the motion picture camera was replaced by video recording systems. Video systems have some distinct advantages over cine systems. Video systems require a much lower radiation dosage level and provide the ability to replay and evaluate the recorded exam immediately. Because cine systems used motion picture film, a developing process was involved. The standard camera speed of a cine unit is 24 frames per second. Standard video recorders function at a slightly faster rate, analogous to 30 frames per second. Although 24–30 frames per second may be sufficient for clinical purposes (Peterson-Falzone et al., 2001), it does not allow for precise documentation of articulatory movements that occur within a shorter time frame. High-speed video systems offering up to 400 frames per second do exist and have been used in research designed to record movement more precisely, but their use in a clinical setting would not be practical.

Recognizing the inability of lateral-view projections to provide information regarding movement in the frontal plane, Skolnick (1969, 1970) introduced the concept of multiview videofluoroscopy. This approach is designed to assess VP function using three separate views (sagittal or lateral, frontal, basal) projecting three anatomic planes (sagittal, coronal, transverse). The lateral view permits visualization of anterior-posterior velar movement and structural relationships between the soft palate and posterior pharyngeal wall. The frontal view permits visualization of lateral pharyngeal wall movement and vertical positioning of VP structures. The basal view permits visualization of the sphincteric component of VP movement (Skolnick, 1970; Watson, Sell, & Grunwell, 2001). Patient positioning for these three views is illustrated in Figure 10.4. For the frontal view, the patient is positioned facing the X-ray tube. For a basal view, the subject lies prone on the fluoroscopy table with the head and shoulders elevated (sphinx position). The three views are filmed consecutively but, when interpreted, provide a composite three-dimensional "picture" of VP structure and function.

Although it is generally accepted that the lateral and frontal views can provide valuable diagnostic information, positioning for the basal view requires considerable hyperextension of the neck. Shelton and Trier (1976) cautioned that the closure phenomenon revealed on a basal view may differ from that revealed on either a lateral or frontal view. Williams

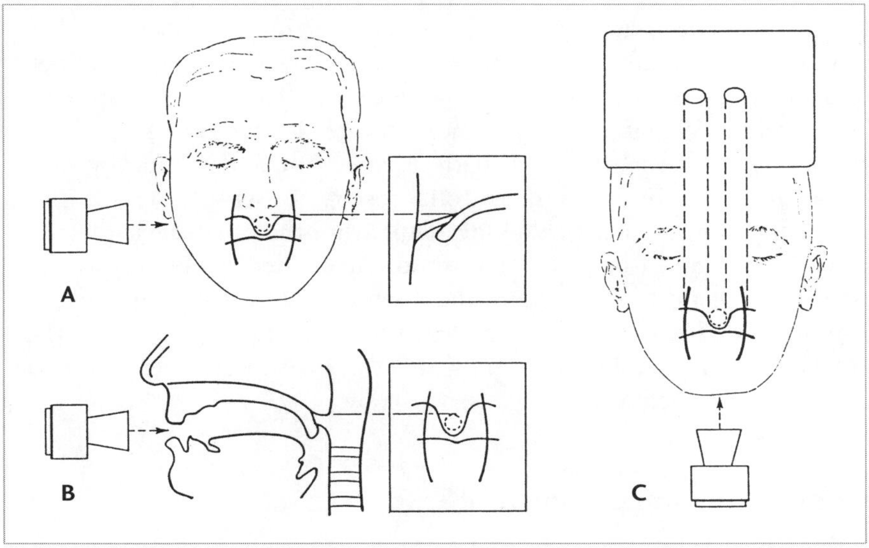


Figure 10.4. Radiographic positioning of patient for (a) lateral, (b) frontal, and (c) basal views of velopharyngeal mechanism. The patient depicted here has a pharyngeal flap. *Note.* From "Velopharyngeal Competence and Incompetence Following Pharyngeal Flap Surgery: Videofluoroscopic Study in Multiple Projections," by L. Skolnick and G. McCall, 1972, *Cleft Palate Journal, 9,* p. 2. Copyright 1972 by American Cleft Palate-Craniofacial Association. Reprinted with permission.

and Eisenbach (1981) agreed and proposed the use of only the lateral and frontal views. While acknowledging these limitations, some (Witt et al., 1998) continue to use the basal view to quantify velopharyngeal orifice cross-sectional area. Omission of the basal view negates the ability to directly observe this sphincteric component of closure. However, combined use of lateral and frontal views still allows for a three-dimension representation of the mechanism. In addition, Stringer and Witzell (1989) assessed the appropriateness of the Towne view (a cross-sectional view of VP function), concluding that it compared well with nasal endoscopic views of the velopharynx.

Multiview videofluoroscopy overcomes many of the disadvantages associated with the lateral-view still radiograph approach. It offers a view of the VP mechanism in motion during connected speech. It depicts, through interpretation of multiple images, the VP mechanism in three dimensions. Multiple viewing techniques, be they two view or three view, are not without liabilities, however. Because the multiple views are obtained consecutively, the patient is exposed to radiation two or three times. In addition, one must assume that the VP mechanism performs the same way each time. Despite these drawbacks, McWilliams et al. (1981) judged multiview videofluoroscopy to be a highly desirable tool. They compared videofluoroscopic data with data collected using manometry and pressure-flow techniques, using perceptual judgments of speech as the standard. Videofluoroscopic findings were "less variable and reflected what was heard in the speech pattern more often than did any of the other measures. In addition, videofluoroscopy provided a visual image of the mechanism that was not available from the other devices" (p. 7). Henningsson and Isberg (1991) also promoted videofluoroscopy as a valuable diagnostic tool. In their study comparing videofluoroscopic images to nasendoscopic images, movements of the lateral pharyngeal walls were observed videofluoroscopically in 33% of the cases, whereas no such movement was detected using nasendoscopy.

## Computed Tomography (CT Scan)

Computed tomography involves the mathematical, computer-assisted reconstruction of a "slice" of anatomy. The input to the mathematical reconstruction process is a series of X-ray transmission measurements made in a number of different directions around the patient, but all located in the tomographic plane or "slice" of interest (Trefler, 1985). Conventional computed tomography produces images that reflect the varying attenuation of X-ray electrons by body tissue of various densities. Sensitive X-ray detectors are mounted in a gantry opposite the X-ray tube and measure the X-ray beam at different points after it has been transmitted through the body. A typical scan requires 2–4 seconds to complete. The patient is required to lay supine on a horizontal table with the head between the X-ray tube above and detector bank below. The obtained image is a view of the target structure in the transverse plane. In the case of the VP mechanism, this would be somewhat analogous to the basal view.

Although not routinely used clinically, CT scanning has been employed by researchers in the study of velopharyngeal form and function. Honjo, Mitoma, Ushiro, and Kawano (1984) reported that using CT scans obtained at rest and during prolongation of a sound, "the dominant component of movement and its grade can be clearly visualized" (p. 624). Honjo et al. also suggested that these scans may be obtained on children if they can phonate a vowel for more than 3 seconds and if the level of VP closure can be determined. Finkelstein, Berger, Nachmani, and Ophir (1996) assessed the variability of the velopharyngeal closure mechanism using axial CT scans obtained at rest. The axial configuration observed correlated well with velopharyngeal closure patterns as observed using nasendoscopy.

The conventional CT scan produces only a static image from a sustained speech sound. Advances in CT imaging technology led to the development of motion picture or cine-computed tomography. The patient is positioned in a fashion similar to that described for conventional CT scans. Prior to the actual scan, a localization scan, consisting of an exposure at each desired level, is obtained to ensure correct positioning. Series of CT scans are then obtained at each level. Each scan represents a single frame of the cine CT "movie," which may be viewed on a video monitor.

The 650-millisecond scan rate reported by Moon and Smith (1987) did not allow for an accurate depiction of movement during ongoing speech. The speech task used by Moon and Smith in their description of this technique was an alternation of (a) inhalation through the nose and (b) a short prolongation of /s/. This task was thought to allow an evaluation of the extremes of movement and possibly some visualization of movement between the extremes. The results of their investigation led Moon and Smith to suggest that

> cine CT technology may have some potential usefulness in the documentation of VP form and function. In its present state of development,

> it allows for visualization of all sides of the velopharynx at different tomographic levels. It also allows, to some degree, visualization of the motion of VP walls during phonatory and non-phonatory events. (p. 230)

Moon and Smith (1987) also commented on a number of liabilities of this system as used for VP function analysis: reduced resolution (as expressed by slice thickness of 8 mm), scan rate, radiation exposure level, possible effects of gravity on the VP mechanism when the patient is supine, and inability to combine simultaneously collected slices to obtain a three-dimensional composite image. Acceptance of CT imaging (static or dynamic) in the assessment of velopharyngeal anatomy and physiology has not materialized to date, most likely because of a lack of significant advances in these liabilities (especially image resolution and radiation exposure).

## Magnetic Resonance Imaging

Application of magnetic resonance imaging, or MRI (see Figure 10.5), to the evaluation of velopharyngeal anatomy and physiology has received significant attention since the 1980s. MRI is based on principles involving magnetic properties of human tissue. Hydrogen nuclei (protons) reside in tissue having some water content. Protons act like spinning magnets that are all aligned when placed in a strong magnetic field, such as that provided by the MRI unit. In response to bombardment with radiofrequency pulses, alignment of the protons becomes perturbed. As they return to equilibrium, they give up energy in the form of radio waves that may be detected with a receiver (Vannier, 1984). These radio signals are decoded and displayed in the form of tomographic images. Contrast between tissues is achieved by using different sequences and timing of radiofrequency pulses (Dunn & Ehrhardt, 1984).

Three principal drawbacks of other imaging techniques (still radiography, videofluoroscopy, CT scanning) are image resolution, radiation exposure, and the two-dimensionality of obtained images. MRI overcomes each of these (Özgür, Tunçbilek, & Cila, 2000). Its ability to image soft tissue easily exceeds that of videofluoroscopy or CT scanning. MRI is capable of producing high-resolution images of velopharyngeal anatomy in all three dimensions without using ionizing radiation and without the need to reposition the patient during image acquisition. From these im-

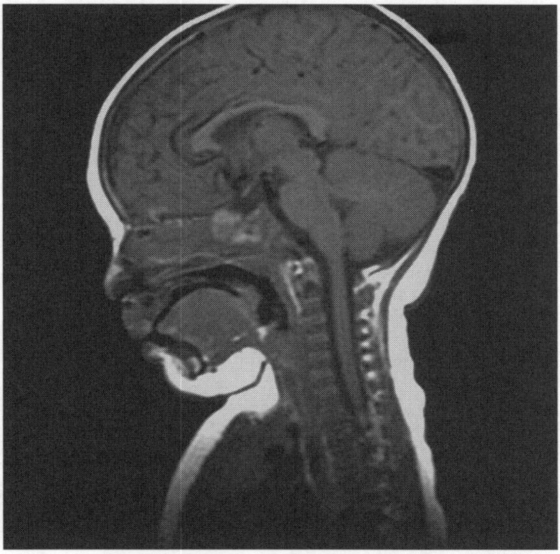

Figure 10.5. Sagittal-view magnetic resonance image of the head.

ages, a variety of anthropometric measures may be made in any of the three planes (Akgüner, 1999).

Technological developments currently being explored will capitalize on the three-dimensionality of MR scanning to reconstruct manipulable three-dimensional renderings of VP anatomy. As envisioned by Witt et al. (2000), clinicians and researchers may be able to "go inside" the anatomy represented in the MR scan, or to observe simulated endoscopic views.

However, its major disadvantage explains why MR imaging has not yet been widely used to study movement of VP structures: The collection of an image requires much more time than is feasible for the analysis of movement. Still, while its application has been limited primarily to the viewing of static rest anatomy, recent technological advances have allowed for imaging during speech. Using turboflash sequencing, Akgüner et al. (1998) were able to form a single image during phonation of /s/ in 3 seconds. While such temporal resolution would not allow the imaging of movement, it does allow for acquisition of high-resolution images of the VP region during speech. Also, advances in MR imaging designed to improve scan rates will allow for multiple images to be acquired during a single phonation (Witt et al., 2000).

As with any new technology, the efficacy of MR imaging during speech production awaits investigation. Given the high costs associated with obtaining these images, the value of any information gained from them must be evaluated relative to perceived benefits and information available from less expensive techniques. An additional drawback of the technique, as with CT scanning, is that images are obtained with the patient in the supine position. Gravitational forces might facilitate closure of the VP mechanism in the supine position and work against closure in the upright position. Indeed, Moon and Canady (1995) reported that VP muscle activation patterns of normal speakers changed when gravitational forces changed. Kuehn, Ray, Ettema, and Barkmeier (2001) suggested that while gravity does not appear to affect rest positioning of the velum in the supine versus upright position, speakers may well employ different motor control strategies to produce speech in one body posture versus the other. Although the functional consequences of gravitational effects may not be significant in the normal population, they may become significant in the speaker with a repaired palatal cleft.

## Ultrasound

The importance of lateral pharyngeal wall movement to the separation of the oral and nasal cavities and the inability of some instrumental techniques to allow visualization of that movement have been discussed earlier. Ultrasound has been investigated as a potentially useful, noninvasive tool for transducing movements of the lateral pharyngeal walls during speech. To assess lateral pharyngeal wall movement, a transducer is placed on the skin below the earlobe and behind the ramus of the mandible (Parush & Ostry, 1986). The transducer employs a crystal that converts electrical signals into acoustic (ultrasound) pulses, which are in turn radiated through the neck skin into the body. When ultrasonic pulses are radiated into body tissue, acoustic echoes or reflections occur at boundaries between nonhomogeneous materials (Ryan & Hawkins, 1976). This is especially true when the pulses meet a volume of air. Reflected pulses are received by the transducer and reconverted into electrical signals for display or recording.

Although ultrasound continues to be used in the study of lower lateral pharyngeal wall motion during speech and swallowing (Miller & Watkin, 1997; Parush & Ostry, 1993), it has not gained acceptance as a diagnostic tool for VP function. Perhaps this is because only lateral pharyngeal wall activity may be viewed, and on only one side at a time. The technical difficulties involved with obtaining consistently useful, interpretable images may also limit its use.

## Endoscopy

The endoscope is an optical instrument that allows for the illumination and visualization of internal body structures not easily visualized by the unaided eye. Light from an external source is passed through the scope via either fiberoptic fibers or a series of lenses to illuminate the area of interest. The image travels through a lens and more fiberoptic fibers to an eyepiece, which may be attached to a still or video camera for recording. Application of endoscopy to the assessment of VP form and function falls into a number of categorizations. In broad terms, these are oral versus nasal endoscopy and flexible versus rigid endoscopy.

Oral endoscopy enjoys limited use for a number of reasons. Karnell and Morris (1985) suggested that the oral perspective might underestimate lateral pharyngeal wall movements in some patients. Insertion of a rigid endoscope into the oral cavity obstructs articulator movement and essentially limits the speech sample to low vowels and bilabial consonants. Also, oral insertion of an endoscope may be quite difficult, if not impossible, in patients with a gag reflex, and especially in children. Karnell and Morris did, however, point out that oral endoscopy and nasal endoscopy led to identification of identical valving patterns in 60% of their cases. Furthermore, they perceived that oral endoscopy resulted in more identifications of Passavant's ridge (anterior movement of the posterior pharyngeal wall) than did nasal endoscopy.

By far the more popular of the two options is nasal endoscopy. This technique involves inserting either a flexible or a rigid endoscope (Figure 10.6) through either the left or right nasal passage in order to view the VP mechanism from above. The rigid endoscope has gained popularity in Great Britain primarily due to the work of Pigott and his colleagues (e.g., Pigott, 1980; Pigott & Makepeace, 1982). In contrast, the end-viewing flexible scope seems to be the instrument of choice in North America. Because of its superior optical characteristics, the rigid scope produces a sharper image than the flexible scope (Pigott, 1980); however, the flexible scope is typically easier to insert (Pigott & Makepeace, 1982).

Pigott's (1980) review of the factors that should be taken into account when conducting endoscopy continues to be applicable today. These

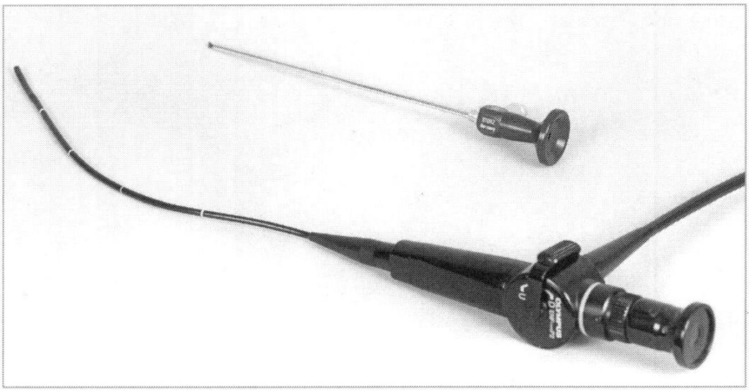

Figure 10.6. Rigid (upper) and flexible (lower) nasal endoscopes.

factors include the exam room and equipment, anesthesia, patient selection, scope insertion, and recording. The majority of endoscopic examinations of the VP mechanism are likely to be conducted on children. As stated by Pigott, it is difficult to anticipate which children will tolerate the technique and which will not. With the trend toward completing corrective surgery at earlier ages, there is growing demand to conduct nasal endoscopy on very young children. Although Lotz, D'Antonio, Chait, and Netsell (1993) reported successful examinations on patients as young as 2 years of age, most practitioners consider between 3 and 5 years as the youngest age appropriate for nasendoscopic evaluation (D'Antonio, Achauer, & Vander Kam, 1993).

The need to have a cooperative patient is of paramount importance. The notion of allowing someone to pass a tube through the nose is undoubtedly terrifying to some children. Little useful information will be obtained from viewing the VP mechanism of a child crying or sobbing uncontrollably who refuses to talk with the scope in place. Endoscopic techniques designed for young children are described in detail by Kummer (2001).

Currently available endoscopes vary in diameter from about 2 to 4 mm, with 3 mm being the most common. Most individuals will not tolerate passage of the scope without topical anesthesia. The patient is typically asked to blow his or her nose to remove any mucous buildup from the nasal passage before applying the anesthetic. The more patent side of the nose can be determined by blocking each side independently and having the patient sniff. A number of approaches can be used to apply the anesthesia. Some clinicians simply spray the nasal passage using an atomizer; others soak a cotton swab or gauze strip in the anesthesia and pass it through the passage along the intended course of the endoscope. The atomizer approach is thought to be simpler and less traumatic by its proponents; however, it results in anesthetization of tissue areas that would not require it. As outlined in the American Speech-Language-Hearing Association (ASHA) policy statement on vocal tract visualization and imaging (1992b) and guidelines for administering topical anesthetics (1992a), application of topical anesthesia and insertion of nasendoscopes fall within the speech pathology scope of practice, given the attainment of a sufficient amount of training.

Assuming that the patient is willing to accept the scope and has been anesthetized (if needed), the insertion path of the scope must also be considered. One of two paths is typically chosen. The easier path is a lower one, along the floor of the nose underneath the inferior turbinate; however, the VP isthmus is then viewed rather obliquely, and a true representation of its function may be difficult to visualize. The optimal path lies just under the middle turbinate, through the middle meatus. By following this path, the viewing end of the fiberscope sits higher in the nasopharynx and can be deflected to look down on the VP mechanism from a more optimal angle (Figure 10.7). Once the scope is positioned, the patient can be instructed to complete any number of speech and nonspeech tasks. The speech sample used varies widely from clinician to clinician. Most samples include prolongations of vowels and fricatives, repetitions of high-pressure consonants (e.g., /pɑ/), sentences loaded with oral consonants, and words and sentences with oral and nasal consonants together (e.g., "hamper," "pimi").

There are many reports in the literature describing both static and dynamic aspects of VP function that may be evaluated using nasal endoscopy prior to and following either surgical or nonsurgical treatment for velopharyngeal incompetence (VPI) (e.g., Finkelstein et al., 1996; Ramamurthy, Wyatt, Whitby, Martin, & Davenport, 1997; Witt et al., 1998; Wu et al., 1996). The procedure may be used to view the presence or absence of an adenoid pad and its contribution to closure, velar movement characteristics (extent, symmetry, consistency), the size of the VP port, the contribution of lateral wall movement to closure, and the presence of any aberrant blood vessels (especially in the posterior pharyngeal wall). One can also look for evidence of bubbling mucus during speech attempts, which may indicate incomplete VP closure. One must realize, however, that the interpretation of data collected using endoscopy is largely

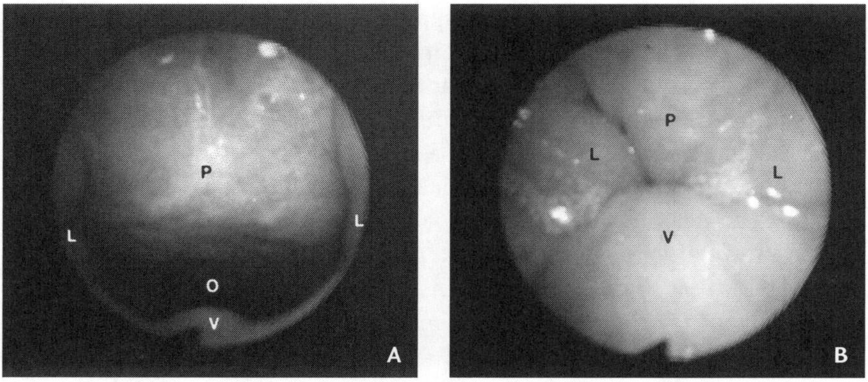


Figure 10.7. View of velopharyngeal region at rest (A) and during production of /s/ (B) using a flexible endoscope. P = posterior pharyngeal wall; L = lateral pharyngeal walls; V = velum; O = velopharyngeal orifice.

subjective in nature. The orientation of the endoscope, its distance from the VP isthmus, and distortion inherent in the endoscopic image itself are possible sources of error in interpretation. In addition, the viewer must also be considered a source of error.

Relatively few attempts have been made to quantify or standardize endoscopic evaluations. Croft, Shprintzen, Daniller, and Lewin (1978) attempted to quantify the size of the VP orifice by inserting catheters of known diameter into the area of VP closure through the airway opposite the endoscope. They compared the diameter of the orifice as viewed through the scope with the known diameter of the catheter, also as viewed through the scope. They then calculated the area of the orifice. Ibuki, Karnell, and Morris (1983) measured velar movement, size of the VP orifice, and extent of lateral pharyngeal wall movement from photographs taken through the endoscope during the production of sustained vowels or fricatives. They concluded that "a trace-and-measure procedure can be used on NPF (nasal endoscope) still photographs that give reliable data" (p. 103). However, measurements of movement of the lateral pharyngeal wall opposite the side of insertion were not reliable. The conclusions reached by Ibuki et al. were criticized by Shprintzen (1983), who pointed out that a side-viewing endoscope (an endoscope with the lens oriented at 90 degrees, which is rarely used clinically) was used in place of an end-viewing endoscope (one with the lens placed directly on the end of the endoscope) and that validity and reliability were assessed against lateral-view cineradiographic images, which do not reflect the three-dimensional nature of the system. Furthermore, Ibuki et al. (1983) admitted that their technique was too cumbersome to be used clinically.

Karnell, Ibuki, Morris, and Van Demark (1983) devised a rating system to standardize judgments of endoscopic images. The VP area was represented as a box, having a lower velar border, two lateral pharyngeal wall borders, and an upper posterior pharyngeal wall border. Movements of each wall were assigned a number based on the extent of movement relative to the total range of movement. The authors concluded that, with some restrictions, judgments of the VP mechanism made from endoscopic images are reliable and valid. Their restrictions included the necessity to obtain a view that encompasses all VP boundaries in a single view and the necessity for the examiner to have prior training in evaluating nasal endoscopic images. These reliability data must be interpreted in the same light as those of Ibuki et al. (1983), because the same side-viewing endoscope was used in both.

Karnell, Linville, and Edwards (1988) tracked velar position over time by measuring soft palate position on a field-by-field basis from nasendoscopic images. They concluded that the technique was reliable and provided useful information regarding within-subject changes in velar position. However, absolute measures of velar movement and position are still not possible.

In 1990, an international working group was formed to attempt to standardize the reporting of nasal endoscopic examinations (Golding-Kushner et al., 1990). This group recommended that movement ratios as opposed to absolute values should be calculated. The group presented standardized qualitative and quantitative approaches to describing velar movement; lateral pharyngeal wall movement; posterior pharyngeal wall and Passavant's ridge; and the size, shape, and location of any velopharyngeal gap (see Figure 10.8).

Endoscopy has grown to be a popular diagnostic tool since its first application to the study of the VP mechanism in the early 1970s. D'Antonio et al. (1993) reported that 90% of cleft palate teams responding to their survey used the technique, and 74% used information gained from nasendoscopy in making management decisions. The continuing popularity of nasendoscopy is undoubtedly due, in part, to the fact that endoscopy offers the diagnostician a direct view of the VP mechanism in motion without the need for exposure to radiation. The main disadvantages of the

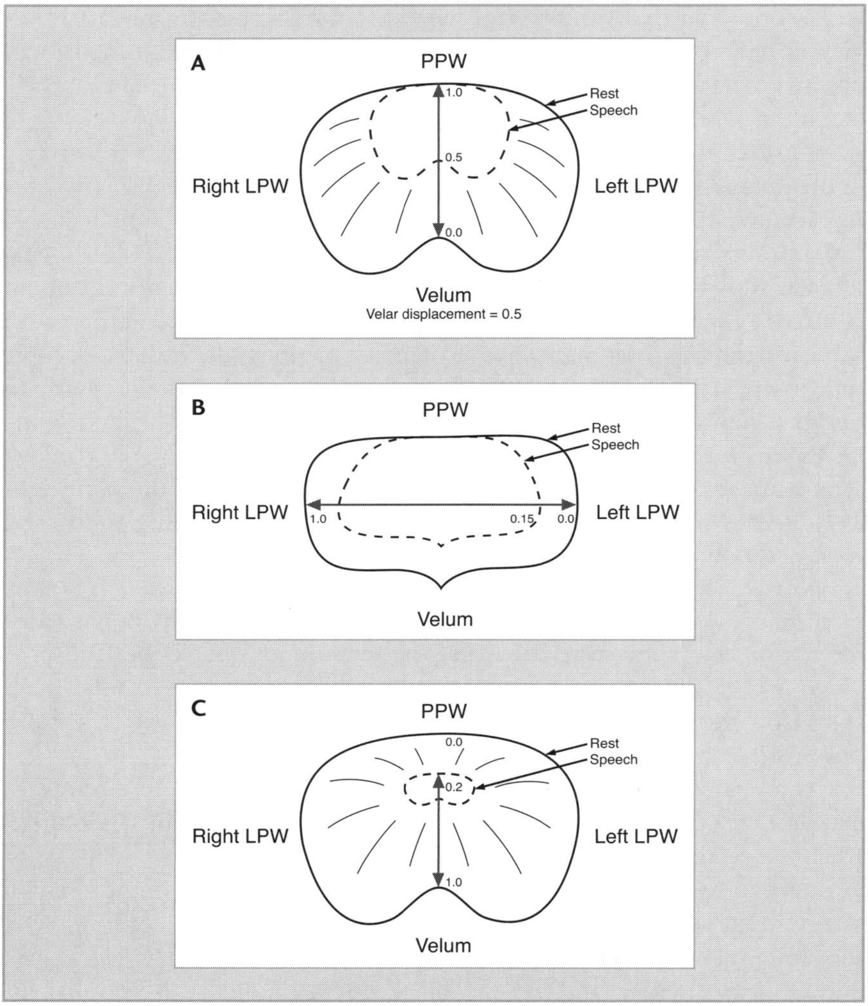


FIGURE 10.8. Examples of standardized system of reporting velopharyngeal form and function as observed endoscopically. (A) Velar displacement. The velum (0.0) moves half the distance to the posterior pharyngeal wall (PPW, 1.0) and, therefore, is scored 0.5. (B) Lateral pharyngeal wall (LPW) displacement. The opposite lateral wall represents 1.0. The left lateral wall moves 0.15 (distance ratio) toward the right lateral LPW. (C) Degree of PPW displacement. In the case of a structurally normal palate, the PPW represents 0.0 while the midline of the musculus uvulae is 1.0. In this case, the posterior wall moves 0.2 of the distance toward the velum at rest. *Note.* From "Standardization for the Reporting of Nasopharyngoscopy and Multiview Videofluoroscopy: A Report from an International Working Group," by K. Golding-Kushner et al., 1990, *Cleft Palate Journal, 27,* pp. 339–341. Copyright 1990 by American Cleft Palate-Craniofacial Association. Reprinted with permission.

technique rest in its invasiveness and the potential difficulties involved with completing the procedure on young children. The fact that interpretation of the data is subjective in nature and remains difficult to quantify must also be considered. However, D'Antonio, Marsh, Province, Muntz, and Phillips (1989) suggested that the judgments made from endoscopic images may be improved by using a panel of experienced clinicians, and Pigott and Makepeace (1982) suggested that endoscopy be used in conjunction with another diagnostic procedure. The latter authors argued that endoscopy and radiography complement each other because endoscopy provides a subjective view of "the real world," whereas radiography provides an objective view of "shadows." Pigott and Makepeace promoted simultaneous recording of nasal endoscopic and radiologic views to take advantage of the complementary information they provide. This view was reinforced by Albery, Bennett, Pigott, and Simmons (1982), who stated that simultaneous measurement will provide information on the size and shape of the orifice and both the proportional and absolute movements of the soft palate and lateral and posterior pharyngeal walls.

# Indirect Primary Approaches

Indirect primary approaches to studying the movement of the VP mechanism include phototransduction, electromyography, movement transduction, and velar closure force.

## Phototransduction

The notion of using photoelectric technology in assessing VP function, as explored by Dalston (1982) and Moon and Lagu (1987), is based on the principles of light transmission through a tube. A light source is placed on one side of the VP opening and a light sensor on the opposite side (see Figure 10.9). The light sensor emits a voltage with magnitude dependent on the amount of light impinging on it. The distance between the light source and detector is held constant.

The device described by Dalston (1982) employs two small (0.75-mm) fiberoptic fibers coupled to a light source and detector electronics, respectively. The fibers are inserted through the nasal cavity until the source

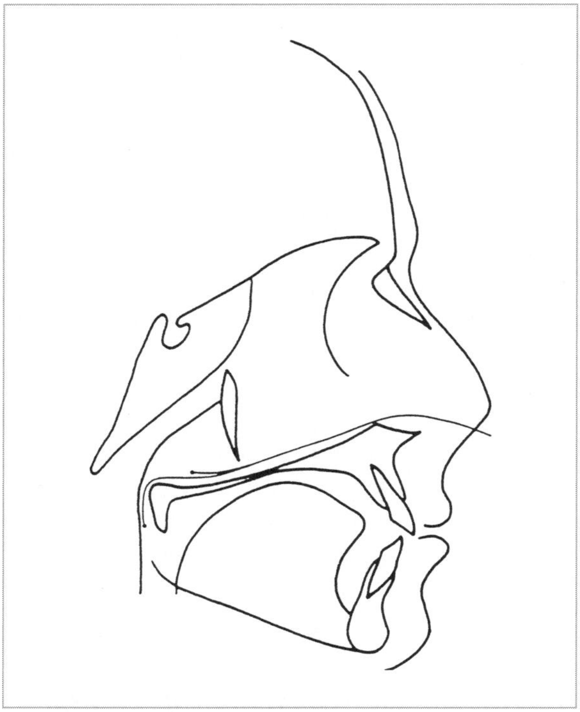

Figure 10.9. Placement of phototransducer. *Note.* From "Photodetector Assessment of Velopharyngeal Activity," by R. Dalston, 1982, *Cleft Palate Journal, 19,* p. 4. Copyright 1982 by American Cleft Palate-Craniofacial Association. Reprinted with permission.

fiber is positioned below the VP port and the detector fiber above. The fibers are small enough that they reportedly produce only slight discomfort when passed through the inferior meatus of the nose. Topical anesthesia is not required in the majority of cases. The fibers weigh less than 1 g and are not thought to interfere with VP function (Dalston, 1982). The fibers do have a rather large bending radius (i.e., stiffness). The effects of this property on function of the mechanism, however, have not been empirically tested. When the velum moves toward closure, the amount of light transmitted through the VP port is diminished, thus reducing the output of the detector. A typical trace is displayed in Figure 10.10.

Data collected using this device are relative; that is, one can interpret the opening size of the VP port in relation to maximal opening size,

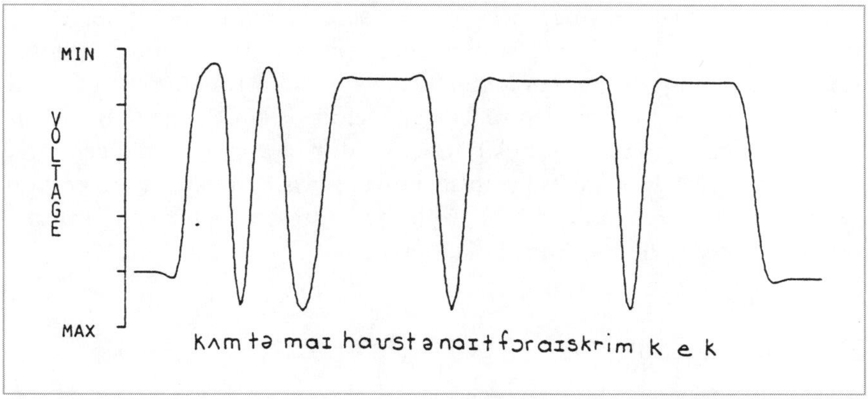


FIGURE 10.10. Sample phototransducer output obtained from normal subject during production of the sentence, "Come to my house tonight for ice cream cake." Minimum and maximum voltage refer to closed and open position, respectively. *Note.* From "A Comparison of Photodetector and Endoscopic Evaluations of Velopharyngeal Functions," by M. Karnell, E. Seaver, and R. Dalston, 1988, *Journal of Speech and Hearing Research, 31,* p. 507. Copyright 1988 by American Speech-Language-Hearing Association. Reprinted with permission.

but not in terms of square millimeter area. Obviously, an important and desirable attribute of this type of device is linearity. Dalston (1982) reported that the device output is related to VP opening size both directly and linearly. This statement is supported by the existence of a high correlation between detector output voltage and known simulated VP orifice areas (Jones & Moon, 1989).

The phototransducer is an interesting development in the battery of VP evaluation instruments. Although not a direct measure of VP movement, it is designed to provide quantifiable data regarding VP movement (e.g., Dalston & Seaver, 1990). It compares quite favorably with other instrumental measures of VP function. Dalston (1982) found a correlation of .907 between phototransducer output and orifice areas as determined using aerodynamic measures (to be discussed later). Zimmermann et al. (1987) evaluated the phototransducer against lateral view cineradiography. They found that (a) the phototransducer output varied with opening and closing movements of the velum as seen on lateral-view cineradiography, (b) most phototransducer output changes occurred within 30 milliseconds of corresponding changes in velar position as seen using cineradiography, and (c) a highly positive relationship ($r > .80$) exists between magnitude of phototransducer output and extent of velar movement as measured from lateral cine traces. While these results are promising, they are based on only 2 subjects. Karnell and Seaver (1993) combined a photodetector assembly with nasendoscopy to evaluate VP function in a patient with marginal VP insufficiency. They concluded that the system was effective in identifying details of VP function during a variety of speech and nonspeech tasks. Despite its promise, however, issues related to toleration by children and reliability will have to be addressed before phototransduction is accepted as a clinical diagnostic tool.

## Electromyography

Electromyography (EMG) involves the study of electrical activity associated with muscle contraction. Electrical activity within the muscle may be detected by inserting very fine wires into the muscle to pick up and conduct the electrical signals to signal-conditioning and -recording equipment outside the body. The wires, referred to as hooked-wire electrodes, are enclosed within a hypodermic needle. The needle is inserted into the muscle and, when removed, leaves the wires behind (see Figure 10.11).

Routine use of EMG as a diagnostic tool has not yet materialized. Although Fritzell (1979) suggested that needle electrode insertion is only minimally discomforting, it is unlikely that children would readily submit to needle insertions in the back of the oral cavity. A second major problem involves electrode placement. The combination of small size, relative inaccessibility, and possible malpositioning of muscles in speakers with cleft

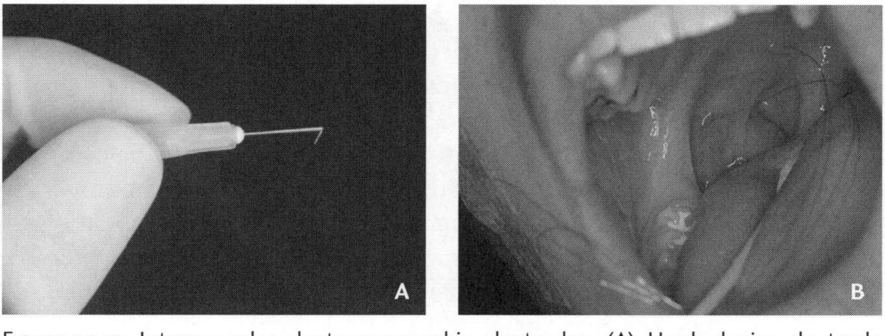


Figure 10.11. Intramuscular electromyographic electrodes. (A) Hooked-wire electrode wire positioned in hypodermic needle prior to insertion. (B) Electrode wires inserted into levator veli palatini and palatoglossus muscles.

palates makes interpretation of EMG signals difficult. Finally, making inferences about movements of the velum based on observed EMG activity is tenuous. As stated by Kuehn, Folkins, and Cutting (1982), direction of muscle forces will undoubtedly change as velar position changes. Until a "quantitative model of velar biomechanics" is developed that takes into account interactions among all of the passive and active forces acting on the VP mechanism, moving from EMG activity to movement patterns of the normal and especially the disordered mechanism cannot be conducted with an appropriate degree of certainty (Kuehn et al., 1982).

Velar muscle electromyography has been used in laboratory settings, however, to learn a great deal about the normal velopharyngeal mechanism (see Figure 10.12 for a typical EMG signal) and the consequences of palatal clefting and repair on VP function. For example, systematic variations in levator veli palatini muscle activation level occur in association with changing body position (supine vs. upright), a finding that may have significance given that imaging procedures such as MRI require the patient to be supine (Moon & Canady, 1995). In response to increased levels of air pressure introduced to the nasal cavity, thereby loading the VP mechanism, normal speakers are able to increase levator muscle activity to maintain velopharyngeal closure during speech without fatiguing (Kuehn & Moon, 2000; Kuehn, Moon, & Folkins, 1993). During normal speaking conditions, levator activation levels are near the lower end of the operating range and speech is a low-effort task (Kuehn & Moon, 1994). For the speakers with repaired palatal clefts studied by Kuehn and Moon (1995), however, levator veli palatini muscle effort was near the upper end of the operating range even when the VP mechanism was not artificially loaded by increased nasal airway pressure. As such, relatively more muscle effort was required by these speakers compared to noncleft speakers. Small increases in velar loading, and hence muscle effort, lead to muscle fatigue and loss of the VP seal (Moon & Kuehn, 1998). These findings have important therapeutic implications.

Kuehn (1991) introduced a new therapy technique based on the premise that the levator veli palatini muscle in speakers with repaired cleft palate is not strong enough to maintain separation between the oral and nasal cavities during speech. Continuous positive airway pressure (CPAP) therapy is designed to strengthen the palatal muscles associated with velopharyngeal closure. By focusing therapy on a specific physiological level thought to be impaired (i.e., muscle strength or endurance), it is hypothesized that the VP mechanism function can be optimized. Research on

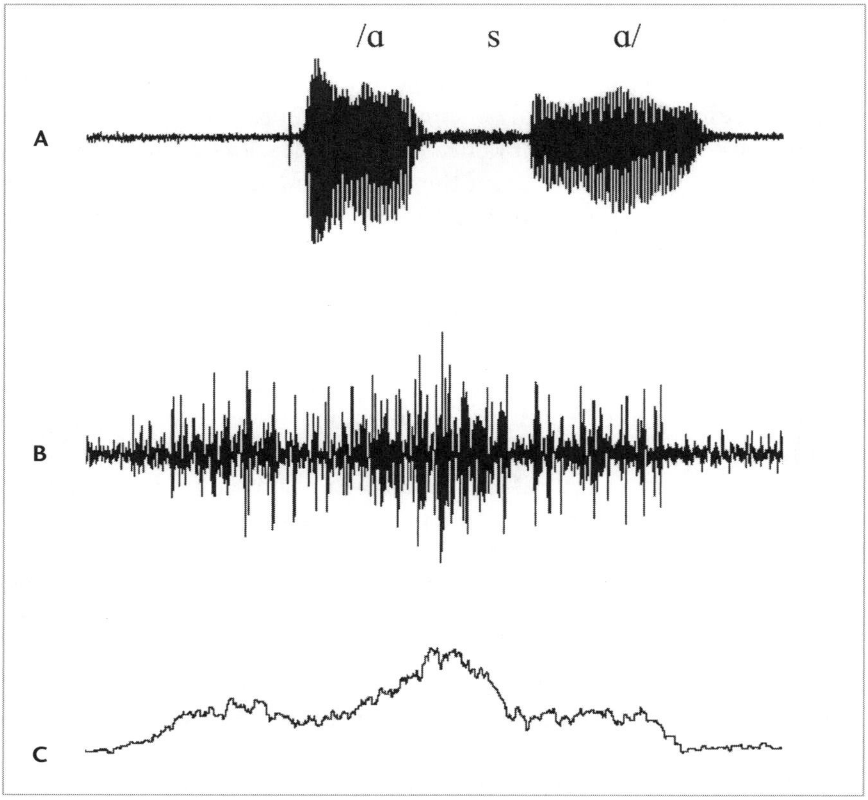


Figure 10.12. Electromyographic (EMG) signal recorded from the levator veli palatini muscle during production of /asa/. A = voice signal; B = raw EMG signal; C = rectified and smoothed EMG signal.

the efficacy of this approach is continuing in both clinic and laboratory settings.

Utilizing EMG recordings from the superior constrictor, palatopharyngeus, and levator veli palatini muscles, Ysunza, Pamplona, Molina, Chacon, and Collado (1999) discovered that closing gestures following sphincter pharyngoplasty appeared due to contraction of the superior constrictor muscle. In a series of studies investigating levator muscle activation patterns following placement of palatal lift prostheses, Tachimura and colleagues (Tachimura, Hohara, Fujiki, Hara, & Wada, 2001; Tachimura, Hohara, Hara, & Wada, 1999; Tachimura, Hohara, & Wada, 2000; Tachimura, Mori, Hirata, & Wada, 2000) found that the assist offered speakers by placement of the prosthesis resulted in lower levels of levator muscle activity. They implied that speakers with repaired palatal clefts wearing a lift appliance might be able to achieve velopharyngeal closure with a level of muscle activity that falls below the muscle fatigue threshold. Velepic, Bonifacic, Lustica, Sasso, and Cvjetkovic (1999) recorded muscle activity from 75 patients with VPI. Velepic et al. asserted that muscle activation patterns can be used to distinguish between patients with and without neurogenic involvement.

It is clear that EMG studies, while still relegated largely to the laboratory, will continue to influence understanding of the physiology of VP function. Although interpretation of EMG patterns must necessarily be made with some caution, this technique also offers an approach to assessing the effectiveness of treatments designed to optimize motor behavior.

## Movement Transduction

A couple of attempts have been made to transduce VP movement using mechanical and electrical devices attached directly to VP structures. Moller, Martin, and Christiansen (1971) and Moller, Path, Werth, and Christiansen (1973) described a strain gauge transducer designed to track velar movement (Figure 10.13a). The device consists of an anchor to a maxillary second molar, and a bar/spring attachment placed into contact with the oral side of the velum in the midline. As the velum elevates, the spring sensor is moved. Velar movement is reflected in the electrical output of the strain gauge resistor. Adaptation to the device in the oral cavity was reportedly achieved readily, normal articulation was not interfered with, and physical discomfort was not a problem. When compared to radiographic measures of velar movement, a high level of agreement was achieved. The device was described as an "unobtrusive intraoral device to record velar moment continuously during speech production" (Moller et al., 1971, p. 275). This displacement transducer system was used as a biofeedback device to increase velar elevation (Moller et al., 1973) but has not been used as an evaluation tool for assessing velar function.

A second mechanical-electrical device designed to collect data on velar position during speech is the velotrace (Bell-Berti & Krakow, 1991; Horiguchi & Bell-Berti, 1987). Whereas the Moller et al. (1971) device was placed intraorally, the velotrace (Figure 10.13b) is passed through the nose after application of topical anesthesia and decongestants. Movements of the velum are translated into linear movements of a push-rod, which, in

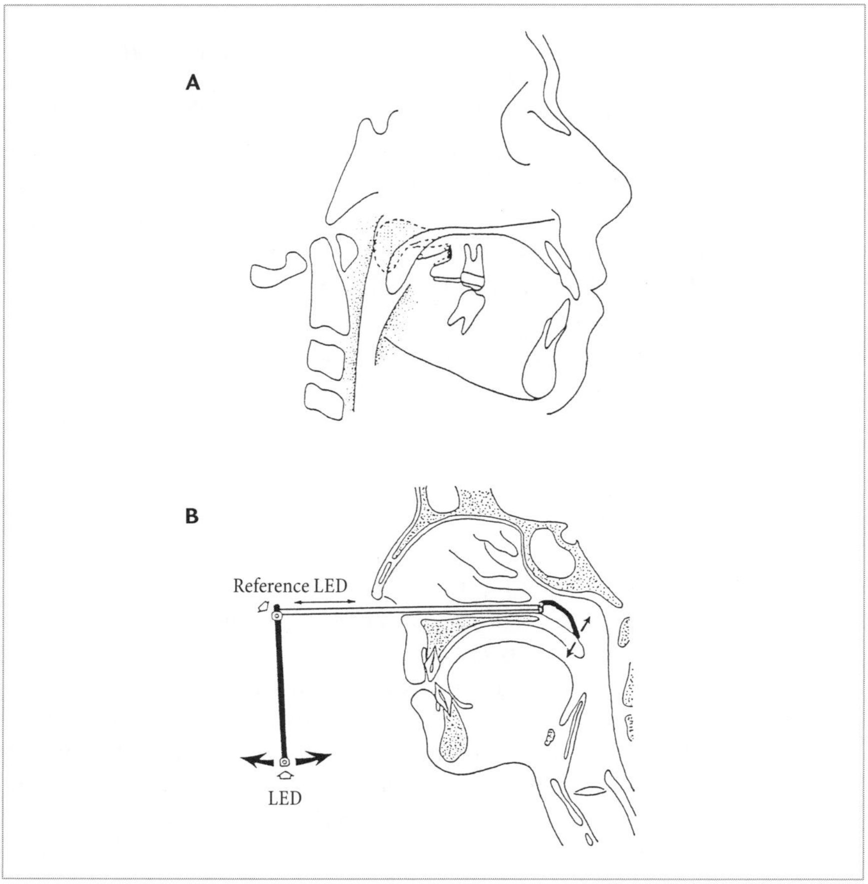


Figure 10.13. Approaches to the transduction of velar movement. (A) Schematic of strain gauge transduction system showing position at rest (solid line) and during production of /s/ (dotted line). *Note.* From "A Technique for Recording Velar Movement," by K. Moller, R. Martin, and R. Christiansen, 1971, *Cleft Palate Journal, 8,* p. 266. Copyright 1971 by American Cleft Palate-Craniofacial Association. Reprinted with permission. (B) The velotrace. *Note.* From "The Velotrace: A Device for Monitoring Velar Position," by S. Horiguchi and F. Bell-Berti, 1987, *Cleft Palate Journal, 24,* p. 105. Copyright 1987 by American Cleft Palate-Craniofacial Association. Reprinted with permission.

turn, are translated into rotational movements of an externally positioned light-emitting diode (LED). A video camera is used to film the LED movement for later analysis. Horiguchi and Bell-Berti (1987) compared velotrace recordings with previously recorded endoscopic views, previously recorded velocity measures, and previously recorded measures of velar moment taken from lateral cineradiography. A different subject was employed for each measure, an approach that undoubtedly added some variability to the comparisons. Nonetheless, the authors concluded that the device accurately reflects velar movement during speech. Reported advantages of the system include no radiation and the ability to analyze movement on a frame-by-frame basis. Horiguchi and Bell-Berti also suggested that the device could be used with children. However, instrument and anatomical sizes obviously become a critical consideration.

Movements of the soft palate also have been transduced using electromagnetic articulography (Engelke, Bruns, Striebeck, & Hoch, 1996; Engelke, Hoch, Bruns, & Striebeck, 1996; Poppelreuter, Engelke, & Bruns, 2000). A small sensor is sutured to the oral side of the velum in the midsagittal plane, and a reference sensor is mounted on the upper incisor. The speaker's head is positioned in the center of a triangular array of three electromagnetic transmitters (see Figure 10.14). As the receiver moves within the electromagnetic fields generated by the transmitter array, an alternating current is induced in each sensor. This current is recorded and

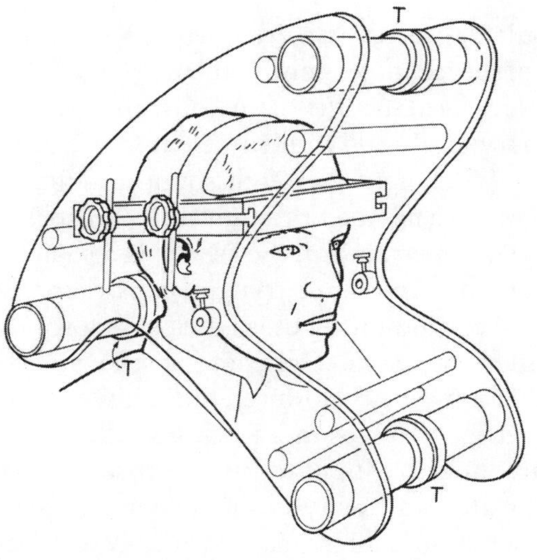


FIGURE 10.14. Electromagnetic articulograph. T = transmitters. *Note.* From "Electromagnetic Midsagittal Articulometer Systems for Transducing Speech Articulatory Movements," by J. Perkell et al., 1992, *Journal of the Acoustical Society of America, 92,* p. 3084. Copyright 1992 by Acoustical Society of America. Reprinted with permission.

used to obtain the distance of each sensor from the three transmitters. In this way, the *x* and *y* coordinates of the sensor can be determined. The device has been used with normal adult speakers to quantify velar trajectories, displacements, and velocities during speech production.

A significant disadvantage of all three of these devices is that they are able to track velar movement only in the sagittal plane. Although many would argue that the most significant and principal movements during VP closure occur in the sagittal plane, it is important to analyze the VP mechanism in all three of its dimensions. The electromagnetic articulograph has recently been used together with transoral video endoscopy in an attempt to quantify the sphincteric activity of the VP mechanism (Engelke, Hoch, et al., 1996; Poppelreuter et al., 2000). These authors argue that "quantification of sphincter morphology and an objective evaluation of VPI is possible within routine examinations" (Poppelreuter et al., 2000, p. 165). However, given its high cost and the extensive signal conditioning required for its use, this technology is unlikely to be used in the near future for routine clinical assessment of VP physiology.

## Velar Closure Force

Control of articulatory forces associated with speech production is a central component of speech motor control theory (Barlow & Bradford, 1992). It is readily acknowledged that the velum must be moved into contact with the posterior pharyngeal wall with sufficient force, or tightness, to seal off the nasal cavity during oral speech sound production. Velopharyngeal closure forces are generated through the coordinated contraction of the muscles of the VP mechanism: the levator veli palatini, palatoglossus, palatopharyngeus, and superior pharyngeal constrictor (Moon, Kuehn, & Huisman, 1994). The monitoring of velar closure force has received little attention because of the inaccessibility of the valve and the lack of an appropriate transduction device. However, the ability to record velar closure force is important for two reasons (Kuehn & Moon, 1997). First, magnitudes of closure force may need to vary to offset mechanical and aerodynamic forces in the oral cavity in order to avoid excessive nasal coupling. Second, velar closure forces may reasonably be adversely affected in anatomically or physiologically impaired mechanisms.

Development of a transducer capable of sensing velar closure force (Moon et al., 1994) allowed for the systematic investigation of VP function on a physiological level not previously addressed. The transducer

(Figure 10.15) is a flattened teardrop-shaped silastic bulb, measuring 5 mm thick and 10 mm wide. The bulb is inserted transnasally and positioned such that it is squeezed between the nasal side of the velum and the posterior pharyngeal wall during velar closing gestures. As the velum is elevated into contact with the posterior pharyngeal wall, the time-varying force of contact is transmitted to the sensing bulb (Figure 10.16). Using this device, Moon et al. (1994) and Kuehn and Moon (1997, 2000) discovered a number of interesting aspects of VP function in both normal speakers and those with repaired palatal clefts. Velar closure forces vary with gender and with phonetic context. It is also evident that closure force is not controlled solely by the levator veli palatini. Further, the ability to achieve and maintain sufficient closure forces can become compromised if the responsible muscles are activated at a level exceeding their threshold of fatigue. This is of particular importance in the case of speakers with repaired palatal clefts (Kuehn & Moon, 2000; Moon & Kuehn, 1998).

The velar closure force bulb has significant potential, both as a diagnostic tool to assess the effects of surgical or behavioral interventions and as a mechanism for providing online feedback about a crucial aspect of VP function during therapy. It allows the researcher or clinician to

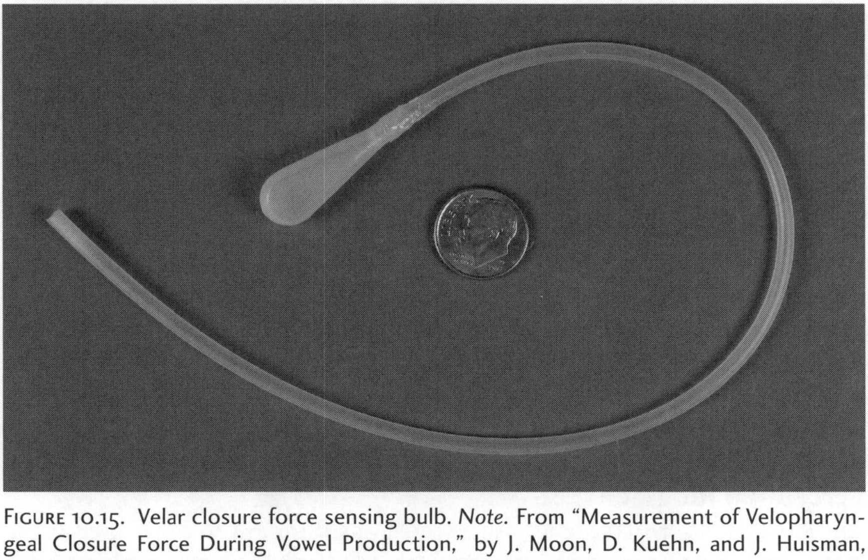

Figure 10.15. Velar closure force sensing bulb. *Note.* From "Measurement of Velopharyngeal Closure Force During Vowel Production," by J. Moon, D. Kuehn, and J. Huisman, 1994, *Cleft Palate-Craniofacial Journal, 31,* p. 357. Copyright 1994 by American Cleft Palate-Craniofacial Association. Reprinted with permission.

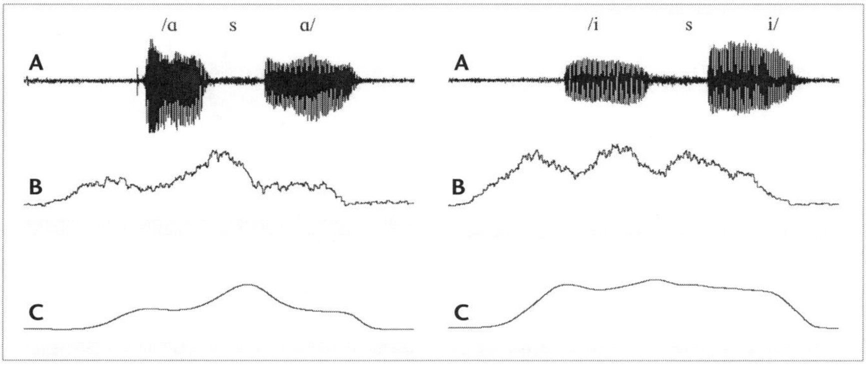


FIGURE 10.16. Velar closure force recorded during production of /ɑsɑ/ (left) and /isi/ (right). A = voice signal; B = rectified and smoothed levator veli palatini EMG signal; C = velar closure force.

directly monitor VP function at a physiological level not accessible using other techniques.

# Secondary Measures

Using the categorization scheme of this chapter, secondary measures all fall under the category of indirect measures; that is, data collected using these techniques may be interpreted to make inferences regarding VP structure and function. They provide data about physiological events that are affected by VP movement. Secondary measures may involve either acoustic or aerodynamic phenomena. Acoustic measures include perceptual judgment, sound spectrography, sound pressure measurement, accelerometry, and acoustic rhinometry. Aerodynamic measures involve analysis of air pressure and airflow patterns in the nasal and oral cavities.

## Acoustic Measures

### Perceptual Judgment

The ear was described earlier as the most basic and, in many respects, the most important diagnostic tool available to provide information about VP function. Although electronic devices have been and continue to be developed to transduce the physiological events associated with movement of the VP mechanism, most clinicians use their ear as the standard against which all other measures are compared.

A number of approaches, ranging in complexity from screening tools to more elaborate multifactorial evaluations, have been used in the perceptual analysis of VP incompetence. Historically, one of the more common screening approaches, sometimes referred to as the Cul-de-Sac test, is to have the patient prolong the vowels /ɑ/ and /i/ while the diagnostician occludes the nostrils (Kummer, 2001). If the VP mechanism is competent, no change in nasality should be perceived compared with the unoccluded condition. When VP valving is inadequate, addition of the nasal cavity to the vocal tract filter will produce a different resonance quality across the two conditions.

Kummer, Curtis, Wiggs, Lee, and Strife (1992) stressed the application of perceptual judgments in predicting the degree of VP insufficiency. Patients with hypernasality were found to have larger VP gaps, as assessed using videofluoroscopy, than those with nasal turbulence or rustle. Kummer (2001) also advocated listening for the perceived force of production of high-pressure consonants as an indication of the adequacy of intraoral air pressure generation. Perceived weakness may be a consequence of VP dysfunction.

A second perceptual screening tool is based on articulatory performance. The *Iowa Pressure Articulation Test* (IPAT; Morris, Spriestersbach, & Darley, 1961) was developed as a tool to discriminate between those with adequate and those with inadequate VP closure. The 43-item test is loaded with fricatives, plosives, and affricates known to require impounding of oral air pressure for correct production. The selection of these items was based on an expectation that performance would reflect "differences in ability to impound such (air) pressure and, inferentially, ability to achieve VP closure" (p. 54). Although children with nasal air escape were likely to do poorly on the IPAT, so were those speakers with an adequate VP mechanism who misarticulated sounds for other reasons (e.g., lateral lisp). McWilliams et al. (1984) cautioned that observation of error type on this test is perhaps more important than the score itself. An additional aspect of this test that warrants comment is that, during test development, grouping of test subjects into adequate and inadequate was based on lateral still radiographs and wet spirometer ratios. Evidence now indicates that performance observed using these approaches might not accurately reflect actual performance during speech. No attempts have been made to re-evaluate the IPAT against performance as observed using other instrumental approaches. The IPAT has been used successfully to differentiate between patients who required secondary management and those who did not (Karnell & Van Demark, 1986).

A more elaborate approach to evaluating VP function perceptually involves evaluating speech performance on a number of parameters to derive a score that reflects adequacy of the VP mechanism for speech (McWilliams et al., 1984; Philips, 1980). Nasal emission, facial grimace, nasal resonance, phonation, and articulation performance are assessed subjectively and scored on a standard form using weighted scores. A weighted score in excess of 7 was interpreted as indicative of VP incompetence.

Although subjective judgments comprise the basic diagnostic approach of many speech-language pathologists, their use has been criticized by numerous investigators. Judgments of nasality made by individual listeners tend to be unreliable (Counihan & Cullinan, 1970). The sources of variability in listener judgments of VP function include lack of a pre-established standard (Counihan & Cullinan, 1970), articulation skills (Dalston & Warren, 1985), vocal pitch and intensity (Hess, 1959), and past experience of the listener (Dalston & Warren, 1985; Starr, Moller, Dawson, Graham, & Skaar, 1984). However, judgment reliability may be expected to improve with training (Philips, 1980) and with the pooling of multiple-judge data (Counihan & Cullinan, 1970). Use of multiple judges may be especially useful when taking into account different listening conditions in which judgments must be made (Moller & Starr, 1984).

Clearly, listener judgments of speech proficiency must play a central role in the assessment of VP function. However, a danger exists in using only a subjective evaluation based on what is heard. Those perceptions need to be supplemented with more standardized and objective views of the mechanism.

## Sound Spectrography

Coupling the nasal cavity to the oral cavity may alter the resonance characteristics of the vocal tract and, hence, the output sound spectrum. Schwartz (1971) described four primary acoustic features associated with nasal-oral coupling during vowel production. The primary and most frequently observed feature in the spectrum of nasalized speech is a reduction in intensity of the first formant. Other features, observed less consistently, include the presence of one or more antiresonances within the spectrum, the presence of extra resonances within the spectrum, and a shift in the center frequency of the formants. Other approaches to analyzing spectral characteristics of speakers with inappropriate nasal-oral coupling have been directed toward more sophisticated computer analyses (Garnier, Gallego, Collet, & Berger-Vachon, 1996; Kataoka, Michi, Okabe, Miura, & Yoshida, 1996). Kataoka et al. (1996) utilized a power spectrum analysis method to quantify energy levels in normalized successive third-octave bands. Increases in power level between the first and second dormants and reduced power level in the second and third formant regions were found to be correlated with perceived hypernasality. Garnier et al. (1996) applied spectral and cepstral analysis procedures to the speech of children with severe velopharyngeal impairment and a normal control group. They were able to discriminate between the two speaker groups using these spectral and cepstral parameters.

Not surprisingly, few speech-language pathologists utilize spectrographic measures in the analysis of VP function. The difficulties involved with such an analysis are numerous. The correlates discussed above occur inconsistently and may not be readily discernible unless the speaker has a highly significant level of VP incompetence. The measurements are time-consuming and are subject to error. While more recent advances in computer-aided acoustic analysis show some promise, these techniques must continue to be classified as experimental.

### Sound Pressure Measurement/Nasometry

Attempts to measure nasal sound pressure level and relate it to oral sound pressure level are based on the premise that changes in the relative magnitudes of oral and nasal sound pressures will reflect the degree to which the oral and nasal tracts are coupled during speech production. Development work completed by Fletcher (1970, 1972) led to The Oral Nasal Acoustic Ratio (TONAR) and TONAR II instrumentation. The device is now commercially available as a computer-based system called the Nasometer.

Simply described, the device consists of two microphones (nasal and oral), separated by a horizontal sound separator (see Figure 10.17). Inputs from the nasal and oral microphones are individually conditioned (amplification, filtering, rectification) before the nasal signal is divided by the combined oral-nasal signal to derive a ratio. Thus, the absence of any nasal signal would result in a ratio of 0, whereas the absence of an oral signal would produce a ratio of 1. The output may be displayed in real time on a computer screen (see Figure 10.18). A special feature built into this device is a filter system that limits the acoustic analysis to the speech frequency spectrum. Fletcher termed this nasal:oral-nasal ratio "nasalance."

Numerous studies have been published about the use of this technology in diagnosing and treating VP dysfunction. Given that varying degrees

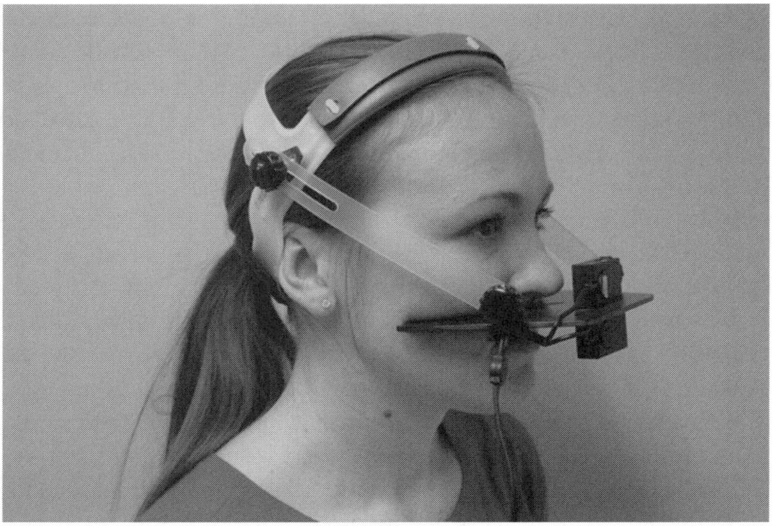

Figure 10.17. The Nasometer in position on the head.

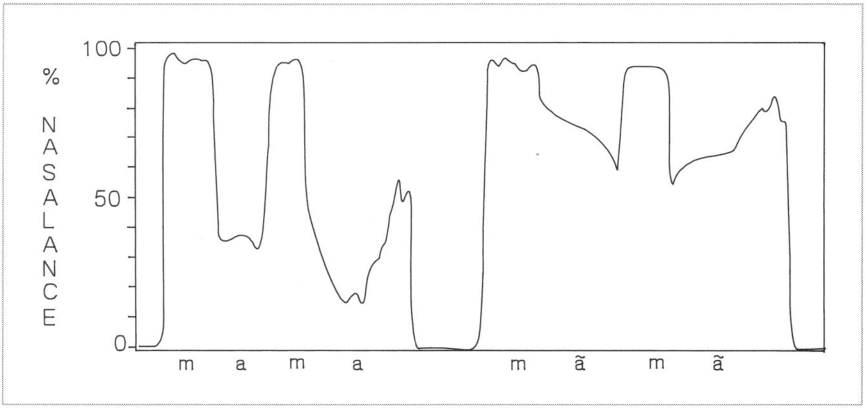


Figure 10.18. Sample output from Nasometer during production of "mama" with normal resonance balance (left) and nasalization of vowels (right).

of nasality are associated with the normal production of speech in different dialects and languages, a number of normative values appear in the literature (Anderson, 1996; Dalston, Neiman, & Gonzalez-Landa, 1993; Haapanen, 1991; Nichols, 1999; Seaver, Dalston, Leeper, & Adams, 1991; Tachimura, Mori, et al., 2000; Van Doorn & Purcell, 1998; Van Lierde,

Wuyts, de Bodt, & van Cauwenberge, 2001; Whitehill, 2001). While standardized stimuli are provided by the device manufacturer, numerous investigators have assessed the effects of phonetic makeup and utterance length on nasalance scores (Bressman, 2005; Karnell, 1995; Laczi, Sussman, Stathopoulos, & Huber, 2005; Lewis, Watterson, & Quint, 2000; Watterson, Hinton, & McFarlane, 1996; Watterson, Lewis, & Foley-Homan, 1999; Watterson, York, & McFarlane, 1994). Fletcher (1976) reported a high degree of agreement between nasalance values and group ratings of nasality ($r = .91$) and concluded that nasalance scores are a valid correlate of perceived nasality. Dalston and Warren (1986) also found a positive relationship ($r = .76$) between TONAR II scores and perceived nasality. Of 118 patients tested, only 3 had TONAR scores that indicated the need for prosthetic or surgical treatment when a speech assessment indicated only mild hypernasality. Three additional patients demonstrated nasalance scores not indicative of additional treatment when speech scores suggested that prosthetic or surgical treatment would be beneficial. However, Warren (1975) and McWilliams et al. (1984) cautioned against use of the device to provide objective data regarding VP function. Fletcher (1978) attempted to relate nasalance values with VP opening as assessed from lateral X-rays. He found a close correspondence between nasalance magnitude and VP closure in the range from touch closure to VP gap $< 2$ mm. Beyond this range (i.e., VP gap $> 2$ mm), "the relationship between the physiological and acoustical measurements became more tenuous" (p. 120).

In a study of 117 patients, Dalston, Warren, and Dalston (1991) compared acoustic (Nasometer), aerodynamic (orifice area calculation), and perceptual measures of VP dysfunction. Using a nasalance cutoff score of 32, they were able to correctly identify the presence of hypernasality 89% of the time (sensitivity) and the absence of hypernasality 95% of the time (specificity). In a similar study, Hardin, Van Demark, Morris, and Payne (1992) proposed using 26 as a nasalance cutoff score to obtain optimal levels of sensitivity and specificity. On the basis of their findings, Dalston et al. (1991) concluded that "the Nasometer can be used with considerable confidence in corroborating clinical impressions of hypernasality in the speech of patients seen for evaluation at craniofacial centers" (p. 187). Hardin et al. (1992) are considerably more cautious in their support for the technique. Nasometry is attractive given its noninvasive interface with the patient and ease of use. However, variations in nasalance scores associated with language, dialect, phonetic content of the speech stimuli, and so forth, necessitate interpreting nasometry data with some caution. Nonetheless, the Nasometer may be found in many clinical settings and does add to the battery of information that may be used to document VP function during speech.

## Accelerometry

As early as 1942, investigators were promoting the use of noninvasive instruments to detect head and neck tissue vibrations (Hultzen, 1942). The use of such instrumentation is based on the observation that acoustic energy present in the nasal cavity not only will be propagated outward into the air but also will tend to vibrate the hard and soft tissues of the nose. Placement of a vibration-sensitive device such as an accelerometer (Stevens, Kalikow, & Willemain, 1975; Stevens, Nickerson, Boothroyd, & Rollins, 1976) over the nasal bone may be employed to "provide a measure of the degree of acoustic coupling through the VP opening" (Stevens et al., 1975, p. 594). Taken a step further, detection of nasal bone vibration in response to the presence of acoustic energy in the nasal cavity has been promoted as an objective correlate of nasality (Horii, 1980).

The accelerometric technique typically used today makes use of two accelerometers. One is placed on the nose (see Figure 10.19). Because this accelerometer must transduce hard and soft tissue vibration, its positioning on the nose is important. Lippmann (1981) compared accelerometer outputs from nine different placements. The position yielding the greatest accelerometer output was located on the upper side of the nose over the lateral nasal cartilage, just in front of the nasal bone. Attachment of the accelerometer to the nose is also important: The sensing surface of the device must remain flat against the nose, adequate (but not excessive) contact pressure must be maintained, and torque on the device must be kept to a minimum. Because the devices are typically quite light, careful use of double-sided tape between the accelerometer and skin is usually sufficient. The second device is placed on the neck, overlying the thyroid lamina (see Figure 10.19). In some cases, a standard microphone is used to obtain the oral signal (Edgerton et al., 1981). The index of nasal coupling is taken as a ratio of nasal to oral or neck transducer output. The neck accelerometer is used as a reference to account for changes in vocal intensity that would elevate nasal accelerometer output without altering nasal coupling magnitude. Accelerometer output gains are adjusted so that, during a sustained production of /m/, a ratio of 1 is obtained—it is assumed that maximal transmission of acoustic energy into the nasal cavity takes place during that speech task. The ratio then may vary between 0 and 1. Various acronyms have been applied to this ratio, including HONC (Horii Oral

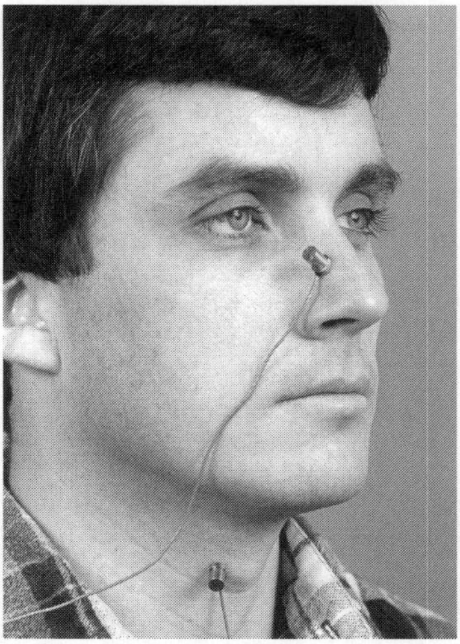

Figure 10.19. Placement of nasal and throat accelerometers for transduction of nasal bone vibration and derivation of nasal/throat accelerometer ratio.

Nasal Coupling; Horii, 1980), NAVI (Nasal Accelerometric Vibrational Index; Redenbaugh & Reich, 1985), and the NRI (Nasal Resonance Index; Edgerton et al., 1981).

During testing, the patient is asked to repeat words, sentences, and so forth. The nasal and oral signals are amplified, rectified, and smoothed before the nasal:oral ratio is calculated. The output of both channels and the resultant ratio (see Figure 10.20) may be displayed in real time on an oscilloscope, computer screen, or other device, and recorded for further analysis if required. Because calculation of this nasality index requires the presence of an oral signal, the ratio will be calculated for vowels and voiced consonants but not typically for unvoiced segments. However, one might see large ratio values if sufficient unvoiced energy occurs in the nasal tract. For example, a nasal snort might be expected to cause some vibration of the nasal soft tissues but little change in oral

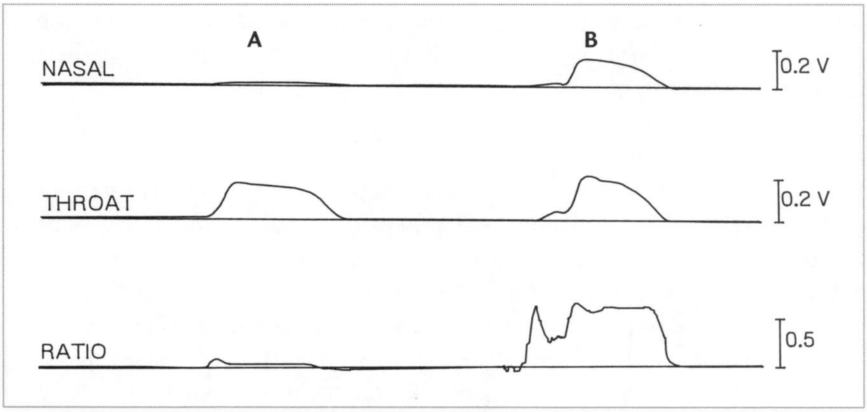


Figure 10.20. Nasal, throat, and nasal/throat accelerometer output recorded during production of /pʌ/. A = normal production; B = simulated hypernasality.

cavity transducer output. Simultaneous audio recordings can prove to be useful in interpreting such signals.

Few comparative studies have been completed in attempts to relate accelerometer data to perceptual ratings of nasality or to other instrumental measures of VP function. Using normal speakers who simulated hypernasal speech, Horii (1983) demonstrated an average correlation of .92 between mean nasal:oral ratios and perceived hypernasality scores. Redenbaugh and Reich (1985) utilized direct magnitude estimation and interval scaling estimates of perceived nasality to relate perceptual measures and accelerometer ratios. Although only 15 children (12 with VP incompetence and 3 normal) were evaluated, moderate to high correlations were obtained. These authors concluded that nasal:oral accelerometer ratios "strongly reflect VP coupling behaviors and the resulting oral/nasal resonance balance" (Redenbaugh & Reich, 1985, p. 280). Jones (2000) utilized the NAVI to determine that temporal patterns of oral-nasal resonance balance might distinguish children with VP insufficiency from those without.

The small amount of data published to date would seem to indicate a significant relationship between accelerometer amplitude ratios and perceived nasality. The diagnostician should, however, be cautioned against interpreting this technique as an indicator of VP movement, as Redenbaugh and Reich (1985) suggested, for the same reasons discussed in the section on TONAR. An additional caution involves determination of nasal patency (Moon, 1990). The anatomic and physiological condition of the nasal passage appears to be an important variable in the detection of nasal tract acoustic energy using the accelerometric technique; that is, nasal:oral accelerometry ratios recorded from the more resistant side of the nose may be larger in magnitude than those recorded from the less resistant side of the nose.

## Acoustic Rhinometry

If a short-duration pulse with a broad frequency spectrum is introduced to a cavity, it will be reflected by changes in acoustic impedance within the tube. Changes in acoustic impedance will occur as a consequence of changes in cross-sectional area or diameter. A comparison of incident and reflected waves can be used to estimate these cross-sectional area changes (Hilberg, Jensen, & Pedersen, 1993). Dalston (1992) introduced the possibility that acoustic rhinometry could be of some use in assessing nasal and velopharyngeal anatomy in patients with craniofacial anomalies. Seaver, Karnell, Gasparaitis, and Corey (1995) assessed the ability of acoustic rhinometry to detect changes in velar position as observed simultaneously using videofluoroscopy. Although only 2 normal adults were assessed, the authors concluded that acoustic rhinometry was capable of detecting changes in velar position during speech. Kunkel, Wahlmann, and Wagner (1999) investigated the nasal airways of 34 adults with unilateral complete cleft lip and palate, further documenting the utility of acoustic rhinometric measures in assessing nasal airway anatomy.

Acoustic rhinometry is a simple, noninvasive tool that preliminary studies have shown to provide some useful information regarding the functional status of the nasal and VP regions of normal speakers as well as speakers with repaired palatal clefts. Clearly, however, more research devoted to study of the reliability and sensitivity of this approach is warranted before conclusions regarding its potential value are reached.

## Aerodynamic Measures

Because speech is an aerodynamic event, measurement of airflows and air pressures associated with both normal and disordered speech production can be expected to provide useful diagnostic information. Measurement of vocal tract aerodynamics is not new; however, technologic advances and refinements in electronic instrumentation have provided more precise and accurate devices that may be used to record airflow and pressure signals during speech production.

### Airflow Detection

Measurement of nasal airflow alone has been used diagnostically for many years. Approaches vary from simple detection of the presence of nasal airflow to measurement of airflow rate and temporal characteristics. Perhaps the least sophisticated approach to studying the aerodynamics of VP function is the mirror test. The rationale for this test is that a lowering of the velum will allow passage of air into the nasal cavity that might serve as an indicator of nasalization (Baken, 1987). The presence of this humidified airstream will fog a mirror placed just under the nares. This crude approach is of questionable utility. Although it may differentiate gross VP incompetence from normal, the more important diagnostic determination of less obvious incompetence is beyond its capability.

An equally crude variation of the mirror test is a device called the See-Scape. A flexible air tube positioned in the patient's naris is connected to a vertically oriented rigid tube housing a small piece of Styrofoam. Air movement in the tube (i.e., nasal airflow) will displace the Styrofoam upward. Like the mirror test, this device is sensitive only to the presence or absence of nasal airflow. It provides no data regarding how much airflow is occurring (other than gross differences), where the air leak is occurring, or how large the air leak is (Glaser & Shprintzen, 1979).

Quantitative measures of airflow rates associated with speech production require the use of more sophisticated equipment. Airflows are typically sensed by placing a known resistance in the airstream and measuring the pressure drop across that resistance. The pressure drop across the constant resistance will be linearly related to the flow through or around the resistance. The most common type of resistance employed is a fine wire-mesh screen, although a honeycomb of narrow tubes has also been used. These resistances are incorporated into a pneumotachograph having an air inlet, an air outlet, a resistance component, and pressure-sensing ports (see Baken, 1987, for a more detailed explanation). The pneumotachograph may be coupled to the subject with some type of mask or with a length of tubing. A number of articles provide examples of different subject-instrument interfaces (e.g., Kastner, Putnam, & Shelton, 1985; Warren, 1984).

Laine, Warren, Dalston, and Morr (1988) demonstrated the use of airflow rate transduction using the pneumotachograph as a screening tool for VP incompetence. Based on data collected from 211 subjects, Laine and colleagues suggested that nasal airflow rates in excess of 125 cc per second during production of /p/ in "hamper" are almost always associated with VP incompetence. Using this criterion, 15% of their diagnoses were considered misses, while only 4% were considered false positives. They did caution, not surprisingly, that this screening approach is not as sensitive with more subtle cases as it is with obvious instances of VP incompetence.

Use of the pneumotachograph assembly, typically coupled to a computer system, allows for the quantification and analysis of nasal airflow signals that may be affected by various aspects of VP dysfunction. A few studies have reported a positive, albeit age- and speech-task-sensitive, relationship between nasal airflow rate measured during speech and perceived nasality (Lohmander-Agerskov, Dotevall, Lith, & Söderpalm, 1996; Warren, Dalston, & Mayo, 1994). Additional research has focused on temporal characteristics of VP function as reflected in nasal airflow data. For example, Dotevall, Ejnell, and Bake (2001) recorded the rate of change of nasal airflow as the soft palate moved from an open posture for nasal sound production to a closed posture for stop sound production. This "maximum flow declination rate" was slower in a group of children with cleft palate than in children without cleft palate.

## Air Pressure Detection

Warren (1979) introduced a VP function screening device utilizing air pressure signals that could be used during speech production. Named the PERCI (Palatal Efficiency Rating Computed Instantaneously), this device calculates the ratio between oral and nasal air pressures recorded during the production of the consonant /p/. Air pressures are transduced with an electronic pressure transducer. The transducer accepts a pressure signal, usually from a small tube placed somewhere in the vocal tract or in close proximity to it, and produces a voltage signal with magnitude linearly related to the magnitude of input pressure (see Baken, 1987, for a more detailed explanation). Based on data collected from over 75 speakers, Warren (1979) concluded that oral:nasal pressure differentials in excess of 3 cm $H_2O$ were associated with adequate VP closure, whereas a pressure difference of less than 1 cm $H_2O$ indicated incomplete VP closure. Differential pressure values between 1 and 3 cm $H_2O$ are associated with borderline VP adequacy. In a follow-up study of 515 patients, Morr, Warren, Dalston, and Smith (1989) demonstrated that pressures greater than 3 cm $H_2O$ were generally associated with adequate closure, whereas pressures less than 3 cm $H_2O$ were generally associated with inadequacy. Like airflow screening, differential pressure screening may be useful in differentiating normal from grossly abnormal but is somewhat less sensitive in borderline or marginal cases, where accurate diagnoses are most important and most difficult to achieve.

## Orifice Area Estimation

The aerodynamic measurement techniques presented thus far provide information only about the presence or absence, and in some cases the magnitude and time course, of airflow or air pressure in the nasal and oral cavities. They do not, however, provide any information about the structure of the VP port itself. Warren and DuBois (1964) first described a pressure-flow technique for estimating the cross-sectional area of the VP orifice. Their technique is based upon a modification of the theoretical hydraulic principle and assumes that the area of an orifice can be determined if the differential pressure across the orifice is measured simultaneously with the rate of airflow through it. Orifice area is calculated using this equation:

$$\text{Orifice Area} = \frac{\text{rate of airflow through orifice}}{k\sqrt{2\left(\frac{\text{orifice differential pressure}}{\text{density of air}}\right)}}$$

Airflow rate is detected using a tube sealed into one naris and connected to a pneumotachograph-pressure transducer system (Figure 10.21). Orifice differential pressure is detected using two small tubes. The reference pressure tube is sealed into the other naris. The second pressure tube is held in the oral cavity. Both tubes are connected to a differential pressure transducer. By referencing oral pressure to pressure in the nasal cavity, the pressure drop across the VP orifice is measured. Patients are typically asked to repeat the CV syllable [pɑ]or the word "hamper." Airflow and

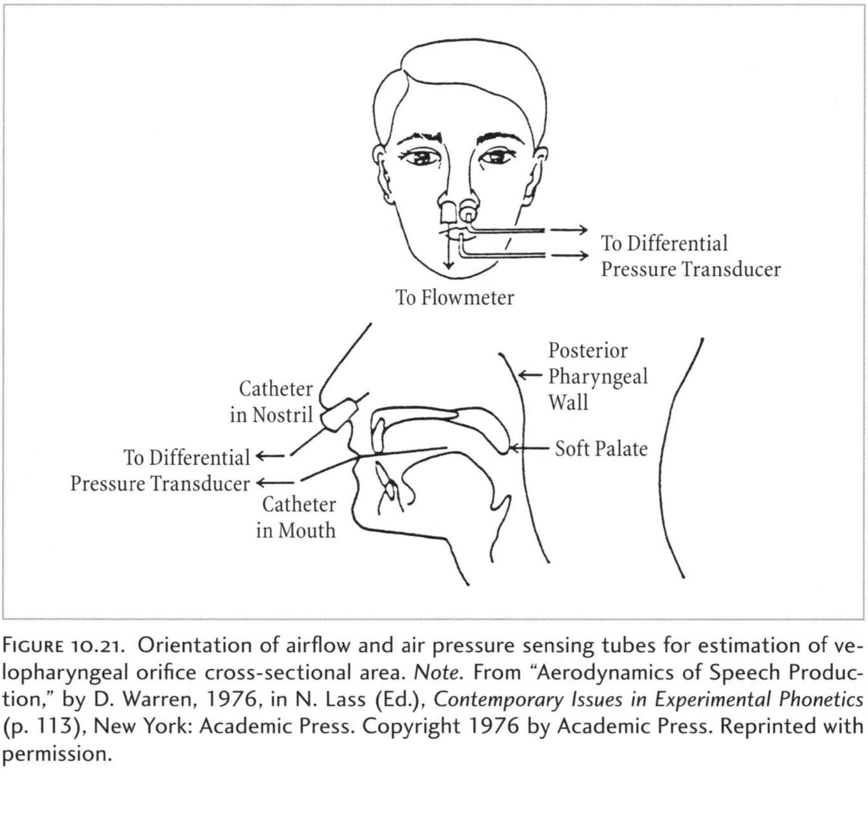


FIGURE 10.21. Orientation of airflow and air pressure sensing tubes for estimation of velopharyngeal orifice cross-sectional area. *Note.* From "Aerodynamics of Speech Production," by D. Warren, 1976, in N. Lass (Ed.), *Contemporary Issues in Experimental Phonetics* (p. 113), New York: Academic Press. Copyright 1976 by Academic Press. Reprinted with permission.

pressure waveforms recorded during production of /pɑ/ with a normal and simulated incompetent VP mechanism are shown in Figure 10.22. Pressure and flow values are measured at the peak of nasal airflow during the bilabial plosive. These values may then be inserted into the equation to calculate cross-sectional area. Area values may also be obtained from a graph or chart, as described by Moon and Weinberg (1985).

Based on orifice area data collected from a large number of patients, Warren (1976) grouped patients into categories of VP function. Patients may be described as having adequate VP closure (areas less than 0.05 $cm^2$), adequate/borderline closure (0.05–0.09 $cm^2$), borderline/inadequate closure (0.10–0.19 $cm^2$), or inadequate closure (greater than 0.20 $cm^2$). An explanation for these cutoff values was provided by Laine et al. (1988). The cutoff of 0.05 $cm^2$ was chosen for adequate closure because normal speakers without clefts do not demonstrate greater areas. The cutoff of 0.20 $cm^2$ was chosen for inadequacy because orifice differential pressure is close to zero above this value. The two categories lying between these extremes were assigned on an arbitrary basis, although Laine and colleagues asserted that they are supported by both aerodynamic and perceptual data.

The pressure-flow technique is a potentially powerful tool in the evaluation of VP incompetence. It is relatively easy to apply and reliable, and it provides quantitative data regarding the functional condition of the VP mechanism (Smith, Moon, & Weinberg, 1984). In general, the technique

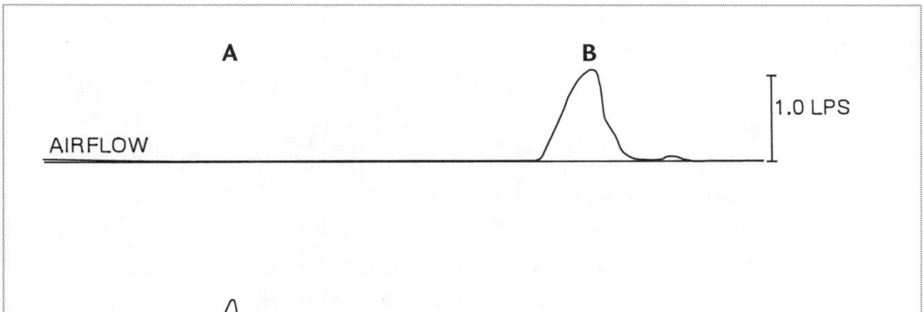


FIGURE 10.22. Nasal airflow and orifice differential pressure traces recorded during production of /pɑ/. A = normal production; B = simulated VP incompetence.

has been proven to provide accurate estimates of cross-sectional VP orifice area, at least in the model. A definitive evaluation of its reliability when applied to the human vocal tract has yet to be completed. Pressure-flow data have been shown to correlate reasonably well with listener judgments of nasality (Warren et al., 1994) and with nasalance scores (Dalston & Warren, 1986).

Aerodynamic measures have proven appealing for the study of speech production. They are noninvasive, typically requiring only a small tube placed in the oral cavity and some type of mask covering the nose, mouth, or both. The systems are easy to calibrate with appropriate equipment and take little time to set up for data collection. They are, however, somewhat expensive. Furthermore, the equipment array may be intimidating to those less experienced in instrumentation.

## Summary

It should be readily apparent from the information presented that VP function is a multifaceted and complex constellation of physiological events. To date, no one tool is available that can evaluate all aspects of VP function. Instead, various devices have been designed to transduce the individual component events that take place during attempts at speech production. As stated at the outset, the bottom line is a perceptual judgment of the functional adequacy of the mechanism. Data collected using supplemental approaches and tools must ultimately be related to that perception and, of equal importance, to the underlying VP events that give rise to that perception.

Assuming for the moment that all of the tools discussed in this chapter are reasonably valid and reliable, one might ask which one is best. McWilliams et al. (1981) suggested that multiview videofluoroscopy is the method of choice. Although this technique might not appeal to everybody, many diagnosticians would probably agree that one of the direct primary approaches would be most useful because they allow visualization of the mechanism. Furthermore, they may be used by the clinician to form a bridge between perception and kinematics. Other tools (e.g., accelerometry, TONAR) provide objective data regarding perceptual phenomena but cannot be used as easily to form the bridge referred to above. Still others (e.g., pressure-flow devices) provide objective data that have been used to infer structural characteristics of the VP mechanism but remain one step removed from observation of the mechanism itself. As discussed earlier, the techniques differ in other features as well. Some involve exposure to ionizing radiation. Some involve insertion of instruments into the oral and/or nasal cavity. Some are attached to an external body surface and are not invasive at all. Some are much more costly than others. Some are much more appropriate only in a medical clinic setting, whereas others might be used in school or other clinic settings.

However, which tool is best is not the important question to ask. The more critical question is, "What combination of different measurements and assumptions will provide the most insight about any particular experimental or clinical question?" (Folkins & Moon, 1991). Stated differently,

> Treatment decisions should not be made on the basis of input from any single source of information concerning patient status. The greater the variety of valid information that can be obtained about patient performance, the more likely it is that an accurate assessment will be made. Of course, it is reasonable to suppose that there is a practical limit beyond which further assessment will provide little or no additional useful information. However, that limit has not yet been identified. (Dalston & Warren, 1986, p. 114)

## References

Akgüner, M. (1999). Velopharyngeal anthropometric analysis with MRI in normal subjects. *Annals of Plastic Surgery, 43,* 142–147.

Akgüner, M., Karaca, C., Barutçu, A., Özaksoy, D., Yurt, A., & Vayvada, H. (1998). Evaluation of velopharyngeal pathophysiology and velopharyngeal insufficiency with magnetic resonance imaging. *European Journal of Plastic Surgery, 21,* 118–128.

Albery, E., Bennett, J., Pigott, R., & Simmons, R. (1982). The results of 100 operations for velopharyngeal incompetence—Selected on the findings of endoscopic and radiologic examination. *British Journal of Plastic Surgery, 35,* 118–126.

American Speech-Language-Hearing Association. (1992a). Sedation and topical anesthetics in audiology and speech-language pathology. *Asha, 34*(Suppl. 7), 41–42.

American Speech-Language-Hearing Association. (1992b). Vocal tract visualization and imaging. *Asha, 34*(Suppl. 7), 37–40.

Anderson, R. (1996). Nasometric values for normal Spanish-speaking females: A preliminary report. *Cleft Palate-Craniofacial Journal, 33,* 333–336.

Baken, R. (1987). *Clinical measurement of speech and voice.* Austin, TX: PRO-ED.

Barlow, S., & Bradford, P. (1992). Measurement and implications of orofacial muscle performance in speech disorders. *Journal of Human Muscle Performance, 1,* 1–31.

Bell-Berti, F., & Krakow, R. (1991). Anticipatory velar lowering: A coproduction account. *Journal of the Acoustical Society of America, 90,* 112–123.

Bensen, J. (1977). A checklist for evaluating palatal closure. *Plastic and Reconstructive Surgery, 60,* 45–48.

Birch, M., Sommerlad, B., Fenn, C., & Butterworth, M. (1999). A study of the measurement errors associated with the analysis of velar movements assessed from lateral videofluoroscopic investigations. *Cleft Palate-Craniofacial Journal, 36,* 499–507.

Bressman, T. (2005). Comparison of nasalance scores obtained with the Nasometer, the NasalView, and the OroNasal System. *Cleft Palate-Craniofacial Journal, 42,* 423–433.

Bzoch, K. (1968, July). Variations in velopharyngeal valving: The factor of vowel changes. *Cleft Palate Journal, 5,* 211–218.

Cassell, M., Moon, J., & Elkadi, H. (1990). Anatomy and physiology of the velopharynx. In J. Bardach & H. Morris (Eds.), *Multidisciplinary management of cleft lip and palate.* Philadelphia: Saunders.

Counihan, D., & Cullinan, W. (1970, January). Reliability and dispersion of nasality ratings. *Cleft Palate Journal, 7,* 261–270.

Croft, C., Shprintzen, R., Daniller, A., & Lewin, M. (1978). The occult submucous cleft palate and the musculus uvulae. *Cleft Palate Journal, 15,* 150–154.

Croft, C., Shprintzen, R., & Rakoff, S. (1981). Patterns of velopharyngeal valving in normal and cleft palate subjects: A multi-view videofluoroscopic and nasendoscopic study. *Laryngoscope, 91,* 265–271.

Dalston, R. (1982). Photodetector assessment of velopharyngeal activity. *Cleft Palate Journal, 19,* 1–8.

Dalston, R. (1992). Acoustic assessment of the nasal airway. *Cleft Palate-Craniofacial Journal, 29,* 520–526.

Dalston, R., Neiman, G., & Gonzalez-Landa, G. (1993). Nasometric sensitivity and specificity: A cross-dialect and cross-culture study. *Cleft Palate-Craniofacial Journal, 30,* 285–291.

Dalston, R., & Seaver, E. (1990). Nasometric and phototransductive measurements of reaction times among normal adult speakers. *Cleft Palate Journal, 27,* 61–67.

Dalston, R., & Warren, D. (1985). The diagnosis of velopharyngeal inadequacy. *Clinics in Plastic Surgery, 12,* 685–695.

Dalston, R., & Warren, D. (1986). Comparison of TONAR II, pressure flow, and listener judgments of hypernasality in the assessment of velopharyngeal function. *Cleft Palate Journal, 23,* 108–115.

Dalston, R., Warren, D., & Dalston, E. (1991). Use of nasometry as a diagnostic tool for identifying patients with velopharyngeal impairment. *Cleft Palate-Craniofacial Journal, 28,* 184–189.

Daniloff, R., Schuckers, G., & Feth, L. (1980). *The physiology of speech and hearing: An introduction.* Englewood Cliffs, NJ: Prentice Hall.

D'Antonio, L., Achauer, B., & Vander Kam, V. (1993). Results of a survey of cleft palate teams concerning the use of nasendoscopy. *Cleft Palate-Craniofacial Journal, 30,* 35–39.

D'Antonio, L., Eichenberg, B., Zimmerman, G., Patel, S., Riski, J., Herber, S., et al. (2000). Radiographic and aerodynamic measures of velopharyngeal anatomy and function following Furlow Z-plasty. *Plastic and Reconstructive Surgery, 106,* 539–549.

D'Antonio, L., Marsh, J., Province, M., Muntz, H., & Phillips, C. (1989). Reliability of flexible fiberoptic nasopharyngoscopy for evaluation of velopharyngeal function in a clinical population. *Cleft Palate Journal, 26,* 217–225.

Dotevall, H., Ejnell, H., & Bake, B. (2001). Nasal airflow patterns during the velopharyngeal closing phase in speech in children with and without cleft palate. *Cleft Palate-Craniofacial Journal, 38,* 358–372.

Dunn, V., & Ehrhardt, J. (1984). Magnetic resonance imaging. *University of Iowa Communication, 1,* 1–5.

Edgerton, M., Sadove, M., Compton, M., Bull, G., Blomain, E., McDonald, W., et al. (1981). Nasal vibration analysis: A noninvasive objective technique to evaluate the speech of patients with palatopharyngeal disorders. *Plastic and Reconstructive Surgery, 68,* 153–157.

Eisenbach, C., & Williams, W. (1984). Comparing the unaided visual exam to lateral cinefluorography in estimating several parameters of velopharyngeal function. *Journal of Speech and Hearing Disorders, 49,* 136–139.

Engelke, W., Bruns, T., Striebeck, M., & Hoch, G. (1996). Midsagittal velar kinematics during production of VCV sequences. *Cleft Palate-Craniofacial Journal, 33,* 236–244.

Engelke, W., Hoch, G., Bruns, T., & Striebeck, M. (1996). Simultaneous evaluation of articulatory velopharyngeal function under different dynamic conditions with EMA and videoendoscopy. *Folia Phoniatrica et Logopaedica, 48*(2), 65–77.

Finkelstein, Y., Berger, G., Nachmani, A., & Ophir, D. (1996). The functional role of the adenoids in speech. *International Journal of Pediatric Otorhinolaryngology, 34*(1–2), 61–74.

Fletcher, S. (1970, April). Theory and instrumentation for quantitative measurement of nasality. *Cleft Palate Journal, 7,* 601–609.

Fletcher, S. (1972). Contingencies for bioelectric modification of nasality. *Journal of Speech and Hearing Disorders, 37,* 329–346.

Fletcher, S. (1976). Nasalance vs. listener judgments of nasality. *Cleft Palate Journal, 13,* 31–44.

Fletcher, S. (1978). *Diagnosing speech disorders from cleft palate.* New York: Grune & Stratton.

Folkins, J. (1988). Velopharyngeal nomenclature: Incompetence, inadequacy, insufficiency, and dysfunction. *Cleft Palate Journal, 25,* 413–416.

Folkins, J., & Moon, J. (1991). Approaches to the study of speech production. In J. Bardach & H. Morris (Eds.), *Multidisciplinary management of cleft lip and palate.* Philadelphia: Saunders.

Fritzell, B. (1979). Electromyography in the study of the velopharyngeal function: A review. *Folia Phoniatrica, 31,* 93–102.

Garnier, S., Gallego, S., Collet, L., & Berger-Vachon, C. (1996). Spectral and cepstral properties of vowels as a means for characterizing velopharyngeal impairment in children. *Cleft Palate-Craniofacial Journal, 33,* 507–512.

Glaser, E., & Shprintzen, R. (1979). See-Scape: Instrument and manual. *Cleft Palate Journal, 16,* 213–214.

Golding-Kushner, K., Argamaso, R., Cotton, R., Grames, L. M., Henningsson, G., Jones, D. L., et al. (1990). Standardization for the reporting of nasopharyngoscopy and multiview videofluoroscopy: A report from an international working group. *Cleft Palate Journal, 27,* 337–348.

Haapanen, M. (1991). Nasalance scores in normal Finnish speech. *Folia Phoniatrica, 43*(4), 197–203.

Hardin, M., Van Demark, D., Morris, H., & Payne, M. (1992). Correspondence between nasalance scores and listener judgments of hypernasality and hyponasality. *Cleft Palate-Craniofacial Journal, 29,* 346–351.

Harrington, J. (1970, January). A cinefluorographic study of the pharyngeal flap mechanism. *Cleft Palate Journal, 7,* 129–138.

Henningsson, G., & Isberg, A. (1991). Comparison between multiview videofluoroscopy and nasendoscopy of velopharyngeal movements. *Cleft Palate-Craniofacial Journal, 28,* 413–417.

Hess, D. (1959). Pitch, intensity, and cleft palate voice quality. *Journal of Speech and Hearing Research, 2,* 113–125.

Hilberg, O., Jensen, F., & Pedersen, O. (1993). Nasal airway geometry: A comparison between acoustic reflections and magnetic resonance scanning. *Journal of Applied Physiology, 75,* 2811–2819.

Honjo, I., Mitoma, T., Ushiro, K., & Kawano, M. (1984). Evaluation of velopharyngeal closure by CT scan and endoscopy. *Plastic and Reconstructive Surgery, 74,* 620–627.

Horiguchi, S., & Bell-Berti, F. (1987). The velotrace: A device for monitoring velar position. *Cleft Palate Journal, 24,* 104–111.

Horii, Y. (1980). An accelerometric approach to nasality measurement: A preliminary report. *Cleft Palate Journal, 17,* 254–261.

Horii, Y. (1983). An accelerometric measure as a physical correlate of perceived hypernasality in speech. *Journal of Speech and Hearing Research, 26,* 476–480.

Hultzen, L. (1942). Apparatus for demonstrating nasality. *Journal of Speech and Hearing Disorders, 7,* 5–6.

Ibuki, K., Karnell, M., & Morris, H. (1983). Reliability of the nasopharyngeal fiberscope (NPF) for assessing velopharyngeal function. *Cleft Palate Journal, 20,* 97–104.

Iglesias, A., Kuehn, D., & Morris, H. (1980). Simultaneous assessment of pharyngeal wall and velar displacement for selected speech sounds. *Journal of Speech and Hearing Research, 23,* 429–446.

Jones, D. (2000). The relationship between temporal aspects of oral-nasal balance and classification of velopharyngeal status in speakers with cleft palate. *Cleft Palate-Craniofacial Journal, 37,* 363–369.

Jones, D., & Moon, J. (1989). *Response characteristics of the velopharyngeal photodetector to known orifice cross-sectional areas.* Paper presented at the annual meeting of the American Cleft Palate Association, San Francisco.

Karnell, M. (1995). Nasometric discrimination of hypernasality and turbulent nasal airflow. *Cleft Palate-Craniofacial Journal, 32,* 145–148.

Karnell, M., Folkins, J., & Morris, H. (1985). Relationships between the perception of nasalization and speech movements in speakers with cleft palate. *Journal of Speech and Hearing Research, 28,* 63–72.

Karnell, M., Ibuki, K., Morris, H., & Van Demark, D. (1983). Reliability of the nasopharyngeal fiberscope (NPF) for assessing velopharyngeal function: Analysis by judgment. *Cleft Palate Journal, 20,* 199–208.

Karnell, M., Linville, R., & Edwards, B. (1988). Variations in velar position over time: A nasal videoendoscopic study. *Journal of Speech and Hearing Research, 31,* 417–424.

Karnell, M., & Morris, H. (1985). Multiview endoscopic evaluation of velopharyngeal physiology in 15 normal speakers. *Annals of Otology, Rhinology and Laryngology, 94,* 361–365.

Karnell, M., & Seaver, E. (1993). Integrated endoscopic/photodetector evaluation of velopharyngeal function. *Cleft Palate-Craniofacial Journal, 30,* 337–342.

Karnell, M., Seaver, E., & Dalston, R. (1988). A comparison of photodetector and endoscopic evaluations of velopharyngeal functions. *Journal of Speech and Hearing Research, 31,* 503–509.

Karnell, M., & Van Demark, D. (1986). Longitudinal speech performance in patients with cleft palate: Comparisons based on secondary management. *Cleft Palate Journal, 23,* 278–288.

Kastner, C., Putnam, A., & Shelton, R. (1985). Custom-fabricated masks for aeromechanical measures. *Cleft Palate Journal, 22,* 197–204.

Kataoka, R., Michi, K., Okabe, K., Miura, T., & Yoshida, H. (1996). Spectral properties and quantitative evaluation of hypernasality in vowels. *Cleft Palate-Craniofacial Journal, 33,* 43–50.

Kuehn, D. (1991). New therapy technique for treating hypernasal speech using continuous positive airway pressure (CPAP). *Plastic and Reconstructive Surgery, 88,* 959–966.

Kuehn, D., Folkins, J., & Cutting, C. (1982). Relationships between muscle activity and velar position. *Cleft Palate Journal, 19,* 25–35.

Kuehn, D., & Moll, K. (1976). A cineradiographic study of VC and CV articulatory velocities. *Journal of Phonetics, 4,* 303–320.

Kuehn, D., & Moon, J. (1994). Levator veli palatini muscle activity in relation to intraoral air pressure variation. *Journal of Speech and Hearing Research, 37,* 1260–1270.

Kuehn, D., & Moon, J. (1995). Levator veli palatini muscle activity in relation to intraoral air pressure variation in cleft palate subjects. *Cleft Palate-Craniofacial. Journal, 32,* 376–381.

Kuehn, D., & Moon, J. (1997). Velopharyngeal closure force and levator veli palatini activation levels in relation to varying phonetic contexts. *Journal of Speech and Hearing Research, 41,* 51–62.

Kuehn, D., & Moon, J. (2000). Induced fatigue effects on velopharyngeal closure force. *Journal of Speech and Hearing Research, 43,* 486–500.

Kuehn, D., Moon, J., & Folkins, J. (1993). Levator veli palatini muscle activity in relation to intranasal air pressure variation. *Cleft Palate-Craniofacial Journal, 30,* 361–368.

Kuehn, D., Ray, R., Ettema, S., & Barkmeier, J. (2001). *The effects of supine versus upright posture on velum and tongue positioning during speech.* Paper presented at annual meeting of the American Cleft Palate-Craniofacial Association, Minneapolis, MN.

Kummer, A. W. (2001). *Cleft palate and craniofacial anomalies: Effects on speech and resonance.* San Diego: Singular Press.

Kummer, A. W., Curtis, C., Wiggs, M., Lee, L., & Strife, J. (1992). Comparison of velopharyngeal gap size in patients with hypernasality and nasal emission, or nasal turbulence (rustle) as the primary speech characteristic. *Cleft Palate-Craniofacial Journal, 29,* 152–155.

Kunkel, M., Wahlmann, U., & Wagner, W. (1999). Acoustic airway profiles in unilateral cleft palate patients. *Cleft Palate-Craniofacial Journal, 36,* 434–440.

Laczi, E., Sussman, J., Stathopoulos, E., & Huber, J. (2005). Perceptual evaluation of hypernasality compared to HONC measures: The role of experience. *Cleft Palate-Craniofacial Journal, 42,* 202–211.

Laine, T., Warren, D., Dalston, R., & Morr, K. (1988). Screening of velopharyngeal closure based on nasal airflow rate measurements. *Cleft Palate Journal, 25,* 220–225.

Lewis, K., Watterson, T., & Quint, T. (2000). The effect of vowels on nasalance scores. *Cleft Palate-Craniofacial Journal, 37,* 584–589.

Lippmann, R. (1981). Detecting nasalization using a low-cost miniature accelerometer. *Journal of Speech and Hearing Research, 24,* 314–317.

Lohmander-Agerskov, A., Dotevall, H., Lith, A., & Söderpalm, E. (1996). Speech and velopharyngeal function in children with an open residual cleft in the hard palate, and the influence of temporary covering. *Cleft Palate-Craniofacial Journal, 33,* 324–332.

Loney, R., & Bloem, T. (1987). Velopharyngeal dysfunction: Recommendations for use of nomenclature. *Cleft Palate Journal, 24,* 334–335.

Lotz, W., D'Antonio, L., Chait, D., & Netsell, R. (1993). Successful nasendoscopic and aerodynamic examinations of children with speech/voice disorders. *International Journal of Pediatric Otorhinolaryngology, 26,* 165–172.

Lubker, J., & Moll, K. (1965). Simultaneous oral-nasal airflow measurements and cinefluorographic observations during speech production. *Cleft Palate Journal, 2,* 257–272.

Lubker, J., & Morris, H. (1968). Predicting cinefluorographic measures of velopharyngeal opening from lateral still X-ray films. *Journal of Speech and Hearing Research, 11,* 747–753.

Mason, R., & Warren, D. (1980). Adenoid involution and developing hypernasality in cleft palate. *Journal of Speech and Hearing Disorders, 45,* 469–480.

McWilliams, B., Glaser, E., Philips, B., Lawrence, C., Lavorato, A., Beery, Q., et al. (1981). A comparative study of four methods of evaluating velopharyngeal adequacy. *Plastic and Reconstructive Surgery, 68,* 1–10.

McWilliams, B., Morris, H., & Shelton, R. (1984). *Cleft palate speech.* Philadelphia: Decker.

McWilliams-Neely, B., & Bradley, D. (1964). A rating scale for evaluation of videotape recorded X-ray studies. *Cleft Palate Journal, 1,* 88.

*Merriam-Webster's collegiate dictionary* (11th ed.). (2003). Springfield, MA: Merriam-Webster.

Miller, J., & Watkin, K. (1997). Lateral pharyngeal wall motion during swallowing using real time ultrasound. *Dysphagia, 12,* 125–132.

Moll, K. (1960). Cinefluorographic techniques in speech research. *Journal of Speech and Hearing Research, 3,* 227–241.

Moll, K. (1964). Objective measures of nasality. *Cleft Palate Journal, 1,* 371–374.

Moller, K., Martin, R., & Christiansen, R. (1971). A technique for recording velar movement. *Cleft Palate Journal, 8,* 263–276.

Moller, K., Path, M., Werth, L., & Christiansen, R. (1973). The modification of velar movement. *Journal of Speech and Hearing Disorders, 38,* 323–334.

Moller, K., & Starr, C. (1984). The effects of listening conditions on speech ratings obtained in a clinical setting. *Cleft Palate Journal, 21,* 65–69.

Moon, J. (1990). The influence of nasal patency on accelerometric transduction of nasal bone vibration. *Cleft Palate Journal, 27,* 266–270.

Moon, J., & Canady, J. (1995). Effects of gravity on velopharyngeal muscle activity during speech. *Cleft Palate-Craniofacial Journal, 32,* 371–375.

Moon, J., & Kuehn, D. (1997). Anatomy and physiology of normal and disordered velopharyngeal function for speech. In K. Bzoch (Ed.), *Communication disorders related to cleft lip and palate* (4th ed.). Austin, TX: PRO-ED.

Moon, J., & Kuehn, D. (1998). *Velopharyngeal closure forces associated with varying phonetic contexts produced by speakers with repaired palatal clefts.* Paper presented at annual meeting of American Cleft Palate-Craniofacial Association, Baltimore.

Moon, J., Kuehn, D., & Huisman, J. (1994). Measurement of velar closure force during vowel production. *Cleft Palate-Craniofacial Journal, 31,* 356–363.

Moon, J., & Lagu, R. (1987). Development of a second-generation phototransducer for the assessment of velopharyngeal activity. *Cleft Palate Journal, 24,* 240–243.

Moon, J., & Smith, W. (1987). Application of cine CT technology to the assessment of velopharyngeal function. *Cleft Palate Journal, 24,* 226–232.

Moon, J., & Weinberg, B. (1985). Two simplified methods for estimating velopharyngeal orifice area. *Cleft Palate Journal, 22,* 1–10.

Morr, K., Warren, D., Dalston, R., & Smith, L. (1989). Screening of velopharyngeal inadequacy by differential pressure measurements. *Cleft Palate Journal, 26,* 42–45.

Morris, H., Spriestersbach, D., & Darley, F. (1961, March). An articulation test for assessing competency of velopharyngeal closure. *Journal of Speech and Hearing Research, 4,* 48–55.

Nichols, A. (1999). Nasalance statistics for two Mexican populations. *Cleft Palate-Craniofacial Journal, 36,* 57–63.

Özgür, F., Tunçbilek, G., & Cila, A. (2000). Evaluation of velopharyngeal insufficiency with magnetic resonance imaging and nasendoscopy. *Annals of Plastic Surgery, 44,* 8–13.

Pae, E., Lowe, A., Sasaki, K., Price, C., Tsuchiya, M., & Fleetham, J. (1994). A cephalometric and electromyographic study of upper airway structures in the upright and supine positions. *American Journal of Orthodontics and Dentofacial Orthopedics, 106,* 52–59.

Parush, A., & Ostry, D. (1986). Superior lateral pharyngeal wall movements in speech. *Journal of the Acoustical Society of America, 80,* 749–756.

Parush, A., & Ostry, D. (1993). Lower pharyngeal wall coarticulation in VCV syllables. *Journal of the Acoustical Society of America, 94*(Suppl. 2), 749–756.

Perkell, J., Cohen, M., Svirsky, M., Matthies, M., Garabieta, I., & Jackson, M. (1992). Electromagnetic midsagittal articulometer systems for transducing speech articulatory movements. *Journal of the Acoustical Society of America, 92,* 3078–3096.

Peterson, G., & Barney, H. (1952). Control methods used in the study of vowels. *Journal of the Acoustical Society of America, 24,* 175–184.

Peterson-Falzone, S., Hardin-Jones, M., & Karnell, M. (2001). *Cleft palate speech* (3rd ed.). St. Louis, MO: Mosby.

Philips, B. (1980). Perceptual evaluation of velopharyngeal competency. *Annals of Otology, Rhinology and Laryngology, 89*(Suppl. 69), 153–157.

Pigott, R. (1980). Assessment of velopharyngeal function. In M. Edwards & A. Watson (Eds.), *Advances in the management of cleft palate.* London: Churchill.

Pigott, R., & Makepeace, A. (1982). Some characteristics of endoscopic and radiological systems used in elaboration of the diagnosis of velopharyngeal incompetence. *British Journal of Plastic Surgery, 35*(1), 19–32.

Poppelreuter, S., Engelke, W., & Bruns, T. (2000). Quantitative analysis of the velopharyngeal sphincter function during speech. *Cleft Palate-Craniofacial Journal, 37,* 157–165.

Ramamurthy, L., Wyatt, R., Whitby, D., Martin, D., & Davenport, P. (1997). The evaluation of velopharyngeal function using flexible nasendoscopy. *Journal of Laryngology and Otology, 111,* 739–745.

Redenbaugh, M., & Reich, A. (1985). Correspondence between an accelerometric nasal/voice amplitude ratio and listeners' direct magnitude estimations of hypernasality. *Journal of Speech and Hearing Research, 28,* 273–281.

Ryan, W., & Hawkins, C. (1976, April). Ultrasonic measurement of lateral pharyngeal wall movement of the velopharyngeal port. *Cleft Palate Journal, 13,* 156–164.

Satoh, K., Wada, T., Tachimura, T., Sakoda, S., & Shiba, R. (1999). A cephalometric study of the relationship between the level of velopharyngeal closure and the palatal plane in patients with repaired cleft palate and controls without clefts. *British Journal of Oral and Maxillofacial Surgery, 37,* 486–489.

Schneider, E., & Shprintzen, R. (1980). A survey of speech pathologists: Current trends in the diagnosis and management of velopharyngeal insufficiency. *Cleft Palate Journal, 17,* 249–253.

Schwartz, M. (1971). Acoustic measures of nasalization and nasality. In W. Grabb, S. Rosenstein, & K. Bzoch (Eds.), *Cleft lip and palate: Surgical, dental, and speech aspects.* Boston: Little, Brown.

Schwartz, M. (1975). Developing a direct, objective measure of velopharyngeal inadequacy. *Clinics in Plastic Surgery, 2,* 305–308.

Seaver, E., Dalston, R., Leeper, H., & Adams, L. (1991). A study of nasometric values for normal nasal resonance. *Journal of Speech and Hearing Research, 34,* 715–721.

Seaver, E., Karnell, M., Gasparaitis, A., & Corey, J. (1995). Acoustic rhinometric measurements of changes in velar positioning. *Cleft Palate-Craniofacial Journal, 32,* 49–54.

Seaver, E., & Kuehn, D. (1980). A cineradiographic and electromyographic investigation of velar positioning in non-nasal speech. *Cleft Palate Journal, 17,* 216–226.

Shaw, R., Folkins, J., & Kuehn, D. (1980). Comparison of methods for measuring velar position from lateral-view cineradiography. *Cleft Palate Journal, 17,* 326–329.

Shelton, R., & Trier, W. (1976). Issues involved in the valuation of velopharyngeal closure. *Cleft Palate Journal, 13,* 127–137.

Shprintzen, R. (1983). An invited commentary on "Reliability of the nasopharyngeal fiberscope (NPF) for assessing velopharyngeal function." *Cleft Palate Journal, 20,* 105–107.

Simpson, R., & Chin, L. (1981). Velar stretch as a function of task. *Cleft Palate Journal, 18,* 1–9.

Skolnick, M. L. (1969). Video velopharyngography in patients with nasal speech, with emphasis on lateral pharyngeal wall motion in velopharyngeal closure. *Radiology, 93,* 747–755.

Skolnick, M. L. (1970, October). Videofluoroscopic examination of the velopharyngeal portal during phonation in lateral and base projections: A new technique for studying the mechanics of closure. *Cleft Palate Journal, 7,* 803.

Skolnick, M. L. (1975). Velopharyngeal function in cleft palate. *Clinics in Plastic Surgery, 2,* 285.

Skolnick, M. L., & McCall, G. (1972). Velopharyngeal competence and incompetence following pharyngeal flap surgery: Videofluoroscopic study in multiple projections. *Cleft Palate Journal, 9,* 1–12.

Skolnick, M. L., McCall, G., & Barnes, M. (1973, July). The sphincteric mechanism of velopharyngeal closure. *Cleft Palate Journal, 10,* 286–305.

Smith, B., Moon, J., & Weinberg, B. (1984). The effects of increased nasal airway resistance on modeled velopharyngeal orifice area estimation. *Cleft Palate Journal, 21,* 18–21.

Starr, C., Moller, K., Dawson, W., Graham, J., & Skaar, S. (1984). Speech ratings by speech clinicians, parents and children. *Cleft Palate Journal, 21,* 286–292.

Stathopoulos, E., & Weismer, G. (1985). Oral air flow and intraoral air pressure: A comparative study of children, youths, and adults. *Folia Phoniatrica, 37,* 152–159.

Stevens, K., Kalikow, D., & Willemain, T. (1975). A miniature accelerometer for detecting glottal waveforms and nasalization. *Journal of Speech and Hearing Research, 18,* 594–599.

Stevens, K., Nickerson, R., Boothroyd, A., & Rollins, A. (1976). Assessment of nasalization in the speech of deaf children. *Journal of Speech and Hearing Research, 19,* 393–415.

Stringer, D., & Witzell, M. (1989). Comparison of multi-view videofluoroscopy and nasopharyngoscopy in the assessment of velopharyngeal insufficiency. *Cleft Palate Journal, 26,* 88–91.

Tachimura, T., Hohara, K., Fujita, Y., Hara, H., & Wada, T. (2001). Change in levator veli palatini muscle activity of normal speakers in association with elevation of the velum using an experimental palatal lift prosthesis. *Cleft Palate-Craniofacial Journal, 38,* 449–454.

Tachimura, T., Hohara, K., Hara, H., & Wada, T. (1999). Effect of placement of a speech appliance on levator veli palatini muscle activity during blowing. *Cleft Palate-Craniofacial Journal, 36,* 224–232.

Tachimura, T., Hohara, K., & Wada, T. (2000). Effect of placement of a speech appliance on levator veli palatini muscle activity during speech. *Cleft Palate-Craniofacial Journal, 37,* 478–482.

Tachimura, T., Mori, C., Hirata, S., & Wada, T. (2000). Nasalance score variation in normal adult Japanese speakers of Mid-West Japanese dialect. *Cleft Palate-Craniofacial Journal, 37,* 463–467.

Thompson, A., & Hixon, T. (1979). Nasal air flow during normal speech production. *Cleft Palate Journal, 16,* 412–420.

Trefler, M. (1985). Computed tomography. In T. Thompson (Ed.), *A practical approach to modern imaging equipment.* Boston: Little, Brown.

Van Demark, D., Kuehn, D., & Tharp, R. (1975). Prediction of velopharyngeal competency. *Cleft Palate Journal, 12,* 5–11.

Van Doorn, J., & Purcell, A. (1998). Nasalance levels in the speech of normal Australian children. *Cleft Palate-Craniofacial Journal, 35,* 287–292.

Van Lierde, K., Wuyts, F., de Bodt, M., & van Cauwenberge, P. (2001). Nasometric values for normal nasal resonance in the speech of young Flemish adults. *Cleft Palate-Craniofacial Journal, 38,* 112–118.

Vannier, M. (1984). Nuclear magnetic resonance imaging. *Postgraduate Medicine, 76,* 159–170.

Velepic, M., Bonifacic, M., Lustica, I., Sasso, A., & Cvjetkovic, N. (1999). The role of electromyography in the diagnosis of velopharyngeal insufficiency: Our experiences. *Acta Medica Okayama, 53,* 127–131.

Wada, T., Yasumoto, M., Ikeoka, N., Fujiki, Y., & Yoshinaga, R. (1970, April). An approach for the cinefluorographic study of articulatory movements. *Cleft Palate Journal, 7,* 506–522.

Warren, D. (1975). The determination of velopharyngeal incompetence by aerodynamic and acoustical techniques. *Clinics in Plastic Surgery, 2,* 299–304.

Warren, D. (1976). Aerodynamics of speech production. In N. Lass (Ed.), *Contemporary issues in experimental phonetics.* New York: Academic Press.

Warren, D. (1979). PERCI: A method for rating palatal efficiency. *Cleft Palate Journal, 16,* 279–285.

Warren, D. (1982). Aerodynamics of speech. In N. Lass, L. McReynolds, G. Northern, & D. Yoder (Eds.), *Speech, language, and hearing.* Philadelphia: Saunders.

Warren, D. (1984). A quantitative technique for assessing nasal airway impairment. *American Journal of Orthodontics, 86,* 306–314.

Warren, D., Dalston, R., & Mayo, R. (1994). Hypernasality and velopharyngeal impairment. *Cleft Palate-Craniofacial Journal, 31,* 267–262.

Warren, D., & DuBois, A. (1964, January). A pressure-flow technique for measuring velopharyngeal orifice area during continuous speech. *Cleft Palate Journal, 1,* 52–71.

Warren, D., & Hofmann, F. (1961, December). A cineradiographic study of velopharyngeal closure. *Plastic and Reconstructive Surgery, 28,* 656.

Watson, A. C. H., Sell, D. A., & Grunwell, P. (2001). *Management of cleft lip and palate.* London: Whurr.

Watterson, T., Hinton, J., & McFarlane, S. (1996). Novel stimuli for obtaining nasalance measures from young children. *Cleft Palate-Craniofacial Journal, 33,* 67–73.

Watterson, T., Lewis, K., & Foley-Homan, N. (1999). Effect of stimulus length on nasalance scores. *Cleft Palate-Craniofacial Journal, 36,* 243–247.

Watterson, T., York, S., & McFarlane, S. (1994). Effects of vocal loudness on nasalance measures. *Journal of Communication Disabilities, 27,* 257–262.

Whitehill, T. (2001). Nasalance measures in Cantonese-speaking women. *Cleft Palate-Craniofacial Journal, 38,* 119–125.

Williams, W., & Eisenbach, C. (1981). Assessing velopharyngeal function: The lateral still technique versus cinefluorography. *Cleft Palate Journal, 18,* 45–50.

Witt, P., Marsh, J., Arlis, H., Grames, L., Ellis, R., & Pilgram, T. (1998). Quantification of dynamic velopharyngeal port excursion following sphincter pharyngoplasty. *Plastic and Reconstructive Surgery, 101,* 1205–1211.

Witt, P., Marsh, J., McFarland, E., & Riski, J. (2000). The evolution of velopharyngeal imaging. *Annals of Plastic Surgery, 45,* 665–673.

Wu, J. T., Huang, G. F., Huang, C. S., & Noordhoff, M. S. (1996). Nasopharyngoscopic evaluation and cephalometric analysis of velopharynx in normal and cleft palate children. *Annals of Plastic Surgery, 36,* 117–122.

Ysunza, A., Pamplona, M., Molina, F., Chacon, E., & Collado, M. (1999). Velopharyngeal motion after sphincter pharyngoplasty: A videonasopharyngoscopic and electromyographic study. *Plastic and Reconstructive Surgery, 104,* 905–910.

Yules, R., & Chase, R. (1971). Secondary techniques for correction of palatopharyngeal incompetence. In W. Grabb, S. Rosenstein, & K. Bzoch (Eds.), *Cleft lip and palate: Surgical, dental, and speech aspects.* Boston: Little, Brown.

Zimmermann, G., Dalston, R., Brown, C., Folkins, J., Linville, R., & Seaver, E. (1987). Comparison of cineradiographic and phototransduction techniques for assessing velopharyngeal function during speech. *Journal of Speech and Hearing Research, 30,* 564–569.

Zwitman, D., Sonderman, J., & Ward, P. (1974). Variations in velopharyngeal closure assessed by endoscopy. *Journal of Speech and Hearing Disorders, 39,* 366–372.

# CHAPTER 11

# Articulation and Phonologic Assessment Procedures and Treatment Decisions

*Judith E. Trost-Cardamone*

Trost-Cardamone discusses the articulation problems of children with cleft palate speech in relation to phoneme acquisition and the occurrence of compensatory misarticulations. She advocates that speech treatment be based on detailed assessment and notes the importance of the status of velopharyngeal closure adequacy in determining treatment strategies.

1. What four speech characteristics cause cleft palate speech to be perceptually deviant and phonetically distinctive?
2. What is the difference between obligatory (passive) speech errors and learned (active) speech errors?
3. The author discusses different patterns of nasal air emission. What are the different sources of these patterns, and why is it important to be able to distinguish and perceptually identify them?
4. What are the main goals of a cleft palate speech evaluation?
5. Why should efforts to correct compensatory misarticulations for stops, fricatives, and affricates include teaching of place of articulation and target-error contrasts?

The most common speech disorder seen in persons with cleft palate is a disordered speech sound system, which frequently impairs speech intelligibility. Disorders that affect speech sound systems have traditionally been labeled in the speech-language pathology literature as *articulation disorders.* However, during the late 1970s and early 1980s, people began to use terms such as *phonological disorders* or *phonological disabilities* to describe problems with the speech sound system.

This change in terminology became more common with the availability of linguistically based procedures for analyzing disordered speech sound systems (e.g., Edwards, 1986; Elbert & Gierut, 1986). Locke (1983a) pointed out that, to some practitioners, this was merely a change in labeling the speech disorder. For others, the term *articulation* referred only to peripheral motor activity, whereas the term *phonological* referred to the speaker's knowledge of the sound system and the rules that governed it. Stoel-Gammon and Dunn (1985) stated that *phonology*

> refers to the organization and classification of speech sounds that occur as contrastive units within a given language, and in another sense it is used as a general term referring to all aspects of the study of speech sounds, including speech perception and production, as well as cognitive and motor aspects of speech. (p. 3)

When clinicians use the term *articulation disorders* for all children with disordered or delayed speech sound systems, it should be assumed their usage of the term extends to all phonological disorders and not only to peripheral production difficulties. It has long been recognized that articulation or phonological disorders can be caused by so-called higher level cognitive or linguistic impairments, as well as by motor control difficulties. An example of such a higher level disorder might be a child who collapses two phonemes into a single sound class because he or she does not make the distinctions needed to separate the phonemes into two sound classes.

At this point, the reader is probably asking, "What is the purpose of such an introduction when the phonological disorders seen in the individual with a cleft palate with or without cleft lip can, in most instances, be assumed to be directly related to structural problems associated with the cleft, and thus be viewed strictly as articulation disorders?" I feel that such a position is too simple an explanation for a complex problem and might often be incorrect. The speech sound system disorders seen in individuals with cleft palate can be labeled and approached as phonological disorders for several reasons:

**1.** The term *phonological disorders* has been accepted as a holistic term that includes both phonetic-articulatory (motor speech gesture) and phonemic-linguistic (rule system) "levels" of impairment, and therefore incorporates both segmental and linguistic or process-based diagnostic and treatment approaches. It is a more inclusive term than *articulation*.

**2.** The child with a cleft palate may have difficulties other than structural problems that may interact and account for the phonological delay or disorder. For example, what effect, if any, does an unoperated cleft have on the baby's early perceptual/sensory speech learning? Does the cleft alter motor speech development? Definitive data are not available on the effects of early chronic middle ear effusions on phonological perception or motor speech learning in children with phonological systems that deviate from the norm. However, published data on the relationship between early otitis media with effusion (OME) and later speech adequacy implicates the auditory effects of OME as a primary source of both delayed and disordered phonological acquisition patterns for some children (Churchill, Hodson, Jones, & Novak, 1988; Luloff, Menyuk, & Teele, 1993; Paden, Novak, & Beiter, 1987; Petinou, Schwartz, Mody, & Gravel, 1999; Rvachew, Slawinski, Williams, & Green, 1999; Shriberg & Smith, 1983). It is probable that several such factors interact to create the misarticulations observed in speakers with cleft palate.

**3.** Some children with cleft palate[1] may have developmental phonological disorders exclusively or in addition to specific speech error patterns associated with structural deviations related to the cleft. Similarly, some children may have problems that are primarily linguistic in nature.

Before leaving this discussion, it is important to point out a couple of caveats. First, the analysis of a child's sound system in terms of phonological patterns or processes provides descriptions of the child's behavior, but does not provide explanations of why it occurs. The identification of phonological processes does not allow one to infer causality or to explain the disorder. When clinicians attempt to ascribe higher linguistic explanations to a child's use of phonological patterns or processes, they should do so with extreme caution. On the other hand, certain error types and patterns in the speech of individuals with phonological disorders can be attributed to phonetic factors and explanations. In the case of individuals with palatal clefts, there are direct causal relationships between phonetic factors and the structural deviations caused by the cleft condition. The observation of nasal emission consistently accompanying pressure

[1]The term *cleft palate* is used throughout this chapter to include palatal clefts, with or without cleft lip.

consonants and excessive and pervasive hypernasality in a child with a documented physically inadequate velopharyngeal closure mechanism is likely to indicate a phonetic problem with a structural explanation. In other instances, a clear causal relationship may be difficult or impossible to determine. For example, the observation that a child with an oronasal fistula deletes stops and fricatives in postvocalic position while substituting glottal stops and pharyngeal fricatives in prevocalic position does not allow an easy phonetic explanation for the pattern of final consonant deletion. In summary, the application of a phonological pattern analysis should be viewed only as a descriptive device and will usually provide very little aid in the explanation of the error pattern. See Chapter 8 by Chapman for further discussion about phonological models used to study speech development in children with cleft palate.

## Speech Production Problems Associated with Cleft Palate

### Early Acquisition

Not all youngsters with cleft palates have speech sound disorders. Normal, or near-normal, speech sound acquisition in children with palatal clefts has become more likely in recent years. Although supporting data are minimal, both speech-language pathologists and plastic surgeons have attributed these results to definitive closure of the cleft palate at earlier ages (often during the second 6 months of life) (Chapman & Hardin, 1992; Chapman, Hardin-Jones, Schulte, & Halter, 2001; Dorf & Curtin, 1982; Kuehn & Trost-Cardamone, 1988; O'Gara & Logemann, 1988, 1990; O'Gara, Logemann, & Rademaker, 1994). Likewise, growing evidence suggests that early surgery using the Furlow (double-opposing) Z-plasty procedure is more successful in mitigating the need for later secondary surgery on the palate (Kirschner et al., 1999; LaRossa et al., 2004). Early surgery, when successful, allows for both a more normal oral structural environment and a competent velopharyngeal closure mechanism, and can be timed to accommodate a child's acquisition of speech sounds in first-word contexts.

A few reports have addressed the importance of surgical closure that is timed to maximize certain sensitive periods in the child's development of phonetic control during the 1st year of life and acquisition of the sound system (Kemp-Fincham, Kuehn, & Trost-Cardamone, 1990; Trost-Cardamone, 1990b). Oller (1980, 2000) outlined several stages in the development of phonetic control during the 1st year of life. The late end of the expansion stage (around 4–6 months) and the canonical stage of reduplicated and variegated babbling (beginning around 6–10 months) are cited as sensitive periods during which the infant gains practice with speech motor control and associated sensorimotor subroutines that underlie coordinated articulatory gestures. An open palate and inadequate velopharyngeal valving mechanism during these stages of development would likely alter the baby's perceptual and motor learning. Chapman et al. (2001) offered some evidence in support of this in their study that compared the vocal development of 9-month-old babies with unoperated cleft palate with that of age-matched peers without clefts. Although the groups were comparable in the overall number of vocalizations, the babies with clefts had smaller canonical babbling ratios and smaller consonant inventories, with fewer stops, glides, and velars.

Likewise, Jones, Chapman, and Hardin-Jones (2003) reported on speech development before and after palatoplasty in this same group of babies. They noted that at 17 months, the babies with cleft palate showed increases in the size of phonetic inventories and in canonical babbling. With regard to expansion of the consonant inventory for oral stops and fricatives, the results were mixed, with some babies (2 of 14) showing no improvement.

The permanence of early speech delays and mislearning and its impact on later representational speech sound acquisition is not well understood. Based on normal acquisition patterns and schedules, compensatory misarticulation patterns are more likely to develop when palate repair is not accomplished successfully by the time a child engages in first-word productions. For some children this may be before 12 months of age, and for others several months later. Based solely on chronological age, palate repair that is delayed beyond 18 months would place most children at risk for developing compensatory strategies that become a part of the child's phonological rule system and may require long-term speech remediation. Hardin-Jones and Jones (2005) studied the speech production of preschoolers with repaired cleft palate in relation to cleft type and age at primary palatoplasty. Their findings suggested that later age at palatoplasty was associated with higher prevalence of (persisting) moderate to severe hypernasality postoperatively, and the authors recommended that palatoplasty be accomplished no later than 13 months of age.

## Speech Deviations Associated with Cleft Palate

Certain speech deviations are commonly observed in individuals with palatal clefts. Four characteristics in particular cause cleft palate speech to be perceptually deviant and phonetically distinctive. These are (a) hypernasal resonance perceived during production of vowels, consonant glides, and liquids; (b) nasal air emission—the nasal airflow that distorts or replaces production of pressure consonants (i.e., stops, fricatives, and affricates); (c) weak pressure consonants associated with diminished intraoral air pressure; and (d) compensatory articulatory gestures observed to occur at several loci in the vocal tract.

It is important to point out that cleft palate speech deviations include both obligatory errors and optional or learned errors (Trost, 1981; Trost-Cardamone, 1987, 1990c; Golding-Kushner, 2001; Peterson-Falzone, Trost-Cardamone, Karnell, & Hardin-Jones, 2006). *Obligatory errors* are due to structural or neurogenic problems and require physical management. *Optional or learned errors* are habituated errors that are the result of early mislearning; they exist/persist despite an adequate velopharyngeal closure mechanism and require speech remediation. The following is an example of an obligatory error: If a child has a structurally insufficient mechanism,[2] there is no way he or she can avoid nasal emission when targeting high pressure consonants, and this will be accompanied by some degree of hypernasality on vowels. By contrast, if a child demonstrates adequate closure and no fistulae, but nasal air escape occurs with high pressure consonants, that suggests the child has *learned to emit high pressure consonants nasally* rather than orally, and that is a result of mislearning. Mislearning is also the source of compensatory misarticulations. That error is more *optional.* Much of the literature out of Europe, especially the United Kingdom and Scandinavia, refers to obligatory errors as *passive* errors and to learned errors as *active* errors (Harding & Grunwell, 1998; Hutters & Brøndsted, 1987; Sell, Harding, & Grunwell, 1998, 1999).

---

[2]In this chapter and in keeping with the author's preferred terminology (see Peterson-Falzone, Trost-Cardamone, Karnell, & Hardin-Jones, 2006), *velopharyngeal inadequacy* (VPI/A) is the generic term that includes all causes of velopharyngeal (VP) impairment. Three main categories are subsumed under VPI/A: *velopharyngeal insufficiency,* where the VP impairment is caused by some type of structural problem (persisting insufficiency after palatal repair, tonsillar interference to closure, etc.); *velopharyngeal incompetency,* where the VP impairment is neurogenic, as in dysarthria; and velopharyngeal mislearning, where inadequate VP closure occurs despite a physically capable closure mechanism, as in learned nasal emission patterns.

Trost-Cardamone (1990a) noted that whereas hypernasal resonance, weak pressure consonants, and nasal air emission accompanying pressure consonants are realized as phonetic *distortions*, compensatory gestures are realized as phonetic *substitutions*. Hypernasal resonance, nasal air emission, and weak pressure consonants are frequently reduced or eliminated by surgical or prosthetic management. In contrast, compensatory misarticulations learned before palatoplasty often persist postoperatively, even when adequate velopharyngeal closure can be achieved. Speech remediation for the speaker with cleft palate requires an appreciation of compensatory productions with respect to their phonetic parameters and error substitution patterns.

Although unanswered questions remain regarding the nature and origins of compensatory misarticulation gestures associated with cleft palate, a sizable body of clinical data is available. These data have revealed the following general characteristics:

1. *Phonetically*, compensatory misarticulations (a) are used as substitutions for pressure consonants and (b) are predominantly errors in place of articulation; the manner of production is usually preserved. The well-known substitutions of glottal stops for stop consonants and pharyngeal fricatives for sibilant fricatives are examples in which manner of production is maintained but place of production is changed.

2. Most compensatory misarticulations represent a pattern of *articulatory* (lingual) *backing* in which the place of articulation tends to be posterior relative to that seen in standard English, and most compensatory misarticulations are non-oral substitutions (Brooks, Shelton, & Youngstrom, 1965, 1966; Lawrence & Philips, 1975; McWilliams & Philips, 1979; Powers, 1962; Trost, 1981). The development and learning of backed articulations has several potential explanations, including (a) pharyngeal and glottal valving of the articulators, where success is more likely because the point of articulation is below the level of the velopharyngeal defect (Bzoch, 1971; Lawrence & Philips, 1975; Morris, 1979); (b) valving in the area of defect, so the tongue is used to occlude the palatal cleft or fistula, establishing a "place compromise" for anterior and posterior pressure consonants (Trost, 1981; Trost-Cardamone, 1987, 2004); (c) attempted use of the tongue as a "lingual assist" to occlude or valve the inadequate velopharyngeal port, causing obligatory backing for many speech sounds (Trost, 1981; Trost-Cardamone & Bernthal, 1993, 2004); and (d) the consequences of early chronic conductive hearing loss associated with OME (Hubbard, Paradise, McWilliams, Elster, & Taylor, 1985; Luloff et al., 1993; Petinou et al., 1999; Trost-Cardamone, 1990c).

Table 11.1 lists eight types of compensatory misarticulations, their general places of production, and corresponding phonetic symbols for transcription. Detailed descriptions of these productions in terms of perceptual speech characteristics, articulatory gestures, and radiographic documentation have been provided elsewhere (Peterson-Falzone et al.,

**Table 11.1**
**Compensatory Misarticulations, Their Places of Production, and Corresponding Phonetic Symbols**

| Compensatory misarticulation | Place of production | Phonetic symbol | |
|---|---|---|---|
| | | Unvoiced | Voiced |
| Glottal stop | Glottis, vocal fold valving | | ʔ |
| Pharyngeal fricative | Lingual base approximates PPW | ʢ | ʕ |
| Pharyngeal affricate | Combines glottal stop and pharyngeal fricative gestures | ʔʢ | ʔʕ |
| Pharyngeal stop | Lingual base contacts PPW to produce stop closure | ʢ̄ | ʕ̄ |
| Velar fricative | Posterior lingual dorsum contacts posterior palate; fricative made in back velar place | χ | ɣ |
| Mid-dorsum palatal stop | Lingual mid-dorsum contacts mid-palate | [k | ɡ] |
| Nasal fricative | Nasal bilabial /m/, tip alveolar /n/, or back velar /ŋ/ production coproduced with nonturbulent nasal frication and release | m̥̃̇ ñ̥̇ ŋ̥̃̇ | |
| Posterior nasal fricative (also called VP fricative)[1] | Velum/uvula approximates PPW of nasopharynx, leaving small gap; back tongue may retract and elevate in attempt to assist in VP closure (produced with turbulent frication/"snorting") | Δ | |

*Note.* PPW = posterior pharyngeal wall; VP = velopharyngeal.

[1]When coproduced with a high pressure consonant, /Δ/ can be used as a superscript or the IPA superscript for turbulence /≈/ can be used.

2006; Trost, 1981; Trost-Cardamone, 1987, 2004). These error types are considered later in this chapter. As a group, compensatory misarticulations tend to occur either as sound replacements (substitutions) or as coproductions. As used here, the term *coproduction* denotes simultaneous articulatory maneuvers. An example of a *compensatory* coproduction would be [$\overset{?}{t}$], where there is one manner of production (stop), with simultaneous valving at two places of production (glottal and tongue tip alveolar), and where the *deviant* place (glottal) is the effective one for manner. In previous publications and presentations, the author has used the term *compensatory coarticulation* for this error type (Trost, 1981; Trost-Cardamone, 1987). In reconsidering this terminology and the phenomena being described, I believe that *coproduction* is a more accurate descriptor. *Coarticulation* should be more strictly applied to mean that "articulation of any one sound is influenced by a preceding or following sound" (Bernthal & Bankson, 1998). Some clinicians and researchers have used the term *double articulation* to describe such a coproduction, particularly with reference to velar-alveolar (stop) double articulations as in [$\overset{?}{t}$, $\overset{?}{k}$] and [$\overset{?}{d}$, $\overset{?}{g}$] (Hardcastle, Barry, & Nunn, 1989; Sell et al., 1998; Whitehill, Stokes, Hardcastle, & Gibbon, 1995).

Trost (1984) reported on certain patterns in compensatory error substitutions and coproductions observed in a group of speakers with repaired cleft palate. Several trends were revealed from these data. Of six types of compensatory misarticulations studied, glottal stops were the most frequently produced and were used to replace all English pressure consonants. Whereas glottal stops, pharyngeal fricatives, and posterior nasal fricatives occurred as substitutions (e.g., /b/ → [ʔ]) *and* coproductions (e.g., /b/ → [$\overset{?}{b}$]), mid-dorsum palatal stops and pharyngeal stops were realized only as substitutions. It follows that compensatory misarticulations were produced more often as substitutions than as coproductions. Pharyngeal fricatives either replaced or occurred as coproductions with the sibilant fricatives. Some speakers produced pharyngeal affricates for the oral affricates as in /tʃ/ → [ʔʕ]. Pharyngeal stops replaced only /k/ and /g/, and mid-dorsum palatal stops replaced only /t/, /d/, /k/, and /g/. Based on these data, Trost concluded that the errors were mainly in-class in terms of manner of production, with the exception of glottal stops, which were used to replace any high pressure consonant—stop, fricative, and affricate. Interestingly, glottal stops have a frequent, but transient, presence in the normal child's phonetic inventory in the second 6 months of life (Locke, 1983b; Stoel-Gammon, 1988). Trost (1984) suggested that in the context of clefting, these aberrant glottal productions could persist and become learned compensatory gestures because of constraints posed by the cleft.

Stopping is a phonological process that occurs in normal phonological acquisition. The presence of glottal stopping in the speech of youngsters with palatal clefts suggests that the young child with a cleft palate may indeed be following the norm, but that the abnormal oral and velopharyngeal structures either prevent the correct phonemic representation(s) from being realized or facilitate an abnormal phonemic representation that does get realized. Either way, the stopping pattern may persist because of the structural problem rather than dropping out as occurs in normal phonological acquisition. Glottal stops in the child with a cleft palate are typically compensatory and sometimes may reflect attempts to use normal phonological (stop) patterns. The data reported by Broen and Moller (1993) appear to support this hypothesis.

In addition to the eight compensatory misarticulations listed in Table 11.1, other atypical backed articulations have been observed in speakers with cleft palates. As a group, these productions are retracted from their normal target place, but still remain oral. Peterson-Falzone et al. have classified these as backed oral productions. They include backing of alveolar and blade palatal fricatives /s, z, ʃ, ʒ to mid-dorsum/ midpalatal and velar place and back velar/uvular substitutions for /n, l, r/, resulting in [ŋ, ʟ, ʁ] articulations, respectively. Posterior shifts of oral targets in the child with a cleft palate may be learned as a result of attempting to "capture" airflow or use the back of the tongue to assist/ help seal the velopharyngeal port. An anterior oronasal fistula or ectopic teeth in the anterior hard palate could also be causative to these types of backed productions. Retracted articulations, particularly velarized /l/ and /r/, also occur in the speech of children and adults without clefts. Their presence cannot always be assumed to represent compensatory behavior.

Other atypical productions classified as compensatory in speakers with cleft palates have been observed to occur in the disordered sound systems of youngsters without clefts. For example, the use of glottal stops to replace some or most consonants, and not merely the high pressure consonants, is not uncommon in the phonetic repertoire of the phonologically deviant child. In fact, glottal replacement and stops substituted for glides have been suggested as idiosyncratic phonological processes in the speech of children with phonological disorders. Likewise, posterior nasal fricatives or "snorts" have been reported in the phonology of speakers without clefts (Edwards & Bernhardt, 1973; Hall & Tomblin, 1975; Trost-Cardamone, 1988). Trost (1981) and Trost-Cardamone (1988, 1990a) described a pattern of a phone-specific nasal emission in speakers without clefts, in which the nasal air escape distorts only certain consonants, especially sibilant fricatives and affricates, in the absence of hypernasality. Peterson (1975) reported similar characteristics in speakers with repaired palatal clefts. Even pharyngeal stops have been documented in the phonetic inventory of a phonologically impaired child without a cleft (Trost-Cardamone, 1985).

## Assessment of the Sound System in Individuals with Cleft Palate

Cleft palate speech assessment requires the speech-language pathologist to have knowledge of the structural deviations in the child's oral cavity that might contribute to deviant articulation patterns (see Chapter 7 by Jones and Seaver and Chapter 10 by Moon). This information includes the status and sphincteric pattern of velopharyngeal speech closure (Croft, Shprintzen, & Rakoff, 1981; Skolnick, McCall, & Barnes, 1973; Skolnick, Shprintzen, McCall, & Rakoff, 1975), the presence of any oronasal fistulae, and the dental and occlusal status. In addition, the palatine tonsils may sometimes cause velopharyngeal inadequacy. Using videonasendoscopy to examine the velopharyngeal sphincter, MacKenzie-Stepner, Witzel, Stringer, and Laskin (1987), Shprintzen, Sher, and Croft (1987), and Finkelstein, Nachmani, and Ophir (1994) all found that tonsillar tissue can grow up and behind the velum and thereby obstruct or impede velopharyngeal closure. Such tonsils, however, may not appear large on intraoral inspection (see Chapter 7). Speakers with consistent hypernasality and nasal air emission who show no obvious intraoral signs of palatal clefting are suspect for such an etiology. The sphincteric pattern of velopharyngeal closure can be determined only by superior or basal views of the port, as obtained through nasendoscopy and/or videofluoroscopy. Discussion of the merits and importance of instrumental assessment is not within the purpose of this chapter, but is discussed in Chapter 10.

The primary clinical task for the speech-language pathologist is to assess the child's speech sound system and then infer the effects of structural deviations on the speech behavior observed. The assessment varies according to the child's chronological age and linguistic and cognitive functioning. Obviously, assessment procedures for a 14-month-old who has acquired approximately 30 words differ from the procedures used with a 2-year-old who is using three- and four-word sentences, or from those used with a 6-year-old child who is using complete sentences.

## A Protocol for Phonological Assessment

This section offers guidelines for assessing the child's phonological status. Although the focus is on the preschool youngster, the suggestions given are intended to be flexible and modifiable according to each patient's age and overall development. Such an assessment usually is done within the context of an overall communication evaluation that includes other aspects of speech and language behavior, such as syntax, pragmatics, semantics, voice, and fluency, as well as hearing testing. A careful orofacial examination is a mandatory component of any cleft palate speech assessment, as data from the perceptual speech assessment often rely on orofacial findings for their accurate interpretation (see Chapter 10 by Moon).

The primary purpose for assessing phonological behavior is to determine whether an individual needs intervention and, if so, the type of intervention. To make these decisions, the clinician samples the client's speech through a variety of sampling procedures and then analyzes the data to determine the need for and possible direction of intervention. Because of the importance that surgical timing may have on influencing the acquisition of speech sounds by a baby with a cleft palate, it is recommended that the speech-language pathologist begin observation/intervention sessions with the child prior to initial palate repair whenever possible, and continue to follow the child until adequate velopharyngeal function and developmentally appropriate phonological behavior are achieved. A goal in evaluation is to distinguish speech errors that are obligatory and due to physically inadequate velopharyngeal closure or other (e.g., orofacial) structural deviations from learned speech errors that persist despite adequate velopharyngeal closure. As with any speech evaluation, developmental errors should be noted and distinguished from cleft-related errors.

## Obtaining the Speech Sample

The type and size of the speech sample that serves as the database for the analysis is extremely important in any phonological assessment. Although a complete discussion of this topic is beyond the scope of the chapter, Edwards (1983) identified a number of issues of potential importance concerning the size and type of the speech sample used to determine phonological status. These still apply. Although not part of Edwards's 1983 publication, these sampling issues can be reorganized into three categories: speech stimuli, speech context, and procedural aspects, as shown in Table 11.2.

This complex issue requires the clinician to make a series of compromises and judgments, especially during clinic visits, where time is often limited. In practice, the speech sampling components must be trimmed to accommodate the numbers of patients and time constraints posed during most cleft palate/craniofacial clinic visits. At the very least, however, speech samples should include several different contexts that are sensitive to capturing cleft palate speech errors. Samples should also be comprehensive enough for making judgments regarding speech intelligibility and acceptability and making a speech diagnosis (Henningsson et al., 2008; Kummer, 2008; Peterson-Falzone et al., 2006). Stimulability testing must also be included.

## Connected Speech

A standard procedure in most assessments is an evaluation of productions during connected or continuous speech. A connected speech sample gives

**Table 11.2**
**Speech Sampling Issues**

| Speech stimuli | Speech context | Procedural aspects |
|---|---|---|
| Phonetic context, word length, complexity, familiarity | Words versus phrases and continuous speech | Spontaneous production versus imitation |
| Specific stimuli versus no set stimuli | Word versus syllable positions | Number of attempts at each sound and number of chances to apply each process |
| Syntactic, pragmatic, prosodic variables | One rendition versus multiple contexts | Size of sample |
| | | Type of transcription |

Modified from M. L. Edwards (1983). Issues in phonological assessment. In J. Locke (Ed.), *Assessing and Treating Phonological Disorders: Current Approaches* (Seminars in Speech and Language, Vol. 4). New York: Thieme-Stratton.

the examiner a notion of the speaker's overall understandability and the consistency of individual speech sound productions, as well as the effect of context and natural prosodic patterns. Some speech-language pathologists recommend a spontaneous speech sample as the exclusive database (Shriberg & Kwiatkowski, 1980; Stoel-Gammon & Dunn, 1985), and others note that spontaneous speech yields the best data for speech understandability and acceptability judgments (Henningsson et al., 2008). The preferred methodology for obtaining a connected speech sample is to engage the child in spontaneous conversation. If this cannot be accomplished, alternative procedures can be used, such as picture description, automatic speech (counting, naming days of the week or months of the year), or rote memory tasks (nursery rhymes, Pledge of Allegiance). For cleft palate speech assessment, a connected speech sample should be a part of the test battery, but other, more controlled samples must also be included.

The size of the corpus is important. Obviously, the clinician needs a sample of sufficient size to obtain a representative and reliable sample of the child's phonology. The sample should contain approximately 100 words in which the child's intended words are known. Note that for the child with marginal velopharyngeal closure, a spontaneous speech sample may demonstrate a velopharyngeal closure problem that can be missed in single-word utterances, which make fewer timing demands on velopharyngeal function. For the unintelligible child, the exclusive use of spontaneous speech sampling may be difficult unless the intended lexical items can be determined. However, for the very young child (18 months or younger), a play situation in which spontaneous speech is sampled in structured play situations may be the only option other than some object naming or imitation following an adult model. Speech sampling with the very young child is difficult to accomplish in a single visit and may be best done through monthly or bimonthly sessions. Assessment should involve the mother or other caregivers to provide guidance on speech-language stimulation and to obtain observations and document speech behaviors in more natural settings, outside of the clinic or office (Hardin-Jones, Chapman, & Scherer, 2006; Peterson-Falzone et al., 2006).

## Sound Inventories

A second useful format is a speech sound inventory in which the child names words in response to picture stimuli. Published inventories typically sample consonants and consonant clusters in word-initial and word-final positions. The specific sounds included in such inventories vary but usually include those sounds that have a high frequency of errors in children's speech. For a child with a cleft palate in whom velopharyngeal closure may be a concern, items should be selected to test the child's performance on pressure consonants (stops, fricatives, and affricates). One instrument that targets high pressure consonants is the *Iowa Pressure Articulation Test,* a subtest of *The Templin-Darley Tests of Articulation* (Templin & Darley, 1969). Another instrument that contains a high percentage of pressure consonants is the *Bzoch Error Pattern Diagnostic Articulation Test* (Bzoch, 2004). In addition, Trost-Cardamone (1990a) and Peterson-Falzone et al. (2006) recommended special sampling contexts and speech tasks that are useful for documenting hypernasality and nasal air emission to determine patterns of phonetic errors. These contexts include

1. sustained phonation of high vowels /u/ and /i/ during nares-unoccluded and nares-occluded (cul-de-sac) productions
2. syllabic (CV [consonant-vowel]) repetitions of obstruent (pressure) consonants
3. single words and sentences loaded with pressure consonants (for capturing compensatory misarticulations and assessing audible nasal air emission)
4. high vowels (for assessing hypernasality), and
5. nasal consonants (for assessing hyponasality).

Such clinical tasks can often distinguish among the various sources of nasal air emission (e.g., velopharyngeal port, anterior or posterior fistulae) and learned phoneme-specific patterns. Syllabic CV serial repetitions of a stop consonant + vowel combination are also particularly useful in hearing and documenting compensatory misarticulations and coproductions. These patterns are discussed in more detail in the later discussion of phonological analysis.

### Stimulability

A third sampling component is stimulability testing. This sampling is based on the child's imitation of an adult model, which may include both auditory and visual cues, and may consist of isolated sounds, syllables, words, or phrases that contain the adult form of the target speech sound. Imitation of sounds may reveal that the child has the necessary articulatory gesture to produce a sound that does not typically appear in his or her phonetic repertoire. In other words, the sound is in the phonetic inventory, but does not enter into spontaneous linguistic usage. Such testing may tap into the child's maximum production capability and provide useful information on where to start therapy.

## Transcription Issues

Although many clinicians continue to use the traditional method of scoring and reporting speech sound error productions as substitutions, omissions, and distortions, it is strongly recommended that the clinician do more in-depth scoring in assessing the speech of children with cleft palates. Specifically, the clinician should use the International Phonetic Alphabet (IPA) and IPA extensions to include diacritics that add detail to the broad phonetic symbols. The reader who desires phonetic notation information in addition to that provided in Tables 11.1 and 11.3 is referred to Edwards (1986), Shriberg and Kent (1987) and Ball, Rahilly, and Tench (1996), and to Peterson-Falzone et al. (2006) for notation of specific cleft type errors. The clinician should record as much phonetic detail as his or her transcription skills allow, but should at least transcribe the target error(s). Phonetic detail can assist the clinician in the differential diagnosis of phonological patterns and speech sound errors that are likely caused by velopharyngeal insufficiency or other structural factors versus learned errors and those not related to the cleft condition.

Table 11.3 lists six possible error productions of the word *show.* These different forms illustrate the importance of careful phonetic transcription. For example, error production 1 in the table reflects an insufficient velopharyngeal mechanism with no fistula present, and other pressure consonants are characterized by nasal emission. Error production 4 documents compensatory replacement of /ʃ/ by a pharyngeal fricative, accompanied by nasal emission that could be due either to true velopharyngeal inadequacy (insufficient closure) or to nasal emission that is caused by the compensatory pharyngeal fricative production. Henningsson and Isberg (1986, 1991) have demonstrated that glottal stop and pharyngeal productions can prevent the velopharyngeal port from closing, thus allowing nasal air escape. The important message from their data is that we cannot assume that glottal stops and other post-uvular and pharyngeal productions are always due to an inability to achieve VP closure. The aberrant compensatory gesture may in fact be the cause of the VP inadequacy.

The clinician should try to record speech samples on videotape and/or audiotape using high-quality equipment so that samples can be played back as often as is required to accurately transcribe the child's utterances and obtain reliability judgments, if possible. High-quality digital video-

**Table 11.3**
**Six Potential Errors in Saying "Show" with Corresponding Phonetic Transcription**

| Target word | Error production | Explanation |
|---|---|---|
| "Show" [ʃoʊ] | 1. [ʃ̃o͠ʊ] | Nasal emission on /ʃ/; hypernasality on /oʊ/ |
| | 2. [ʕoʊ] | Pharyngeal fricative substitution for /ʃ/ |
| | 3. [$\overset{ʕ}{ʃ}$oʊ] | Pharyngeal fricative coproduction with /ʃ/ |
| | 4. [ʕ̃o͠ʊ] | Pharyngeal fricative substitution for /ʃ/; nasal emission on /ʕ/; hypernasality on /oʊ/ |
| | 5. [ñ̥oʊ] | Substitution of nasal fricative for /ʃ/ |
| | 6. [t̃o͠ʊ] | Substitution of /t/ for /ʃ/ (phonologic process of stopping); nasal emission on /t/; hypernasality on /oʊ/ |

taping will provide maximum production information. Included on the recording should be a "gloss" of what the clinician believes the child intended to say. Recordings of the child will be of value not only in obtaining accurate transcriptions but also as a baseline measure to assess change in the child's speech and language following intervention.

Finally, the clinician should establish a standard protocol for assessment. A standard protocol is a useful tool to establish a baseline for later assessment. A comparison of the child's speech production on the same stimuli pre- and postintervention is critical in assessing surgical outcome, as well as other interventions. This advice has merit with all types of disorders, but is most compelling with the population of individuals with cleft palates.

In summary, it is recommended that the phonological test battery include a connected speech sample, special controlled speech sampling contexts and tasks sensitive to cleft palate speech errors, a standard picture or word articulation test, if time permits, and a test of stimulability. The phonetic transcription should be done live, whenever possible, and should include at least the target error and ideally whole-word transcriptions with as much phonetic detail as the clinician can provide. All samples should be videotaped and/or audiotaped for further transcription refinement and to assure a baseline record of the child's phonological status.

## Analyzing the Speech Sample

Following administration of the assessment protocol, the clinician analyzes the data to determine (a) the presence of cleft palate misarticulations and any noncleft (developmental or other) contributions to the disorder; (b) whether the child should be seen for speech treatment, and the direction it should take; (c) the need for instrumental assessment; and (d) whether (further) physical management is indicated.

### Overall Intelligibility

One of the clinician's first analysis procedures is to make a perceptual judgment of overall speech intelligibility or understandability. Speech intelligibility is a subjective judgment made by a listener and is the most frequent factor cited by listeners when rating speech. Speech intelligibility ratings are influenced by a variety of factors, including hypernasal resonance and nasal air emission, but a major influence is the percentage of words in a speech sample understood by the listener. Speech intelligibility represents a continuum ranging from *unintelligible*, where the message is not understood at all, to *totally intelligible*, where all words in the message are understood. The intelligibility ratings of a child with a cleft palate are affected by a number of factors that do not typically affect the child with disordered speech and a normal vocal tract. For example, the child with velopharyngeal inadequacy is likely to have speech characterized by hypernasal resonance, compensatory misarticulatory gestures, audible nasal emission of air, and weak pressure consonants. These factors tend to make the child's speech less understandable. In fact, a low intelligibility rating may be less of a factor in determining whether this child should receive speech instruction than would such a rating in the case of a child with a normal speech mechanism. For example, the child who is scheduled for pharyngeal flap surgery in the future may not be a candidate for speech instruction until after the surgical procedure even though the child's speech intelligibility might be relatively low.

When compensatory misarticulations coexist with velopharyngeal inadequacy, however, caution is in order. As noted earlier, data suggest that in some individuals compensatory gestures may actually interfere with velopharyngeal closure. The videofluoroscopic data of Henningsson and Isberg (1986, 1991) showed that the use of glottal stops can alter otherwise adequate velopharyngeal speech closure. This can be understood as *compensatory misarticulation-induced* or, in this example, *glottal stop-induced* velopharyngeal inadequacy. Pharyngeal fricative, glottal stop, or other compensatory misarticulation-induced velopharyngeal inadequacy warrants speech remediation, whereas true, physically based velopharyngeal inadequacy requires physical management. This data on compensatory misarticulation behavior underscores the importance of examining the correlation between the perceptual speech data and instrumental findings. Moreover, data from clinical studies in which videonasendoscopy has been applied in biofeedback therapy have shown that instrumental biofeedback therapy has good potential to modify the closure pattern from inadequate to adequate closure (Hoch, Golding-Kushner, Siegel-Sadowitz, & Shprintzen, 1986; Witzel, Tobe, & Salyer, 1988). Collectively, these data support the use of visual imaging instrumental assessment prior to making decisions concerning secondary surgery. Discussion of the merits and importance of instrumental assessment is not within the purpose of this chapter, but is covered in Chapter 10 by Moon.

### Comparison of Productions to Developmental Norms

A second factor that is frequently used to determine whether a child is a candidate for speech intervention is the appropriateness of the sound productions relative to the child's age. Traditionally, norms have been used to compare a child's speech sound productions with those of normally developing children to determine whether the speech sound productions are typical for the child's age. More recently, the presence of phonological patterns or processes in a child's speech has been compared with the ages at which such patterns tend to no longer be used by a normal child during the phonological acquisition period. A comparison of performance against a normative standard is important for the child with a cleft palate, but the way in which such data are interpreted must be modified in some instances. For example, a child with a cleft may not produce bilabial stops (usually mastered early in the developmental sequence) because he or she is unable to build up the necessary intraoral air pressure because of an anterior palatal fistula. In this case, developmental data on bilabial stops would not be a significant factor in deciding whether to provide speech services to that child. The clinician should also keep in mind that in using the data from any large group study, individual subject data are obscured. Nevertheless, certain sound segments tend to be mastered earlier than others, and if segments normally acquired early are not present and their absence cannot be attributed to the structural deviation, developmental data will contribute to the treatment decisions.

## Phonetic Inventory

The clinician should identify all consonant targets that the child produced correctly in the samples. All correct productions should be documented by position in words, the speech context in which such productions occurred (syllables, words, sentences, conversation), and the consistency with which such productions occurred. In the case of segments that were produced in a manner or place that did not match the adult standard, the clinician should record the position and context in which they occurred, the consistency with which they occurred, and the exact phonetic description of the error.

## Phonological Pattern Analysis

An essential part of the analysis procedure is the organization of the speech sound errors into a meaningful picture. The clinician should review the test data and categorize errors according to commonalities or patterns. Frequently, these error patterns affect entire sound classes. For example, the child with an existing anterior oronasal fistula may have an error pattern that distorts production of anterior obstruents, such as /p, b, f, v, s, z/. On the other hand, a pattern of gliding of liquids, as in /w/ for /r/, is unlikely to be related to structural problems associated with the cleft. These analysis procedures are important to understanding a child's phonological status and determining treatment needs.

A difficult issue for the clinician is to distinguish between those error patterns that are developmental in nature and those that may have a structural or physical explanation as a result of the cleft. The clinician must be aware of common patterns that may have a physical basis in children with cleft palate. The following patterns are sometimes seen in children with cleft palates and are not typically seen in children with structurally intact and functional oral and pharyngeal mechanisms.

1. *Consonants distorted by nasal emission*—It is feasible to differentiate three error patterns associated with nasal emission, and different interventions may be in order for each.

   - *Audible nasal emission because of persisting velopharyngeal insufficiency.* When nasal emission is due to velopharyngeal insufficiency, the speaker exhibits nasal emission during production of all pressure consonants in the inventory. The nasal emission is pervasive and continuous. Additionally, there typically is pervasive hypernasality heard in production of vowels and the vocalic consonants /l/, /r/, /j/, and /w/.

- *Audible nasal emission due to an oronasal fistula.* When nasal emission is the result of an oronasal fistula, there is a relationship between the location of the fistula and the consonants affected (Peterson-Falzone et al., 2006; Trost-Cardamone, 1986, 1990a). When the fistula is located posteriorly near the juncture between the hard and soft palates, /k/ and /g/ are likely to be produced with nasal emission, and there may be little effect on the production of consonants produced in the anterior portion of the oral cavity. When a fistula is located in the anterior portion of the oral cavity, such as in the area of the incisive foramen, the more anterior pressure consonants, especially /t/, /d/, /s/, and /z/, are likely to be accompanied by nasal emission. If the fistula is nasolabial, located in the area of the labial sulcus, consonants /p/ and /b/ will be affected. In both instances, airflow is diverted into the nasal cavity because place of articulation of the target consonant and location of the fistula are the same.
- *Audible nasal emission that is phoneme specific.* This pattern may occur in the absence of clefting or other velopharyngeal impairment (Peterson-Falzone & Graham, 1990; Peterson-Falzone et al., 2006; Trost-Cardamone, 1988). Phoneme-specific nasal emission (PSNE) is *selective* nasal emission. It typically affects the sibilant fricatives, especially /s/ and /z/, and possibly /ʃ/ and the affricates /tʃ/ and /ʤ/, while the remainder of the high pressure consonants in the inventory are produced with normal/adequate oral airflow. Also, PSNE rarely has hypernasality associated with it so the selective nasal emission is the key perceptual characteristic. The nasal emission may be turbulent or nonturbulent and may either accompany the target phoneme or replace it, resulting in nasal fricative or posterior nasal fricative substitutions. PSNE is the result of faulty learning and does not require surgical intervention. It can usually be treated with traditional speech therapy (Peterson-Falzone & Trost-Cardamone, 2001; Peterson-Falzone et al., 2006; Ruscello, Shuster, & Sandwisch, 2001; Trost-Cardamone, 1988, 2004). PSNE is a very important pattern to understand and perceptually identify. Unfortunately, this pattern is not always diagnosed appropriately, and the nasal emission is mistakenly assumed to be due to a submucous cleft

palate or other form of true VPI. Such youngsters may undergo unnecessary (and unsuccessful) surgery or prolonged and unprofitable speech instruction. Other terms that have been used to describe this error pattern are *phone-specific* and *sound-specific* nasal emission.

- *Nasal emission that persists postoperatively.* This refers to persisting nasal emission in youngsters who have had their cleft palates repaired and appear to have adequate VP closure capability, but who continue to use early-learned patterns of nasal air emission on some or many high pressure consonants. This is a learned speech error that requires instrumental confirmation and speech remediation to teach and train oral direction of airflow.

In contrast to the pervasive nasal emission that characterizes VP insufficiency or incompetency, nasal emission that is due to a fistula or to VP mislearning (PSNE or persisting postoperatively) is perceived as more intermittent. Because of the distinctly different treatments required in relation to these sources of nasal air escape, it is critical that the speech-language pathologist be able to identify and distinguish among these etiologically different error patterns.

**2.** *Vowel distortions secondary to hypernasality*—These patterns warrant little discussion or explanation. It is important for the clinician to separate the hypernasal resonance deviations on vowels and vocalic consonants from the aerodynamic consequences of deficient velopharyngeal closure on pressure consonants (i.e., nasal airflow and weak pressure consonants).

**3.** *Compensatory misarticulations*—Several types of compensatory misarticulations were presented earlier in this chapter. With respect to treatment planning and in order to select appropriate intervention procedures, the clinician should be able to distinguish between productions that are used as substitutions and those that occur as coproductions.

**4.** *Atypical backed articulations*—These patterns also have been addressed earlier in this chapter. The presence of such productions in the speaker's inventory, with or without coexisting compensatory misarticulations, should be analyzed to determine whether they are part of a phonological pattern of backing or whether they represent selective articulatory substitutions.

Phonological analysis procedures have been published by several authors (Hodson, 2004; Ingram, 1981; Khan & Lewis, 1986; Shriberg & Kwiatkowski, 1980). In these procedures, error patterns are described as phonological processes. Phonological patterns or processes are defined as systematic sound changes or simplifications that affect a class of sounds. The specific patterns or processes identified with these assessment procedures vary, and process-based approaches often yield little useful data on structural-organic or physically based disorders. For compensatory misarticulations in particular, and organic disorders in general, a place-manner-voicing analysis procedure similar to that described by Elbert and Gierut (1986) is recommended.

Broen and Moller (1993) and the report by Estrem and Broen (1989) provide data on phonological patterns observed in young children with cleft palate. In addition to the material presented here, those data can be used by the clinician to help determine whether the phonological patterns identified in a particular child are characteristic of those seen in children with normally developing phonology, or in children with developmentally delayed phonology, or in children with cleft palate. Severe limitations are inherent in any attempt to describe the organization of the phonological system, even in structurally intact 11- to 15-month-old children who have relatively few words. Until a child has a working vocabulary of at least 50 words, the identification of the child's phonological patterns and phonetic inventory of English speech sounds is usually unreliable. Even normally developing children differ substantially in their phonetic preferences, word selection, and stability of word shapes (Vihman, 1988).

The assessment of toddlers may require several sessions and/or audio- or videotapings of the parent-child interactions in the home. Phonological status often cannot be determined until the child has some amount of connected speech. The stops are the earliest class of pressure consonants in the infant's inventory and are usually present in the speech of structurally and cognitively intact children at 10–14 months of age. In contrast, the fricatives and affricates—speech sounds that constitute more than half of the consonants most likely to be replaced by compensatory productions by children with clefts—are mostly absent even in phonologically normal children at the beginning of the 2nd year. However, none of the pressure consonants (obstruents) in English are normally produced in association with nasal air emission at any age. Therefore, the baby who undergoes palatal repair at a young age; whose consonant output consists primarily of stops, nasals, and glides; and whose word shapes are predominantly open (CV) syllables ("car" → [kɑ]) and syllable reduplications ("water" → [wɑwɑ] or "cookie" → [kʊki]) should not have nasal emission of air during pressure consonant production if there is structural and functional integrity of the mechanism.

A judgment of the adequacy of velopharyngeal closure and reasonable judgments concerning the need for secondary surgery usually can be made in toddlers who produce oral stops and fricatives. Judgments of compensatory misarticulations and the permanence of the phonetic inventory are difficult to make and may not be reliable in the young child. For example, some youngsters may not yet be targeting sibilant fricatives and affricates, so the absence of pharyngeal fricatives or affricates is not informative. However, some youngsters may have a sizable pressure consonant inventory and appear to demonstrate velopharyngeal inadequacy. In such instances, the possible interaction between compensatory gestures and velopharyngeal closure needs to be carefully evaluated, usually with the aid of instrumental imaging assessment, as soon as the child can cooperate.

In choosing phonological patterns and target segments for the initiation of treatment, the clinician should be aware of normal acquisition data because these data have application to children who have clefts (Chapman et al., 2001; Grunwell, 1981; Hodson & Paden, 1981; Locke, 1983b; Prather, Hedrick, & Kern, 1975; Smit, 1986; Stoel-Gammon, 1987; Stoel-Gammon & Dunn, 1985). Unfortunately, there is meager reliable information concerning phonological acquisition in children with cleft palate with or without cleft lip. Broen and Moller (1993) discussed these issues and have reported data on phonological patterns in children with clefts. They also made a plea for the collection of additional data on early phonological development in children with cleft palate. (See Chapter 8 by Chapman for additional recent data.) Several characteristics of normal phonological development appear to be established:

1. Open syllables (CV) and syllable reduplication are common phonological patterns that modify syllable structures used by children. Final consonant deletion and syllable reduplication are also common patterns in young children with cleft palates. These patterns are not usually seen in the phonologically normal child after about 30 months.
2. Singleton consonants are usually produced correctly by the child before consonant clusters. However, sometimes a specific cluster may facilitate production of a single consonant.
3. Most nasals, stops, and glides are acquired fairly early. Fricatives, affricates, and liquids are usually acquired later, and the time required for mastery is usually longer than for nasals, stops, and glides.

4. Generally, front placements precede back placements, labials precede alveolars, alveolars precede palatals, and velars are typically acquired last.
5. Stops are typically used in word-initial position before word-final or word-medial positions.
6. Many fricatives are produced correctly in word-final position prior to correct production in word-initial or word-medial positions.
7. Phonetic productions that are non-phonemic (for English) drop out of the child's consonant production repertoire toward the end of the 1st year.
8. Vowels are usually mastered by age 3, and by age 4 the normal child is producing most consonant sounds correctly.
9. Young children vary a great deal in their phonetic preferences, their word selection, and the stability of their word shapes. Children's patterns trend toward uniformity with age and increased knowledge of the language.

# Speech Treatment Decisions

## Establishing Diagnostic Baselines

Effective speech management depends upon comprehensive and reliable assessment. In the child with cleft palate or related velopharyngeal inadequacy, assessment involves both clinical and instrumental procedures (see Chapter 10 by Moon). The assessment should provide data on the status and potential of the velopharyngeal closure mechanism, any oral structural deviations (including fistulae), hearing status, and a comprehensive speech analysis. Based on this diagnostic baseline data, appropriate speech treatment decisions can be made. Malocclusion and specific dental deviations are secondary agents of impaired articulation in youngsters with cleft palate with or without cleft lip, and the resulting speech impairments usually are relatively minor (Trost-Cardamone, 1990b). Frequently, they are resolved through developmental (growth) changes in dentofacial relationships and by direct orthodontic, prosthodontic, and/or orthognathic surgery interventions.

The main focus in the remainder of this chapter is the treatment of compensatory misarticulations and the efficacy of various treatment alternatives for cleft palate misarticulations, since these are exceptional, somewhat idiosyncratic characteristics that distinguish the treatment of misarticulating children with cleft palate from their noncleft peers with phonological impairments. The following discussion presumes that any nasal air emission caused by oronasal fistulae is either minimal or has been eliminated by surgery or prosthetic obturation and that otologic and hearing problems have been documented and are being appropriately managed.

## Speech Errors: Deciding How to Treat Them

### Velopharyngeal Closure and Phonological Error Patterns

In a child with repaired cleft palate, the relationship between velopharyngeal closure and phonological error patterns can take several forms. Understanding this relationship is essential to appropriate choice of treatment. Table 11.4 presents hypothetical cases and outlines several of the more common speech error pattern and velopharyngeal closure relationships seen in individuals with cleft palate, and corresponding recommended treatments. As shown in the table, postoperative velopharyngeal closure can be adequate, inadequate, inconsistently (questionably) adequate, or marginal. Associated speech patterns can vary from compensatory substitutions and no perceptible hypernasality or nasal emission, to pervasive nasal emission and hypernasality with no compensatory misarticulations, to velopharyngeal inadequacy specifically associated with compensatory postures and not observed on oral consonant productions, and so forth. This table is not meant to be used as a menu for a "cookbook approach" to treatment. (As in treatment for other communication disorders, one size does not fit all.) Rather, the examples in the table are offered as a guide for considering these important physiological relationships. In particular, the reader is urged to note how the different treatment alternatives vary in relation to the interaction between velopharyngeal closure status and articulatory error patterns.

An additional treatment variable is the presence or absence of compensatory misarticulations. Hoch et al. (1986) and Golding-Kushner (2001) extended the instrumental findings of Henningsson and Isberg (1986, 1991). They pointed out that the postoperative velopharyngeal insufficiency in patients who use pharyngeal and glottal compensatory misarticulations differs in pattern and consistency from that observed in speakers with repaired clefts and no compensatory misarticulations whose

**Table 11.4**

**Treatment Decisions Based on Velopharyngeal Status and Phonological Error Patterns**

| Velopharyngeal status | Phonologic error pattern(s) | Recommended treatment(s) |
|---|---|---|
| Case 1. Repaired and adequate | Compensatory substitutions; no hypernasality or nasal emission | Articulation instruction to modify compensatory placements |
| Case 2. Repaired (or no cleft) and adequate | Phone-specific nasal air emission affecting /s, z, ʃ/ ± /tʃ, ʤ/ | Behavioral (articulation) instruction to eliminate pattern<br>Biofeedback therapy, using videonasendoscopy, if necessary (Witzel, Tobe, & Salyer, 1988) |
| Case 3. Repaired and inadequate | Pervasive and moderate to severe hypernasality and nasal emission across phonetic contexts; no compensatory misarticulations | Further physical repair, surgical or prosthetic<br>Postoperative reassessment |
| Case 4. Repaired and inconsistently (questionably) adequate | Compensatory misarticulations accompanied by nasal emission; marginal or adequate closure on orally articulated pressure consonants | Articulation instruction to modify compensatory misarticulation placements; watch for changes in nasal emission with establishment of oral placements<br>Pre- and posttreatment videonasopharyngoscopy<br>Nasopharyngoscopy biofeedback instruction to modify pharyngeal and/or glottal compensatory articulations<br>Speech training appliance to close velopharyngeal port and facilitate compensatory misarticulation modifications |
| Case 5. Repaired and marginally adequate | Mild nasal emission and hypernasality across phonetic contexts; no compensatory misarticulations | Videonasopharyngoscopy biofeedback instruction to modify sphincteric closure pattern (Siegel-Sadowitz & Shprintzen, 1982)<br>Combined videonasopharyngoscopy and bulb reduction instruction to close velopharyngeal gap (McGrath, 1988) |

hypernasality and nasal emission accompany oral pressure consonant productions. They recommended the use of speech therapy instruction in the attempt to modify some compensatory gestures prior to making decisions regarding secondary surgery. Depending upon its severity, submucous cleft palate (occult or classical) could present articulatory patterns similar to those presented in Table 11.3 for Cases 3, 4, or 5. Likewise, velopharyngeal insufficiency associated with tonsillar obstruction or with postoperative adenoidectomy might show articulatory patterns similar to those described in Cases 3 and 5. Often, tonsillectomy or secondary surgery, such as pharyngeal flap or sphincter pharyngoplasty, is necessary in such cases where the problem exceeds marginal closure and mild speech severity levels.

## Modifying Compensatory Misarticulations

Although it is not known to what extent early oral structural deviations associated with cleft palate interfere with acquisition of underlying phonological representations, the child with compensatory substitutions has problems with place features at the surface level. For this reason, the clinician should focus instruction on teaching place contrasts within the vocal tract, for the stops, fricatives, and affricates (Peterson-Falzone et al., 2006). Correction of compensatory misarticulations frequently involves shifting or expanding the child's places of articulation. Typically, this includes moving posterior and inferior (post-uvular) placements forward and upward, as, for example, in modifying a pharyngeal fricative for /s/ substitution, or glottal stop for /b/ substitution. Some children who lack the articulatory gestures for correct productions or do not have the sound in their phonetic inventory will need to be taught how to make the target sound, using phonetic placement techniques. Based on data from very young children, Estrem and Broen (1989) suggested that some speakers with cleft palate prefer to articulate at the peripheral ends of the vocal tract, making little or no speech use of the middle and posterior hard palate. Thus, in remediation, auditory modeling alone usually does not provide sufficient cues to facilitate the desired placement modifications. Mirror work, tactile cues, and even schematic or diagrammatic visual representation of target sound placement information are useful treatment strategies, especially in the early stages of speech management. Figure 11.1 shows place of production for all high pressure consonants. This type of diagram is a useful therapy tool. It can be modified to map *desired* target places depending on the child's error sounds and patterns. Likewise, it can be modified to teach the place contrast between the desired oral target

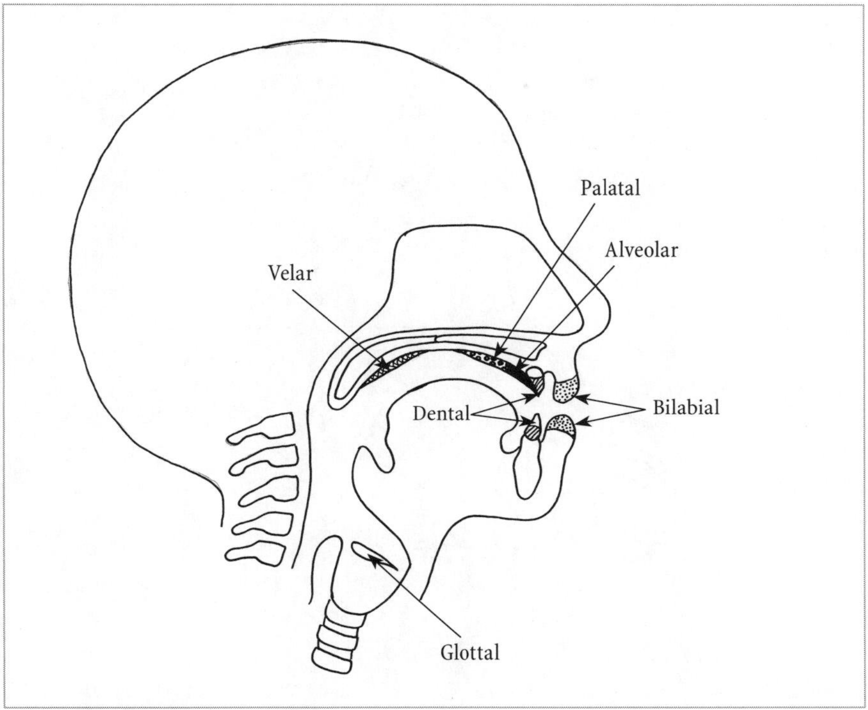


FIGURE 11.1. Mapping places of articulation.

and the glottal, pharyngeal, or backed oral error production. Figure 11.2 illustrates the place difference for bilabial /b/ versus glottal/vocal fold /ʔ/ place of production.

Direct work on place of articulation to modify articulatory gestures is a motor-phonetic activity. Once the desired articulatory placement has been established in the child's production repertoire, then mastery of the phonemic pattern (voicing, airflow) may be an appropriate goal. Treatment can be delivered through a number of approaches or combinations of approaches, including traditional segmentally based treatment (Bernthal & Bankson, 2004; Peterson-Falzone et al., 2006). When multiple errors occur, treatment based on pattern analysis (Elbert & Gierut, 1986; Hodson & Paden, 1981) may be preferred. If compensatory coproductions exist, it is recommended that establishing correct oral placement be the first step in therapy. For example, when a child makes a coproduced glottal stop + bilabial closure coproduction for /b/, the clinician should first

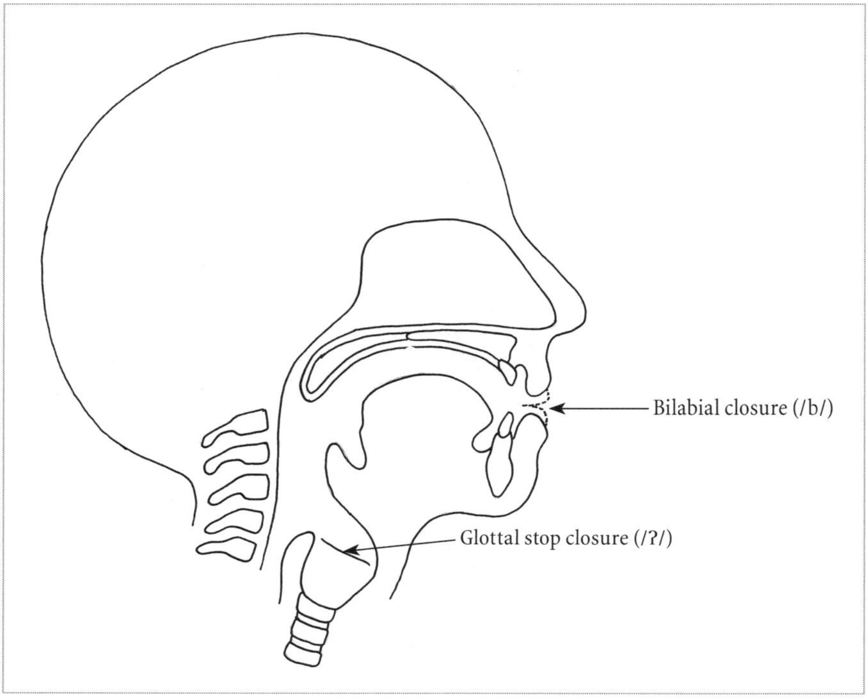


FIGURE 11.2. Place contrast for [b] versus [ʔ].

work to establish oral place (bilabial) closure. Once oral place has been isolated from the bilabial-glottal coproduction and oral place closure has been established, the airflow component can be added. In establishing oral stops, teaching the voiceless, homorganic oral fricative first has been reported to be a useful technique for breaking up compensatory coproductions (Peterson-Falzone & Trost-Cardamone, 2001; Peterson-Falzone et al., 2006; Trost, 1981). For example, in the case of [$\overset{ʔ}{b}$] coproduction, once bilabial place has been established, bilabial fricative production can be taught and drilled to facilitate oral airflow to bilabial place, and ultimately stop production.

Irrespective of the type of compensatory substitution or coproduction used by the child, the management goals and procedures are usually similar. The goals of placement work are threefold: (1) to teach the child (speaker) where to produce the correct target, (2) to establish internal mechanisms for correct target selection and perceptual-motor self-monitoring, and (3) to facilitate learning generalization and carryover.

Hoch et al. (1986) described techniques for eliminating compensatory errors associated with velopharyngeal insufficiency. With respect to target phoneme selection, they recommended that training begin with phones that are stimulable, have an anterior place of production, are highly visible, and are developmentally appropriate. In keeping with Morley (1970), they also recommended (a) that voiceless phones be established before voiced, particularly when error patterns involve glottal stop substitutions, and (b) that whispered speech be used to facilitate oral valving and reduce or eliminate glottal valving.

In addition to developmental considerations, it is recommended that the clinician select target segments or focus on error patterns that contribute most to reduced intelligibility (Peterson-Falzone et al., 2006). Less priority may be given to developmental norms. For example, if a 5-year-old uses pharyngeal fricative to replace /s/, and also produces glottal stops for /k/ and /g/ and substitutes /w/ for /r/ (gliding of liquids), /s/ might be an early focus because of its high frequency of occurrence and important grammatical role in spoken English. Even if the child at first only produces a (developmentally acceptable) /θ/ and /ð/ frontal lisp pattern on /s/ and /z/, the interdental fricative makes speech more understandable and more acceptable than the compensatory pharyngeal or glottal substitution, and can be further shaped to /s/ and /z/.

Compensatory substitution patterns tend to be fairly consistent across phonetic contexts, with minimal variability across word contexts. This is in marked contrast to the normally developing speech of 2- and 3-year-olds and to the impaired speech of the structurally intact but phonologically delayed child. These children frequently show a wide range of phonetic ability to produce targets, but their phonemic behavior typically displays variability across contexts.

## Summary

The treatment of children with cleft palate involves special considerations when compared with that of phonologically delayed children who have structurally intact speech mechanisms. A major consideration for the child with a cleft is the interaction of velopharyngeal closure and the phonological patterns observed. This relationship frequently influences the nature of phonological management. For example, when velopharyngeal closure is inadequate and nasal emission and hypernasality are present, additional physical management, surgical or prosthetic, may be the most appropriate treatment decision, with speech instruction delayed until physical management is completed. In contrast, for the youngster who has a repaired cleft with adequate velopharyngeal closure, but still has nasal emission of air on selected sounds (a phone-specific pattern), treatment utilizing a traditional phonetic approach to instruction that focuses on phonetic placement and/or biofeedback using videonasendoscopy may be the treatment of choice (Peterson-Falzone et al., 2006). A second area for treatment that is a frequent target for children with clefts is the modification of compensatory articulations, which usually requires moving the place of articulation forward and upward. Once oral articulatory placements have been established, then the focus of treatment usually is on error pattern analysis and elimination. The approaches used are similar to those used with the phonologically delayed child who has a structurally intact oral mechanism. For some youngsters who present with both velopharyngeal inadequacy and glottal and pharyngeal compensatory articulations, speech instruction with or without the use of velopharyngeal biofeedback techniques may eliminate the use of compensatory articulations and satisfactorily modify velopharyngeal closure. For others, both speech treatment and physical management may be required.

## References

Ball, M. J., Rahilly, J., & Tench, P. (1996). *The phonetic transcription of disordered speech.* San Diego: Singular.

Bernthal, J. E., & Bankson, N. W. (Eds.). (2004). *Articulation and phonological disorders* (5th ed.). Englewood Cliffs, NJ: Prentice Hall.

Broen, P., & Moller, K. (1993). Early phonological development and the child with cleft palate. In K. Moller & C. Starr (Eds.), *Cleft palate: Interdisciplinary issues and treatment* (pp. 219–249). Austin, TX: PRO-ED.

Brooks, A. R., Shelton, R. L., & Youngstrom, K. A. (1965). Compensatory tongue-palate-posterior pharyngeal wall relationships in cleft palate. *Journal of Speech and Hearing Disorders, 30,* 166–173.

Brooks, A. R., Shelton, R. L., & Youngstrom, K. A. (1966). Tongue-palate contacts in persons with palatal defects. *Journal of Speech and Hearing Disorders, 31,* 14–25.

Bzoch, K. R. (1971). Categorical aspects of cleft palate speech. In W. C. Grabb, S. W. Rosenstein, & K. R. Bzoch (Eds.), *Cleft lip and palate: Surgical, dental and speech aspects.* Boston: Little, Brown.

Bzoch, K. R. (2004). A battery of clinical perceptual tests, techniques and observations. In K. R. Bzoch (Ed.), *Communicative disorders related to cleft lip and palate* (5th ed.). Austin TX: PRO-ED.

Chapman, K. L., & Hardin, M. A. (1992). Phonetic and phonological skills of 2-year-olds with cleft palate. *Cleft Palate-Craniofacial Journal, 29,* 535–543.

Chapman, K. L., Hardin-Jones, M., Schulte, J., & Halter, K. A. (2001). Vocal development of 9-month-old babies with cleft palate. *Journal of Speech, Language, and Hearing Research, 44,* 1268–1283.

Churchill, J. D., Hodson, B. W., Jones, B. W., & Novak, R. E. (1988). Phonological systems of speech disordered clients with positive/negative histories of otitis media. *Language, Speech and Hearing Services in Schools, 19,* 100–107.

Croft, C. B., Shprintzen, R. J., & Rakoff, S. J. (1981). Patterns of velopharyngeal valving in normal and cleft palate subjects: A multi-view videofluoroscopic and nasendoscopic study. *Laryngoscope, 91,* 265–271.

Dorf, D. S., & Curtin, J. (1982). Early cleft repair and speech outcome. *Plastic and Reconstructive Surgery, 70,* 74–79.

Edwards, M. L. (1983). Issues in phonological assessment. *Seminars in Speech and Language, 4.*

Edwards, M. L. (1986). *Introduction to applied phonetics: Laboratory workbook.* Austin, TX: PRO-ED.

Edwards, M. L., & Bernhardt, B. (1973). *Phonological analyses in the speech of four children with language disorders.* Unpublished manuscript, Stanford University, Stanford, CA.

Elbert, M., & Gierut, J. (1986). *Handbook of clinical phonology: Approaches to assessment and treatment.* Austin, TX: PRO-ED.

Estrem, T., & Broen, P. A. (1989). Early speech productions of children with cleft palate. *Journal of Speech and Hearing Research, 32,* 12–23.

Finkelstein, Y., Nachmani, A., & Ophir, D. (1994). The functional role of tonsils in speech. *Archives of Otolaryngology, Head and Neck Surgery, 120,* 846–851.

Golding-Kushner, K. (2001). *Therapy techniques for cleft palate speech and related disorders.* San Diego: Singular/Thompson Learning.

Grunwell, P. (1981). The development of phonology: A descriptive profile. *First Language, 3,* 161–191.

Hall, P., & Tomblin, J. (1975). Case study: Therapy procedures for remediation of a nasal lisp. *Language, Speech and Hearing Services in Schools, 6,* 29–32.

Hardcastle, W., Barry, R. M., & Nunn, M. (1989). Instrumental articulatory phonetics in assessment and remediation: Case studies with the electropalatograph. In J. Stengelhofen (Ed.), *Cleft palate: The nature and remediation of communication problems.* Edinburgh, Scotland: Churchill Livingstone.

Hardin-Jones, M., Chapman, K., & Scherer, N. (2006). Early intervention in children with cleft palate. *The ASHA Leader, 11.*

Hardin-Jones, M. A., & Jones, D. L. (2005). Speech production of pre-schoolers with cleft palate. *Cleft Palate-Craniofacial Journal, 42,* 7–13.

Harding, A., & Grunwell, P. (1998). Active versus passive cleft-type speech characteristics: Implications for surgery and therapy. *International Journal of Language and Communication Disorders, 33,* 329–352.

Henningsson, G. E., & Isberg, A. M. (1986). Velopharyngeal movement patterns in patients alternating between oral and glottal articulation: A clinical and cineradiographical study. *Cleft Palate Journal, 23,* 1–9.

Henningsson, G. E., & Isberg, A. M. (1991). A cineradiographic study of velopharyngeal movements for deviant versus non-deviant articulation. *Cleft Palate-Craniofacial Journal, 28,* 115–117.

Henningsson, G., Kuehn, D., Sell, D., Sweeney, T., Trost-Cardamone, J., & Whitehill, T. (2008). Universal parameters for reporting speech outcome in individuals with cleft palate. *Cleft Palate–Craniofacial Journal, 45,* 1–17.

Hoch, L., Golding-Kushner, K. J., Siegel-Sadowitz, V. L., & Shprintzen, R. J. (1986). Speech therapy. *Seminars in Speech and Language, 7,* 313–325.

Hodson, B. W. (2004). *The Hodson assessment of phonological patterns* (3rd ed.). Austin, TX: PRO-ED.

Hodson, B. W., & Paden, E. P. (1981). Phonological processes which characterize unintelligible and intelligible speech in early childhood. *Journal of Speech and Hearing Disorders, 46,* 369–373.

Hubbard, T., Paradise, J., McWilliams, B. J., Elster, B., & Taylor, F. (1985). Consequences of unremitting middle ear disease in early life: Otologic, audiologic and developmental findings in children with cleft palate. *The New England Journal of Medicine, 312,* 1529–1534.

Hutters, B., & Brøndsted, K. (1987). Strategies in cleft palate speech—With special reference to Danish. *Cleft Palate Journal, 24,* 126–136.

Ingram, D. (1981). *Procedures for the phonological analysis of children's language.* Baltimore: University Park Press.

Jones, C., Chapman, K., & Hardin-Jones, M. (2003). Speech development of children with cleft palate before and after palatal surgery. *Cleft Palate Craniofacial Journal, 40,* 19–31.

Kemp-Fincham, S. I., Kuehn, D. P., & Trost-Cardamone, J. E. (1990). Speech development and the timing of primary palatoplasty. In J. Bardach & H. L. Morris (Eds.), *Management of cleft lip and palate* (pp. 736–745). New York: Grune & Stratton.

Khan, L. M., & Lewis, N. P. (1986). *Khan-Lewis phonological analyses.* Circle Pines, MN: American Guidance Service.

Kirschner, R. E., Wang, P., Jawad, A. F., Duran, M., Cohen, M., Solot, C., et al. (1999). Cleft-palate repair by modified Furlow double-opposing Z-plasty: The Children's Hospital of Philadelphia experience. *Plastic and Reconstructive Surgery, 104,* 1998–2010.

Kuehn, D. P., & Trost-Cardamone, J. E. (1988). *Speech development and the timing of primary palatoplasty.* Paper presented at the annual meeting of the American Cleft Palate Association, Williamsburg, VA.

Kummer, A. W. (2008). *Cleft palate and craniofacial anomalies* (2nd ed.). Clifton Park, NJ: Thompson Delmar Learning.

LaRossa, D., Jackson, O. H., Kirschner, R. E., Low, D. W., Solot, C. B., Cohen, M. A., et al. (2004). The Children's Hospital of Philadelphia modification of the Furlow double-opposing Z-plasty: Long-term speech and growth results. *Clinics in Plastic Surgery, 31,* 243–249.

Lawrence, C., & Philips, B. J. (1975). A telefluoroscopic study of lingual contacts made by persons with palatal defects. *Cleft Palate Journal, 12,* 85–94.

Locke, J. L. (1983a). Clinical phonology: The explanation and treatment of speech sound disorders. *Journal of Speech and Hearing Disorders, 48,* 339–341.

Locke, J. L. (1983b). *Phonological acquisition and change.* New York: Academic Press.

Luloff, A. K., Menyuk, P., & Teele, D. W. (1993). Effect of persistent otitis media on the speech sound repertoire of infants. In D. J. Lim, C. D. Bluestone, J. O. Klein, P. D. Nelson, & P. L. Ogra (Eds.), *Recent advances in otitis media: Proceedings of the fifth international symposium* (pp. 531–533). Philadelphia: Decker.

MacKenzie-Stepner, K., Witzel, M. A., Stringer, D., & Laskin, R. (1987). Velopharyngeal insufficiency due to hypertrophic tonsils. *International Journal of Pediatric Otolaryngology, 14,* 57–63.

McGrath, C. O. (1988). *Prosthetic management strategies for velopharyngeal dysfunction.* Study session given at the annual meeting of the American Cleft Palate Association, Williamsburg, VA.

McWilliams, B. J., & Philips, B. J. (1979). Velopharyngeal incompetence. In *Audioseminars in speech pathology.* Philadelphia: Saunders.

Morley, M. E. (1970). *Cleft palate and speech* (7th ed.). London: Churchill Livingstone.

Morris, H. L. (1979). Abnormal articulation patterns. In K. R. Bzoch (Ed.), *Communicative disorders related to cleft palate* (2nd ed.). Boston: Little, Brown.

O'Gara, M. M., & Logemann, J. A. (1988). Phonetic analyses of the speech development of babies with cleft palate. *Cleft Palate Journal, 25,* 122–134.

O'Gara, M., & Logemann, J. A. (1990). Phonological development in children with cleft lip and palate. In J. Bardach & H. L. Morris (Eds.), *Multidisciplinary management of cleft lip and palate.* Philadelphia: Saunders.

O'Gara, M. M., Logemann, J. A., & Rademaker, A. W (1994). Phonetic features by babies with unilateral cleft lip and palate. *Cleft Palate-Craniofacial Journal, 31,* 446–451.

Oller, D. K. (1980). The emergence of the sounds of speech in infancy. In G. H. Yeni-Komshian, J. F. Kavanagh, & C. H. Ferguson (Eds.), *Child phonology: Volume 1. Production.* New York: Academic Press.

Oller, D. K. (2000). *The emergence of the speech capacity.* Mahwah, NJ: Erlbaum.

Paden, E. P., Novak, M. A., & Beiter, A. L. (1987). Predictors of phonological inadequacy in young children prone to otitis media. *Journal of Speech and Hearing Disorders, 52,* 232–242.

Peterson, S. J. (1975). Nasal emission as a component of the misarticulation on sibilants and affricates. *Journal of Speech and Hearing Disorders, 40,* 106–114.

Peterson-Falzone, S., & Graham, M. (1990). Phoneme-specific nasal emission in children with and without palatal anomalies of the velopharyngeal mechanism. *Journal of Speech and Hearing Disorders, 55,* 132–139.

Peterson-Falzone, S. J., & Trost-Cardamone, J. E. (2001). *Speech therapy for cleft palate misarticulations.* Miniseminar at the annual convention of the American Speech-Language-Hearing Association, New Orleans.

Peterson-Falzone, S. J., Trost-Cardamone, J. E., Karnell, M. P., & Hardin-Jones, M. A. (2006). *The clinician's guide to treating cleft palate speech.* St. Louis, MO: Elsevier.

Petinou, K., Schwartz, R. G., Mody, M., & Gravel, J. S. (1999). The impact of otitis media with effusion on early phonetic inventories: A longitudinal prospective investigation. *Clinical Linguistics and Phonetics, 13,* 351–367.

Powers, G. (1962). Cinefluorographic investigation of articulatory movements of selected individuals with cleft palate. *Journal of Speech and Hearing Research, 5,* 59–69.

Prather, E. M., Hedrick, D. L., & Kern, C. A. (1975). Articulation development in children aged two to four years. *Journal of Speech and Hearing Disorders, 40,* 179–191.

Ruscello, D., Shuster, L., & Sandwisch, A. (1991). Modification of context-specific nasal emission. *Journal of Speech and Hearing Disorders, 34,* 27–32.

Rvachew, S., Slawinski, E. B., Williams, M., & Green, C. L. (1999). The impact of early onset otitis media on babbling and early language development. *Journal of the Acoustical Society of America, 105,* 467–475.

Sell, D., Harding, A., & Grunwell, P. (1998). *Speech assessment GOS.SP.ASS. 94 and 98—A training video of speech characteristics (with accompanying manual).* Huttersfield, England: Chatsworth Group.

Sell, D., Harding, A., & Grunwell, P. (1999). GOS.SP.ASS. 98: An assessment for speech disorders associated with cleft palate and/or velopharyngeal dysfunction (revised). *International Journal of Language and Communication Disorders, 34,* 17–33.

Shprintzen, R. J., Sher, A., & Croft, C. B. (1987). Hypernasal speech caused by tonsillar hypertrophy. *International Journal of Pediatric Otolaryngology, 14,* 45–56.

Shriberg, L. D., & Kent, R. D. (1987). *Clinical phonetics* (2nd ed.). Boston: Allyn & Bacon.

Shriberg, L. D., & Kwiatkowski, J. (1980). *Natural process analysis.* New York: Wiley.

Shriberg, L. D., & Smith, A. J. (1983). Phonological correlates of middle ear involvement in speech delayed children: A methodological note. *Journal of Speech and Hearing Research, 26,* 293–297.

Siegel-Sadowitz, V. L., & Shprintzen, R. J. (1982). Nasopharyngoscopy of the normal velopharyngeal sphincter: An experiment of biofeedback. *Cleft Palate Journal, 19,* 194–200.

Skolnick, M. L., McCall, G. N., & Barnes, M. (1973). The sphincteric mechanism of velopharyngeal closure. *Cleft Palate Journal, 10,* 286–305.

Skolnick, M. L., Shprintzen, R. J., McCall, G. N., & Rakoff, S. J. (1975). Patterns of velopharyngeal closure in subjects with repaired cleft palate and normal speech: A multiview videofluoroscopic analysis. *Cleft Palate Journal, 12,* 369–376.

Smit, A. B. (1986). Ages of speech sound acquisition: Comparisons and critiques of several normative studies. *Language, Speech and Hearing Services in Schools, 17,* 175–186.

Stoel-Gammon, C. (1987). Phonological skills of 2-year-olds. *Language, Speech and Hearing Services in Schools, 18,* 323–329.

Stoel-Gammon, C. (1988). Prelinguistic vocalizations of hearing impaired and normal hearing subjects: A comparison of consonantal inventories. *Journal of Speech and Hearing Disorders, 53,* 302–315.

Stoel-Gammon, C., & Dunn, C. (1985). *Normal and disordered phonology in children.* Austin, TX: PRO-ED.

Templin, M. C., & Darley, F. L. (1969). *The Templin-Darley tests of articulation* (2nd ed.). Iowa City: University of Iowa, Bureau of Educational Research and Service.

Trost, J. E. (1981). Articulatory additions to the classical description of the speech of persons with cleft palate. *Cleft Palate Journal, 18,* 193–203.

Trost, J. E. (1984). *Compensatory articulations: Error types, patterns, and treatment approaches.* Paper presented at the annual meeting of the American Cleft Palate Association, Seattle, WA.

Trost-Cardamone, J. E. (1985). *Phonological process analysis: Its role in the diagnosis of the child with cleft palate.* Paper presented at the annual meeting of the American Speech-Language-Hearing Association, Washington, DC.

Trost-Cardamone, J. E. (1986). Effects of velopharyngeal incompetency on speech. *Journal of Childhood Communication Disorders, 10,* 31–49.

Trost-Cardamone, J. E. (1987). *Cleft palate misarticulations: A teaching tape* [Videotape]. Northridge: California State University, Instructional Media Center.

Trost-Cardamone, J. E. (1988). *Phone-specific nasal emission: A cleft palate sound-alike.* Paper presented at the annual meeting of the American Cleft Palate Association, Williamsburg, VA.

Trost-Cardamone, J. E. (1990a). The development of speech: Assessing cleft palate misarticulations. In D. A. Kernahan & S. W. Rosenstein (Eds.), *Cleft lip and palate: A system of management* (pp. 340–349). Baltimore: Williams & Wilkins.

Trost-Cardamone, J. E. (1990b). Speech: Anatomy, physiology and pathology. In D. A. Kernahan & S. W. Rosenstein (Eds.), *Cleft lip and palate: A system of management* (pp. 432–437). Baltimore: Williams & Wilkins.

Trost-Cardamone, J. E. (1990c). Speech in the first year of life: A perspective on early acquisition. In D. A. Kernahan & S. W. Rosenstein (Eds.), *Cleft lip and palate: A system of management* (pp. 204–213). Baltimore: Williams & Wilkins.

Trost-Cardamone, J. E. (2004). Diagnosis of specific cleft palate speech error patterns for planning therapy or physical management needs. In K. R. Bzoch (Ed.), *Communicative disorders related to cleft lip and palate* (5th ed., 463–492). Austin, TX: PRO-ED.

Vihman, M. M. (1988). Early phonological development. In J. E. Bernthal & N. W. Bankson (Eds.), *Articulation and phonological disorders.* Englewood Cliffs, NJ: Prentice Hall.

Whitehill, T., Stokes, S., Hardcastle, W. J., & Gibbon, F. (1995). Electropalatographic and perceptual analysis of the speech of Cantonese children with cleft palate. *European Journal of Disorders of Communication, 30,* 193–202.

Witzel, M. A., Tobe, J., & Salyer, K. (1988). The use of nasopharyngoscopy biofeedback therapy in the correction or velopharyngeal closure. *International Journal of Pediatric Otolaryngology, 75,* 137–142.

# CHAPTER 12

# Behavioral Approaches to Treating Velopharyngeal Dysfunction and Nasality

*Leslie E. Glaze*

*This chapter is dedicated to Clark D. Starr, our mentor, colleague, and friend, whose professional career was dedicated to the quest for clinical evidence to support improved assessment and rehabilitation for individuals with cleft palate, craniofacial anomalies, and voice disorders.*

As a member of the interdisciplinary team, the speech-language pathologist is responsible for delivering effective behavioral treatment for velopharyngeal dysfunction and nasality. The speech-language pathologist also has primary responsibility for recommending the benefits of a behavioral approach to be used instead of or in conjunction with physical management of velopharyngeal closure. Glaze outlines the rationale, selection criteria, procedures, special considerations, and clinical evidence that support the use of behavioral therapy to improve communication skills in children and adults with velopharyngeal inadequacy for speech. Glaze promotes a functional approach to improving speech production and intelligibility toward a larger goal of socially acceptable communication competence.

1. Glaze supports the view of contemporary master clinicians and researchers who collectively reject the use of nonspeech oral-motor tasks (blowing, whistling, sucking, etc.) to modify velopharyngeal function for speech. What evidence is available to support this current understanding that nonspeech tasks will not facilitate improved velopharyngeal closure to reduce hypernasality or audible nasal air emission?

2. What is the role of behavioral therapy within the context of interdisciplinary team management? How do clinicians select and prioritize various approaches to improving velopharyngeal closure, especially choices between behavioral, surgical, and prosthodontic management?
3. List the physical, cognitive/learning, and social variables that form optimal selection criteria for recommending behavioral treatment for velopharyngeal dysfunction or nasality. Even when these selection criteria are only partially met, what rationale might justify a trial of behavioral therapy?
4. Outline both specific speech tasks and broader communication targets that contribute to an optimal treatment plan to improve velopharyngeal closure. Besides these aspects, what other variables help individualize a treatment plan, to ensure positive outcomes?
5. Develop a list of speech-based treatment activities suitable for reducing hypernasality and audible nasal air emission in a preschooler, including a range of task levels from imitated speech sounds to spontaneous connected speech. Then, vary these activities to incorporate multiple communication partners in functional communication contexts. Finally, adapt these activities to suit a school-age child, an adolescent, and an adult speaker.

## Role of the Speech-Language Pathologist on the Interdisciplinary Team

Speech-language pathologists are the professionals who provide behavioral treatment for individuals with cleft palate, craniofacial anomalies, or other disorders that affect speech due to an abnormal velopharyngeal valve. Starr (1993) defined behavioral approaches broadly, as promoting a patient's ability to "develop control over velopharyngeal closure and nasality by making use of the structures and functions available" (p. 338). These treatment approaches seek to modify voluntary speech behaviors to improve resonant quality, presumably by increasing velopharyngeal closure. The treatment may include any elicited change that actively modifies speech control cued by a variety of facilitative methods, such as self-monitoring using visual or auditory feedback to improve resonance and reduce audible nasal air emission. Thus, behavioral therapy is distinct from other surgical and prosthodontic techniques because the patient must participate actively in this process by learning to detect, discriminate, and adapt speech directly. Consequently, behavioral approaches will not be successful for every patient because of the potential physical limits that may be present in cleft and craniofacial disorders, as well as the cognitive and learning challenges that may accompany select disorders that affect the velopharynx. The behavioral approach will also vary based on the patient's psychosocial motivation and compliance, attendance in therapy, social communicative support, and other environmental factors.

## When Is Behavioral Treatment Appropriate?

As discussed by Moller in Chapter 1, the speech-language pathologist's role within the interdisciplinary team is to evaluate and appraise the patient's potential to make behavioral speech changes that will improve resonant quality, intelligibility, or social communication competence. When contemplating a recommendation for behavioral treatment for velopharyngeal closure, the speech-language pathologist is responsible for gathering sufficient clinical evidence from informal observation and structured assessment to understand exactly what behavior(s) will be targeted for change. For example, the goal may be to increase velopharyngeal function, improve speech resonance, or enhance speech intelligibility. Often, the behavioral targets to improve resonance overlap with targets in speech sound production (articulation), as described by Trost-Cardamone in Chapter 11. Certainly, the behavioral goal at the outset is always to achieve the best possible speech, although the professional may not know exactly how much progress can be made, or how quickly, using behavioral techniques alone. Thus, the challenge is to predict realistic outcomes of behavioral therapy, based on the patient's ability to modify and control spontaneous speech.

For many patients, a behavioral approach alone may be insufficient, in which case speech therapy may serve as an important adjunct to alternative surgical or prosthodontic management. Speech therapy may occur beforehand as a trial course to determine the maximal benefits attainable through behavioral strategies. Also, speech therapy may follow surgery to help the patient adapt most effectively to the altered velopharyngeal mechanism. Finally, speech therapy may occur at distributed intervals, as developmental changes in communication competence covary with the patient's physical growth and the timing of possible physical management. For example, a 2-year-old whose intelligibility is limited by distracting audible nasal air emission due to an anterior fistula may require therapy throughout the period of speech sound development, to monitor and foster correct articulatory placements before surgery while the team awaits optimal timing to close the fistula. A school-age patient whose nasality worsens despite compliance with behavioral therapy may require physical management followed by sufficient therapy to generalize target speech skills. Finally, an adult who experiences acquired velopharyngeal inadequacy following cancer excision in the velopharynx may require a short course of postsurgical therapy to maximize intelligibility despite an altered velopharyngeal port. As noted throughout this text, speech-language pathologists are most likely to arrive at the correct decision for the timing and duration of behavioral therapy when they operate within a team, with full knowledge of the availability and the acceptability of allied approaches to physical management, including plastic surgery and prosthodontic alternatives (see Chapter 1 by Moller).

## Principles of Behavioral Treatment for Velopharyngeal Dysfunction

Behavioral speech treatment is an indirect treatment for an underlying physical problem—that is, lack of control or movement of the speech articulators, including the velum. The goal is to improve the perceptual quality of speech resonance, and possibly to improve the precision and accuracy of other speech articulation skills under conditions of better velopharyngeal closure (see Chapter 7 by Jones and Seaver). These targets cannot be addressed directly through behavioral therapy, in the sense that the velopharynx cannot be easily seen, felt, manipulated, or measured. Thus, behavioral approaches seek to improve the perceptual quality of speech production and resonance. The speech-language pathologist identifies specific attributes of the speech signal that can be modified, such as aberrant hypernasal resonance, audible nasal air emission, and other articulation errors, including maladaptive compensations for velopharyngeal inadequacy (e.g., glottal stops). The overarching goal is to facilitate socially competent communication skills, including readily intelligible speech. Accordingly, clinical outcomes are judged by the consistency of speech gains made in resonance, intelligibility, and overall communication skills. Further enfolded is the wish to have the patient learn enough about his or her own speech skills that he or she can self-monitor and correct errors, and, in effect, become the therapist by recognizing, anticipating, and spontaneously producing the target behaviors for optimal speech.

Prior to behavioral treatment of speech problems related to cleft palate and craniofacial anomalies, the interdisciplinary team assesses the structural adequacy of the physical mechanism, such as the velum and velopharyngeal closure. These factors are key indicators of the potential for a speaker to reduce hypernasality, audible nasal air emission, or other distortion errors. Indeed, anecdotal evidence using flexible nasendoscopy has shown that following successful behavioral treatment, some patients exhibit apparent improvements in the coordination, range, rate, or consistency of velopharyngeal movement and closure. However, one may not assume that successful treatment for speech resonance relies exclusively on improved (or even changed) velar timing and range of motion. Surprisingly, the association between the adequacy of velar structure and function and anticipated speech performance may be low. In discussing the predicted impact of improved velopharyngeal closure, Tomes, Kuehn, and Peterson-Falzone (1997) wrote, "It is often presumed but not stated that reaching these goals [for velopharyngeal closure] should result in improvements in conversational speech" (p. 159). Indeed, this is not always the case.

The methods used to attain behavioral speech goals have varied tremendously through history. Despite the lack of sufficient evidence-based practice in this area, the profession's understanding of speech therapy for velopharyngeal closure has evolved. The current view is that to improve speech performance, the clinician must target changes in *speech* itself (Kuehn & Moller, 2000). For several decades, hopeful, but ultimately ineffective, treatment approaches presumed falsely that velopharyngeal closure in other nonspeech contexts might, with behavioral effort, transfer or generalize to speech. Old and now refuted clinical models attempted to stimulate increased velar muscle activity using indirect nonspeech approaches, such as blowing, sucking, whistling, swallowing, gagging, and other tasks (Ruscello, 1982; Shprintzen, McCall, & Skolnick, 1975). These exercises were presumed inaccurately to promote increased velopharyngeal strength, timing, coordination, and control. Powers and Starr (1974), for example, investigated the utility of nonspeech tasks in a prospective treatment study. Four subjects with repaired clefts and significant residual hypernasality performed a sequence of blowing, swallowing, and gagging exercises three times a day over a 6-week period. Outcomes were measured using lateral still radiographs to observe changes in gap size and speech recordings to assess changes in perceptual resonant quality. After the 6-week period, no changes were evident in either gap size or nasality. This study has been cited repeatedly as a classic example of the lack of evidence for these well-intended but misguided nonspeech treatment approaches.

In her excellent text, *Therapy Techniques for Cleft Palate and Related Disorders*, Golding-Kushner (2001) listed nonproductive "evaluation and therapy techniques to avoid" (pp. 133–135). She argued against the utility of nonspeech oral-motor exercises, including yawning, blowing, and whistling, and sensory techniques that have been used to stimulate a response in the velopharynx, such as gagging, sucking, swallowing, and icing. Unfortunately, based on current evidence, these and the other nonspeech techniques mentioned above will not affect or improve speech quality. Speech-language pathologists now understand that many critical aspects of movement are different for speech and nonspeech velopharyngeal closure patterns, including timing, range, and even neural control mechanisms (Clark, 2003; Dworkin, Marunick, & Krouse, 2004; Forrest, 2002; Lof, 2003; Weismer, 2006; Yorkston et al., 2001).

Nonetheless, there remains in many clinical communities an unfortunate and unjustified attempt to use oral-motor exercises (usually nonspeech gestures) to alter velar muscle strength or timing as a presumed means of improving velopharyngeal closure for speech. Some clinicians are lured into well-marketed, but spurious, treatment protocols that target velopharyngeal strengthening. For example, one vendor promotes a velar muscle training paradigm using a series of blowing instruments with increased resistance. The notion is attractive to some, because the devices are inexpensive, are easy to use at home and in the clinic, are fun for children, and appear to make sense if one believes that strong oral pressure for blowing might carry over to increased oral pressure for speech. Although the concept is alluring, it is flawed on several counts. First, muscle strength cannot be measured directly, and no clinically practical tools are available to measure velar coordination and timing discretely. Electromyographic (EMG) recordings can display the presence or absence of motor unit activation in the velum but will not provide reliable measures of velar length, strength, or movement planes. The technique requires needle sensor probes to be placed in the velum, so electromyography is usually reserved for ruling out neurological disease or injury or for experimental protocols (Baken & Orlikoff, 1999). Second, to learn more about neural control of speech and nonspeech gestures in the velum, Kuehn and Moon (1994) recorded EMG motor unit signals from the levator veli palatini muscle during blowing (nonspeech) and oral plosive (speech) tasks. Findings revealed that both the magnitude and range of EMG data were different for blowing than for oral plosive productions. These data support the idea that there are different neural control mechanisms underlying muscle movements for speech as compared to nonspeech activities.

Thus, professionals can neither measure the presumed changes in muscles that control velar movements nor verify that a specific treatment task impacts the velar muscle targeted for change. Even if such a measure existed, there is no evidence that changes in discrete muscle strength or coordination would improve following nonspeech exercises. Finally, there is no reason to expect that muscle activity produced for nonspeech acts will influence muscle activity for speech production. I recommend that all speech treatment for velopharyngeal dysfunction use real speech stimuli exclusively.

Fortunately, behavioral treatment for velopharyngeal inadequacy has progressed beyond nonspeech oral-motor tasks, toward functional interventions that employ varied speech and language stimuli in natural communication contexts. Indeed, the evolution of behavioral speech treatment from isolated single-sound and word repetitions to more ecologically valid conversational models is a welcome innovation. Kuehn and Moller (2000) promoted using methods that reinforce successful speech performance in as many communicative environments as possible. Support for this notion was reinforced by Pamplona and Ysunza (2000), who examined treatment progress in a group of children with cleft palate. Those who were treated for language delays with their mothers present and participating actively in the treatment outperformed a control group that received similar therapy with the speech-language pathologist alone. This important finding underscores at least three important recognitions:

1. the need to promote behavioral speech treatment using holistic approaches that incorporate ecologically valid experiences by including stimuli, tasks, and functional contexts that are immediately relevant to the patient's communication needs;
2. the valuable contributions possible from the patient's family members, teachers, or peers who can prompt the patient in natural communication settings; and

3. the rationale for home programming, which extends the frequency, consistency, and relevance of treatment tasks as a link to generalization.

Ultimately, the speech-language pathologist's charge is to teach the patient to produce the target changes accurately and then quickly apply and stabilize that new skill in his or her communication environment. Professionals can facilitate those behavioral changes by working directly with the patient, the family, and others in the environment who can support and encourage speech improvement. For example, classroom teachers may indirectly but successfully stimulate increased oral speech intelligibility by requesting a repetition (e.g., "Sorry, could you say that again more clearly?"). Similarly, parents and siblings might effectively stimulate improved speech patterns by encouraging the patient to use his or her "best speech" or to practice a certain speech technique (e.g., "Bobby, remember, make the air come out your mouth"). Effective speech programs engage clear support and monitoring from caregivers and siblings in a home program and provide a similar classroom consultative plan for teachers and classmates or peers. This requires the speech-language pathologist to have provided clear directives beforehand to discriminate among the patient's acceptable, emerging, and unacceptable speech behaviors so that listeners can detect and prompt the patient independently. For example, a parent may require a child to produce known targets accurately in conversation at the dinner table. Clearly, external feedback must be delivered with tact, patience, and encouragement. Otherwise, the speaker may perceive a listener's supportive prompts negatively. Nonetheless, whenever possible, having the patient practice speech in natural settings with various listening partners is an important adjunct to individual therapy. The greater the network of communicative partners who can monitor appropriate speech targets, the more likely it is that the patient can generalize "best speech" skills outside the treatment room and acquire the ability to self-correct. In an ideal behavioral treatment program, discharge criteria are met when the patient and his or her communication partners effectively *become* the clinician.

## Candidates for Behavioral Speech Treatment

Master clinicians with experience treating velopharyngeal dysfunction endorse the benefits of speech therapy only when it is appropriate to expect that the patient has the potential to improve speech production through behavioral techniques (Golding-Kushner, 2001; Kuehn & Moller, 2000; Kummer, 2001b; Peterson-Falzone, Hardin-Jones, & Karnell, 2001; Ruscello, 1982, 2004; Starr, 1993). Despite uncertainty that improvement will be possible, the team may wish to attempt speech therapy before enlisting more invasive and costly physical management. Certainly, patients who are judged to have mild and inconsistent resonance distortion, with or without nasal air emission, are excellent candidates for trial therapy. Kummer, Curtis, Wiggs, Lee, and Strife (1992) and Kummer, Briggs, and Lee (2003) reported that patients with nasal turbulence due to a small velopharyngeal gap were also promising candidates for behavioral therapy. Tomes et al. (1997) identified other specific patient profiles that may be most likely to benefit from behavioral treatment, including individuals with inconsistent or borderline velopharyngeal closure or phoneme-specific nasal air emission, and those who have recently undergone secondary palatal surgery. If the speech-language pathologist can verify that the patient has the potential to achieve closure in some contexts, the patient may be a good candidate for trial therapy, at the minimum.

To augment listener perceptions, most state-of-the-art clinics rely on visual evidence from flexible nasendoscopy or videofluoroscopy examinations (see Chapter 10 by Moon). Velopharyngeal imaging assists both the clinician and the patient in understanding what might be possible physically, and what voluntary speech gestures might facilitate velopharyngeal closure (Karnell, 1994). Although flexible nasendoscopic examinations must be conducted and interpreted carefully to avoid common recording or instrumental artifacts, securing visual evidence of velopharyngeal closure or near-closure is invaluable for behavioral treatment planning and prognosis. Furthermore, visual biofeedback from periodic flexible endoscopic examinations may serve as a primary treatment tool within the treatment course for compensatory articulation errors (Brunner, Stellzig-Eisenhauer, Pverres, & Komposch, 2005; Ysunza, Pamplona, Femat, Mayer, & Garcia-Velasco, 1997).

Determining whether an individual is a good candidate for behavioral intervention may begin with a short, focused, and intensive course of speech therapy. The goal is to determine whether behavioral speech changes can produce *measurable* and *sustainable* improvement. Both the observable change and the persistence of that change across time are essential. Even when the patient appears initially stimulable in behavioral speech trials, he or she may not be able to sustain those positive changes across time, in diverse speech environments, and under more demanding communicative demands. For example, a patient with questionable velopharyngeal closure may be able to reduce hypernasality in the treatment room and in limited speech tasks, such as sentences. However, if speech improvement deteriorates repeatedly under longer or more complicated tasks, the team may well conclude that behavioral treatment alone is insufficient. When a trial of *appropriate* speech therapy produces negligible, inconsistent, or unsustainable improvements, then that individual may not be a good candidate for behavioral treatment.

How long is an appropriate trial? Because other factors such as the patient's age, cognitive abilities, compliance, and motivation, as well as the size of the velopharyngeal gap, will influence the prognosis for improvement with behavioral treatment, the time needed to assess treatment gains will vary across patients. Generally, measurable speech gains occur within 3–6 months of active, consistent speech-based treatment, assuming that the patient is compliant and cooperative. Again, clinical experience indicates that even with the advantages of velopharyngeal imaging, acoustic and nasometry evaluations, and perceptual judgments, professionals cannot always predict from the outset which patients will respond optimally to behavioral therapy.

## Goals for Behavioral Speech Treatment

The central purpose in behavioral therapy is to improve the intelligibility and social acceptability of oral communication. However, it may be helpful to consider five separate treatment goals that can underlie a wide range of specific techniques. These five goals are not mutually exclusive and do not constitute an exhaustive list. Rather, they provide a framework for selecting specific targets that in combination will form a comprehensive treatment plan that addresses quality, accuracy, and intelligibility of the speech signal, social communication acceptability, and self-monitoring. These are the five goals of behavioral speech therapy:

1. Alter resonance characteristics to achieve perceptually normal speech. Usually, this involves reducing or eliminating hypernasality in connected speech production, but it may also involve modifying other forms of aberrant resonance such as cul-de-sac or rare cases of functional hyponasality (DeMarco & Moller, 2004).

2. Alter other speech production targets to improve intelligibility generally, by improving the accuracy and consistency of articulatory placements; increasing intraoral pressure and oral airflow during stop, fricative, and affricate sounds; and increasing speech precision (see Chapter 11 by Trost-Cardamone).
3. Eliminate or reduce maladaptive compensations that may be related to velopharyngeal inadequacy, including glottal stopping, pharyngeal frication, and nasal grimacing or snorting. Some cases of inconsistent audible nasal air emission may also be amenable to behavioral techniques.
4. Develop strategies that enhance communication competence and confidence by promoting speech practice in real contexts, with actual communication partners at home, school, work, and casual social settings.
5. Develop self-monitoring skills that allow the patient to detect, discriminate, and modify speech sounds and resonance patterns to improve overall signal quality. For some patients, this compensatory awareness will be so refined that the speaker may avoid producing faulty speech. For others, compensation may be limited to the ability to self-correct productions after initial communication breakdowns (i.e., "Sorry, what did you say?).

## Establishing Treatment Plans

Behavioral treatment attempts to "close the gap" (literally and figuratively) between what a patient *does* and what a patient *can do.* The ideal candidate for behavioral therapy should exhibit at least borderline velopharyngeal closure capabilities, because of a small or inconsistent velopharyngeal gap (Golding-Kushner, 2001; Kuehn & Moller, 2000; Kummer, 2001b; Kummer et al., 2003; Kummer et al., 1992; Peterson-Falzone et al., 2001; Starr, 1993). If the potential for velopharyngeal closure is established, the prognosis for improving speech resonance, reducing audible nasal air emission, and increasing overall speech intelligibility is stronger. If clinical findings reveal that the patient is unable to "close the gap," then the target goals must be adjusted to reflect what the patient can reasonably accomplish, such as a reduction in aberrant secondary behaviors (e.g., nasal grimacing or glottal stopping). In these cases, behavioral treatment refocuses on near-best compensations that produce socially acceptable communication (see Chapter 11 by Trost-Cardamone).

Evaluating the status of velopharyngeal closure has been discussed by Moon in Chapter 10, and those same tools are also useful early in treatment to help establish goals, and later as intermittent probes and biofeedback monitors. Velopharyngeal imaging, acoustic, and aerodynamic measures all provide clinical evidence of velopharyngeal status, but it is essential that the treatment probes be obtained during real speech tasks in a context that is as natural and spontaneous as possible, given the limits of the treatment circumstance.

An optimal treatment plan will specify (a) the target task that the patient will learn, (b) the clinical evidence that justifies a positive prognosis for change, and (c) the predicted communication outcome. Treatment plans must also consider multiple factors that characterize not only the speaker's current abilities, but also the potential for learning and personal motivation to use new speech skills, as well as other external circumstances that may influence the treatment outcome. By attending to the patient's physical limits, cognitive and learning aptitude, and social communication competence, the speech-language pathologist increases the likelihood of selecting realistic goals and devising an effective individualized treatment program.

## Methods of Behavioral Speech Treatment

The traditional approach to speech therapy is time honored for its logical, stepwise approach from simplest to most complex, as patients progress from early inconsistencies to stable production in isolation, followed by gradually more difficult speech contexts. Elements of a typical progression may include imitated versus spontaneous target production; targets in isolation versus words, phrases, or sentences; and generalization to targets in reading passages and unscripted connected speech. However, clinical evidence from the dysarthria literature has suggested that a macroscopic focus on overall naturalness of speech rate, prosody, and intonation may provide stronger benefits for overall intelligibility and communication competence than a traditional reductionist hierarchy from sound to syllable to word to phrase, and so forth (Weismer, 2006). Whereas a "bottom-up" approach may facilitate focal skill acquisition, the "top-down" approach targets general speech features, such as the impact of prosody or loudness on intelligibility. Regardless of the method, the patient must achieve and maintain control over the target speech behavior. To explore the stability of this control, the clinician may challenge the performance in a negative practice exercise (e.g., "Say it the *old* way; now the *new* way"). If the patient can demonstrate this level of voluntary discrimination and control, he or she will be able to generalize the target in more challenging natural speech contexts.

Clinical evidence from motor speech disorders and motor skill acquisition literatures indicates that motor learning occurs most rapidly following massed trials, but that new skills are retained and generalized following distributed practice (Schmidt & Young, 1998). This means that different but complementary treatment targets are addressed simultaneously using diverse approaches. The clinician can create effective distributed practice opportunities by using varied tasks and contexts to target increased loudness, varied speech prosody/contrastive stress, stronger intraoral pressure, and improved resonance. These same targets can be applied both within and outside of the treatment room, as in a home program or classroom consultative model. Because all of these approaches may facilitate velopharyngeal closure, professionals may not know which of these multiple treatment cues will be most helpful. Nonetheless, there are distinct advantages to distributed practice. First, this approach ensures that the patient is exposed to a variety of functional speech challenges that are more likely to be engaging, despite the need for many repetitions. Also, distributed practice provides the clinician with an expedient opportunity to determine which cues and targets are most readily achievable for the patient and which are most difficult. Finer observations may reveal whether speech breakdown occurs in specific tasks or, conversely, whether select contexts promote carryover and generalization.

In addition to selecting multiple treatment targets, the clinician will find it useful to employ those targets in a variety of activities. For children, activities may include speech games using cards, puzzles, picture books, puppets, rhymes, and trail games that require verbal exchange. Older children may enjoy role plays, reading passages, phonetically loaded poems and limericks, spontaneous storytelling, and even speech rate challenges (e.g., "Name as many 'b' words as you can in 1 minute, using your *best speech*. Ready? GO!"). Adolescents and young adults may take advantage of communication opportunities in the environment, through phone calls, role plays, and informational requests, and by practicing specific speech targets in communication at school, on the job, or in social situations. Thus, the overarching approach is to promote therapy strategies that employ functional speech cues in natural communication contexts.

## Compensatory Techniques

Not all patients will be able to modify speech sounds, and some who do acquire the targets will not be able to use them consistently. Professionals may have those patients practice "on demand" speech skills that serve as functional compensations. Often, clinicians elicit broader speech changes that are thought to improve speech intelligibility. For example, McHenry (1997) used pressure flow measures to determine that young adults with velopharyngeal problems, including hypernasality and audible nasal air emission, were able to decrease estimated orifice size by using louder voice, although audible nasal air emission increased slightly. However, clinicians who teach louder voice as a strategy for improved speech must ensure that patients use appropriate breath support to avoid vocal hyperfunction, which adds a risk for nodules (D'Antonio, Muntz, Province, & Marsh, 1988; McWilliams, Lavorato, & Bluestone, 1973).

Compensatory changes in speech may be effective in functional communication if a speaker can modify but not eliminate other mild or inconsistent speech errors. We see children in our clinic who slow their speech rate slightly and increase vocal loudness when speaking to new or unfamiliar listeners to compensate for mild, inconsistent audible nasal air emission. Similarly, an adolescent with habitually mild hypernasal resonance may increase articulatory precision to bolster speech intelligibility while reading aloud in class without eliminating the resonance problem completely. Thus, these compensatory strategies can yield effective treatment outcomes if they sufficiently improve the speech quality when needed, as in difficult listening environments, with unfamiliar listeners, or during special presentations. These compensatory skills are ideal for patients who have mild, residual, and inconsistent hypernasality or nasal air emission, but who are not candidates for physical management, due to medical or surgical risk factors (for surgical management) or dental hazards (for prosthodontic alternatives).

Compensatory skills are also useful for patients who can produce a target but do not use it consistently. These patients know how to achieve "perfect" speech but choose to demonstrate these skills only as needed. For example, school-age patients may relax speech precision in familiar conversations with close friends but alter their speech performance when ordering fast food or answering the telephone. Adults may selectively bolster speech performance on a job interview or when meeting new people. The essential component that elevates this outcome from random and unreliable performance to variable but competent skills is the patient's ability to internally anticipate, self-monitor, and adjust speech performance to accommodate pragmatic communication needs.

## Biofeedback and Delayed Cues: Auditory, Visual, and Tactile

*Biofeedback* is defined classically as a technique that "permits an individual to gain control over physiologic processes of which he is ordinarily unaware by arranging for these to produce easily perceived stimuli which can be monitored" (*Churchill's Medical Dictionary,* 1989). Thus, any biofeedback tool used for the purposes discussed in this chapter must provide readily observable, real-time knowledge of the adequacy of velopharyngeal closure or resonant voice quality. Biofeedback might also signal the magnitude of an aberrant speech pattern (e.g., presence of audible nasal air emission or nasal grimacing).

Although little research has been done on biofeedback in children, Higgins, McCleary, and Schulte (2000) determined that preschoolers with cochlear implants could make use of visual feedback in a speech therapy paradigm. Volin (1998) reported positive gains using visual biofeedback in young adults who were learning a novel respiratory task. Biofeedback was most effective for participants who were not readily stimulable for the task, which suggests that biofeedback may help patients who cannot readily imitate a desired target in learning the new skill.

In studying velopharyngeal dysfunction and nasality, various reports by Garber and Moller (1979), Peterson-Falzone and Graham (1990), and Ruscello, Shuster, and Sandwisch (1991) have demonstrated that visual, auditory, or combined biofeedback strategies that monitor nasalization or nasal air emission can be helpful in modifying speech production, especially when the errors are phoneme specific. For treatment purposes, not all tools used in research will be feasible, but both high- and low-technological instruments are available to offer audio, visual, or tactile biofeedback as an adjunct to behavioral treatment. These tools have the advantage of providing this feedback *during* connected speech. Additionally, other monitoring devices provide slightly delayed information about the adequacy of speech after the production. Each tool has assets, limitations, and potential artifacts, and none of the techniques is adaptable to external communication settings.

## Nasal Occlusion

The nasal flutter, an example of biofeedback, is a useful task for discriminating hypo- and hypernasality, and for observing the extent to which a patient can modify his or her resonance quality. When the patient's nares are occluded during speech, both the patient and the clinician can often perceive resonance characteristics more easily in both isolated syllables and connected speech. Suppose that a clinician occludes the nares of a patient with velopharyngeal inadequacy as the patient produces oral sentences, such as "Buy Bobby a puppy." The patient may *feel* kinesthetic sensations of intraoral air pressure build up as air pressure and airflow are diverted and blocked in the nasal cavity. The clinician may simultaneously *detect* hypernasal resonance on vowels due to amplified acoustic energy in the nasal cavity. Ideally, this technique will supply an important auditory and proprioceptive/kinesthetic model for target productions, especially oral plosives, fricatives, and affricates. The approach is especially helpful as a cue to eliminate or reduce audible nasal air emission. Nares occluded on oral phrases ("We were away a year ago") and on oral pressure consonants ("This is the house that Jack built," "basketball," "chocolate chip cookie," "Buy Bobby a puppy," "patty cake," "buttercup," etc.) will reveal hypernasality whenever velopharyngeal closure is incomplete. To clarify the presence of hyponasality, the clinician can occlude the nares as the patient says nasal consonants in phrases such as "Mommy made me," "Man in the moon," "eeny meeny miney mo," and so forth. In these nasal contexts, normal speakers exhibit aberrant cul-de-sac or mixed resonance due to the amplification of vowel hypernasality with simultaneous denasalized consonants when the nares are closed. Under similar conditions, hyponasal speakers will sound virtually the same with nares open or closed, because their nasopharynx or nasal passageways are already obstructing and dampening the normal amount of nasal resonance required for some vowels and nasal consonants.

Nasal flutter can facilitate changes in perceptual speech characteristics by stimulating different oral resonance in speakers who have not achieved this contrast independently. This simple task may also teach patients to discriminate between speech with and without hypernasality or with and without audible nasal air emission. Thus, nasal flutter tasks are useful as a primary treatment technique as well as a diagnostic tool. However, there are several important caveats. First, many children "play" with nasal voices by holding nares closed. The clinician should not misjudge a child's potential for normal resonance just because the child is making a funny nasal sound in the first few trials. Rather, if hypernasality is present, the clinician must follow up with a clear model (e.g., "Can you make it sound the same, just like this?"). If a child speaks quietly, the presence of hypernasality may be masked on a nasal flutter task. To verify, the clinician needs to prompt the child to speak louder. Because children and adults will always perform better on structured elicited imitations than in spontaneous speech, it is useful to introduce longer, more complex oral contexts, such as "This is the house that Jack built," "Sister Sue shopped for sixty-six shoes," and so forth. In therapy, nasal flutter tasks can be used periodically to add kinesthetic and auditory cues that can augment the patient's ability to self-monitor resonance and velopharyngeal closure. The nasal flutter feedback can help ensure that treatment targets generalize to more challenging connected speech practice using oral phonetic contexts. The nasal flutter task is especially useful for teaching three specific speech goals:

1. eliminating or reducing phoneme-specific audible nasal air emission,
2. adding increased intraoral pressure to speech target production, and
3. preventing the aberrant development of nasal fricative substitutions in children who acquire early fricatives (e.g., /f, s/)

Golding-Kushner (2001) described a gentle treatment approach to use with babies and toddlers to stimulate oral plosion by placing both index fingers gently against the nares and repeating simple consonant-vowel syllables, such as "pa, pa, pa," in rhymes, songs, and other vocal play. When the child imitates, use nasal occlusion to stimulate oral plosives using phoneme-loaded oral plosives, such as *puppy, baby, tiptop, daddy, kitty,* and *gobble.*

## Feedback for Resonance

***Delayed Auditory Feedback.*** Tape recordings or loops that replay the patient's speech trials may also provide useful, albeit asynchronous, auditory feedback. As always, there are perceptual confounds when listening to one's own voice, which is filtered by the recording and playback equipment and the listener's ear. Initially, it may be helpful for the patient to listen to other speaker samples of normal, hyponasal, and hypernasal resonance before attempting to discriminate his or her own speech productions.

Another technique that may promote recognition of perceptual contrasts between accurate and faulty speech productions is to practice exploring (or even exaggerating) the range of possible targets (e.g., most hypernasal vs. most hyponasal). Sometimes, it is easier to isolate correct oral productions when the speaker has had a chance to conduct negative practice trials, thereby revealing the patient's perceptual range of hypernasal and hyponasal capabilities. For practice, the clinician can have developmentally appropriate lists of oral, nasal, and oral-nasal (mixed) words, phrases, and sentences available for practice (see Appendix 12A). These stimuli are useful for exploring the maximal contrasts between a patient's "in-nose" versus "stuffed-up" trials. A tape recording can document these opposing perceptual endpoints and provide a follow-up model for treatment goals to detect, discriminate, and produce resonance targets accurately. Audiotapes also provide effective models for home practice. Ideally, practice with discriminating audio samples will improve the patient's ability to self-monitor and improve resonant quality. Eventually, it is critical that patients learn to accurately perceive differences between correct and faulty productions, if they are to self-monitor speech resonance independently.

***Simultaneous Visual Feedback for Resonance.*** Two clinical instruments are available to record the speech signal and derive a ratio of oral to nasal acoustic energy to create a nasalance score, which is thought to correlate to perceived (hyper-)nasal resonance (Fletcher, 1976; Fletcher, Adams, & McCutcheon, 1989). Both the Nasometer II, Model 6400 (see the KayPentax Web site for more information: www.kayelemetrics.com/Product%20Info/6400/6400.htm), and the NasalView (see the Dr. Speech Web site for more information: www.drspeech.com/NasalView.html) provide real-time visual feedback of this acoustic measure through specialized recording hardware and software programs. Normative data for nasalance values have been collected across ages and standardized connected speech samples for comparison (Awan, 1997; Kummer, 2001a). Although correlations between listener judgments and nasalance measures have varied across study conditions, languages, and speech samples, in general, excessive nasalance is intended to indicate hypernasality, while low nasalance scores may reflect hyponasality (Bressman et al., 2000).

Both devices use specialized headsets with dual oral and nasal microphones separated by a baffle to isolate recordings of oral and nasal acoustic energy. These signals are processed, analyzed, and displayed in real time on a computer monitor. As the patient speaks, the acoustic energy is displayed as a scrolling line moving horizontally across the screen. The NasalView displays the speaker's oral, nasal, and a derived nasalance acoustic curve on the monitor, with average statistics indicated below. The Nasometer II displays the nasalance in relative height to an optional referent bar. The clinician may select this bar under the Options menu and designate an incentive level, usually just below the current average nasalance percentage. For example, one might set the referent bar at 30% for a patient whose mean nasalance score on the Zoo passage is 35%, then gradually decrease the criterion toward the normative range (A. Baylis, personal communication, 2006). Patients may use that display to monitor and adjust speech to accomplish lower nasalance levels. Having this nasalance feedback available during running speech targets and can assist the patient in learning to self-monitor and correct as speech task complexity increases in generalized contexts. When the visual display is covered, the clinician can observe the patient's ability to rely on internal kinesthetic or acoustic auditory-perceptual cues to produce speech accurately. As with all instruments, the interpretation of findings must be considered carefully, with a clear understanding of the potential artifacts posed by the patient, the device, calibration error, and other caveats (Vallino-Napoli & Montgomery, 1997). For example, the simultaneous presence of nasal air emission may present as additive noise that confounds the summary nasalance score (Cassidy, 2003). If this nasal flow is associated with phoneme-specific contexts, it may be possible to circumvent the artifact by constructing a speech sample that excludes difficult sound combinations to achieve "best" nasalance data as a patient-specific benchmark.

### Feedback for Nasal Air Emission

***Simultaneous Auditory Feedback for Nasal Airflow.*** A useful low-tech feedback device is a simple, flexible tube with soft bulbs on either end connecting the patient's naris to his or her own ear. Riski (1984), Kummer and Lee (1996), and Kummer (2001b) reported a similar approach using a bendable drinking straw held at the naris and positioned by the ear to detect nasal air emission. When nasal air is present, the rustle of turbulence through the tube is audible and provides an alert to the presence of nasal air emission during connected speech. Initially, the patient must learn to identify and discriminate the presence of the turbulence and learn when nasal air is appropriate (e.g., during nasal speech contexts) and inappropriate (e.g., during oral speech contexts). Later, the feedback is intended to help shape the physical maneuvers necessary to modify audible nasal air emission across a range of short phrases, longer sentences, and spontaneous conversational speech. For all patients, it is important to verify that the tube is sealed in the naris and that the end is placed close enough to the ear to hear this feedback. Patients who have hearing loss may not be able to use this technique successfully.

***Simultaneous Visual Feedback for Nasal Airflow.*** The See-Scape tube (available from PRO-ED; www.proedinc.com) is a clever and portable instrument that provides visual feedback for nasal air emission by attaching to one naris a nasal bulb that is connected to a clear tube and vertical cylinder. If air from the naris enters the tube, it elevates a light Styrofoam float within the cylinder. This float varies in height with the flow entering the tube as a gross visible indicator that nasal air is present. This device allows the patient and clinician to view the presence, timing, and relative displacement of the float due to nasal air emitted during various speech contexts. Similar to the listening tube, the See-Scape's feedback is useful for detecting both excessive and insufficient nasal air, so the device is used most commonly with patients who have slight velopharyngeal gaps as a feedback tool to reduce inappropriate nasal flow in oral speech tasks.

There are several caveats to using the See-Scape. First, the presence of nasal air emission can only be detected in one naris at a time, so if the patency of left and right nasal passages differs, it is essential to couple the nasal bulb to the side with greater nasal escape. Second, the nasal bulb must fit comfortably, but snugly, against the naris to prevent artifacts. Third, because some patients exhale through the nose at the end of utterances, the nasal flow readings are most reliable during the middle portion of the speech task. Finally, children who use the See-Scape are tempted to make the float *rise* in the cylinder, because they seem to enjoy "blowing" it up the tube, which is counterproductive to the goal of preventing the float from rising (A. Baylis and A. Thurmes, personal communication, 2006). Clinicians may take advantage of that interest by allowing younger patients to discriminate between "old" and "new" speaking patterns by contrasting inappropriate nasal flow (old way) with no flow (new way).

A less common use of the See-Scape is as a feedback device for those who have excessive or phoneme-specific hyponasal speech that is modifiable. These patients may use the visual float to increase nasal flow slightly in select nasal speech contexts. However, clinicians must be aware that hyponasality is often structurally based due to a deviated septum, hypertrophic or congested nasal tissues, or chronic allergies. In these cases, denasal productions will not change using behavioral treatment alone.

*Delayed Visual Feedback for Nasal Air.* A nasal mirror held below the nares is a useful, portable, low-tech tool that detects the presence of nasal air emission by displaying condensation whenever air flows through the nares. If this visible nasal fogging (produced in oral contexts) is a correlate to audible nasal air emission, then the mirror can provide useful visual feedback. Often, the visual cues are more feasible for clinician guidance, as it is usually difficult for the patient to observe the nasal mirror while speaking. Similar to the See-Scape, the nasal mirror is also a helpful indicator for patients with hyponasality who can use the nasal fogging cue to increase nasality during nasal speech tasks. As mentioned previously, clinicians should be aware that nasal flow is common due to exhalation at the end of sentences. To avoid this artifact, the clinician should sample nasal flow during the middle portion of the speech sample.

### Feedback for Velopharyngeal Closure

***Simultaneous or Delayed Visual Feedback During Transnasal Endoscopy of the Velopharynx.*** Both videofluoroscopy and transnasal endoscopic imaging of the velopharynx allow the examiner to observe the movement of the velum during connected speech. Because of the added radiographic exposure, most clinics restrict videofluoroscopy to diagnostic procedures. In contrast, flexible nasendoscopy is less invasive, does not require X-ray exposure, and is less costly. Where permitted by state licensing boards and institutional guidelines, a trained speech-language pathologist may conduct the transnasal endoscopy independently in a medical setting (American Speech-Language-Hearing Association, 2004). Under these circumstances, the visual feedback can be acquired periodically in probes across treatment sessions. For school-age children and older patients who can tolerate the procedure easily, the view of velopharyngeal closure as it occurs during short connected speech samples may be invaluable. Often, visual evidence may help clinicians to determine whether an individual even has the potential for velopharyngeal closure. If it appears that velopharyngeal length, timing, or range of movement may produce successful closure, clinicians may attempt a trial of behavioral therapy alone (Ysunza et al., 1997). Videoendoscopic feedback may also serve as a primary treatment tool to help patients with borderline or intermittent velopharyngeal closure achieve closure consistently.

There are both rigorous precautions and important artifacts associated with nasendoscopy of the velopharynx, as described by Moon in Chapter 10 and reviewed in outstanding detail by Karnell (1994). Our assessment team has developed a slow, gentle approach that works well with children. If possible, we work in pairs so that one clinician can interact with the child while the other operates the equipment. We schedule sufficient time to describe every step of the procedure to the patient in child-friendly but accurate terms. By orienting the patient and his or her caregivers directly and calmly, we can verify that they understand and support the need to gather visual evidence. Most patients relax when we explain that the endoscopy takes only 3–5 minutes. We outline each step of the preparation carefully: Two cotton swabs with decongestant and topical anesthetic are inserted gently and slowly into the nasal passage, followed by the endoscope. Children who are reluctant may respond to rewards during as well as after the technique. For example, we might provide a sticker page with six blank squares (a few extras!) to provide a framework for the potential number of "steps" in the process. We award the first sticker after the sound recording, the second after advancing the first cotton swab, a third after the second swab, and another after the endoscope. We may also unwrap a sucker to let the child hold and instruct, "Some kids think this medicine tastes funny, so here's a sucker in case you do, too. Then, we'll save the rest for later." We may use visual cues or pictures to help us explain the task. We have the child practice the words and phrases that will be elicited during the procedure beforehand, to familiarize the child with speech samples required during the examination (see Appendix 12A for a representative sample). Finally, I allow the child (within reason) to indicate when he or she is "ready to begin," often by giving a choice of talking to parents first or getting out of the chair sooner. If a child begins to cry during the nasendoscopy, I gently remind him or her, "As soon as you can take a breath and say these words without crying, we'll be done!"

Typically, children above age 5 or 6 are able to tolerate nasendoscopy easily, especially as they become comfortable with the brief time needed for the procedure. In school-age children who can demonstrate intermittent velopharyngeal closure, I may attempt to use the visual image for biofeedback in therapy. Although the overall speech goal is to improve resonance or reduce audible nasal air emission, I use visual nasendoscopic feedback to help the patient learn speech gestures required to achieve velopharyngeal closure consistently. Usually, there is only a short window of time (e.g., 5 minutes or less) to practice these trials. I position the patient so that he or she can view the video monitor. I then ask the patient to view the velopharynx as he or she is speaking and familiarize him or her with key physical signs, such as changes in velar elevation during oral versus nasal contrasts, the dark hole indicating a velopharyngeal gap, and air bubbling or rippled mucosa during nasal leakage through the velopharyngeal port. Using structured oral and nasal stimuli, this treatment is similar to approaches used with other feedback strategies, with an added visual element that is directly related to the status of velar movement (Brunner et al., 2005; Ysunza et al., 1997). We incorporate oral, nasal, and mixed stimuli, and contrast trials with successful velopharyngeal closure and with incomplete closure (e.g., negative practice) to demonstrate control, if possible.

Brunner and colleagues (2005) reported promising clinical outcomes in a prospective treatment study using videoendoscopic feedback with 11 participants, ranging in age from 7 to 30 years. Each individual had already received conventional speech therapy but had not improved. In this multiple-baseline single-subject design, investigators used nasopharyngoscopic feedback of patients' velopharyngeal closure efforts as a treatment stimulus. Patients observed two feedback trials, 6 weeks apart, for each target sound. Velopharyngeal closure was assessed after treatment and again at a 6-month follow-up. In both probes, participants achieved and retained velopharyngeal closure. Moreover, gains identified in word production had also generalized to sentences. These important findings support the rationale for including visual feedback of velopharyngeal closure in treatment protocols.

## Direct Intervention Using Continuous Positive Airway Pressure

The Continuous Positive Airway Pressure (CPAP) device is a close-fitting nasal mask coupled to a filtered air compressor that delivers variable airflow into the nares. Although CPAP is not a behavioral technique, its application has produced interesting and potentially useful findings over a decade of clinical investigation (Kuehn & Moller, 2000). The purpose of CPAP is to alter the strength of the velar muscles by stimulating the velum to work against progressive resistance in a hierarchy of real speech trials, which the patient must perform consistently and repeatedly to create a benefit. The CPAP regimen relies on select principles of neuromuscular (re)training. These include principles of *overloading*, or applying increased intensity over typical workload, as airflow rate and pressure exceed the inertia of the velum in habitual speech under atmospheric conditions. A second principle is *progressive resistance*, which employs a gradual increase in intensity of airflow and time using CPAP across trials and sessions. Finally, the principle of *specificity* applies, as CPAP is thought to activate the exact and correct muscles and corresponding neural pathways during speech that are needed to increase (velar) muscle strength (Kuehn et al., 2002). It is not possible, however, to determine whether pre- versus post-treatment differences represent actual changes in muscle strength, as no direct measure for this variable is available at present.

In a review of the efficacy of an 8-week prospective treatment study with cleft palate subjects, Kuehn et al. (2002) revealed that although many participants were judged by independent expert listeners to have reduced nasality, the response was highly variable across individuals. The authors speculated that compliance might be an influencing variable, because subjects from one site unaccountably performed worse than those from other centers. Expanded clinical treatment research is needed to clarify the efficacy of this treatment regimen and how patient selection criteria relate to optimal outcomes. Because many patients with velopharyngeal problems may also exhibit central or peripheral neurological deficits, there is certain potential for highly variable individual responses to CPAP in future trials of this technique. Although it is premature to predict the benefits of CPAP in these special populations, as more data and experience are reported, professionals will understand its role in the clinical spectrum of treating resonance and velopharyngeal dysfunction efficiently and effectively.

## Special Considerations for Special Patients: Case Studies

Clinicians recognize the need for behavioral therapy to be engaging, functional, and meaningful for patients. This final section considers variables that support a successful treatment plan. The underlying philosophy is holistic: Each patient is treated in the context of his or her communication demands, interests, and listening partners. The treatment materials target the goals, and are realistic and inviting samples of the patient's communication environment. School-age children may use microphones and video recordings to increase the "fun factor" in speech practice, followed by telephone assignments for generalization. Adults may practice skills that are most troublesome for them, such as delivering a sales promotion. Preschoolers with an affinity for animals or action heroes may find an entire home program geared around those stimuli. Adolescents struggling with social confidence may practice a job interview. Throughout, the goal is to attend not only to communicative *competence*, but also to social communication *confidence*. This is especially important in light of recent studies that have explored the social and communicative quality-of-life challenges facing adolescents with craniofacial differences (Kapp-Simon, McGuire, Long, & Simon, 2005; Lahll & Rochet, 2000; Slifer et al., 2004; Topolski & Edwards, 2005). Although these principles and approaches are not exclusive to behavioral therapy for velopharyngeal function, to illustrate these concepts in behavioral treatment plans, I have included five case studies of patients without acceptable velopharyngeal closure, ranging from preschool age to adult. These cases highlight the physical, cognitive, and sociocommunicative variables that may influence treatment outcomes in behavioral therapy for velopharyngeal dysfunction and nasality.

## Case Study 1

A preschooler with a repaired cleft palate is developing age-appropriate language and articulation placements, but displays consistent audible nasal air emission with weak pressure consonants during connected speech, as noted during a periodic evaluation at the interdisciplinary cleft palate team visit. Following the clinician's model, she produces strong pressure consonants on anterior sounds (/p, b, t, d/) when speaking single words, such as "puppy," "baby," "tiptoe," and "daddy" during nasal flutter tasks (i.e., speech stimulus contrasts with nares closed). With nares open, she also reduces the amount of air visible on a nasal mirror when asked to "make the sound come out of your mouth," following a clinician model.

### Target Task

The patient will reduce audible nasal air emission and increase oral pressure in plosive consonants (criterion to be determined by clinician) in spontaneous speech using picture descriptions, requests for toys, and role-plays with her mother and sister. Treatment will begin with single words, expanding to carrier phrases and full sentences, to teach correct productions. Picture cards, toys, and real objects will be employed in labeling games such as "Go Fish," and "I Spy," coupled with auditory (listening tube), visual (See-Scape), and social communicative feedback ("Here you go!" vs. "What did you ask for?") in a parent-patient picture request task.

## Clinical Evidence

Physical: The patient appears to be able to accomplish velopharyngeal closure in some speech contexts, based on flexible nasendoscopic examination.

Cognitive/Learning: She is learning language and speech sounds spontaneously, and all other developmental milestones are age appropriate. She is described as a bright, curious child and appears to be a normal learner.

Social Communicative: She appears to enjoy naming pictures with the clinician and parents, and her parents describe her as a "chatterbox," though they cannot understand all that she says. She does not appear to be self-conscious about her speech.

## Communication Outcome

This patient improved speech intelligibility by reducing audible nasal air emission and increasing intraoral pressure for speech. She was eager to play speech games in a home program with her mother and sisters and learned to modify her speech productions even with simple visual cues from her mother (e.g., pointing to her own nose). Her social confidence may have helped her to achieve these changes. Although she maintained positive speech changes for about 3 years, she reappeared in our clinic 4 years later, due to recurring concerns about her hypernasality, which was noted by her second-grade teacher. Her speech placements were correct, and audible nasal emission was negligible. Flexible endoscopy revealed that velopharyngeal closure was achieved inconsistently and diminished with longer and more complex utterances. A second course of trial behavioral therapy was only partially helpful, and later that year, physical management was recommended to improve velopharyngeal closure for speech.

## Case Study 2

A kindergartner developed sudden onset of audible nasal air emission and hypernasality following a tonsillectomy and adenoidectomy, and these symptoms have persisted for 6 months. Initially, the parents were advised that speech would improve after a few months. Recently, his parents became more concerned because he has not adjusted well to a new school, where peers do not understand him. The child has started to either withdraw or become angry when listeners ask, "What did you say?" A flexible nasendoscopy reveals a short soft palate that makes inconsistent touch closure with the pharyngeal wall. The parents are reluctant to consider surgery because the child had a mild postoperative complication (excessive bleeding) following the tonsillectomy.

### Target Task

The target speech goals are to explore the patient's potential to reduce hypernasality and audible nasal air emission using behavioral techniques alone. A second overlaid target is to restore and promote communication confidence, so that he can communicate effectively and avoid the negative social consequences of decreased intelligibility. Treatment involves teaching the patient to use supportive visual cues (e.g., gestures, contextual cues) as well as direct speech changes (e.g., louder voice, increased articulatory precision). Treatment will include some sessions with peers, who can provide realistic listening models during intelligibility probes (e.g., barrier games).

### Clinical Evidence

Physical: The patient demonstrates inconsistent velopharyngeal closure, but he does have the potential to achieve complete closure. This therapy trial will determine whether behavioral treatment can achieve the desired changes.

Cognitive/Learning: His speech is characterized by moderate and consistent hypernasality, affecting his overall speech intelligibility despite the fact that language and articulatory placements are accurate across all speech sounds.

Social Communicative: He speaks with unfamiliar listeners when needed but is starting to respond negatively when he is not understood. He has been diagnosed with attention-deficit/hyperactivity disorder and may be at risk for difficulty with social interactions.

### Communication Outcome

The clinician targeted improved speech intelligibility and more consistent velopharyngeal closure, if possible. Moreover, select treatment routines were used to teach the patient how to repair speech breakdowns effectively, first in the treatment room, followed by experiences in natural environments. The clinician used these communicative successes as a strategy for restoring the patient's social communication confidence. The patient had many opportunities to practice these speech targets in a school-based social skills classroom. He improved his communication confidence by learning to speak louder, which simultaneously increased intelligibility. He also improved oral plosion and reduced audible nasal air emission with careful attention. However, hypernasality persisted, especially when he was tired, upset, or less attentive to his speech patterns. After a 3-month trial period of behavioral speech therapy, he could still not sustain complete velopharyngeal closure. Because he was over 1 year post-tonsillectomy and adenoidectomy, there was little expectation of further spontaneous recovery. Consequently, a speech prosthesis was recommended to provide more consistent velopharyngeal closure, with the hope that he might be able to train out of the device through systematic reduction (see Chapter 18 by Leeper, Charles, and Sills).

## Case Study 3

A sixth grader with velocardiofacial syndrome and mild learning disabilities is experiencing increased social communicative difficulties, based on his teacher's report that he "mumbles" and "can't be heard easily." He has already received a pharyngeal flap to reduce hypernasality. The nasendoscopic exam reveals that although velar timing is slightly irregular, complete closure is demonstrated. His parents report that he has experienced some teasing from peers and is reluctant to initiate communication outside of his immediate family members and a couple of friends. His speech is characterized by reduced intelligibility due to mild hypernasality, reduced loudness and prosody, minimal articulatory pressure despite correct speech placements, and intermittent audible nasal air emission. Following the clinician's model, he increases loudness and speech plosion surprisingly well, but he cannot produce these changes spontaneously.

## Target Task

The patient will increase speech intelligibility (criterion to be determined by clinician) in a spontaneous speech sample using a story-retelling task. Intelligibility will be measured by two unfamiliar listeners' word-for-word transcriptions of the 100-word sample without visual cues. Treatment will address six rotating, yet integrated, goals, practiced in a variety of elicited and spontaneous connected speech tasks:

1. Increase speech loudness using increased breath support and larger mouth movements: facilitated by barrier exercises such as increased physical distance, blocked facial/visual cues, overcoming low levels of background noise, and functional role plays that elicit louder speech ("Sorry, I couldn't hear you").
2. Expand speech prosody: facilitated by contrastive stress and intonation exercises, including emotional contexts ("Oh, no! Watch out for the car!") or variable emphasis sentences ("WHAT did HE BUY at the STORE?").
3. Increase articulatory precision: facilitated by shaping from slower, more careful articulation placements, then stabilizing those targets at a typical speech rate; use negative practice (e.g., "mumbled" vs. "precise" speech) to demonstrate precise articulation, accurate self-monitoring, and control.
4. Reduce hypernasality: facilitated by using visual biofeedback (Nasometer).
5. Eliminate inconsistent audible nasal air emission: facilitated by using visible biofeedback with the See-Scape.
6. Increase communication competence using social communication practice challenges outside the treatment room: examples include calling restaurants to secure price bids on pizza, asking the clinic receptionist for directions, rehearsing a short classroom

presentation in front of a few unfamiliar listeners, and other pragmatic communication tasks.

### Clinical Evidence

Physical: The patient has a pharyngeal flap that has the potential to accomplish complete velopharyngeal closure. Inaccurate or delayed velar timing inhibits complete closure at times.

Cognitive/Learning: His learning deficits suggest that treatment may require longer and more consistent practice routines, with deliberate practice and generalization at home and school (e.g., answering the home telephone, ordering a meal at restaurants, answering questions in the classroom).

Social Communicative: He is reluctant to speak with unfamiliar listeners, and speech quality tends to deteriorate with increased social stress or cognitive load. Speech practice will include a set of communication experiences with unfamiliar listeners, after learning strategies for repairing listener breakdowns (e.g., visual cues, louder voice).

### Communication Outcome

The patient improved speech intelligibility most effectively by increasing speech loudness and prosody, although his oral resonance during connected speech remained inconsistent. He required occasional cues to maintain best productions. Treatment focused on social support and education regarding velocardiofacial syndrome (VCFS); he practiced, then presented information on VCFS to his class in a disabilities unit. Gradually, he and his mother reported increased social communication confidence, as he made new friends and reported feeling happier at school. At discharge from behavioral speech treatment, he was referred for counseling to address peer interactions and self-identity.

## Case Study 4

An 18-year-old male has a history of cleft palate and has undergone two secondary surgeries to reduce hypernasality. His speech is readily intelligible, but residual mild hypernasality persists, which he dislikes. Interestingly, the presence of hypernasality is not confined to a consistent set of speech contexts. He is unwilling to have another surgery and wishes to explore behavioral alternatives. Flexible endoscopy reveals a small, inconsistent velopharyngeal gap that does close during some pressure consonant productions.

### Target Task

The patient will reduce or eliminate mild hypernasality using Nasometer biofeedback to provide a learning opportunity for internal calibration and speech adjustment. This patient has the potential to modify his hypernasal resonance but has not been able to generalize that skill. The visual feedback provided by the Nasometer will help the patient identify the speech variables that appear to coincide with his intermittent hypernasality, including phonetic and coarticulatory contexts, prosody and loudness, utterance length, and others.

### Clinical Evidence

Physical: The patient has a small, inconsistent velopharyngeal gap, but can achieve full closure.

Cognitive/Learning: He is a college freshman and has no apparent learning challenges.

Social Communicative: He speaks competently, but this hypernasality is a distracter and he dislikes the sound of his resonance.

### Communication Benefit

The patient practiced varied speech productions using visual nasalance feedback to produce and replicate speech with consistent oral-nasal balance. Although he was never able to explain to the clinician exactly what internal adjustment(s) he made, after several sessions of experimentation using the visual biofeedback, he was able to produce appropriate resonance on demand. During one stretch of apparent relapse into hypernasal quality, he excused himself from the session, took a short break, and returned able to achieve correct oral-nasal balance again. Eventually, he stabilized this set of internal kinesthetic and auditory cues and reduced nasalance scores to a normal level in virtually all speech contexts. To reinforce his ability to self-monitor correct targets, he practiced speech phrases with the visual monitor covered. At the conclusion of treatment, he conceded that he was not likely to use this strategy 100% of the time, but planned to maintain the skill to apply when he wished to "sound my best." He also agreed to return to the clinic for single sessions during college breaks, as needed, for "recalibration." At 3- and 6-month follow-up visits, he was able to produce satisfactory resonance quality and achieve normal nasalance scores.

## Case Study 5

A 36-year-old male immigrated to the United States from Mexico 7 years ago. He speaks near-fluent English. He has a 30-year history of velopharyngeal inadequacy following a traumatic injury to the palate as a young child. His speech is characterized by reduced intelligibility due to moderate to severe hypernasality, reduced loudness, minimal articulatory pressure despite correct speech placements, and intermittent audible nasal air emission. He received a pharyngeal flap 6 weeks ago, and videonasendoscopy reveals an intact flap, but velopharyngeal closure is not accomplished due to lack of movement of the lateral pharyngeal walls.

### Target Task

Increase velopharyngeal closure and reduce audible nasal air emission during connected speech production.

### Clinical Evidence

Physical: The patient has consistent lateral velopharyngeal openings following pharyngeal flap surgery and is not using the flap effectively during speech production.

Cognitive/Learning: He has normal language and learning capabilities.

Social Communicative: He has learned to speak with unfamiliar listeners, when needed, but has always been embarrassed about his speech quality due to severe hypernasality that decreases his overall speech intelligibility. His articulatory placements are accurate. As a child, he was teased often about the sound of his voice and nicknamed "Snort," presumably due to audible nasal emission.

### Communication Outcome

The patient practiced pressure consonant drills with nares closed and open and acquired velopharyngeal closure for oral speech sounds. At first, this closure was highly inconsistent, so he used three separate sessions of videonasendoscopy feedback to practice closing the port voluntarily, including negative practice to demonstrate contrasts and control over the target. At home, he used both nasal flutter and a nasal mirror to stimulate oral plosion and monitor a reduction of nasal air emission. Using short, functional speech reading tasks (e.g., reading the newspaper headlines aloud to his wife), he learned to reduce hypernasality and consistently eliminate audible nasal air emission. His employment setting had few speech demands, but he reported improved social communication confidence and increased intelligibility in other situations, such as speaking on outings with friends, from another room (e.g., without visual cues), and in noisy listening conditions.

## Summary

Effective behavioral treatment for velopharyngeal closure is both challenging and rewarding. There remains a great need to develop and study clinical approaches that reduce hypernasality and audible nasal air emission in speakers of all ages. Clinicians must use techniques that are grounded in a small but growing body of evidence-based practice drawn from speech motor control, skill acquisition literature, and outcomes of interdisciplinary teams that care for cleft palate and craniofacial anomalies. Successful outcomes range from complete mastery over resonance and intelligibility deficits to compensatory strategies that enable better communication in certain conditions. My treatment philosophy highlights the need to consider the functional communicative needs of each individual to establish appropriate goals to achieve communication competence and confidence.

## Acknowledgments

To Adriane Baylis, Kelly Nett Cordero, Karlind Moller, and Anna Thurmes for sharing their wisdom and experience so generously and for helpful comments on previous versions of this chapter.

# APPENDIX 12A

# Practice Words and Phrases to Assess Nasal and Oral Sounds

| Nasals | Mixed | Oral |
|---|---|---|
| **Practice words** | | |
| man | nickel | puppy |
| mine | monkey | pickle |
| mama | pumpkin | papa |
| money | sample | baby |
| morning | napping | Boy Scout |
| mummy | magazine | tiptoe |
| no no | banana | ticket |
| nanny | hamper | tipsy |
| noun | napkin | daffy duck |
| noon | ninety | kitty cat |
| nine | nap time | slippery soap |
| ring | beanbag | sticky spaghetti |
| song | flimsy material | fifty-five fish |
| | shiny pennies | shoes for sale |
| | train on time | choo choo track |
| | | Jack built this house |
| | | chocolate chip cookies |
| **Practice phrases and sentences** | | |
| Mama makes muffins. | No, Nancy, don't go. | Please pat the puppy. |
| Man in the moon. | Buy Bobby a banana. | Pick up the kickball. |
| No no, not now. | Give me a nickel. | Put the baby by the tub. |
| Many men make money. | Bring me a pumpkin. | Take out the trash. |
| My mama made me. | Don't go down the drain. | Talk to the teacher. |
| Nan went away a year ago. | Ginny gave me a gumball. | How hard did he hit? |
| Now we're really zooming | Morning bells are ringing. | Who heard her holler? |

# References

American Speech-Language-Hearing Association. (2004). Vocal tract visualization and imaging: Technical report. *Asha*(Suppl. 24), 140–145.

Awan, S. N. (1997). Analysis of nasalance: Nasalview. In W. Ziegler & K. Deger (Eds.), *Clinical phonetics and linguistics* (pp. 518–525). London: Whurr.

Baken, R. J., & Orlikoff, R. (1999). *Clinical measurement of speech and voice.* San Diego: Singular.

Bressman, T., Sader, R., Whitehill, T. L., Awan, S. N., Zeilhofer, H., & Horch, H. (2000). Nasalance distance and ratio: Two new measures. *Cleft Palate-Craniofacial Journal, 37,* 248–256.

Brunner, M., Stellzig-Eisenhauer, A., Pverres, R., & Komposch, G. (2005). The effect of nasopharyngoscopic biofeedback in patients with cleft palate and velopharyngeal dysfunction. *Cleft Palate-Craniofacial Journal, 42,* 649–657.

Cassidy, T. M. (2003). *The effect of summary knowledge of results on reducing nasalance values in a speaker with hypernasality.* Unpublished master's thesis, University of Minnesota.

*Churchill's Medical Dictionary.* (1989). New York: Churchill Livingstone.

Clark, H. M. (2003). Neuromuscular treatments for speech and swallowing: A tutorial. *American Journal of Speech-Language Pathology, 12,* 400–415.

D'Antonio, L., Muntz, H., Province, M., & Marsh, J. (1988). Laryngeal/voice findings in patients with velopharyngeal dysfunction. *Laryngoscope, 98,* 432–438.

DeMarco, A. L., & Moller, K. T. (2004). *The use of nasometric biofeedback in a rare case of functional hyponasality.* Paper presented at the annual meeting of the American Cleft Palate-Craniofacial Association, Chicago.

Dworkin, J. P., Marunick, M. T., & Krouse, J. H. (2004). Velopharyngeal dysfunction: Speech characteristics, variable etiologies, evaluation techniques, and differential treatments. *Language, Speech, and Hearing Services in Schools, 35,* 333–352.

Fletcher, S. G. (1976). Nasalance vs. listener judgments of nasality. *Cleft Palate Journal, 13,* 31–44.

Fletcher, S. G., Adams, S. E., & McCutcheon, M. J. (1989). Cleft palate speech assessment through oral-nasal acoustic measures. In K. Bzoch (Ed.), *Communicative disorders related to cleft lip and palate* (pp. 246–257). Boston: College Hill Press.

Forrest, K. (2002). Are oral-motor exercises useful in the treatment of phonological/articulatory disorders? *Seminars in Speech and Language, 23,* 15–25.

Garber, S. R., & Moller, K. T. (1979). The effects of feedback filtering on nasalization in normal and hypernasal speakers. *Journal of Speech and Hearing Research, 22,* 321–333.

Golding-Kushner, K. J. (2001). *Therapy techniques for cleft plate and related disorders.* San Diego: Singular Thomson Learning.

Higgins, M. B., McCleary, E., & Schulte, L. (2000). Use of visual feedback to treat negative intraoral air pressures of preschoolers with cochlear implants. *American Journal of Speech-Language Pathology, 9,* 21–35.

Kapp-Simon, K. A., McGuire, D. E., Long, B. C., & Simon, D. J. (2005). Addressing quality of life issues in adolescents: Social skills interventions. *Cleft Palate-Craniofacial Journal, 42,* 45–50.

Karnell, M. P. (1994). *Videoendoscopy: From velopharynx to larynx.* San Diego: Singular.

Kuehn, D. P., Imrey, P. B., Tomes, L., Jones, D. L., O'Gara, M. M., Seaver, E. J., et al. (2002). Efficacy of continuous positive airway pressure for treatment of hypernasality. *Cleft Palate-Craniofacial Journal, 39,* 267–276.

Kuehn, D. P., & Moller, K. T. (2000). *Speech and language issues in the cleft palate population: The state of the art* [Electronic version]. *Cleft Palate-Craniofacial Journal, 37,* 348-1–348-35.

Kuehn, D. P., & Moon, J. B. (1994). Levator palatini muscle activity in relation to intraoral air pressure variation. *Journal of Speech and Hearing Research, 37,* 1260–1270.

Kummer, A. W. (2001a). Nasometry. In A. W. Kummer (Ed.), *Cleft palate and craniofacial anomalies: The effects on speech and resonance.* Clifton Park, NY: Thomson Delmar.

Kummer, A. W. (2001b). Speech therapy for effects of velopharyngeal dysfunction. In A. W. Kummer (Ed.), *Cleft palate and craniofacial anomalies: The effects on speech and resonance.* Clifton Park, NY: Thomson Delmar.

Kummer, A. W., Briggs, M., & Lee, L. (2003). The relationship between characteristics of speech and velopharyngeal gap size. *Cleft Palate-Craniofacial Journal, 40,* 590–596.

Kummer, A. W., Curtis, C., Wiggs, M., Lee, L., & Strife, J. L. (1992). Comparison of velopharyngeal gap size in patients with hypernasality, hypernasality and nasal emission or nasal turbulence (rustle) as the primary speech characteristic. *Cleft Palate-Craniofacial Journal, 29,* 152–156.

Kummer, A., & Lee, L. (1996). Evaluation and treatment of resonance disorders. *Language, Speech, and Hearing Services in the Schools, 27,* 271–281.

Lahll, A. K., & Rochet, A. P. (2000). The effect of information on listeners' attitudes toward speakers with voice or resonance disorders. *Journal of Speech, Language, and Hearing Research, 43,* 782–795.

Lof, G. L. (2003, April). *Oral motor exercises and treatment outcomes. Perspectives: Special Interest Division 1, Languages and Learning.* Rockville, MD: American Speech-Language-Hearing Association.

McHenry, M. A. (1997). The effect of increased vocal effort on estimated velopharyngeal orifice area. *American Journal of Speech-Language-Hearing, 6*(4), 55–61.

McWilliams, B. J., Lavorato, A. S., & Bluestone, C. D. (1973). Vocal cord abnormalities in children with velopharyngeal valving problems. *Laryngoscope, 11,* 1745–1753.

Pamplona, M. C., & Ysunza, A. (2000). Active participation of mothers during speech therapy improved language development of children with cleft palate. *Scandinavian Journal of Plastic and Hand Surgery, 34,* 231–236.

Peterson-Falzone, S. J., & Graham, S. (1990). Phoneme-specific nasal emission in children with and without physical anomalies of the velopharyngeal mechanism. *Journal of Speech and Hearing Disorders, 55,* 132–139.

Peterson-Falzone, S. J., Hardin-Jones, M. A., & Karnell, M. P. (2001). *Cleft palate speech* (3rd ed.). St. Louis, MO: Mosby.

Powers, G., & Starr, C. (1974). The effects of muscle exercises on velopharyngeal gap and nasality. *Cleft Palate Journal, 11,* 28–35.

Riski, J. E. (1984). Functional velopharyngeal incompetence: Diagnosis and management. In H. Winitz (Ed.), *Treating articulation disorders: For clinicians by clinicians.* Baltimore: University Park Press.

Ruscello, D. M. (1982). A select review of palatal training procedures. *Cleft Palate Journal, 19,* 181–193.

Ruscello, D. M. (2004). Considerations for behavioral treatment of velopharyngeal closure for speech. In K. R. Bzoch (Ed.), *Communicative disorders related to cleft lip and palate* (5th ed., pp. 763–795). Austin, TX: PRO-ED.

Ruscello, D. M., Shuster, L. I., & Sandwisch, A. (1991). Modification of context-specific nasal emission. *Journal of Speech and Hearing Research, 34,* 27–32.

Schmidt, R. A., & Young, D. E. (1998). Methodology for motor learning: A paradigm for cinematic feedback. *Journal of Motor Behavior, 23,* 13–24.

Shprintzen, R. J., McCall, G. M., & Skolnick, L. (1975). A new therapeutic technique for the treatment of velopharyngeal incompetence. *Journal of Speech and Hearing Disorders, 40,* 69–83.

Slifer, K. J., Amari, A., Diver, T., Hilley, L., Beck, M., Kane, A., et al. (2004). Social interaction patterns of children and adolescents with and without oral clefts during a videotaped analogue social encounter. *Cleft Palate-Craniofacial Journal, 41,* 175–184.

Starr, C. D. (1993). Behavioral approaches to treating velopharyngeal closure and nasality. In K. T. Moller & C. D. Starr (Eds.), *Cleft palate: Interdisciplinary issues and treatment* (pp. 337–356). Austin, TX: PRO-ED.

Tomes, L. A., Kuehn, D. P., & Peterson-Falzone, S. J. (1997). Behavioral treatment of velopharyngeal impairments. In K. R. Bzoch (Ed.), *Communicative disorders related to cleft lip and palate* (4th ed.). Austin, TX: PRO-ED.

Topolski, T. D., & Edwards, T. C. (2005). Quality of life: How do adolescents with facial differences compare with other adolescents? *Cleft Palate-Craniofacial Journal, 42,* 25–32.

Vallino-Napoli, L. D., & Montgomery, A. A. (1997). Examination of the standard deviation of mean Nasalance scores in subjects with cleft palate: Implications for clinical use. *Cleft Palate-Craniofacial Journal, 34,* 512–519.

Volin, R. A. (1998). A relationship between stimulability and the efficacy of visual biofeedback in the training of a respiratory control task. *American Journal of Speech-Language Pathology, 7,* 81–90.

Weismer, G. (2006). Philosophy of research in motor speech disorders. *Clinical Linguistics & Phonetics, 20,* 315–349.

Yorkston, K. M., Spencer, K., Duffy, J., Beukelman, D., Golper, L. A., & Miller, R. (2001). *Journal of Medical Speech Language Pathology, 9,* 257–274.

Ysunza, A., Pamplona, M. C., Femat, T., Mayer, I., & Garcia-Velasco, M. (1997). Videonasendoscopy as an instrument for visual biofeedback during speech in cleft palate patients. *International Journal of Pediatric Otorhinolaryngology, 41,* 291–298.

# CHAPTER 13

# Psychological Characteristics Associated with Cleft Palate

*Lynn C. Richman and Michele J. Eliason*

Richman and Eliason discuss the profession of psychology and the role of the psychologist on the interdisciplinary team. They review literature related to parents' reactions to the birth of children with clefts and parent-child interactions. They discuss the effect of physical attractiveness on attitudes and behaviors of others, as well as current knowledge about intellectual abilities, academic achievement, behavior, and personality development of children with clefts and their status as adults.

1. How might the distortion of facial appearance affect a patient's ability to communicate?
2. What are the four common concerns of parents who have children with clefts? According to Richman and Eliason, how should they be dealt with?
3. In what ways do teachers' and parents' perceptions of the behavior of children with clefts appear to differ?
4. How do children with and without clefts appear to differ on IQ and reading test scores? What is the explanation?
5. According to the authors, what two types of language learning disabilities appear to be present in children with clefts?
6. Is there a high incidence of psychopathology in persons with clefts? Do they have unique personalities?
7. Based on studies reviewed by the authors, how do adults with clefts differ from their peers in relation to marriage, education, and vocational attainment?

## The Profession of Psychology and the Role of the Psychologist on a Cleft Palate and Craniofacial Team

Identifying an appropriately trained psychologist to serve on a cleft palate and craniofacial team requires some awareness of the profession of psychology in general. Practicing psychologists are trained in many different specialty programs, such as clinical, counseling, school, rehabilitation, and health psychology. A psychologist involved with a cleft palate and craniofacial team will need to serve the developmental, cognitive, emotional, and educational concerns relevant to craniofacial anomalies. Any of the above mentioned psychology specialties may provide an individual psychologist with a knowledge background appropriate for a cleft team; however, most important are the individual's intern and postdoctoral training experiences. Psychological aspects of the cleft or craniofacial condition, for example, will require experience with early parent concerns regarding guilt and acceptance of a child with a chronic medical condition; training in early childhood development (especially related to speech, language, and intellectual development); and experience treating emotional responses of the patient, family, peers, and others to possible physical differences. Furthermore, reading and learning problems related to speech and/or language impairment, as well as inhibitions regarding class discussions or volunteering in class, frequently present significant educational and social problems. Therefore, it is important to identify a psychologist with training and experience with these types of psychological problems.

A relatively new specialty in psychology is health psychology, which is frequently identified as pediatric psychology in child health settings or hospitals. This specialty provides training in clinical, educational, and developmental psychology, as well as supervised experience within a health care setting. A health psychologist or pediatric psychologist is especially appropriate to serve on a cleft palate and craniofacial team because the individual will have prior training and experience evaluating and treating children with chronic medical and developmental problems. However, psychologists from any of the mentioned applied psychology programs may have obtained similar expertise through internship and postdoctoral training. The psychologist should be trained in evaluating infants and toddlers, since parents of children with craniofacial anomalies often have concerns regarding developmental and intellectual status. The psychologist should also have expertise in evaluation techniques used to assess children with speech, language, and hearing problems. For example, it is beneficial to know that use of traditional tests of cognitive ability, which are usually verbal, may result in an underestimate of intellectual ability for children with speech and language disorders. Furthermore, evaluation of emotional responses to an observable disability requires training and experience in behavioral and personality assessment of individuals with chronic health-related conditions.

The American Psychological Association, the primary national organization of psychologists, is divided into over 40 specialty divisions. Divisional membership usually identifies special areas of interest and professional expertise. Pertinent divisions for individuals participating on a craniofacial team might include, but are not restricted to, the following: child clinical, pediatric, children and youth, educational, school, clinical, and health psychology. The clinical practice of psychology is governed in most states and provinces by formal licensure and usually requires a doctoral degree, as well as supervised clinical training at the postdoctoral level. Although credentials provide a general index for evaluating a qualified psychologist for a craniofacial team, experience and training in the assessment and treatment considerations previously mentioned are equally important. Psychologists with doctoral training have experience in research methodology and statistics because these are integral components in the measurement of human behavior, intelligence, learning, and emotions. The role of the psychologist on the cleft and craniofacial team will be partially dependent on the makeup of the team. However, typical roles might include the following:

- Consultation with parents who have an adverse emotional reaction to the birth of a child with a craniofacial anomaly
- Developmental assessment during preschool years, especially when a delay in development may be related to speech and/or language deviation, hearing loss, or emotional withdrawal
- Educational assessment during early elementary and adolescent years
- Evaluation of behavior and emotions when children respond negatively to teasing or lack of acceptance by others
- Personality evaluation, especially during adolescence or early adulthood, when withdrawal or acting out may be a response to the disability

In addition, the psychologist's input is frequently important in management decisions. For example, the timing of surgical intervention might be clarified by the psychologist's evaluation of emotional response to appearance. The psychologist may be asked to assist in the differential diagnosis of developmental disability, language disability, and severe emotional withdrawal when verbal skills are delayed. Another patient management decision that may involve the psychologist's input is parental or patient noncompliance with recommended treatment. The psychologist also provides objective assessment of development, behavior, intelligence, and personality to assure that management decisions are based on reliable measurement of the child's functioning rather than on assumptions of parents, teachers, or others.

## Overview of Psychological Aspects of Cleft Lip and Palate

Children with cleft lip and palate are at risk for the development of psychological problems because of several factors. They often have a visible facial deformity, which may elicit negative reactions from parents, siblings, peers, teachers, and others. The face is a significant source of communication that provides the initial stimulus for the expression of the speaker's emotions, character, and personality (Cohen, 1982). Atypical facial appearance may impair the ability of others to accurately interpret facial expression as a source of nonverbal communication. Another risk factor for cognitive and psychosocial concerns includes a high incidence of early middle ear infections, with resulting fluctuating hearing sensitivity and hearing loss, along with frequent hospitalizations, separation from family and friends, and possible speech deviations. A third risk factor is the high frequency of speech problems, including articulation and resonance difficulties. These speech disorders are related to factors that require habilitation, including surgery for palatal problems, dental intervention, and speech treatment. The speech difficulties may result in being misunderstood or being teased and are often accompanied by self-perception concerns, decreased self-esteem, and social withdrawal, which may warrant psychological intervention. All of these risk factors may be related to secondary psychological factors, including behavioral inhibition, lower school achievement, and self-consciousness regarding the perceptions of others. Psychosocial problems secondary to the disability may also adversely influence the final habilitative process more than the primary disability does (Lencione, 1980). There is a need for awareness of these psychological factors because an individual's behavior may be influenced more by self-perception of facial appearance and speech than by the "objective" assessment of these by professionals. These psychological influences may create learning, emotional, and social effects throughout life (Millard & Richman, 2001; Richman & Eliason, 1986a, 1986b).

The following discussion of psychosocial aspects is divided into these areas: (a) early parental reactions and developmental concerns, (b) parent-child interactions, (c) physical attractiveness variables, (d) intellectual ability and school achievement, (e) behavior and personality, and (f) psychological adjustment of adults with cleft lip and palate. Throughout this chapter, the term *children with clefts* will refer generically to all types of clefts and related craniofacial conditions.

## Early Parental Reactions and Developmental Concerns

Giving birth to a child with an observable medical condition can be a traumatic, guilt-laden event. A wide variety of negative emotions have been described in parents' responses to an infant with a cleft: grief, anxiety, confusion, depression, shock, anger, disbelief, inadequacy, resentment, withdrawal, and frustration (Clifford, 1987). Cohen (1982) categorized five stages of parental reaction, beginning with shock or disbelief, followed by sadness, denial, equilibrium, and finally reorganization. It has been suggested that the stress of the birth of a child with a disability may lead to family disintegration in some cases, but may actually strengthen family bonds in others. Although the duration of the initial crisis period has been reported to vary from family to family, most studies, usually based on retrospective interviews, have found that rapid dissipation of the negative feelings occurred within a short period (Clifford, 1987). For a comprehensive review of these early psychosocial factors, see Eder (1995).

The resolution of early negative reactions can be facilitated by professional intervention. Although most parents are informed about the cleft at birth, some learn about it later, especially when the infants have cleft palate only. It has been hypothesized that the parents of a child with a cleft may not fulfill the usual social rituals associated with a new baby, such as encouraging family and friends to meet the infant. Also of concern is the finding that mothers of infants born with cleft palate may show varying face-to-face interactions with their infant (Endriga & Speltz, 1997). However, this is not always directly related to appearance per se and may be related to other parent or child characteristics.

The following are some areas of parental concern expressed shortly after the birth of a child with a cleft:

1. The child's appearance
2. Feeding
3. Desirability of immediate surgery
4. Speech development
5. Reaction of the spouse
6. Reaction of siblings
7. Reaction of friends and family
8. Intellectual development
9. Recurrence of the defect in yet unborn children

These concerns have been reported by several investigators (Benson, Gross, Messer, Kellum, & Passmore, 1991; Eliason, 1991; Endriga & Kapp-Simon, 1999; Richman & Eliason, 2001).

Appearance variables are frequently the major concern of parents and are discussed in a separate section. The desire for immediate surgery and concern over reactions of others are likely related to the child's appearance. Although speech development is a legitimate concern for parents, some parents with no prior knowledge of the cleft condition have expressed the belief that the child would not learn to speak or would be unintelligible. It is important to be alert to the fact that parents often mistakenly associate defective speech with the possibility of lowered intelligence. It is important to assess the parents' knowledge concerning cleft lip and palate shortly after birth and provide them with realistic expectations. Continued effort should be made to monitor parents' expectations and knowledge of various treatment considerations throughout the habilitation years.

Feeding problems may present psychological concerns because feeding a baby is usually a time of closeness and attachment for mother and infant. The nontraditional feeding methods required for some children with clefts may initially produce anxiety for mothers; however, in the majority of cases, feeding is rarely a long-term problem. For extremely difficult to feed infants, it may be important to supplement the mother and child's bonding experience independent of the feeding time, when physical closeness can be a more pleasant interaction. This is especially important for those parents who may experience negative social interaction behaviors such as less face-to-face contact or less eye contact with their infant (Langlois, 1995).

Another problem not frequently encountered in parents' reports, but likely to be a source of some concern, is the high incidence of middle ear infections. The additional stress on parents frequently awakened by an infant with ear pain may exacerbate other sources of stress in managing a child with a chronic medical condition. In addition, the child needs close monitoring of hearing status and perhaps repeated placement of ventilation tubes, thus adding to the frequency of clinic visits. The time-off needed from work and the expense of this management may create further parental difficulties.

A frequently felt but often unexpressed parental concern is who might be responsible for the defect. Parents may think of other, perhaps quite distant, family members with the disorder and worry about whether their spouse will blame them. Less frequent, but quite dramatic when it occurs, is the mother's concern that she may have done something during pregnancy to create the condition. Although genetic counseling and information regarding reproduction and fetal developmental are beneficial, it is also important to assess the emotional response to this information. Many examples of parents' thoughts and feelings are provided by intensive interviews reported by Spriestersbach (1973). Based on these reports, it is apparent that positive yet direct questioning is needed to elicit these underlying thoughts. Sensitivity to these parental concerns may provide a pathway to assist the family toward relative normalization of the parent-child relationship (Clifford, 1987).

Some parents are concerned that the child may have brain damage or mental retardation. This may be (a) based on misconceptions related to perceptions of people who have other syndromic conditions that affect both brain and face or (b) due to the physical proximity of the defect to the brain. Providing assurance regarding the incidence of mental retardation in the cleft population may not be compelling if the parent has psychological fears related to many of society's superstitions. Introducing parents to other families who have children with clefts and normal intelligence and development may be more reassuring than professional counseling. Also, a professional proactive approach that points out the more common and milder developmental risks and how these can be treated may provide the reassurance often associated with a knowledgeable and sensitive cleft and craniofacial team.

Because parents experience a variety of emotional reactions to the child with a cleft and have continued developmental concerns, it is important for the professional to determine which of these are realistic and typical. Parental concerns regarding appearance, surgical interventions, speech, and feeding are so common that counseling regarding these areas should occur with almost every parent of a child who has a cleft lip and palate. Even though a parent may not verbalize a concern, underlying feelings can affect treatment. It is especially important for the professional to provide a direct but supportive interview regarding sensitive parental feelings that may have the potential to create long-term emotional problems, including possible negative reactions of a spouse, anxiety related to the nature of intercourse, and guilt regarding maternal care during fetal development. These are the least likely feelings to be expressed due to the sensitivity of the subjects. However, if such feelings exist and remain unresolved, the effects may be disastrous to the family. The professional must also be alert to the possibility of denial of parental negative feelings toward the child, because this may lead to projection of blame onto the child, a subtle form of rejection. Fortunately, the literature indicates that most parents of children with cleft or other craniofacial anomalies adjust to the management problems and are realistic in their concerns for their child. This process of adaptation can be facilitated by proactive counseling and information sharing by knowledgeable professionals rather than waiting until problems are expressed by parents.

## Parent-Child Interactions

Attachment is defined as a unique relationship between two people that is specific and enduring. A mother must first accept her baby before an attachment or bond can occur. Eye contact, touching, and holding of the child are important factors in forming the mother-infant bond, as are the compatibility of the mother's and child's temperaments. Although the fear of having a baby with an anomaly is experienced by many pregnant women, few are prepared for the emotional shock involved with the reality of an infant with a craniofacial anomaly.

In spite of many early concerns, parents of children with clefts generally demonstrate satisfactory adjustment and form positive parent-child attachments. Perhaps the process of healthy adjustment is aided by improvements in early medical-surgical interventions, increased emphasis on public awareness of the condition, and parental knowledge of other families with children who have clefts. McDonald (1979) suggested that parental needs and stresses are variable during different periods in the child's development. Stressful periods include the birth experience and initial hospitalization, the beginning of expressive language, entry into school, and the adolescent years. In most cases, periods of relative calm are interspersed with the traumatic events. It is interesting to note that the life events reported by MacDonald produce mild stress for parents of any child; however, the intensity of stress may be exacerbated for parents of a child with a facial anomaly. Although some early reports suggested that facial impairment might decrease parental attachment, it has been shown that parents of children with cleft lip and palate showed more involvement with their infant than parents of children with cleft palate only and less facial anomaly (Endriga & Speltz, 1997). Thus, it is important to consider parental factors as well as infant factors beyond the face when assessing maternal-child attachment.

Several studies have examined parenting characteristics of parents of children with clefts beyond the early infancy stage. One study found that parents of children with clefts were more permissive of acting-out behavior (Tobiasen & Hiebert, 1984). Speltz, Morton, Goodell, and Clarren (1993) also found a higher incidence of acting out in children with clefts. However, acting-out behavior has not been a prominent feature of most school-age and older children with clefts. Rather, overinhibition is a more typical long-term behavior, with acting out being more transient (Richman & Millard, 1997). In a study of older children, Richman and Harper (1978a) compared parental child-rearing practices as reported by children with clefts versus a group of control children without clefts. The children reported their perceptions of the parenting techniques used by their parents. The study examined reports of 68 children with clefts ranging in age from 9 to 18, and 68 matched controls. Findings revealed no significant differences between children with clefts and controls on parental acceptance/rejection or firm control/lax control measures. However, males with clefts perceived their mothers as exerting greater psychological control or intrusiveness than did male controls, suggesting some degree of overprotectiveness by mothers of males with clefts.

In summary, though many factors could interfere with healthy parent-child interactions, such as the stress of dealing with an "imperfect" baby, frequent hospitalizations, and visible anomaly, the majority of families appear to experience healthy interactions. Many impaired parent-child interactions may be due to factors other than the cleft and may only be exacerbated by this condition. Objective information regarding parent-child interactions is sparse. Most reports are based on parental interview or, in some cases, interview of the child. The most comprehensive data are based on reports of both parent and child (Spriestersbach, 1973). The findings reveal many areas of concern that warrant further investigation. These include examination of family dynamics by comparing the behavior of the parents toward their child with a cleft and toward their other children. Further research is also needed to determine how concerns expressed by parents affect their behavior toward a child with a cleft compared with behavior of parents of a child without a cleft. One question that needs further research is how noncleft variables, including parent and family variables, affect psychological outcomes of children with clefts (Speltz & Richman, 1997). An important question is whether the parents' expressed concerns affect parent-child interaction. If so, are these exaggerated effects of normal parent concerns regarding birth, appearance, development, and so forth, or are they unique to the parent-child interactions of the family with a child with a cleft? A comprehensive review of these issues can be found in Eder (1995).

## Physical Attractiveness Variables

### Subjects Without Physical Differences

Physical appearance variables often convey as much information about an individual as actual behavior and personality traits. Research in social psychology has revealed the strength of physical attractiveness in forming opinions about others (Bull & Rumsey, 1988; Langlois, 1995). Children without physical anomalies but of lesser attractiveness were rated by teachers as having lower achievement, less chance at higher education, and fewer peer relationships than attractive peers (Clifford & Walster, 1973). Female college students rated an unattractive child who had committed a serious transgression more harshly than an attractive child who had committed the same act (Dion, 1972). Children rate unattractive peers as less friendly, not as smart, and less desirable playmates (Dion, 1973; Langlois & Stephan, 1977). Research on stereotyping based on appearance has shown that less attractive children were more likely to be blamed for behavioral infractions and more likely to be referred by their teachers for psychological and educational services. Research on children with clefts has shown effects similar to those seen in noncleft studies. Children with bilateral clefts have been rated more negatively on behavioral characteristics than those with unilateral clefts, who were rated more negatively than children without clefts (Schneiderman & Harding, 1984). Also children with clefts were rated more negatively on personality characteristics than children without clefts (Richman, 1978a; Tobiasen, 1987).

Observations of unattractive children in play suggest that they behave according to others' expectations (Snyder, Tanke, & Berscheid, 1977) or play with others of the same attractiveness level (Langlois & Downs, 1979). Langlois and Downs also found unattractive preschoolers to be more aggressive and active than attractive children. Dion and Berscheid (1974) reported that unattractive male preschoolers were considered more aggressive, and unattractive female preschoolers more fearful, than attractive peers. Some studies have found no significant relationship between school achievement and attractiveness; however, Lerner and Lerner (1977) found a low, but significantly positive correlation between attractiveness and grade point average. However, there may be a stronger relationship between achievement and attractiveness for individuals with observable physical anomalies. If attractiveness variables influence interactions of individuals without anomalies, a facial anomaly may create even greater difficulty in social interactions.

One problem with much of the research on facial disfigurement and perception of others is that most of the research has been based on facial photographs, which omits aspects of facial movement and expression. One study that used more realistic videotapes of children with and without a facial disfigurement (port-wine stain) found that peers' judgments of personality, attractiveness, and socialization were more complex than just the disfigurement per se (Demellweek, Humphris, Hare, & Brown, 1997). For more extensive review of the perception of facial disfigurement and social judgment, see Bull and Rumsey (1988).

## Attitudes Toward Children with Physical Disabilities

Livneh (1982) discussed the origins of negative attitudes toward people with physical disabilities and listed several possible factors in the development and maintenance of these negative reactions. These factors include:

1. Sociocultural conditioning, with society's emphasis on beauty, youth, athletic prowess, productivity, and achievement.

2. Childhood influences, which involve parental beliefs, both verbal and behavioral, and child-rearing practices that emphasize health and normalcy.
3. Psychodynamic explanations of negative attitudes, including the requirement of mourning, whereby people with disabilities should grieve the lost part or function and are expected to suffer. Disability is sometimes associated with punishment for sin, or fear of social ostracism from being seen in the company of someone with a disability and guilt over being able-bodied.
4. Disability-related factors, including whether the disorder is functional or organic, level of severity, degree of visibility of the handicap, degree of cosmetic involvement, contagiousness, affected body part, and degree of curability.
5. Other miscellaneous factors, including aesthetic aversion, threat to body image, attitudes toward minority groups in general, and demographic and personality variables.

In a famous series of studies, Richardson (1970, 1971a, 1971b) reported on investigations of children with and without handicaps at a summer camp. Children ranked drawings of children based on preference for friendship in the following order: (1) no handicap, (2) crutches and brace on one leg, (3) wheelchair bound, (4) hand missing, (5) facial disfigurement, and (6) obesity. These rankings were relatively consistent over age, sex, and socioeconomic status. Females tended to rate facial disfigurement more negatively, whereas males rated functional disability more negatively (Richardson, 1970, 1971a). Unfortunately, Richardson (1971b) found that even after peers had interacted with children with handicaps during the summer camp experience, the rankings did not change.

## Individuals with Cleft Lip and Palate

Podol and Salvia (1976) examined stereotypes associated with a cleft. Sixty speech pathology students, all of whom read the same case study of a 9-year-old female with a repaired cleft (type unspecified) viewed one of two pictures, one showing a cleft lip scar and one retouched to remove the scar. Those who saw the picture with a lip scar while listening to speech judged the speech as more nasal and were more likely to recommend speech therapy than those who listened to the same speech while observing the picture with the lip scar removed.

Teachers' judgments of the abilities of children are affected by the severity of facial disfigurement. Richman (1978a) divided children with cleft lip and palate into two groups: one with relatively normal facial appearance and one with moderate to severe disfigurement. The groups were formed on the basis of independent ratings by five professionals prior to the study. All children had also received individual intelligence tests prior to the study, and the teachers did not know the results. Teachers underestimated the ability of bright children with significant disfigurement and overestimated the ability of slower children with significant disfigurement. Children with relatively normal facial appearance received quite accurate estimates of intellectual ability by their teachers. It is not clear what effect unrealistic teacher expectations may have on actual child behavior, although some studies have suggested that less attractive individuals receive more punishment, have lower achievement, and are less friendly (Berscheid & Walster, 1974; Clifford & Walster, 1973; Dion, 1972, 1973).

Richman, Holmes, and Eliason (1985) compared two groups of adolescents with both cleft lip and cleft palate who were divided by parent ratings on a behavior checklist into a well-adjusted group ($n$ = 18) and a poorly adjusted group ($n$ = 18). In addition to parents' ratings of behavior, the adolescents' teachers were asked to rate their facial appearance. The adolescents also completed self-ratings of behavior and appearance. It was found that well-adjusted adolescents' ratings of appearance and behavior were similar to those of teachers and parents, suggesting a realistic perception. The poorly adjusted group rated themselves as more attractive than did teachers and rated their behavior as more "normal" than did their parents. The authors suggested that poorly adjusted adolescents were not realistic in their perceptions, perhaps due to denial of facial disfigurement and resultant social withdrawal.

## Summary

Although little research is available on peers', teachers', and others' perceptions of children with cleft lip and palate, research with other populations with physical stigmata suggests that a subtle negative reaction may impair the judgment of others in estimating ability and behavior. The research available regarding children with cleft lip and palate indicates that teachers rate the children's behavior as more inhibited than parents do (Richman, 1978b), and teachers underestimate the intellectual ability of bright children with cleft lip and palate who have significant facial disfigurement (Richman, 1978a). Furthermore, the research suggests that school-age children are less likely to choose a child with a cleft lip and palate as a friend than children with other physical anomalies. The relationships cited above do not provide enough evidence to determine specific effects of facial disfigurement on the judgment of others.

It is extremely difficult to isolate the possible negative effects of facial disfigurement on others because judgments of others are based on many complex aspects of appearance and behavior. Many of the research paradigms used in nondisabled populations appear to be appropriate, such as examining judgments of the same individual under different facial appearance conditions while holding all other conditions constant. This, of course, is an extremely difficult task to design and must be done with picture alteration. One study that examined appearance along with other variables on the adjustment of children with cleft found that appearance did have a significant relationship to adjustment, at least in some cleft subgroups (Millard & Richman, 2001).

## Intellectual Ability and School Achievement

There is a high frequency of grade retention, lower achievement, and learning disability in children with clefts (Broder, Richman, & Matheson, 1998). Although many early studies suggested that children with clefts showed lower than average intellectual ability, later studies have disputed this finding (Richman & Eliason, 1986b). There are several hypothesized causes of intellectual delay and learning problems for these students. These include speech and language problems, hearing loss, social withdrawal, and language-based learning disability (Richman & Eliason, 2001). Even when matched to controls by IQ, children with clefts have been shown to have lower achievement (Richman, 1976; Richman & Harper, 1978b). In fact, Richman (1980) showed that approximately 50% of a group of children with clefts who had average IQ were below average in reading. Another study showed low written expression and syntax in a group of children with clefts who had average and above intelligence (Kommers & Sullivan, 1979). Two studies have suggested a sex × cleft type interaction with IQ (Eliason & Richman, 1987; Lamb, Wilson, & Leeper, 1973). Those children in the lowest frequency by occurrence groups (females with cleft lip and palate and males with cleft palate only) were more likely to be "language deficient." It has also been proposed that younger children with clefts have impaired language skills that improve with age (Musgrave, McWilliams, & Matthews, 1975). This interpretation is based on data showing lower verbal ability for younger children with cleft lip and palate and higher verbal ability for older children. However, this explanation does not account for the cleft type × sex differences in verbal ability. There has also been a report indicating that language skills of children with clefts decline with age (Kommers & Sullivan, 1979); however, this study was based on measures of written language and, therefore, cannot be compared to the other studies that used measures of spoken language.

Some studies have attempted to isolate specific cognitive disabilities in children with cleft lip and palate. Brantley and Clifford (1979) compared a group of adolescents with cleft palate, a group with obesity, and a control group on several cognitive measures of language, memory, and visual perception, and found no significant differences. However, there is some question as to whether all these tasks were actually intellectual or cognitive style measures, and the effects of IQ were not controlled. In general, it is recognized that most of the cognitive deficits seen in cleft populations are related to language-based learning problems (Lamb, Wilson, & Leeper, 1972; Richman, 1980; Richman & Eliason, 1984; Richman & Ryan, 2000). Specific language deficits may even account for some findings of poor visual-perceptual skills because some picture tasks require naming skill and some strategies used to solve visual-perceptual tasks rely on verbal mediation.

Several studies by Richman have suggested at least two types of language learning disability in children with cleft lip and palate who demonstrate verbal deficits. Richman (1980) examined 57 children with clefts who had Verbal IQs less than Performance IQs. This study included examination of results from the *Hiskey-Nebraska Test of Learning Aptitude,* a test originally developed for deaf children which requires no spoken language on the part of the examiner or the child. However, it does test nonverbal language mediation skills and short-term memory. One group of children with clefts displayed average performance on the Hiskey, indicating a specific verbal expressive deficit. The other group, however, demonstrated poor associative reasoning (verbal mediation) on the Hiskey, reflecting a general language disability. This group included a high number of males with cleft palate only who also displayed a significant degree of academic underachievement.

A later study compared 24 children with cleft palate only (CPO) and 24 children with cleft lip and palate (CLP) (ages 8–12 years) who were matched for age, sex, and Verbal, Performance, and Full Scale IQs (Richman & Eliason, 1984). The sample consisted of 14 males and 10 females in each group. The Hiskey and cognitive measures of associative reasoning, memory, visual-perceptual skills, and reading achievement were administered. Results supported the finding that children with CPO are more likely to have pervasive language disability, whereas children with CLP have a milder verbal expressive deficit and higher reading achievement. The type of reading errors also differed between groups. The CPO group tended to make more whole-word, gestalt-type errors and demonstrated poorer performance on guessing a word based on its initial letter. Children with CLP were more likely to make phonetic errors reflecting peripheral speech problems interfering with phonics performance. Despite the lack of any finding of neuropsychological deficits, children with CLP had lower reading achievement than expected, reflecting the effects that even a mild disability can have on reading.

In a survey of the incidence of reading disability in a large sample of children with clefts (Richman & Eliason, 1985), the overall incidence of reading disability in the sample was 36%, compared with estimated figures of 10%–20% in the general population. Children with CPO had an incidence of 48% compared with about 30% in children with CLP. This finding of more significant language and reading problems for children with CPO than for those with CLP has received further support (Richman, Eliason, & Lindgren, 1988). In this latter study of 172 children, the children with CPO had a high rate of reading disability at all ages, whereas the children with CLP had decreasing rates of reading disability from ages 6 to 13. A two-center comparison study also reported a 30%–40% incidence of learning disorder in cleft populations (Broder et al., 1998).

Several recent reports have analyzed the type of reading disabilities and the underlying cognitive deficits of children with clefts. In one study, models of dyslexia were applied to 154 children, ages 7–11, with nonsyndromic CLP (Richman & Ryan, 2002). Of those children screened, 30% met criteria for reading disability. The models of dyslexia that were examined were (a) phonemic awareness disorder, (b) dysphasia (verbal expression deficit), and (c) dysnomia (word finding deficit). These three models were investigated comparing two groups of children with clefts, one group with and one group without reading disability. The reading disability was related most to dysnomia. Dysnomia in children with clefts is often associated with short-term verbal memory deficits. This deficit is not related only to early speech problems because it persists after speech has improved.

Findings of recent studies suggest that there may be a more basic neurodevelopmental difference in some children with clefts. Further studies of neuropsychological and neuromaturation functions of children with clefts are indicated. One study suggested possible neurological volume differences in adult males with CPO, based on neuroimaging (Nopoulos et al., 2000). Several related studies found that there is an increased incidence of corpus collosum or midline brain anomalies in adult males with nonsyndromic cleft (Nopoulos et al., 2001). Furthermore, brain imaging has shown atypical structural brain abnormalities in adult males with clefts of the lip and palate, and these occur in areas associated with language and reading functions (Nopoulos et al., 2002). Another study suggests that in children with clefts, dysnomia (naming deficits) can occur independent of speech problems or social anxiety, suggesting that dysnomia may have more of a biological base (Richman & Ryan, 2000).

In summary, although early studies suggested that children with clefts have lower IQs than the general population, in most cases this can be attributed to only a verbal deficit. No other specific cognitive deficits have been consistently identified. The verbal deficit has been identified in two subtypes of children with clefts who have language disabilities. One form involves only a mild verbal expressive deficit characterized by word finding problems (dysnomia) and short-term memory deficit with some effect on reading. This problem may be developmental in nature, similar to mild developmental dyslexia. The other subtype involves a more pervasive language disorder with more profound effects on overall school achievement.

School achievement deficits have consistently been identified in children with cleft lip and palate, and remedial intervention, such as special reading assistance, is required for these children. More children (especially males) with CPO demonstrate a more pervasive language disorder that warrants more extensive language evaluation and therapy. Further research in language and other neuropsychological functions of children with clefts is warranted to determine if there are indications of neurological impairment, especially in certain cleft type $\times$ sex subgroups.

## Behavior and Personality

Studies in several areas of disability have attempted to identify specific personality patterns related to specific types of disability; however, this has not been successful (Shontz, 1975). In the area of cleft palate, there have been no reports of significant psychopathology. Although some studies have noted subtle variations of normal behavior, there are some inconsistencies in the findings. Elementary-age children with clefts have been found to have lower self-concept than controls (Broder, Smith, & Strauss, 1994; Broder & Strauss, 1989; Kapp-Simon, 1986; Kapp-Simon, Simon, & Kristovich, 1992), but adolescents with clefts were found to have higher self-concept than controls in one study (Brantley & Clifford, 1979). However, the different age groups and different self-esteem measures make comparisons among these studies difficult. Overall, there is increasing evidence that the relationships among cleft-related risk variables (speech, facial appearance) and adjustment variables (self-esteem, inhibition) are complex and may be different for different cleft subtypes (Millard & Richman, 2001). Millard and Richman (2001) found that facial appearance was an important predictor of adjustment in children with CLP, but speech was a more important predictor of adjustment for children with CPO.

In a study of *Minnesota Multiphasic Personality Inventory* (MMPI) results from 52 adolescents with clefts, Harper, Richman, and Snider (1980) found no significant psychopathology. The authors did note that the adolescents with clefts displayed excessive inhibition of impulse, increased self-concern, and ruminative self-doubts over interpersonal relationships. Females with clefts expressed more dissatisfaction with their life situation than did males. Richman (1983) also examined 30 adolescents with clefts and 30 controls (ages 15–18) regarding their self-perceived adjustment and concerns related to speech, social, and appearance factors. The MMPI and a structured interview were administered. No significant difference was found between the control group and the entire cleft sample on perceived educational satisfaction or social satisfaction. MMPI results showed that 16 of the profiles of adolescents with clefts were normal and 14 were abnormal. The adolescents with abnormal profiles expressed more concern over school, social, and appearance variables. Even well-adjusted adolescents expressed some concern over facial appearance, suggesting that facial concerns were related to normal adolescent concern over appearance and body image. Results indicated that younger adolescents may be more concerned with speech, whereas older adolescents may worry more about appearance. Beder and Weinstein (1980) found that adolescents with orofacial anomalies scored higher than the norms on the Inadequacy, Anger, and Sensitivity scales of the *Cornell Medical Index*. A study of younger children with clefts (who were in elementary school) also showed excessive inhibition of impulse (Richman & Harper, 1979). In an important

8-year longitudinal study, Richman and Millard (1997) found that although there may be transient periods of acting out, behavioral inhibition is constant over the childhood years for many children with clefts. Another important finding of this study was that adolescent females with clefts showed increased behavioral inhibition and acting out, which may suggest more serious psychological discomfort.

Spriestersbach (1973), using structured parent interviews, found that parents perceived their children with clefts as less independent, less aggressive, and less confident than control children. Richman (1976, 1978b) and Richman and Harper (1978b), using behavior checklists, and Richman and Harper (1979), using self-rated personality measures, supported those findings. These studies indicated that children with clefts tend to score higher than noncleft children on internalizing factors (withdrawal, inhibition of impulse).

Richman (1978b) found a difference between teacher and parent ratings of children with CLP. Teachers viewed both male and female children with clefts as more inhibited in the classroom than other children, whereas parents rated their children's behavior as comparable to that of other children. This finding could be related to different behaviors in the different settings, or it could indicate that parents do not perceive inhibited behavior as a problem. A child's parents tended to show good agreement with each other.

There appears to be some relationship between cleft severity and certain measures of personality. Children with milder degrees of facial deformity showed greater inhibition of impulse than children with more severe disfigurements (Harper et al., 1980). This finding is contrary to the common assumption that more severe deformity leads to more withdrawal and passivity. It may be that the less severe disability creates more behavioral withdrawal in order to avoid calling attention to oneself, whereas more severe disfigurement is more noticeable and not likely to be overlooked.

The reasons for age, sex, and cleft type variations in behavior remain unclear, and further examination of these relationships is warranted. A study by Millard and Richman (2001) provided a suggestion of some of these relationships. This study examined 65 children, ages 8–17 years, who were placed into three groups: unilateral cleft lip and palate, bilateral cleft lip and palate, and CPO. The findings indicated that the children with CPO showed more problems of anxiety, depression, and school learning than the other groups. Also, these problems for the CPO group were related the most to speech problems. The other two groups showed fewer problems, with the unilateral group showing the fewest problems.

Also, these latter two groups showed a greater relationship of adjustment problems to facial appearance rather than to speech.

Few studies have examined interventions to improve social skills and decrease the inhibition of children with clefts. However, it has been shown that social skills may be related to appearance and behavioral inhibition, suggesting the need for social skills training (Kapp-Simon et al., 1992).

In summary, although the cleft palate population exhibits no increased incidence of psychopathology, several studies do indicate excessive inhibition. This pattern may be even more pronounced in mildly affected individuals than in those with more severe deformities. Furthermore, behavioral manifestations may be related to age, sex, and cleft type, without clear support for consistent generalizations. Children and adolescents with clefts appear to experience normal developmental stresses, which may be exacerbated by physical disfigurement, speech problems, and social responses of others.

## Psychological Adjustment of Adults with Cleft Lip and Palate

The same factors that contribute to maladjustment of children or adolescents with clefts—parental reactions, physical appearance variables, lowered academic expectations and school achievement, and behavioral inhibition— may also affect the adjustment of adults with clefts. However, there are very few reports on the psychological adjustment of adults with cleft. Clifford, Crocker, and Pope (1972) evaluated 98 adults who had undergone surgery by the same surgeon 22–27 years prior to the interview. Their satisfaction with employment, marriage, and accomplishments was high, although they had some continued concerns about appearance and speech. In general, however, this group perceived their clefts as having little influence on their lives.

In a comprehensive adult study, Peter and associates presented a four-part discussion of adult functioning in 196 individuals (ages 24–54) with cleft lip and/or palate, 190 of their siblings, and 209 random controls. Questionnaire data were gathered in four major areas: marriage, education, vocational and economic aspects, and social integration. Peter and Chinsky (1974a) reported that adults with clefts marry at a significantly lower rate than siblings or controls; 26.5% of the cleft group, 8.9% of the siblings, and 8.6% of the controls had never married. There was also a difference in age at first marriage; adults with clefts marry later (age 24.2) than siblings (21.7) or controls (21.2). Individuals with CLP marry later than individuals with CPO, perhaps reflecting the effects of cosmetic appearance. Although the divorce rate was highest for controls (who also married the earliest), the divorce rate for individuals with clefts was higher than for their siblings. Individuals with clefts also had significantly fewer children per marriage and were more likely to remain childless than siblings or controls.

Peter and Chinsky (1974b) found that general educational attainment and school dropout rates did not differ between cleft and noncleft groups, although other studies have suggested a higher dropout rate for individuals with clefts (McWilliams & Paradise, 1973). Of the 196 persons with clefts, 26% had attended 1 or more years of college, compared to 29% of the siblings and 34% of the controls. This was not a statistically significant difference. Individuals with CLP were more likely to complete college than persons with CPO. Questionnaire responses comparing educational aspirations with actual educational attainment indicated that a significantly greater number of persons with clefts had aspired to higher education than they actually obtained. Of those aspiring to higher education, individuals with CLP had lower aspirations than controls, whereas those with CPO did not differ from controls. Additionally, the rate of college attendance was slightly lower for individuals with clefts than for siblings or controls, but the rate of completion of college was comparable.

Peter, Chinsky, and Fisher (1975a) examined vocational and economic conditions of individuals with cleft lip and palate. In this phase of the study, the socioeconomic status (SES) scales of the U.S. Census were used to judge economic status of the groups. No differences were found in mean SES levels or occupational and educational status; however, income status did differ. Individuals with clefts earned less than siblings, although they did not differ from controls. Persons with clefts also earned less gross family income than either siblings or controls. Employment stability (continuous employment in one job) did not differ by overall groups; however, periods of unemployment were more frequent and of greater duration for persons with clefts than for either siblings or controls. Controls felt more suited to their jobs, but the groups did not differ in job satisfaction. Individuals with clefts tended to have higher aspirations for getting a better job than did controls. These results suggest that adults with clefts may experience less job satisfaction and income than others even when they have similar educational levels. It is unclear whether this difference is related to objective work productivity differences or possible prejudices of employers.

Peter, Chinsky, and Fisher (1975b) evaluated the family and social integration of adults with clefts. Family interdependence measures showed that persons with clefts, regardless of marital status, were more likely to live with relatives and, of those who lived away from home, to visit relatives more often than siblings or controls. They were also more likely to settle in the same geographic area as their parents. When home activities were categorized as active or passive, individuals with clefts were more likely to engage in passive activities and reported more difficulty in meeting new people, reported fewer close friendships, and belonged to fewer community organizations than siblings or controls.

Peter and associates warned against literal interpretation of their results for several reasons. Self-report questionnaires of this type may be misleading due to a possible discrepancy between self-perceptions of behavior and actual behavior or to a social desirability effect, whereby individuals provide favorable interpretations of their situation. However, even with limitations of the method, it seems that, like children with cleft lip or palate, adults with clefts differ from controls in subtle ways. Although these adults report more social isolation, they express no significant signs of emotional maladjustment. For example, Richman and Harper (1980) found that young adults with clefts (mean age 18.5) experience less self-doubt and concern over social interactions than do adolescents with clefts (Harper & Richman, 1978). However, these young adults had received ongoing team care since infancy, which may have assisted them in developing maximum physical and psychological adjustment. In one study of middle-age adults with clefts, Richman (1997) found self-reports of more internalizing characteristics, but no significant personality disorder.

## Summary and Conclusions

This chapter discussed the major areas of psychological concern for individuals with clefts. Early concerns are largely parent based and include problems related to coping with the birth of a child with a cleft and learning to adjust to a long-term disability. Parents are concerned about the infant's appearance and how others will react. They are concerned about feeding, speech, and intellectual development. They worry about how they will cope financially with the numerous surgeries and extensive orthodontic treatments, and they fear that subsequent children will be born with clefts. Many of these concerns can be dealt with effectively by the cleft and craniofacial team. Most parents quickly adjust to different feeding methods and can be reassured regarding speech and mental development. Financial concerns are often overcome by insurance or state support. Genetic counseling provides the parents with empirical information about the nature of clefting and risk figures for having another child with a cleft.

The issue of physical appearance is frequently not dealt with satisfactorily. All team members need to be sensitive to the variations of physical appearance that may remain for many patients, even after extensive treatment. Professionals should discuss realistic management goals with parents and children regarding appearance and speech performance. As many studies have shown, even minor deviations from normal appearance or speech may influence other people's perceptions of the child. These perceptions can result in the child's having more difficulty with social interactions and in lessened expectations by others (teachers, parents, employers). Use of pictures or real-life models after treatment may help persons with clefts and their families to establish realistic goals. It is also important for professionals to be aware that objective measures of appearance and speech may be less influential on the child's adjustment than self-perception of these variables. Hypersensitivity to minor deviations and denial of disfigurement need to be identified and dealt with.

Another issue that needs to be addressed by cleft palate management teams is the problem of underachievement and learning disability in children with clefts. Parents should be alerted to watch for signs of learning problems (especially reading), and teachers should be informed of the child's abilities in order to avoid possible detrimental expectations related to the physical attractiveness stereotype. Because teachers may underestimate the ability of children with facial disfigurement, they may attribute lower achievement to perceived lower ability level and, therefore, may not seek further diagnosis or treatment. Routine screening of a child's reading ability is a cost-effective means of identifying reading problems early and instituting remediation before the problem becomes more severe.

Behavioral symptoms of inhibition of impulse, which are frequent characteristics of children with clefts, may contribute to lower school achievement and less satisfactory social relations. Helping the child to cope with an altered facial appearance at an early age may aid later social adjustment. Cleft type, age, and sex seem to influence behavior, although these relationships need further study. In general, children with clefts show relatively good adjustment to their disability, with only minor variations of normal behavior. Adults with clefts appear similar to controls in social relationships, college completion rates, and levels of employment. Further studies are needed to examine those individuals with clefts who demonstrate adjustment problems, to determine more specific factors related to these problems.

In conclusion, the psychologist serves a vital function on a cleft and craniofacial team in the areas of developmental, intellectual, and personality assessment; parent and/or child counseling; liaison work with schools; monitoring of possible psychological consequences of disability; and fostering an atmosphere sensitive to normal child behavior. Although children's feelings, self-concepts, and school achievement difficulties may not be obvious in the clinic setting, these may be major factors in the habilitation process. For optimal results from treatment, the total child must be considered.

## Acknowledgment

This chapter was supported in part by PHS Grants DE 00853, DE 05837, and DE 13076, from the National Institute of Dental Research.

## References

Beder, O., & Weinstein, P. (1980). Explorations of the coping of adolescents with orofacial anomalies using the Cornell Medical Index. *Journal of Prosthetic Dentistry, 43,* 565–567.

Benson, B. A., Gross, A. M., Messer, S. C., Kellum, G., & Passmore, L. A. (1991). Social support networks among families of children with craniofacial anomalies. *Health Psychology, 10,* 252–258.

Berscheid, E., & Walster, E. (1974). Physical attractiveness. In L. Gerkowitz (Ed.), *Advances in experimental social psychology* (Vol. 7). New York: Academic Press.

Brantley, H., & Clifford, E. (1979). Cognitive, self-concept, and body-image measures of normal, cleft, and obese adolescents. *Cleft Palate Journal, 16,* 177–182.

Broder, H., Richman, L., & Matheson, P. (1998). Learning disability, school achievement and grade retention among children with cleft: A two center study. *Cleft Palate-Craniofacial Journal, 31,* 429–435.

Broder, H., Smith, F. B., & Strauss, R. P. (1994). Effects of visible and nonvisible oral-facial defects on self perception and adjustment across developmental eras and gender. *Cleft Palate-Craniofacial Journal, 31,* 429–435.

Broder, H., & Strauss, R. P. (1989). Self concept of early primary school children with visible and invisible defects. *Cleft Palate Journal, 26,* 114–117.

Bull, R., & Rumsey, N. (1988). *The social psychology of facial appearance.* New York: Springer-Verlag.

Clifford, E. (1987). *The cleft palate experience: New perspectives on management.* Springfield, IL: Thomas.

Clifford, E., Crocker, E., & Pope, B. (1972). Psychological findings in the adulthood of 98 cleft palate children. *Journal of Plastic and Reconstructive Surgery, 50,* 234–237.

Clifford, M., & Walster, E. (1973). The effect of physical attractiveness on teacher expectations. *Sociology of Education, 46,* 248–258.

Cohen, M., Jr. (1982). *The child with multiple birth defects.* New York: Raven Press.

Demellweek, C., Humphris, G., Hare, M., & Brown, J. (1997). Children's perceptions of and attitude toward unfamiliar peers with port wine stains. *Journal of Pediatric Psychology, 22,* 471–485.

Dion, K. (1972). Physical attractiveness and evaluation of children's transgressions. *Journal of Personality and Social Psychology, 24,* 207–213.

Dion, K. (1973). Young children's stereotyping of facial attractiveness. *Developmental Psychology, 9,* 183–188.

Dion, K., & Berscheid, E. (1974). Physical attractiveness and peer perception among children. *Sociometry, 37,* 1–12.

Eder, R. A. (Ed). (1995). *Craniofacial anomalies: Psychological perspectives.* New York: Springer-Verlag.

Eliason, M. (1991). Cleft lip and palate: Developmental effects. *Journal of Pediatric Nursing, 6,* 107–113.

Eliason, M., & Richman, L. (1987). *Behavioral characteristics of cleft children related to age, sex, and cleft type.* Paper presented at the annual meeting of the American Cleft Palate Association, San Antonio, TX.

Endriga, M. C., & Kapp-Simon, K. A. (1999). Psychological issues in craniofacial care: State of the art. *Cleft Palate-Craniofacial Journal, 36,* 3–11.

Endriga, M. C., & Speltz, M. L. (1997). Face to face interaction between infants with orofacial clefts and their mothers. *Journal of Pediatric Psychology, 22,* 439–453.

Harper, D., & Richman, L. (1978). Personality profiles of physically impaired adolescents. *Journal of Clinical Psychology, 34,* 636–642.

Harper, D., Richman, L., & Snider, B. (1980). School adjustment and degree of physical impairment. *Journal of Pediatric Psychology, 5,* 377–383.

Kapp-Simon, K. (1986). Self-concept of primary school age children with cleft lip, cleft palate or both. *Cleft Palate Journal, 23,* 24–27.

Kapp-Simon, K., Simon, D. J., & Kristovich, S. (1992). Self perception, social skills, adjustment, and inhibition in young children with craniofacial anomalies. *Cleft Palate-Craniofacial Journal, 29,* 352–356.

Kommers, M., & Sullivan, M. (1979). Written language skills of children with cleft palate. *Cleft Palate Journal, 16,* 18–85.

Lamb, M., Wilson, F., & Leeper, H. (1972). A comparison of selected cleft palate children and their siblings on the variables of intelligence, hearing loss, and visual-perceptual-motor skills. *Cleft Palate Journal, 9,* 218–228.

Lamb, M., Wilson, F., & Leeper, H. (1973). The intellectual function of cleft palate children compared on the basis of cleft type and sex. *Cleft Palate Journal, 10,* 367–377.

Langlois, J. (1995). The origins and functions of appearance-based stereotypes: Theoretical and applied implications. In R. A. Eder (Ed.), *Developmental perspectives on craniofacial problems.* New York: Springer-Verlag.

Langlois, J., & Downs, A. (1979). Peer relations as a function of physical attractiveness: The eye of the beholder or behavioral reality? *Child Development, 50,* 409–418.

Langlois, J., & Stephan, C. (1977). Effects of physical attractiveness and ethnicity on children's behavioral attributions and peer preferences. *Child Development, 48,* 1694–1698.

Lencione, R. (1980). Psychosocial aspects of cleft lip and palate. In M. Edwards & A. Watson (Eds.), *Advances in the management of cleft palate.* New York: Churchill Livingstone.

Lerner, R., & Lerner, J. (1977). Effects of age, sex, and physical attractiveness on child-peer relations, academic performance, and elementary school adjustment. *Developmental Psychology, 13,* 585–590.

Livneh, H. (1982). On the origins of negative attitudes toward people with disabilities. *Rehabilitation Literature, 43,* 338–345.

McDonald, S. (1979). Parental needs and professional responses: A parental perspective. *Cleft Palate Journal, 16,* 188–192.

McWilliams, B., & Paradise, L. (1973). Educational, occupational, and marital status of cleft palate adults. *Cleft Palate Journal, 10,* 223–229.

Millard, T., & Richman, L. C. (2001). Different cleft conditions, facial appearance and speech: Relationship to psychological variables. *Cleft Palate-Craniofacial Journal, 38,* 68–75.

Musgrave, R., McWilliams, B., & Matthews, M. (1975). A review of the results of two different surgical procedures for the repair of clefts of the soft palate only. *Cleft Palate Journal, 12,* 281–290.

Nopoulos, P., Berg, S., Canady, J., Richman, L., Vandemark, D., & Andreasen, M. C. (2000). Abnormal brain morphology in patients with isolated cleft lip, cleft palate or both: A preliminary analysis. *Cleft Palate-Craniofacial Journal, 37,* 441–446.

Nopoulos, P., Berg, S., Canady, J., Richman, L., VanDermark, D., & Andreasen, N. C. (2002). Structural brain abnormalities in adult males with clefts of the lip and palate. *Genetics in Medicine, 4*(1), 1–9.

Nopoulos, P., Berg, S., VanDermark, D., Richman, L., Canady, J., & Andreasen, N. C. (2001). Increased incidence of midline brain anomaly in adult males with nonsyndromic clefts of the lip and/or palate. *Journal of Neuroimaging, 11,* 1–7.

Peter, J., & Chinsky, R. (1974a). Sociological aspects of cleft palate adults: I. Marriage. *Cleft Palate Journal, 11,* 295–309.

Peter, J., & Chinsky, R. (1974b). Sociological aspects of cleft palate adults: II. Education. *Cleft Palate Journal, 11,* 443–449.

Peter, J., Chinsky, R., & Fisher, M. (1975a). Sociological aspects of cleft palate adults: III. Vocational and economic aspects. *Cleft Palate Journal, 12,* 193–199.

Peter, J., Chinsky, R., & Fisher, M. (1975b). Sociological aspects of cleft palate adults: IV. Social integration. *Cleft Palate Journal, 12,* 304–310.

Podol, J., & Salvia, J. (1976). Effects of visibility of a prepalatal cleft on the evaluation of speech. *Cleft Palate Journal, 13,* 361–366.

Richardson, S. (1970). Age and sex differences in values towards physical handicaps. *Journal of Health & Social Behavior, 11,* 207–214.

Richardson, S. (1971a). Children's values and friendships: A study of physical disability. *Journal of Health and Social Behavior, 12,* 253–258.

Richardson, S. (1971b). Handicap, appearance, and stigma. *Social Science and Medicine, 5,* 621–628.

Richman, L. (1976). Behavior and achievement of cleft palate children. *Cleft Palate Journal, 13,* 4–10.

Richman, L. (1978a). The effects of facial disfigurement on teachers' perception of ability in cleft palate children. *Cleft Palate Journal, 15,* 155–160.

Richman, L. (1978b). Parents and teachers: Differing views of behavior of cleft palate children. *Cleft Palate Journal, 15,* 360–364.

Richman, L. (1980). Cognitive patterns and learning disabilities in cleft palate children with verbal deficits. *Journal of Speech and Hearing Research, 23,* 447–456.

Richman, L. (1983). Self-reported social, speech, and facial concerns and personality adjustment of adolescents with cleft lip and palate. *Cleft Palate Journal, 20,* 108–112.

Richman, L. (1997). *Personal adjustment of adults with cleft.* Paper presented at the American Cleft Palate-Craniofacial Association Annual Meeting, New Orleans, LA.

Richman, L., & Eliason, M. (1984). Type of reading disability related to cleft type and neuropsychological patterns. *Cleft Palate Journal, 21,* 1–6.

Richman, L., & Eliason, M. (1986a). Development in children with cleft lip and/or palate. *Seminars in Speech and Language, 7,* 225–239.

Richman, L., & Eliason, M. (1986b). Psychological characteristics of cleft lip and palate children. *Cleft Palate Journal, 19,* 249–258.

Richman, L., & Eliason, M. (2001). Disorders of communication, developmental language disorders and cleft palate. In C. E. Walker & M. C. Roberts (Eds.), *Handbook of clinical child psychology* (Rev. ed.). New York: Wiley.

Richman, L., Eliason, M., & Lindgren, S. (1988). Reading disability in children with cleft lip and palate. *Cleft Palate Journal, 25,* 21–25.

Richman, L., & Harper, D. (1978a). Observable stigmata and perceived maternal behavior. *Cleft Palate Journal, 15,* 215–219.

Richman, L., & Harper, D. (1978b). School adjustment of children with observable disabilities. *Journal of Abnormal Child Psychology, 6,* 11–18.

Richman, L., & Harper, D. (1979). Self-identified personality patterns of children with facial or orthopedic disfigurement. *Cleft Palate Journal, 16,* 257–261.

Richman, L., & Harper, D. (1980). Personality profiles of physically impaired young adults. *Journal of Clinical Psychology, 36,* 668–671.

Richman, L. C., Holmes, C. S., & Eliason, M. J. (1985). Adolescents with cleft lip and palate: Self-perceptions of appearance and behavior related to personality adjustment. *Cleft Palate Journal, 22,* 93–96.

Richman, L. C., & Millard, T. (1997). Cleft lip and palate: Longitudinal behavior and relationships of cleft conditions to behavior and achievement. *Journal of Pediatric Psychology, 22,* 487–494.

Richman, L. C., & Ryan, S. (2000, April). *The relationship of anxiety and verbal expression deficits to social and emotional adjustment.* Paper presented at the American Cleft Palate-Craniofacial Association Annual Meeting, Atlanta, GA.

Richman, L. C., & Ryan, S. (2002). Do the reading disabilities of children with cleft fit into current models of developmental dyslexia? *Cleft Palate-Craniofacial Journal, 40,* 154–157.

Schneiderman, C., & Harding, J. (1984). Social ratings of children with cleft lip by school peers. *Cleft Palate Journal, 21,* 219–223.

Shontz, F. (1975). *Psychological aspects of physical illness and disability.* New York: Macmillan.

Snyder, M., Tanke, E., & Berscheid, E. (1977). Social perception and interpersonal behavior: On the self-fulfilling nature of social stereotypes. *Journal of Personality and Social Psychology, 35,* 656–666.

Speltz, M. L., Morton, K., Goodell, E. W., & Clarren, S. K. (1993). Psychological functioning of children with craniofacial anomalies and their mothers. *Cleft Palate-Craniofacial Journal, 30,* 482–489.

Speltz, M. L., & Richman, L. C. (1997). Psychological study of craniofacial anomalies. *Journal of Pediatric Psychology, 22,* 433–438.

Spriestersbach, D. C. (1973). *Psychosocial aspects of the "cleft palate problem"* (Vols. 1 & 2). Iowa City: University of Iowa Press.

Tobiasen, J. M. (1987). Social judgments on facial deformity. *Cleft Palate Journal, 24,* 323–327.

Tobiasen, J. M., & Hiebert, J. M. (1984). Parents' tolerance for the conduct problems of the child with cleft lip and palate. *Cleft Palate Journal, 21,* 82–85.

# PART IV

# Interdisciplinary Medical, Surgical, and Dental Concerns and Treatment

# CHAPTER 14

# Surgical Repair of the Cleft Lip and Palate

## Procedures and Issues

*Marie-Claire Buckley and George H. Landis*

Buckley and Landis recognize the value and importance of interdisciplinary team decisions in successful surgical outcome for the patient with cleft lip and palate. Following the primary or initial lip and palate repair, the surgeon and team discuss the need for and benefits of additional surgical procedures to improve the form (appearance) and function of the lips, nose, mouth, palate, and velopharyngeal management for improved speech production.

The authors present a timetable and rationale for consideration of the more common or anticipated surgical procedures consistent with the child's facial growth and development and speech and language development. They discuss specific approaches and procedures with focus on goals, timing, and issues and controversies.

1. What do Buckley and Landis say about feeding a child born with a cleft lip or with a cleft palate? How does this information compare to guidelines presented by Breen, Chibbaro, and Hopper in Chapter 6?
2. What is meant by the "rule of 10s" when planning for initial lip repair?
3. The authors discuss a procedure called nasoalveolar molding. What is that designed to accomplish for the surgeon? How does it benefit the child?
4. Buckley and Landis state two goals of cleft palate repair that relate to speech production. What are they?

5. List two surgical options (procedures) for secondary surgical improvement of velopharyngeal closure for speech. For each, state the anatomical and physiological requirements for successful speech outcome. What are some risks for each procedure?

Surgical repair of cleft lip and palate deformities is best accomplished as part of a comprehensive team approach involving interdisciplinary diagnosis, evaluation, and treatment planning for long-range management of persons born with cleft lip and palate. The reconstructive plastic surgeon is one of many team members who contribute to the best possible aesthetic and functional outcome. As pointed out by Moller in Chapter 1, the most successful approach to cleft lip and palate treatment must be a patient-oriented rather than a specialty-oriented effort.

As a member of the cleft team, the reconstructive plastic surgeon has undergone a minimum of 3–5 years of general surgical training in addition to 2–3 years of plastic surgery residency. An extra year of subspecialty training in a pediatric or craniofacial fellowship is optional. This specialized training prepares the plastic surgeon to repair or remodel a variety of tissue types (skin, muscle, bone, nerves) in all areas of the body, including the face, that are deformed by tumor and trauma as well as congenital anomalies. The restoration of form and function is the ultimate goal that guides the reconstructive plastic surgeon in the care of the cleft patient.

When a family is faced with the news that their new baby has a cleft lip or palate, whether diagnosed by prenatal ultrasound or at the time of birth, the reconstructive plastic surgeon may be the first member of the team to see the baby, meet the family, and discuss the treatable nature of the cleft, including the general timeline for typical surgical procedures. A more individualized treatment plan is tailored dependent on team consensus and the child's physical and psychosocial growth and development.

Early referral to the interdisciplinary cleft clinic team can help to allay some of the family's fears and concerns about clefts, as well as provide assurance and information on additional services and resources available to meet their child's needs during the coming months and years. In collaboration with other members of the cleft team, the reconstructive plastic surgeon helps to coordinate necessary surgical procedures based on the child's speech and hearing development, as well as maxillofacial and dental growth.

# Feeding

Before any surgery is contemplated, adequate feeding and nutrition must be established to maximize healing potential and minimize anesthetic risks of surgery. There are still misconceptions, even within the medical community, about feeding the child with a cleft. An isolated cleft lip rarely creates feeding difficulties. If there is a problem with "latching on," the lip can be "sealed" with a finger or tape or the breast mound itself.

Even a cleft palate may not interfere with feeding if the defect is unilateral, or if special bottles and nipples can help overcome the difficulties of developing an adequate sucking mechanism. It is very unusual that a child would require a nasogastric feeding tube, but if the child fails to gain weight, this option should be seriously considered. The diagnosis of a cleft should never deter attempts to breast or bottle feed. Lactation specialists have many techniques for finding the most effective feeding methods for each individual baby.

A thorough discussion about feeding issues and early pediatric care is found in Chapter 6 by Breen, Chibbaro, and Hopper. Once the goals for adequate nutrition and acceptable weight gain and growth are being met, surgical repair can proceed.

# Surgical Timing/Staging

The basic timing of surgical repairs depends on the cleft type and severity as well as surgeons' preferences. Generally speaking, the lip and nose are addressed first, followed by the palate. While plastic surgery attempts to restore both appearance and function, surgeons must balance the effects of postsurgical scarring with the child's facial growth and development.

Although cleft lips have been repaired as early as the first few days of life, or even attempted in utero in animal models, traditional teaching has proposed the "rule of 10s"—waiting until the child has reached the age of 10 weeks, a weight of 10 pounds, and a hemoglobin of 10. Although there are many exceptions to the rule, this delay helps to minimize the risk of general anesthesia, maximize the child's nutritional status and healing capacity, and facilitate the technical aspects of surgical repair based on the child's size. Of course, if there is a need for presurgical premaxillary molding, repair may be further delayed.

Cleft nasal deformities traditionally have been repaired "secondarily" prior to school age or during the teen years, but now are often initiated at the time of primary lip repair. If there is wide clefting of the alveolus (dental ridge) in addition to a cleft lip, nasoalveolar molding procedures may begin as early as 4 weeks, depending on the technique used; these will be discussed later in this chapter.

Clefts of the alveolus (part of the primary palate) can be repaired either after molding is completed with a gingivoperiosteoplasty at the time the lip is repaired, or just before eruption of certain permanent teeth, between ages 6 and 9 years (see Chapter 17 by Swift). Clefts of the secondary palate are typically repaired between 6 and 18 months of age, but ideally (from a speech-language pathologist's standpoint) prior to early speech development. Ventilation (pressure equalization) tubes are often placed in the eardrums by an otolaryngologist at the time of palate repair or earlier to prevent the sequela of inadequate middle ear ventilation (see Chapter 15 by Sidman).

Usually by age 2, the basic lip and palate repairs have been completed. Revisions, or stages of repair, to the lip and nose can be done anytime after that. However, these may often be delayed until after alveolar bone grafting or midface orthognathic (jaw) surgery provides a more anatomically correct and solid foundation.

If the child has velopharyngeal inadequacy despite aggressive speech therapy, a pharyngeal flap, sphincteroplasty, or other surgical procedure may be necessary to improve speech intelligibility as early as 4 years old.

Deficiencies in midface growth due to postsurgical scarring or hypoplasia may be addressed with midface advancement, usually during the early teens. Further septorhinoplasty for nasal airway compromise due to a deviated septum and residual nasal tip deformities is most frequently done during the mid- to late teens. Table 14.1 illustrates a general timeline for the various stages of cleft surgery.

## Nasoalveolar Molding

Nasoalveolar molding and/or presurgical premaxillary/maxillary repositioning is a technique that attempts to bring the cleft lip, nose, and alveolar components into closer proximity prior to definitive repair. For wide cleft lips without involvement of the alveolus, taping methods can often

**Table 14.1**
**Timeline of Surgical Procedures**

| Defect | Procedure | | | | | | | | | | | | | | | |
|---|---|---|---|---|---|---|---|---|---|---|---|---|---|---|---|---|
| Cleft lip only | Definitive cleft lip repair | | | | | | | | Lip revisions → | | | | | | | |
| Nose | Definitive nose repair | | | | | | | | (Optional) Columellar lengthening, **if bilateral cleft lip** → | | | Tip rhinoplasty → | | | Septorhinoplasty (unilateral clefts, usually) → | |
| Wide cleft lip and alveolus | Presurgical nasoalveolar molding | | Definitive cleft lip repair | | | | | | | (Optional) Alveolar bone graft **if insufficient bone or fistula** → | | | | (Optional) Midface advancement or distraction osteogenesis **if malocclusion** → | | |
| | | Lip adhesion and primary gingivoperiosteoplasty | | | | Definitive cleft lip repair | | | | | | | | | | |
| Cleft palate (one- and two-stage surgeries) | | | | One-stage: Definitive cleft palate repair (hard and soft palate) | | | | | | (Optional) Later procedure, **if VPI:** Pharyngeal flap, Sphincter pharyngoplasty, or Palatal lengthening (conversion to Furlow Z-plasty) | | | | | | |
| | | Two-stage: 1. Primary veloplasty (soft palate only) | | | | 2. Hard palate repair | | | | | | | | | | |
| | Age | | | | | | | | | | | | | | | |
| Surgical repair | 1 mo. | 2 mos. | 3 mos. | 4–5 mos. | 6–8 mos. | 9–11 mos. | 12–17 mos. | 18–23 mos. | 2–3 years | 4–5 years | 6–7 years | 8–9 years | 10–11 years | 12–13 years | 14–17 years | 18+ years |

*Note.* // = nonlinear time units.

"stretch" the lip edges closer to each other prior to repair. With complete clefts of the lip and alveolus or primary palate, there is often misalignment between the premaxilla and the alveolar ridges as well as deformity of the nose. If the cleft is particularly wide, with the alveolar cleft greater than 0.5 cm, there may be increased tension on the tissues, resulting in a widened scar or even possible dehiscence when the lip is repaired. Molding misshapen or misplaced structures into a more normal anatomic position helps to minimize possible complications and the need for future surgeries, while providing improved aesthetic results.

A number of techniques have been developed over time to manage the protuberant and malpositioned premaxillary segment in bilateral clefts of the primary palate (see Figures 14.1a and 14.1b). Although there was a historical period in cleft surgery when the premaxilla was actually fractured and "set back" or even excised completely, surgeons soon realized the importance of preserving the premaxilla for soft tissue support, dental development, and midface growth and projection, and they looked for other ways to facilitate lip closure. External molding with a head bonnet and strap across the lip dates back to the 1760s, but is difficult to maintain and tolerate. Lip adhesion is essentially a form of external alveolar molding, bringing the mucosal edges of the lip together to reposition the premaxilla and stretch the tissues prior to definitive repair with reapproximation of the orbicularis oris muscle. The disadvantages of this technique are scarring and an additional surgical procedure (see Figure 14.1c).

Although many surgeons have avoided the risk of tissue dehiscence by first performing a lip adhesion, some feel that the orthopedic effects of lip adhesion are less controlled compared to nasoalveolar molding. Molding has the added benefit of better alveolar alignment to facilitate primary gingivoperiosteoplasty—a primary repair of the alveolar cleft—if this particular procedure is practiced by the surgeon.

Current presurgical orthopedic appliances use intraoral palatal molds to actively "pull" or passively direct growth to guide the premaxilla into alignment with the lateral palatal shelves (Grayson, Santiago, Brecht, & Cutting, 1999). There are several basic models being used in major cleft centers. As described by Berkowitz, Mejia, and Bystrik (2004), Latham and Georgiade developed a pin-retained prosthesis adjusted daily by a screw-driven spring gauge to expand the lateral palatal shelves and retract the premaxilla (see Figure 14.2). Papay, Morales, Motoki, and Yamashiro (1995) developed a similar pin-anchored palatal retainer requiring weekly tightening of elastic chains attached to a premaxillary plate (see Figure 14.3). These palatal prostheses accomplish what a lip ad-

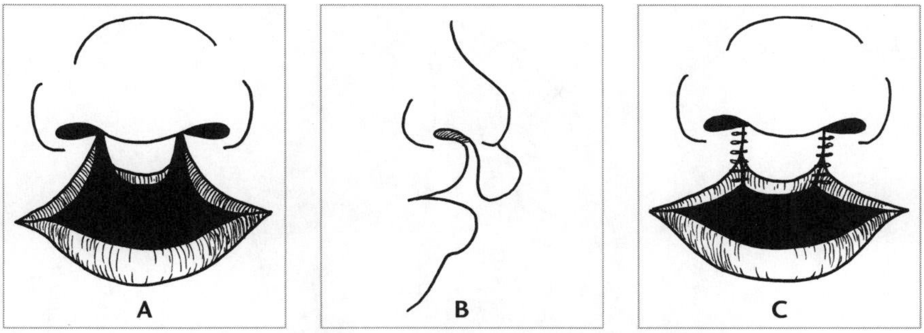


FIGURE 14.1. (A) Coronal view: Bilateral cleft lip. (B) Lateral view: Detached prolabium associated with bilateral cleft lip. (C) Suture lines following bilateral lip adhesion.

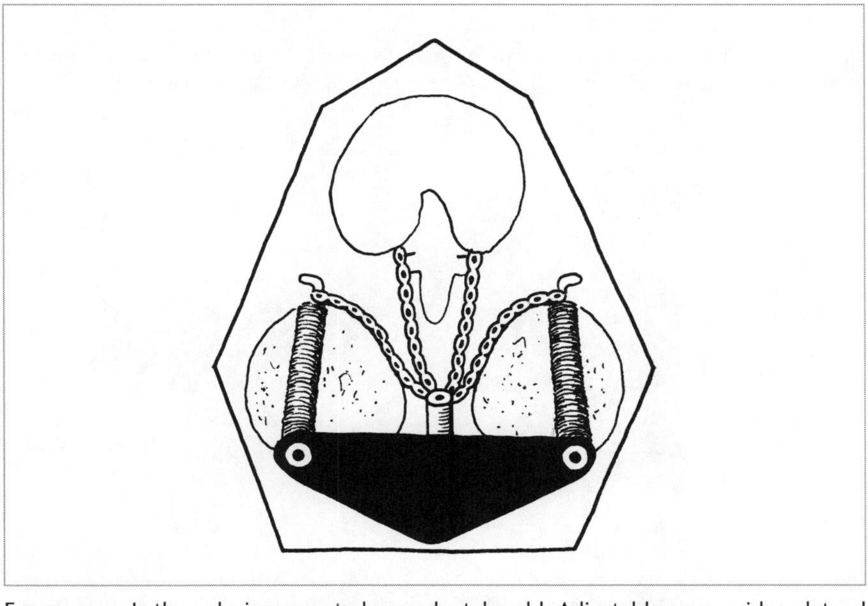

FIGURE 14.2. Latham device mounted on a dental mold. Adjustable screw widens lateral palatal shelves and pulls the premaxilla posteriorly.

hesion does without lip scarring, and facilitate gingivoperiosteoplasty, if desired. The "passive" model used by Cutting (2000) can also add a nasal extension to the palatal prosthesis to help mold the affected nostril by stretching the shortened columella and rounding out the flattened lower lateral alar cartilage (see Figure 14.4).

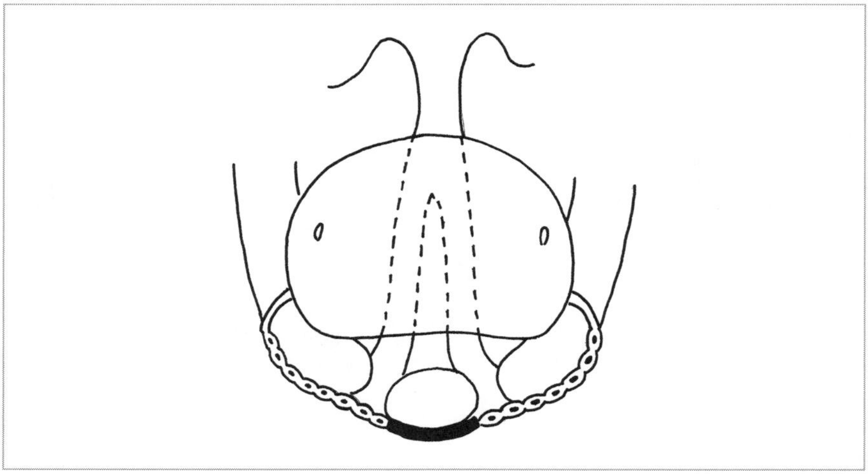

FIGURE 14.3. Yamashiro-Morales palatal prosthesis. Elastic chains attached to small premaxillary metal plate pull premaxilla posteriorly to align with the alveolar ridge.

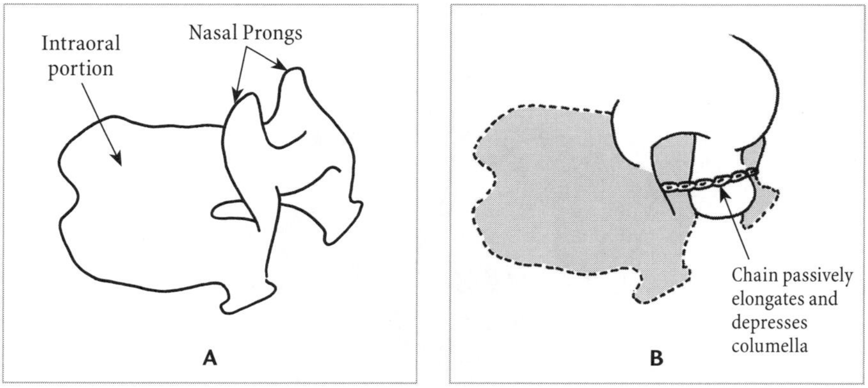


FIGURE 14.4. (A) Nasoalveolar molding device (prosthesis) with bilateral nostril prongs. (B) Nasoalveolar molding device, which passively elongates columella, rounds flattened alar rims, and repositions premaxilla posteriorly.

## Timing

The palatal mold for the prosthesis is usually made when the child is 4–6 weeks of age, either in the clinic or during a short general anesthetic. The active, pin-retained models require a second anesthetic for insertion.

Repositioning or molding then takes place over the next 4–6 weeks, with daily or weekly adjustments, until the alveolar segments are within 2 mm for possible gingivoperiosteoplasty. By repositioning the premaxilla, the soft tissues of the lip are also brought closer together to allow for an easier repair.

### Controversies

Nasoalveolar molding or premaxillary repositioning requires a skilled dental specialist (pediatric dentist, orthodontist, prosthodontist), considerable parental cooperation, frequent adjustments, delayed definitive lip repair, and possible additional anesthesias and procedures. Although some surgeons feel that neither lip adhesion nor premaxillary molding is necessary, there has been a trend toward molding, with or without gingivoperiosteoplasty. Lip adhesion remains an important technique for children with wide cleft lip and alveolus, if palatal prostheses are unavailable.

## Cleft Lip

### Anatomy

There are certain anatomical landmarks of the normal lip that are important to re-establish when repairing a cleft lip: the vermilion border, the philtral columns, the nasal columella, and Cupid's bow with peaks (see Figure 14.5).

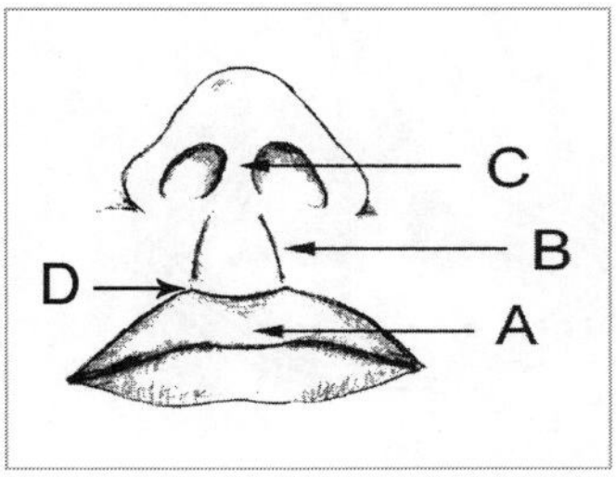


FIGURE 14.5. Normal lip anatomy: (A) vermilion; (B) philtral column; (C) columella; (D) Cupid's bow with peak.

### Characteristics

A cleft lip is thought to be due to a lack of mesodermal migration or ingrowth resulting in the dissolution of the overlying ectoderm. The orbicularis oris muscle does not meet its contralateral counterpart, and instead becomes aberrantly attached to the lateral alar base. In the lip, this results in a loss of landmarks on the affected side, such as Cupid's peak, the philtral column, and continuity of the vermilion border. In the nose, the columella is shortened and the lower alar cartilage is depressed, resulting in an asymmetric nasal tip (see Figure 14.6). In the bilateral cleft lip, the columella is short, the nostrils are depressed, and the central prolabial segment is short and devoid of any muscle.

## Classification

There are varying degrees of cleft lip deformity, ranging from mild microform (forme fruste) to a severe cleft involving the floor of the nose. Any of these can be seen as unilateral or bilateral, or in any combination (see Figure 14.7).

## Goals and Timing of Repair

The goals of cleft lip repair are to restore a more normal appearance through the re-creation of landmarks, to restore functional continuity of the orbicularis oris muscle, and to restore nasal symmetry. This is most often done between the ages of 6 weeks and 3 months, although there is no age limit to when a cleft lip can be fixed. Definitive lip repair may be

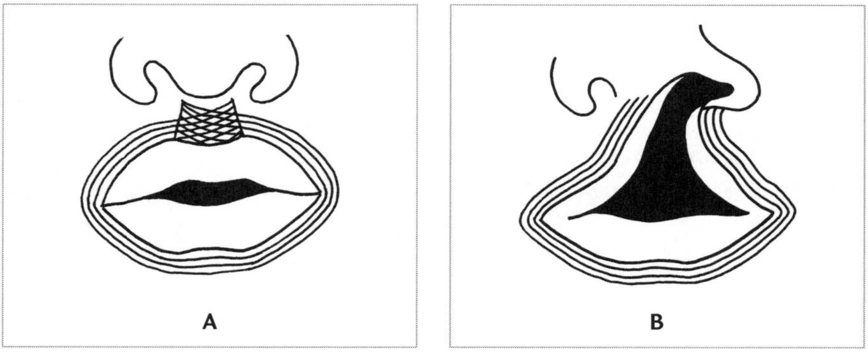


Figure 14.6. (A) Normal orbicularis oris muscle interdigitation. (B) Cleft lip with abnormal attachment of orbicularis oris to alar base.

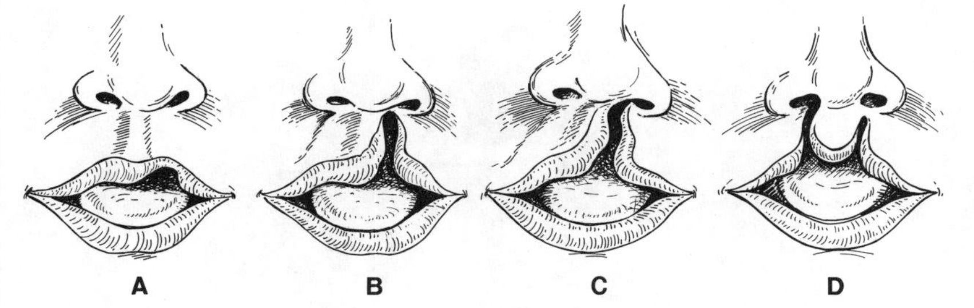


FIGURE 14.7. Varieties of lip clefts. Views A, B, and C show unilateral or one-sided clefts, which vary in severity. The bilateral cleft seen in view D is more severe on the right side. *Note.* From *A Parent's Guide to Cleft Lip and Palate* (p. 11), by K. T. Moller, C. D. Starr, & S. A. Johnson, 1990, Minneapolis: University of Minnesota Press. Copyright 1990 by Regents of the University of Minnesota. Reprinted with permission.

delayed due to any additional surgical steps, such as premaxillary molding or lip adhesion, as discussed previously.

Although numerous methods of repair have been proposed since the first recorded repair in 390 A.D. China, three general categories of cleft lip repair are practiced most often today: (1) the rotation-advancement repair developed by Millard, (2) the triangular flap by Tennison-Randall, and (3) straight-line techniques, which are usually reserved for microform or mild incomplete clefts (Byrd, 1997).

The rotation-advancement technique has the advantage of camouflaging the scars along the philtral column and the nasal alar groove. This repair is probably used most often by surgeons today. The medial segment is rotated downward to lower Cupid's peak. The lateral segment is then advanced into the resultant defect at the base of the columella to add length to the lip and keep the peak level with the normal side (see Figure 14.8).

The Tennison-Randall repair corrects the discrepancy in lip length between medial and lateral segments by inserting a small triangular flap from the lateral lip to the shorter medial side. While this is particularly useful in very severe clefts, the triangular flap crosses the philtral column more visibly (Schendel, 2000) (see Figure 14.9).

For bilateral cleft lips, the Millard technique is most popular, but may result in a short, narrow philtrum/upper lip and a tethered nasal tip (Mulliken, 2000) (see Figure 14.10).

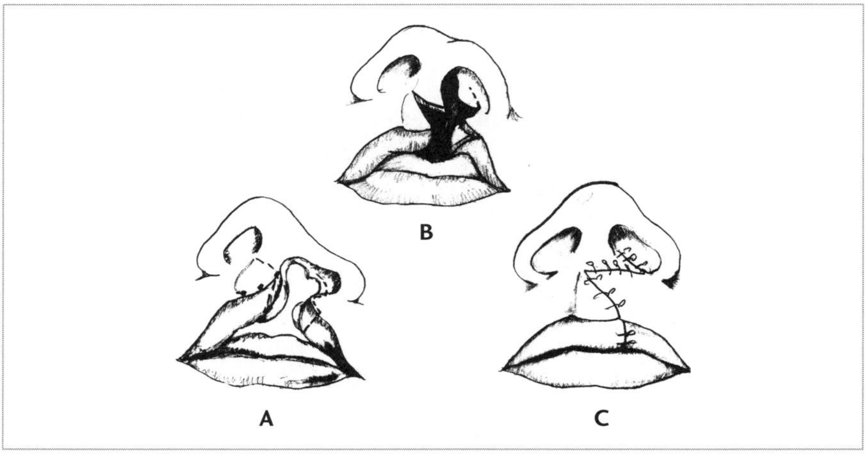


FIGURE 14.8. Millard rotation-advancement repair: (A) surgical incisions; (B) tissue flap rotation; (C) suture lines.

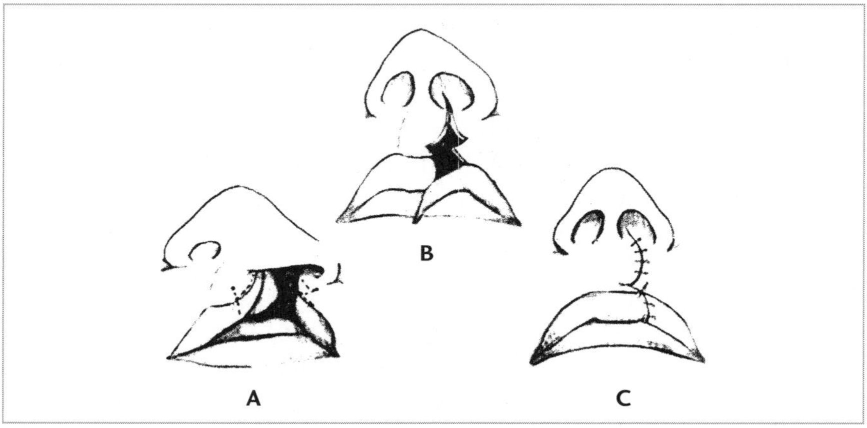


FIGURE 14.9. Tennison-Randall triangular repair: (A) surgical incisions; (B) tissue flap rotation; (C) suture lines.

## Controversies

Aside from a surgeon's preference for a particular technique, the real controversy lies in the timing of cleft lip repair. A few surgeons have tried repair within the first few days of a child's life, and even intrauterine repair

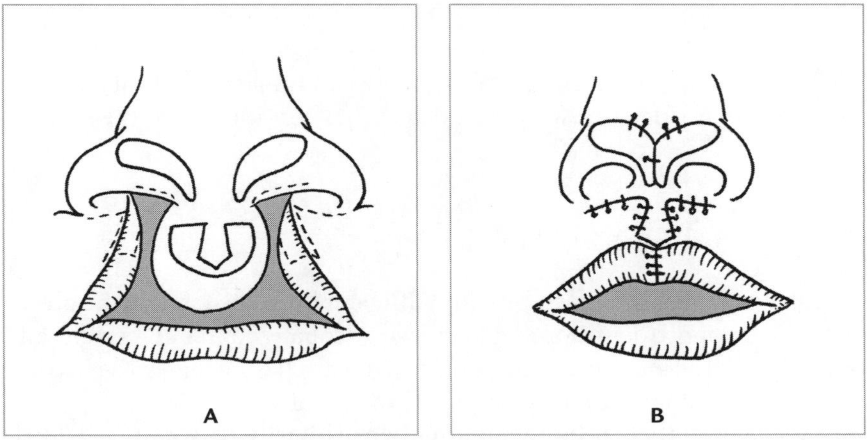


FIGURE 14.10. Millard bilateral cleft lip repair: (A) surgical incisions; (B) suture lines.

in animal models, but these attempts are limited by small structures to work with and increased anesthetic risk. Although the cleft lip defect is the most visible and socially stigmatizing, surgeons are beginning to realize that the very treatment intended to make patients look more normal during infancy may actually lead to the scarring that inhibits future midface growth and the characteristic cleft facies (Kuijpers-Jagtmann & Long, 2000). While many cultures places importance on early repair, there are some developing parts of the world where clefts go unrepaired even into adulthood. In these cases, studies have shown that there is nearly normal midface growth without surgery (Will, 2000). Despite that fact, early normalization of appearance trumps future hypoplasia that can be corrected with orthognathic surgery, and very few practitioners would propose delayed lip repair. Any remaining irregularities or asymmetries after primary repair can be revised at any time, although they are often postponed until after alveolar bone grafting or later.

## Alveolar Clefts

Although surgical repair of the alveolar cleft will be discussed in greater detail by Swift in Chapter 17, we will briefly comment on the topic here.

## Classification

Clefts of the alveolus of the primary palate can range from a subtle notch in the alveolar ridge to a wide cleft defect that continues into the secondary palate.

## Goals and Timing of Repair

Alveolar cleft repair aims to provide sufficient bone to stabilize the alveolar ridge, support dentition, and achieve adequate dental alignment and occlusion. Additionally, closure of the alveolar cleft occludes the accompanying nasolabial fistula and supports the nasal sill.

Alveolar clefts can be repaired either primarily or secondarily. Primary repair includes either primary bone grafting or primary gingivoperiosteoplasty at the time of lip repair, facilitating spontaneous local bone formation. Gingivoperiosteoplasty was mentioned previously when discussing nasoalveolar molding. Secondary repair is the more frequent approach, grafting the bony defect with cancellous cranial or iliac crest (hip) bone between ages 5 and 9 years to provide adequate bony support for erupting teeth adjacent to the cleft.

Primary bone grafting has fallen out of favor due to the high rate of midface hypoplasia. Gingivoperiosteoplasty is becoming more popular with premaxillary repositioning, but may still require additional bone grafting later if there is insufficient bone growth present to support dentition. Gingivoperiosteoplasty has the benefit of closing any nasolabial fistulae early, and can be extended posteriorly to close the anterior palate prior to any definitive palate repair. While this appears to be a promising technique, with up to 60% bone formation, there are few long-term studies to evaluate the possible effects on midface growth (Pantaloni & Hollier, 2000).

# Cleft Palate

## Anatomy

The primary palate involves the lip and alveolus anterior to the incisive foramen, and the secondary palate refers to the hard and soft palate posterior to the incisive foramen (see Figure 14.11).

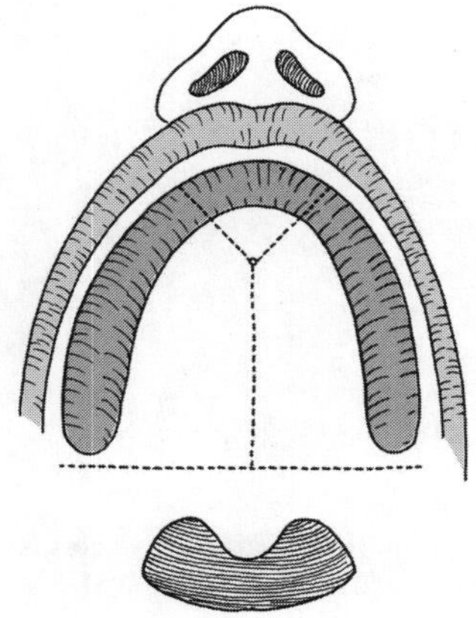

FIGURE 14.11. Normal palatal anatomy. Note incisive foramen between primary and secondary palate, and junction of secondary hard and soft palate. *Note.* From *A Parent's Guide to Cleft Lip and Palate* (p. 8), by K. T. Moller, C. D. Starr, & S. A. Johnson, 1990, Minneapolis: University of Minnesota Press. Copyright 1990 by Regents of the University of Minnesota. Reprinted with permission.

## Characteristics

Palatal clefts can involve the alveolus, hard palate, and/or soft palate.

- *Alveolar cleft*—The premaxilla fails to fuse with one or both anterior lateral palatal shelves. Edges of alveolar bone are covered by gingival mucosa.
- *Hard palate cleft*—The lateral palatal shelves do not fuse in the midline with the vomer or the primary palate.
- *Soft palate cleft*—The tensor and levator veli palatini muscles fail to fuse in the midline to form the normal soft tissue sling or "hammock." Instead, the muscles are attached to the posterior hard palate, resulting in an inability to elevate the soft palate to close off the nasopharynx (see Figures 14.12 and 14.13). Abnormal muscle attachments also prevent the Eustachian tubes from adequately ventilating the middle ear, resulting in negative pressure in the middle ear space that can cause fluid buildup, infection, and reduced hearing. See Chapter 15 by Sidman and Chapter 9 by Carlstrom and Nelson.

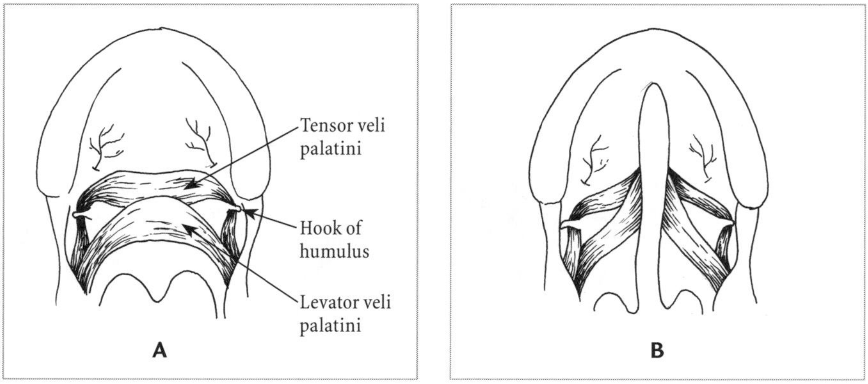


FIGURE 14.12. (A) Normal anatomy of the palatini muscles, showing bilateral attachments at midline. (B) Abnormal palatal muscles in cleft palate, attached to posterior edge of hard palate.

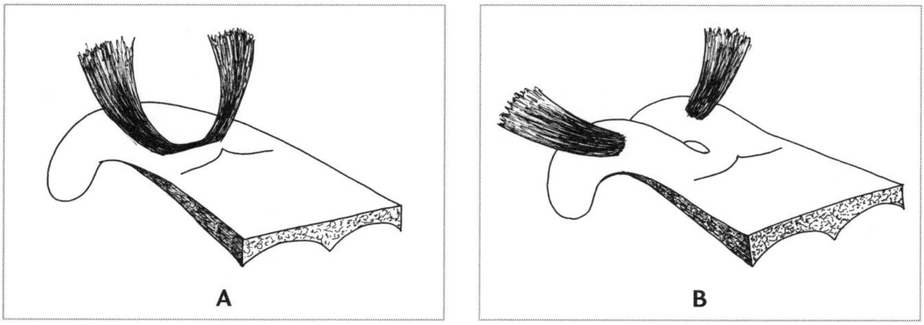


FIGURE 14.13. (A) Muscle sling of normal soft palate. (B) Abnormal attachment of cleft palate muscles, which widens cleft opening and prevents velopharyngeal closure.

## Classification

Similar to cleft lips, cleft palates can be complete or incomplete, involving only the soft palate or the soft palate and hard palate. Also, clefts involving the hard palate can be unilateral or bilateral depending upon lateral bony shelf attachment to the vomer (see Figure 14.14). Of particular importance is the submucous cleft involving the soft palate. While the oral mucosal layer is intact, the underlying muscles have failed to fuse and the soft palate tissue may appear thin and bluish in color (zona pellucida).

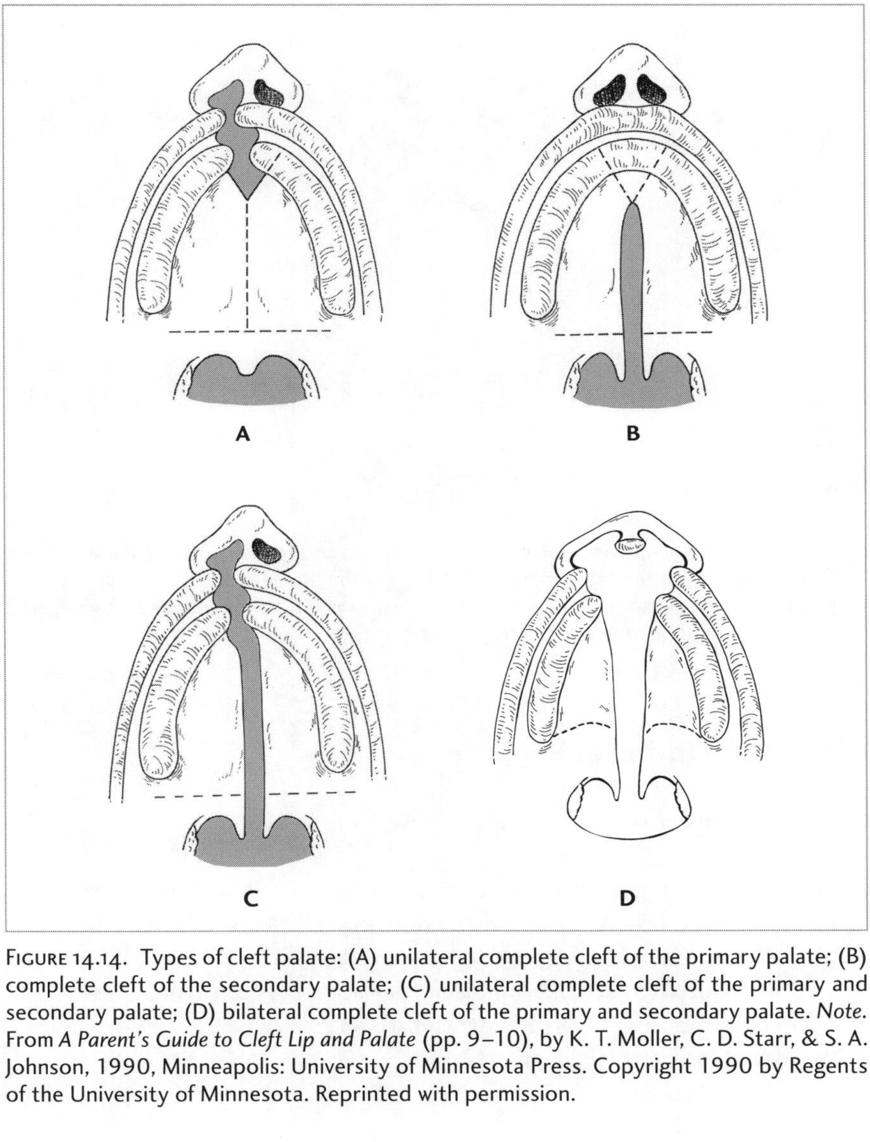


FIGURE 14.14. Types of cleft palate: (A) unilateral complete cleft of the primary palate; (B) complete cleft of the secondary palate; (C) unilateral complete cleft of the primary and secondary palate; (D) bilateral complete cleft of the primary and secondary palate. *Note.* From *A Parent's Guide to Cleft Lip and Palate* (pp. 9–10), by K. T. Moller, C. D. Starr, & S. A. Johnson, 1990, Minneapolis: University of Minnesota Press. Copyright 1990 by Regents of the University of Minnesota. Reprinted with permission.

A notch in the posterior border of the hard palate is also often present. Another indication of a possible submucous cleft is the presence of a bifid or cleft uvula (see Figure 14.15). Not infrequently, submucous clefts are underdiagnosed, unless there are issues with velopharyngeal closure and speech.

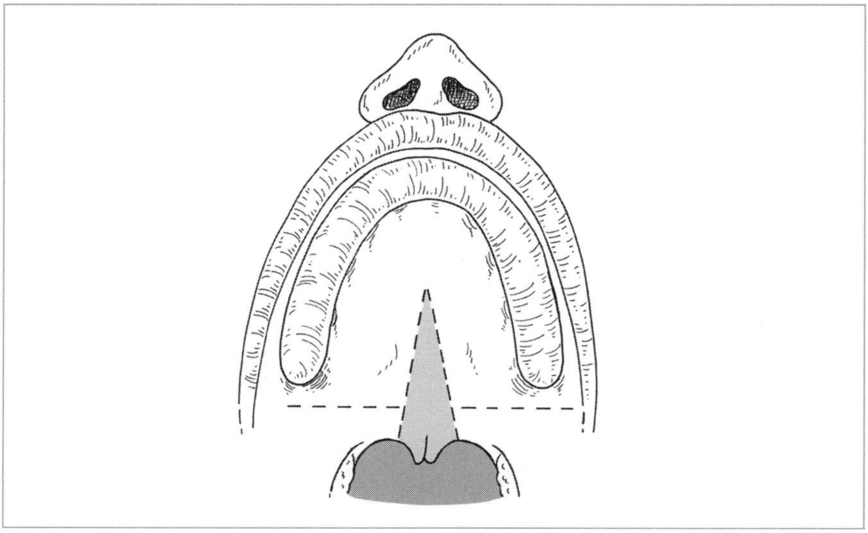

FIGURE 14.15. Submucous cleft palate. Note bifed uvula and zona pellucida (shaded). *Note.* From *A Parent's Guide to Cleft Lip and Palate* (p. 10), by K. T. Moller, C. D. Starr, & S. A. Johnson, 1990, Minneapolis: University of Minnesota Press. Copyright 1990 by Regents of the University of Minnesota. Reprinted with permission.

## Goals and Timing of Repair

Cleft palate repair serves several purposes:

- To restore a separation between the nose and mouth in the hard palate area and restore the soft tissue sling for functional velopharyngeal closure during acceptable speech production
- To provide an intact anterior palatal surface for speech articulation
- To obtain closure of any nasolabial fistulae
- To facilitate normal dental occlusion
- To facilitate hearing

Cleft palate repair is usually done between 6 and 18 months, hopefully prior to significant speech development. Concern that "early" palatal repair may interfere with midfacial and maxillary growth remains controversial.

The soft and hard palate is usually repaired in a single stage. Some surgeons repair the palate in two stages, starting with the soft palate (primary veloplasty) at age 6 to 12 months, followed by second-stage repair of the hard palate defect at age 4. Although staged repairs presumably narrow the residual hard palate defect, few attempts have been made to obturate the anterior hard palate cleft to prevent speech problems from developing prior to the second stage. Neither single nor staged repairs address any alveolar cleft or nasolabial fistula(e) until secondary alveolar bone graft is performed.

> Normal speech should be the most important consideration in the therapeutic plan. Growth disturbance should be minimized, but not at the expense of speech impairment, because the facial distortion can be satisfactorily managed with further surgery whereas speech impairment can often be irreversible. (Pantaloni & Hollier, 2000, p. 12)

## Surgical Techniques

Von Graefe is credited with the first soft palate (velar) cleft repair in 1816. Today, there are three commonly practiced techniques:

- Von Langenbeck's bilateral bipedicled mucoperiosteal flaps (developed in 1861). This procedure is traditionally done without levator reconstruction (see Figure 14.16).

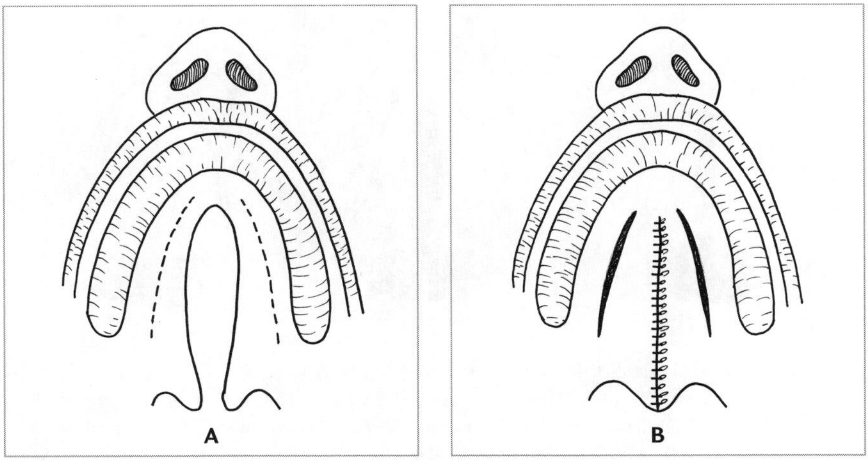


Figure 14.16. Von Langenbeck repair: (A) surgical incisions; (B) suture lines.

- Veau-Wardill-Kilner V-Y pushback (developed in 1937). This procedure includes lateral relaxing incisions, bilateral flaps based on posterior palatine arteries, separate nasal layer closure, separate muscle layer closure, hamulus fracture, and VY soft palatal lengthening (see Figure 14.17).
- Furlow double-opposing Z-plasty (developed in 1986). This procedure re-creates the muscle sling posteriorly, lengthens the soft palate, and avoids a theoretical midline scar contracture (see Figure 14.18).

## Controversies

Despite having only three basic techniques for cleft palate repair, there are numerous opinions as to which one is the "best" technique with regard to (a) true lengthening or "pushback" of the soft palate, (b) effectiveness in avoiding velopharyngeal inadequacy for speech and the need for secondary surgery, (c) minimizing exposure of the hard palate and the effects on facial growth, and (d) whether staged repair is an acceptable alternative to the more traditional single-stage approach. Ultimately, the choice of technique belongs to the surgeon and what works best in his or her experience (LaRossa, 2000).

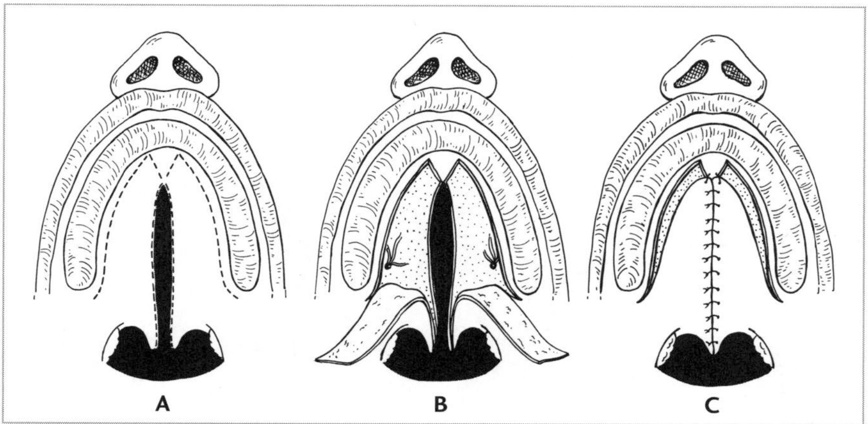


FIGURE 14.17. Veau-Wardill-Kilner V-Y pushback repair: (A) surgical incisions; (B) tissue flap rotation; (C) suture lines. *Note.* From *A Parent's Guide to Cleft Lip and Palate* (p. 31), by K. T. Moller, C. D. Starr, & S. A. Johnson, 1990, Minneapolis: University of Minnesota Press. Copyright 1990 by Regents of the University of Minnesota. Reprinted with permission.

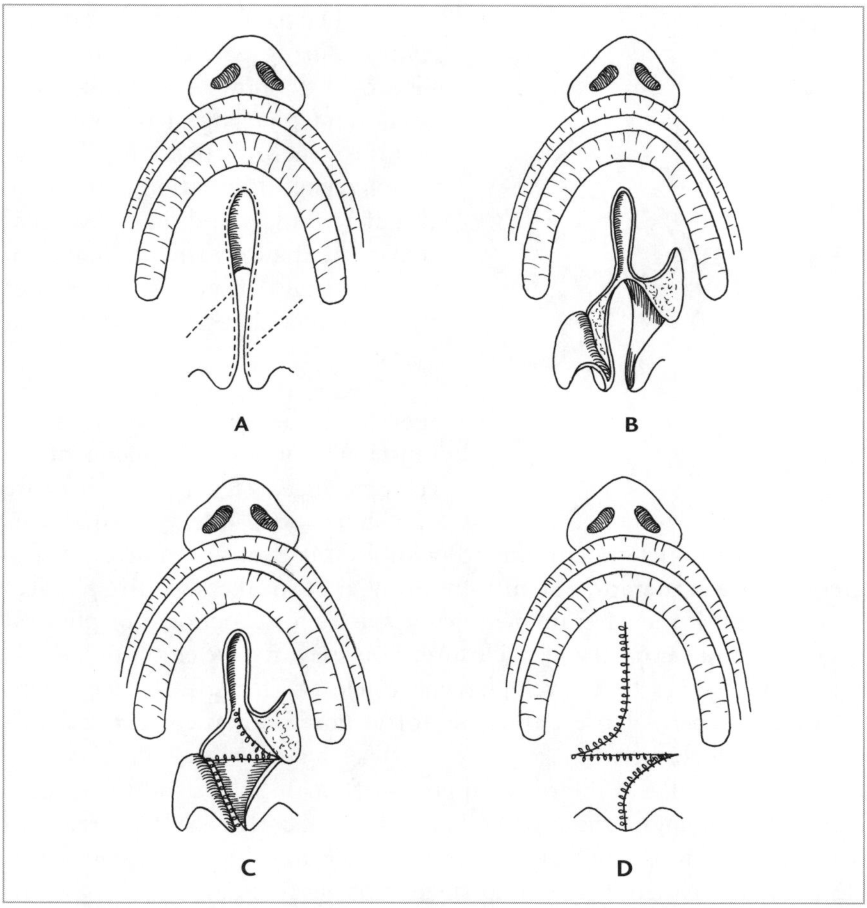


FIGURE 14.18. Furlow repair: (A) Surgical incision lines create two layers of tissue for repair. (B) Oral tissue flaps are elevated. (C) Nasal tissue flaps rotated and sutured to close. (D) Oral flaps are sutured to complete closure.

# Velopharyngeal Inadequacy

Approximately 80%–85% of patients will develop acceptable speech following primary cleft palate repair. However, many of them will require speech therapy to develop acceptable speech. The remaining 15%–20% of patients will require secondary physical management of velopharyngeal closure. Velopharyngeal inadequacy (VPI) is the inability to accomplish

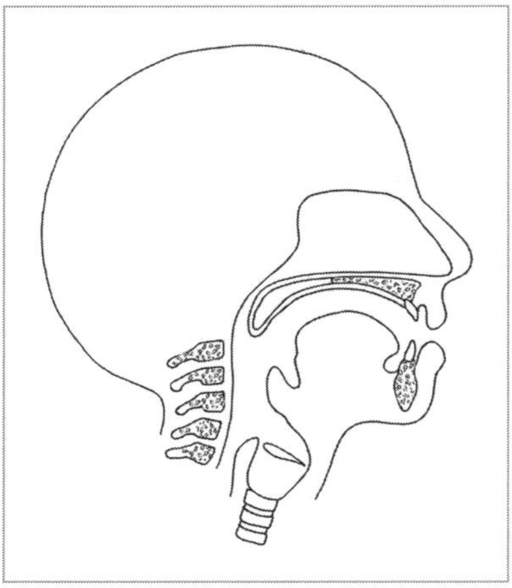

FIGURE 14.19. Sagittal view of normal palate structures.

closure between the nasal and oral spaces during speech production. Figure 14.19 shows the normal soft palate and pharyngeal relationships and the structures that contribute to velopharyngeal function. For more complete understanding and discussion of the anatomy and physiology of velopharyngeal function, the reader is referred to Chapter 7 by Jones and Seaver.

Velopharyngeal dysfunction for speech can occur because of neuromuscular (mobility) problems of the velopharyngeal structures or because of a short soft palate following healing after cleft palate repair, due to possible scar contracture. Despite aggressive speech therapy, a significant number of speakers require physical management if they are unable to compensate for functional or physical deficiencies in velopharyngeal closure. This may involve either prosthetic speech appliances to aid velopharyngeal closure for speech (see Chapter 18 by Leeper, Charles, and Sills) or a more permanent surgical improvement of closure.

Members of the interdisciplinary cleft team, such as the speech-language pathologist and prosthodontist, work closely with the surgeon to determine the most effective and practical way to achieve velopharyngeal closure at the patient's particular stage of physical and behavioral growth and development. Nasendoscopy and videofluoroscopy provide valuable information regarding the anatomy and function of the velopharyngeal structures to determine the most appropriate approach. Additionally, if the surgical approach is judged to be the most appropriate for a given speaker, the endoscopic and radiographic imaging will be valuable for the surgeon to choose the best operation for success.

## Surgical Options for VPI

### Pharyngeal Flap

In pharyngeal flap surgery, a flap of tissue is taken from the posterior pharyngeal wall and brought forward and attached to the soft palate as a permanent "bridge" across the velopharyngeal portal, leaving lateral openings or ports. This flap depends on inward or medial movement of the lateral pharyngeal walls to close the lateral ports for successful closure during speech (see Figure 14.20).

## Dynamic Sphincteroplasty (Sphincter Pharyngoplasty)

In dynamic sphincteroplasty, palatopharyngeus muscle flaps from the posterior tonsillar pillars are brought together with a short posterior pharyngeal wall flap to create a smaller central port that can be closed during speech if the soft palate is sufficiently mobile (see Figure 14.21).

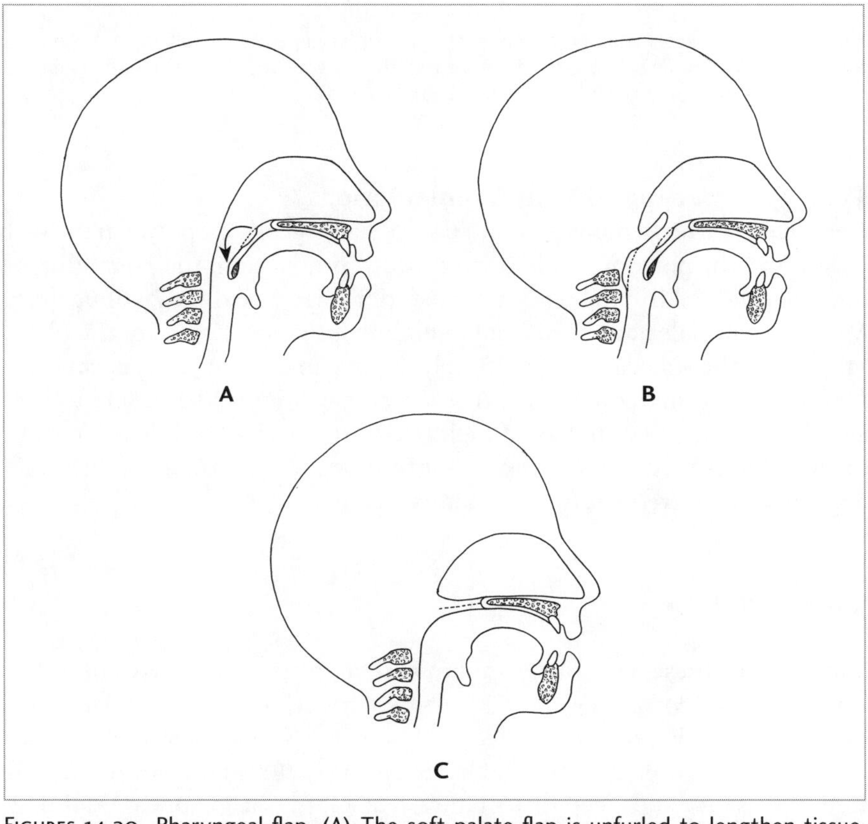


FIGURES 14.20. Pharyngeal flap. (A) The soft palate flap is unfurled to lengthen tissue. (B) Pharyngeal tissue is elevated from the posterior wall and rotated superiorly. (C) Posterior pharyngeal and soft palate flaps are sutured to create a "bridge" across the velopharyngeal gap.

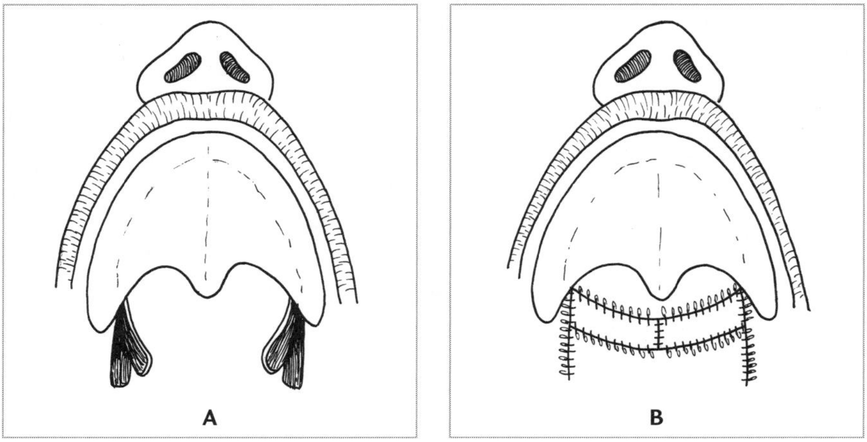


FIGURE 14.21. Dynamic sphincteroplasty. (A) Palatopharyngeus muscle flaps are elevated bilaterally. (B) The muscle flaps are sutured to the soft palate. The attached segments decrease the area of the central velopharyngeal port.

### Posterior Pharyngeal Wall Augmentation

For speakers who demonstrate small velopharyngeal gaps between the soft palate and the posterior wall during speech production, the possibility of augmenting ("plumping out") the posterior pharyngeal wall is appealing. Various materials have been used to augment the soft tissues of the pharynx where the soft palate most closely approximates the pharyngeal wall. Unfortunately, many materials that are currently considered safe to use, such as fat and collagen, have a high rate of resorption, or it is difficult to localize the exact place to augment for best closure. For these reasons, this approach is not frequently used at most centers.

## Controversies

With any of these surgical procedures, there is always the risk of either under- or overcorrecting the VPI. Undercorrection leaves persistent hypernasality, which occurs in 3%–20% of cases. Overcorrection may occur in 4%–18% of cases (Pantaloni & Hollier, 2000) and can often lead to hyponasality and sleep disturbances (including sleep apnea), and may require surgical revision or modification.

In patients who have had a previous straight-line closure resulting in an immobile, scarred, and shortened soft palate, surgeons may also consider "converting" to a Furlow Z-plasty to lengthen the soft palate and avoid a more permanent alteration of the velopharyngeal port with a pharyngeal flap (Sloan, 2000).

## Nose

Cleft nose deformities usually correlate with the severity of the cleft lip deformity. Forme fruste and some incomplete cleft lips have relatively minimal nostril asymmetry that may not require any surgical correction.

The classic cleft nose deformity seen with complete unilateral cleft lip has the following characteristics, as illustrated in Figure 14.22.

- Alar base—wide
- Alar rim—flattened, concave
- Columella—shortened on affected side
- Dome—asymmetric
- Tip—wide
- Septum—deviated toward the cleft side, narrowing normal airway
- Nasal sill—absent

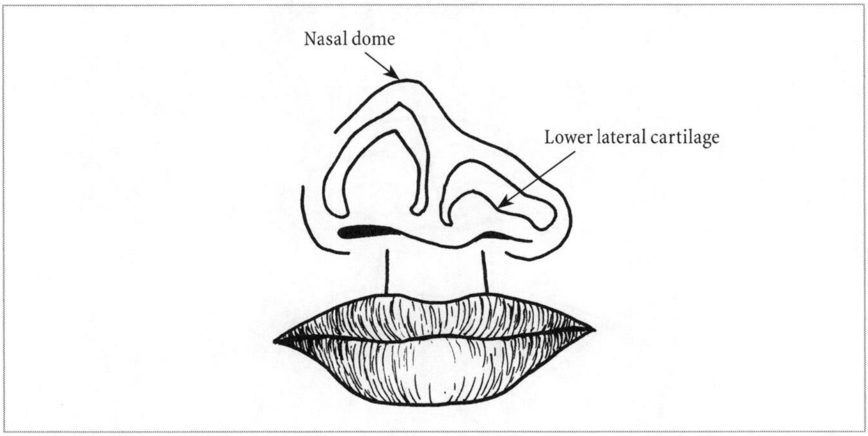


FIGURE 14.22. Unilateral cleft nose deformity. Note wide nostril floor, deviated columella and nasal tip, and buckling lateral alar cartilage.

The nasal deformity in a bilateral complete cleft lip is even more pronounced, with the following additional characteristics, as illustrated in Figure 14.23.

- Columella—extremely short or almost nonexistent
- Prolabium—short and narrow philtral lip length and lack of vermilion

## Techniques

The traditional approach to cleft nose deformities has been secondary repair of the tip and nostril, usually after alveolar bone grafting has provided more support to the nasal sill. In the last 10–20 years, the emphasis has shifted to primary rhinoplasty—that is, at the time of definitive lip repair—or even presurgical nasoalveolar molding for better symmetry. With molding, soft tissue lengthening of the columella and nostril reshaping can be achieved without surgical scarring.

Primary rhinoplasty affords a more symmetric-looking nose at an earlier age, although secondary revisions may still be necessary. With secondary rhinoplasty, more asymmetric growth has occurred, and additional cartilage grafts may be required to create tip projection and round out the affected nostril for more symmetry.

Whether primary or secondary rhinoplasty is performed, the goals are the same: to bring in the widened alar base, to free the lower lateral cartilage from the abnormal orbicularis oris attachments, to round out

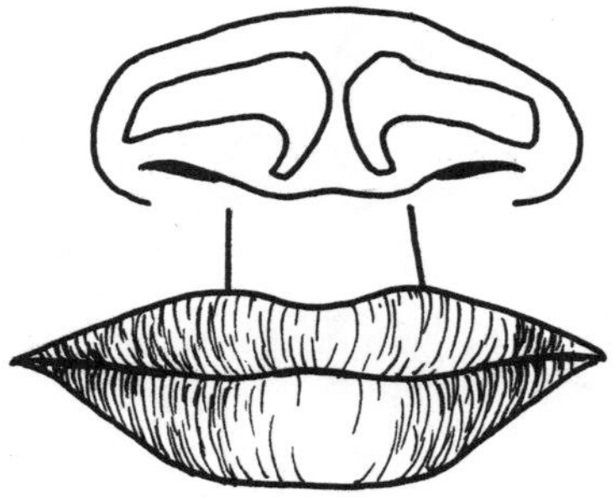

FIGURE 14.23. Bilateral cleft nose deformity. Note wide alar bases, flattened and separated domes, and short columella.

the affected nostril by freeing the depressed lower lateral alar cartilage, and to narrow the tip and provide more projection by lengthening the columella.

Septoplasty of the unilateral deviated septum is usually postponed until the mid- to late teen years, when facial growth has reached near-adult stage. If there is symptomatic obstruction of the contralateral airway, removal of hypertrophic turbinates (turbinectomy) may also be indicated.

## Secondary Procedures

After primary repair of the cleft lip, nose, and palate, patients may require secondary procedures or revisions for persistent irregularities in both appearance and function. Postsurgical scarring and/or a shortage of soft tissues may result in asymmetric growth, altered anatomical landmarks, or even ineffective closure of cleft defects. These secondary surgeries are usually done during the teen years or as needed, if the individuals have any related psychosocial or functional problems.

### Abbe Flap (Lip Switch/Cross-Lip Flap)

In bilateral cleft lip repairs, there is usually deficient philtral length and width, which is even more noticeable when compared to a full lower lip. To achieve better balance between the upper and lower lips, as well as a "less tight" upper labial sulcus (vestibule), an Abbe cross-lip flap may be considered beneficial. This procedure involves transposing a full-thickness wedge of tissue from the lower lip, based on the labial artery. While the flap is developing a new blood supply from the upper lip inset site, there is a tissue bridge across the lips carrying the labial artery that is divided at 10–21 days. This creates a more full and normal looking upper lip with a minimally visible donor site on the lower lip (Salomon & Hobar, 1997) (see Figure 14.24).

### Palatal Fistulae

Palatal fistulae occur in about 6% of cases (Pantaloni & Hollier, 2000). The most common locations are either at the junction of the hard and

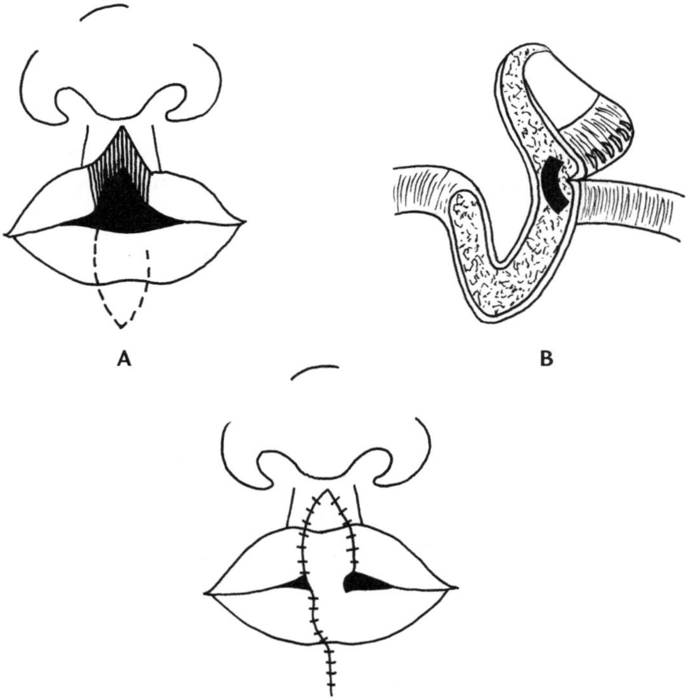


FIGURES 14.24. Abbe cross-lip flap to widen philtrum using central lower lip tissue. (A) Surgical incisions are made. (B) Lower lip flap is elevated and rotated, preserving blood supply from the labial artery. (C) Lower lip flap inset stays attached to vascular pedicle from labial artery for 2–3 weeks before separation.

soft palate or at the incisive foramen (the junction between primary and secondary palate). Although very small fistulae may not need closure, larger defects may cause nasal regurgitation of liquids and food and contribute to nasal air escape during pressure consonant sounds during speech. If simple "reclosure" of a palatal fistula is not possible due to scar tissue, it may become necessary to import healthy tissue from adjacent structures, such as the buccal sulcus or cheek mucosa, or even the tongue, to effectively close the defect. The timing of palatal fistula repair can be as early as age 3–4 years as decisions are being made regarding the best methods for optimizing speech.

## Conclusion

For the person with cleft lip and palate, the surgical care and repair of cleft defects is but one part of the interdisciplinary cleft team approach. The goal is to tailor the best possible care for the patient throughout all stages of growth and development. As new parents become more aware of the surgical options and specialty resources available to cleft patients, they too can and must become active members of the team to help their child develop the confidence needed to reach his or her full potential in life.

## References

Berkowitz, S., Mejia, M., & Bystrik, A. (2004). A comparison of the effects of the Latham-Millard procedure with those of a conservative treatment approach for dental occlusion and facial aesthetics in unilateral and bilateral complete cleft lip and palate: Part I. Dental occlusion. *Plastic and Reconstructive Surgery, 113*(1), 1–18.

Byrd, H. S. (1997). Cleft lip I: Primary deformities. *Selected Readings in Plastic Surgery, 8*(21), 13–21.

Cutting, C. (2000). Secondary cleft lip nasal reconstruction: State of the art. *Cleft Palate-Craniofacial Journal, 3,* 538–541.

Grayson, B. H.., Santiago, P. E., Brecht, L. E., & Cutting, C. B. (1999). Presurgical nasoalveolar molding in infants with cleft lip and palate. *Cleft Palate-Craniofacial Journal, 36,* 486–498.

Kuijpers-Jagtmann, A. M., & Long, R. E. (2000). The influence of surgery and orthopedic treatment on maxillofacial growth and maxillary arch development in patients treated for orofacial clefts. *Cleft Palate-Craniofacial Journal, 37,* 527-1–527-12.

LaRossa, D. (2000). The state of the art in cleft palate surgery. *Cleft Palate-Craniofacial Journal, 33,* 225–228.

Moller, K. T., Starr, C. D., & Johnson, S. A. (1990). *A parent's guide to cleft lip and palate.* Minneapolis: University of Minnesota Press.

Mulliken, J. B. (2000). Repair of bilateral complete cleft lip and nasal deformity—State of the art. *Cleft Palate-Craniofacial Journal, 37,* 342–347.

Pantaloni, M., & Hollier, L. (2000). Cleft palate and velopharyngeal incompetence. *Selected Readings in Plastic Surgery, 9*(23), 1–38.

Papay, F. A., Morales, L., Jr., Motoki, D. S., & Yamashiro, D. K. (1995). Presurgical orthopedic premaxillary alignment in cleft lip and palate reconstruction. *Cleft Palate-Craniofacial Journal, 32,* 353–355.

Salomon, J., & Hobar, P. C. (1997). Cleft lip II: Secondary deformities. *Selected Readings in Plastic Surgery, 8*(22), 1–29.

Schendel, S. A. (2000). Unilateral cleft lip repair—State of the art. *Cleft Palate-Craniofacial Journal, 37,* 335–341.

Sloan, G. M. (2000). Posterior pharyngeal flap and sphincter pharyngoplasty: The state of the art. *Cleft Palate-Craniofacial Journal, 37,* 112–122.

Will, L. A. (2000). Growth and development in patients with untreated clefts. *Cleft Palate-Craniofacial Journal, 37,* 523–526.

# CHAPTER 15

# Pediatric Otolaryngology

## Management of the Ear, Nose, Throat, and Airway

*James D. Sidman*

The otolaryngologist on the interdisciplinary cleft palate team is primarily responsible for the health of the patient's ears, nose, and throat and the associated functions of hearing; breathing passages in the nose, mouth, and throat; voice and speech production; and swallowing. Increasingly, otolaryngologists with specialized training are also performing primary repairs of the cleft lip or palate. Sidman describes the scope of practice, training experience, and clinical issues that encompass the practice of pediatric otolaryngologists who diagnose and treat patients with cleft lip or palate and other craniofacial anomalies. Sidman also reviews select clinical etiologies and management approaches for airway obstruction, early feeding and swallowing issues, and hearing concerns that are common in this population.

1. There are many possible sources of airway obstruction due to structural anomalies of the nose and throat in infants and children with cleft palate. Identify these structural sources and explain how they are identified and managed clinically.
2. Describe the sequence of embryologic events that lead to cleft palate in patients diagnosed with Robin sequence. How do these structural anomalies create an airway threat for these infants? What nonsurgical and surgical management options are available to protect the airway in these young patients?
3. Describe the impact of enlarged adenoid tissue on breathing and on velopharyngeal closure in patients with a short soft palate. How might enlarged adenoid tissue affect speech resonance positively or negatively? List the medical considerations for performing

an adenoidectomy in children with cleft palate and explain the potential influence on speech production.

4. Define the signs and symptoms of sleep apnea. What might predispose children with cleft palate to this disorder? What testing and measures are available to describe and document sleep apnea?
5. What are the various feeding strategies used to accommodate babies born with cleft lip or palate? How does the lack of strong suck alter the newborn's ability to feed normally?
6. Explain why eustachian tube dysfunction is common in children with cleft palate. Describe the benefits and hazards of pressure equalization (PE) tube placement, including the impact on hearing acuity, the tympanic membrane, speech and language development, and future ear disease.

Otolaryngology is the medical and surgical specialty concerned with the ears, nose, throat, and head and neck surgery. Accordingly, the specialty is sometimes called ENT. The field includes the diagnosis and treatment of disorders, diseases, or other problems related to ears, eustachian tubes, pharynx, palate, larynx, upper esophagus, breathing passages (from the nose, sinus cavities, and mouth to the lungs), and other soft tissues of the neck and the skull base. The otolaryngologist also diagnoses and treats etiologies that create functional problems, such as disorders of smell, hearing, speech, voice, and swallowing. Usually, the otolaryngologist does not treat brain diseases, vision problems, or conditions that affect the spine. A notable aspect of the otolaryngologists' scope of practice is that their treatments may include medical, surgical, or a combination of approaches. Therefore, on the cleft palate and craniofacial team, the otolaryngologist with specialized training may address any medical or surgical problems that affect the function of the ears, nose, palate, pharynx, or larynx.

An otolaryngologist is a physician who has completed medical school and 5–6 additional years of residency training in otolaryngology head and neck surgery. This residency includes both clinical and surgical experience in managing disorders of the ear, nose, and throat, and diseases of the head and neck. Although not all otolaryngology residency-training programs provide specialty experience in surgical repair of the cleft lip and palate, that emphasis is increasing.

After completing the otolaryngology residency, the physician may choose to take an additional 1–2 years of subspecialty fellowship training in areas such as pediatric otolaryngology, facial plastic and reconstructive surgery, otology, neuro-otology, head and neck surgery, or sinus surgery. General otolaryngologists, pediatric otolaryngologists, and specialists in facial plastic and reconstructive surgery are often members of cleft palate and craniofacial teams. They are trained to evaluate and treat the varied ear, nose, and throat problems in cleft and craniofacial patients, which may be different from the common otolaryngologic conditions seen in the noncleft population. Most of these problems develop due to the unique anatomic relationships seen in cleft palate and craniofacial anomalies. For example, deformities in the oronasopharynx or trachea may produce breathing problems or obstruction. Incomplete velopharyngeal closure may contribute to feeding or swallowing problems. Ear malformations may contribute to hearing loss. Anomalies of the tongue, pharynx, or larynx may create problems with airway protection or speech development. While each patient is unique, the otolaryngologist who is specialty trained in managing cleft palate and craniofacial anomalies will be prepared to recommend suitable medical or surgical alternatives for each of these issues.

## Role of the Otolaryngologist on the Cleft Palate and Craniofacial Team

In the early part of the 20th century, pediatric surgeons performed the cleft surgeries in North America. Later, plastic surgeons managed the cleft repairs. Currently, otolaryngologists conduct cleft palate repairs in many regions, if they have had the specialty training that qualifies them to perform these procedures.

Traditionally, the general otolaryngologist has performed the role of diagnosing and treating middle ear disease in patients with clefts. Due to the anatomy associated with clefting of the primary or secondary palate, virtually all patients with cleft palate have middle ear disease early in life because of disrupted palatal muscles. The otolaryngologist has both medical and surgical options for remediating the problem. For example, prescription antibiotic drugs may eliminate middle ear infections. Surgically, the otolaryngologist may place pressure equalization (PE) tubes or repair the tympanic membrane (eardrum) to relieve middle ear disease. Following any treatment, the child's middle ear must be monitored consistently to verify that treatment has been adequate. The otolaryngologist will also recommend hearing testing by the audiologist to confirm that any impact of the middle ear disease on the child's hearing has resolved. (See also Chapter 9 by Carlstrom and Nelson for a description of hearing tests and procedures.)

A second area of focus for the otolaryngologist on the cleft palate and craniofacial team is the management of breathing problems that are related to nasal or oral obstruction, problems at the level of the tongue base or larynx, or tracheal-bronchial obstruction. Other medical specialists manage intrinsic respiratory diseases of the lung, such as premature lung disease or cystic fibrosis. Otolaryngologists may select either medical treatment (pharmaceutical agents such as decongestants, steroids, or other drugs that treat symptoms of upper airway congestion) or surgery, if the obstruction is a structural anomaly that interferes with patent airflow. When children with cleft lip and palate have breathing problems in conjunction with swallowing difficulties, these are diagnosed and treated by the otolaryngologist in collaboration with a speech-language pathologist or occupational therapist.

A third concern of the otolaryngologist on the cleft palate and craniofacial team is the child's communication development, including speech, voice, and hearing. The otolaryngologist is responsible for diagnosing medical disorders of the velum (soft palate) or larynx that may contribute to speech problems. For example, hypernasal resonance may be related to a variety of physical anomalies that result in incomplete velopharyngeal closure, such as a short or adynamic soft palate or a submucous cleft palate. Persistent or recurrent hoarseness in children may signal a range of possible laryngeal pathologies, including nodules, congenital cysts, laryngeal web, papilloma, or idiopathic paralysis. These conditions may require surgical management to improve speech or voice quality. As described in Chapters 8 (Chapman), 11 (Trost-Cardamone), and 12 (Glaze), some speech and voice disorders may respond positively to behavioral interventions. Thus, the otolaryngologist works closely with the speech-language pathologist in diagnosing and treating these disorders and advocating for appropriate behavioral, medical, or surgical intervention(s), as needed. Similarly, as described by Carlstrom and Nelson in Chapter 9, hearing problems are managed cooperatively by the otolaryngologist, who will provide the medical or surgical management of ear disease, and the audiologist, who will conduct behavioral testing and may provide aural (re)habilitation. Early diagnosis and intervention are critical to establishing effective communication skills for children with cleft palate or craniofacial anomalies, who are often at risk for speech, voice, or hearing impairments.

In addition to managing ear, nose, and throat concerns, in recent years many otolaryngologists have been performing primary cleft lip and palate repairs in infants, as well as other reconstructive revisions of the nose, lip, and palate later in childhood and the teenage years. Not all otolaryngologists will perform these procedures, but the number of practitioners who have completed additional training in facial plastic reconstruction or who have expanded residency-training experience in cleft palate are increasing nationally (Mann & Sidman, 1994).

## Airway Management

Anomalies in the size or spatial relationships of the nose, mouth, tongue, jaw, pharynx, and larynx may create challenging airway problems for some infants with cleft palate or craniofacial conditions. Airway concerns are a critical focus for the otolaryngologist, who may be responsible for managing early challenges to breathing and feeding caused by structural or functional defects of the upper airway. The extent and nature of airway issues are difficult to predict due to the large number of varied syndromes associated with cleft palate and micrognathia (small jaw) (Sidman, Sampson, & Templeton, 2001). Following is a description of some representative examples of airway issues in infants with cleft palate and craniofacial anomalies.

### Cleft Lip and Palate

Whenever a newborn has trouble breathing or gaining weight, consideration must be given to possible structural breathing problems and an otolaryngologist should be consulted. Possible problems that lead to upper airway obstruction in children with or without cleft lip or palate include rhinitis (inflamed nasal passages), choanal atresia (bony or soft tissue obstruction of the posterior nasopharynx), deviated nasal septum from birth trauma, and laryngomalacia (floppy and collapsible supraglottic laryngeal tissues). Children with cleft lip and palate with syndromes and children with other craniofacial anomalies can present with an even larger array of abnormalities of multiple etiologies. For example, infants with G/BBB (Opitz-Frias) syndrome often present with cleft lip and palate, midline brain abnormalities, laryngeal clefting, and other anomalies (Bershof, Guyuron, & Olsen, 1992). The cleft larynx is almost always associated with either airway obstruction or chronic aspiration.

To diagnose and treat these airway anomalies, the otolaryngologist will perform a direct laryngoscopy and bronchoscopy to visually examine the infant's pharynx, larynx, trachea, and mainstem bronchi under anesthesia (see Figure 15.1). Various diagnostic imaging techniques are also available to help define and diagnose airway anomalies by providing precise delineation of the deep hard and soft tissues. Computerized tomography (CT) scans are most helpful for observing bony and cartilage structures of the upper airway (i.e., spine, trachea, jaw, palate, mandible, and septum), but sometimes require contrast agent by injection. Newer

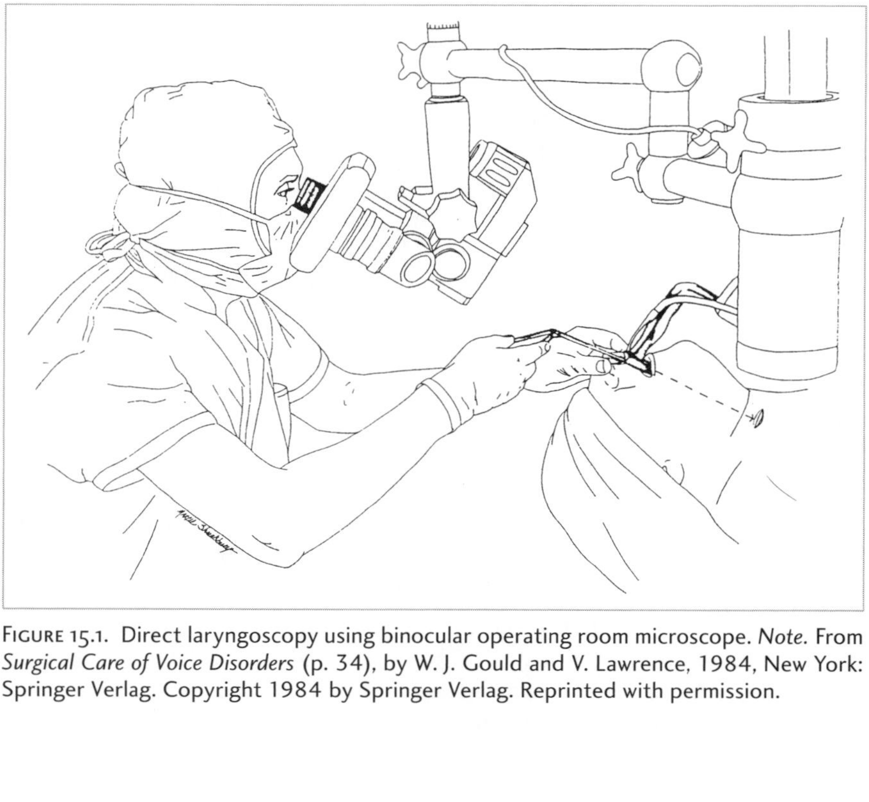

FIGURE 15.1. Direct laryngoscopy using binocular operating room microscope. *Note.* From *Surgical Care of Voice Disorders* (p. 34), by W. J. Gould and V. Lawrence, 1984, New York: Springer Verlag. Copyright 1984 by Springer Verlag. Reprinted with permission.

CT scanners do not require prolonged sedation or high levels of radiation exposure. In infants, plain X-ray films can be of some benefit in observing skeletal and cartilage structures more quickly. Magnetic resonance imaging (MRI) scans provide superior images of soft tissues and do not expose the patient to radiation, but do require longer periods of sedation to obtain accurate scans. Fluoroscopy can be used to define airway and swallowing passages during real-time movements (e.g., breathing and swallowing) (Altman, Wetmore, & Mahboubi, 1998). For all procedures, the goal is to identify the extent of the defect and its current impact on the infant's airway patency, protection, and swallowing, all of which are essential to early growth and development.

## Robin Sequence

A special case of cleft palate is seen in children diagnosed with Robin sequence. Individuals with Robin sequence present with a triad of symptoms: a U-shaped cleft palate, micrognathia, and glossoptosis (tongue falling backwards into the throat). Robin sequence is considered to be a sequence and not a syndrome because the events leading up to these findings are related and understood (Prows & Bender, 1999). Prenatally, the tongue was positioned back and into the palatal area, presumably inhibiting palatal closure and creating a signature U-shaped cleft palate (Cohen, 1999), which is distinct from the more common V-shaped cleft palate. The posterior tongue positioning, which is maintained even after birth and often through early childhood, can lead to associated problems with breathing and swallowing.

Robin sequence can be part of a syndrome or can be found in isolation without any associated syndrome. The earliest signs of this disorder are often difficulty breathing shortly after birth or difficulty feeding and gaining weight in the first months of life. Importantly, the feeding problems are almost always secondary to breathing problems, and not the other way around (Sidman et al., 2001). If a baby cannot breathe well, then he or she will not be able to feed well enough to gain adequate weight. These children may be incorrectly diagnosed with "failure to thrive" if the deleterious impact of the airway obstruction goes unrecognized. As these babies try to breathe, it is easy to mistake the movement of the chest rise and fall as successful respiration. In fact, they may be trying to breathe against an obstructed airway and may not be moving any air at all. Usually, alleviating the airway obstruction will also resolve the feeding problem. Thus, treating the feeding problem alone is not sufficient, if there are underlying complications with breathing.

Micrognathia in Robin sequence results in the posterior positioning of the tongue. The muscles of the tongue are attached to the front of the mandible and hold the tongue in its normal resting position. If the mandible is deficient (i.e., has limited anterior dimension), then the tongue will sit farther back in the throat, attached to the small jaw. In some children, it can even be difficult to see the tongue due to its posterior position of rest in the pharynx. Thus, the problem of obstructed breathing in Robin sequence is due to the tongue falling backwards into the throat and blocking the breathing space.

Treating airway obstruction in the infant with Robin sequence is complex, especially when managing the interaction between breathing and feeding. The simplest approach is to place the infant in a prone position and support the jaw during feeding. In the prone position (lying on the abdomen), the tongue will often fall forward and open up the airway in the pharynx. During feeding, the caregiver can put two fingers behind the angle of the infant's jaw and give mild forward pressure to push the tongue and jaw forward and open up the airway. If further measures are necessary, then long nasal breathing tubes can be inserted through the nose and into the pharynx to displace the tongue forward in the mouth and provide a patent airway from the nares to the pharynx (Heaf, Helms, Dinwiddie, & Mathew, 1982). These nasal tubes are invasive and must be changed frequently as they can easily become blocked with secretions.

Surgical intervention in babies with Robin sequence is necessary if conservative treatments fail. As a temporary measure, gastrostomy (feeding tube placed through the abdominal skin into the stomach) or nasogastric (feeding tube placed through the nose into the stomach) tube feedings can be used to establish nutrition and maintain growth. However, these techniques only treat the symptom of poor feeding and do not resolve the underlying problem of airway obstruction, which may require one of several surgical management approaches.

Because the airway obstruction is based on the posterior placement of the tongue, some surgeons perform tongue-lip adhesions. This operation attempts to pull the tongue forward by surgically stitching it to the front of the mandible (Li, Lo, Chen, Wong, & Chang, 2002). Most airway specialists have abandoned this procedure as being ineffective for children in whom conservative management fails (Myer, Reed, Cotton, Willging, & Shott, 1998) due to the other negative complications of this treatment.

First, the tongue repositioning may not be sufficient to ensure a patent airway in the posterior pharynx. Second, the adhesion must remain in place for several months, until the child outgrows the micrognathia or vertical growth dimensions increase, dropping the tongue lower in the oropharynx. During this treatment, the tongue is anchored and not able to develop normal movements for feeding, swallowing, and speech sound development (e.g., babbling).

Instead, the "gold standard" for managing the obstructed airway in an infant with Robin sequence is a tracheostomy. This procedure creates a surgical opening in the neck, just below the larynx, to bypass the obstructed upper airway and allow adequate ventilation through the tracheostomy tube. The "trach tube" must remain in place until the child outgrows the airway obstruction, usually by 6–18 months of age, following significant mandibular growth that allows the tongue to rest anteriorly, out of the pharynx and airway (Daskalogiannakis, Ross, & Tompson, 2001; Vegter, Hage, & Mulder, 1999).

If a child does not outgrow the micrognathia, then surgery can be considered, to lengthen the mandible to bring the tongue forward in the mouth. The newest technique to accomplish mandibular lengthening is distraction osteogenesis. The procedure is aptly named, as the bone is cut and ends are systematically separated (distracted) to allow new bone growth (osteogenesis) to fill in the intervening gap. Once the mandible is cut on both sides, pins are placed into the bone and attached to a device that can be used to gradually separate the bone segments at the surgical cut. This device gradually pulls the bony segments apart, approximately 1.5 mm per day. The slow separation of the bony segments stimulates natural bone regrowth that fills the space and lengthens the bone. The process is continued until sufficient new bone growth and lengthening has been achieved. It is possible to gain as much as 10–15 mm of new mandible length over time. Distraction osteogenesis has been applied to infants with airway obstruction secondary to micrognathia and has been successful in either preventing the need for tracheotomy or allowing earlier removal of the tracheotomy tube (Sidman et al., 2001).

## Nasal Congestion and Obstruction

Older children with cleft lip and palate often have symptoms of chronic nasal congestion and obstruction. This condition can arise following surgery for cleft lip repair or surgery for velopharyngeal closure, or from an underlying nasal deformity. Surgery to close a cleft lip may create nasal valve stenosis, especially if the segments are far apart or there is limited tissue to create the closure (Trenite, Paping, & Trenning, 1997). A deviated septum is almost always found in patients who have a cleft palate, and is not necessarily related to the surgery. A deviated septum with significant nasal obstruction is common in patients with unilateral and bilateral cleft palate, especially if the hard palate was involved in the cleft (Drake, Davis, & Warren, 1993; Warren, Drake, & Davis, 1992). Repair of the deviated septum is usually deferred until the teenage years to avoid damaging the potential for midfacial growth, which is closely related to growth of the nasal septum. If the problem is severe, limited septoplasty can be accomplished in younger children.

Posteriorly, choanal atresia may be present unilaterally or bilaterally. The obstruction is due to bony or soft tissue blockage, which must be removed surgically and held open with stents to create a patent airway. If the obstruction is bilateral, the surgical repair may be necessary in the newborn period, because most newborns are obligate nasal breathers and will suffocate without an adequate nasal airway. Choanal atresia is seen with some craniofacial syndromes but is rare in patients with isolated cleft lip or palate.

## Tonsils and Adenoids

As children grow, airway obstruction from growing tonsils or adenoids can cause increased snoring. Although medical therapy with antibiotics or topical nasal steroids has been described to alleviate snoring, it is rarely helpful in the long term. Persistent snoring is not normal in children and should be evaluated by the otolaryngologist to rule out sleep apnea (loss of oxygen). Sleep apnea affects children negatively by depriving them of adequate rest due to disruptions in the normal sleep pattern. Sleep apnea is suspected whenever parents report that a child exhibits symptoms of loud, prolonged, and obstructive snoring; daytime drowsiness; restless sleep; and other behavioral or health problems (Messner, 2003). Recent studies suggest that many behavioral manifestations of attention deficit can be attributed to obstructive sleep apnea in some children (Mitchell & Kelly, 2007; Wei, Mayo, Smith, et al., 2007). These behavioral problems are thought to be caused by lack of consistent deep sleep, so the children are essentially deprived of good quality rest through the night. Sleep apnea can be assessed directly during a clinical sleep study, which monitors and records the child's breathing patterns, respiratory rate, apneic episodes, and oxygenation ($CO_2$ and $O_2$ levels) by observing chest wall motion in combination with pulse oximetry fluctuations, and using other measures.

Enlarged adenoids are commonly seen in children as young as 6 months old and can be a problem until the teenage years, when the adenoids gradually regress. The diagnosis of adenoid enlargement is made either with nasal endoscopy or with lateral neck X-rays to examine soft tissue. The presence of enlarged adenoids increases the potential for nasal obstruction or recurrent upper respiratory infections. Common symptoms of this problem include chronic runny nose, snoring, frequent colds, and mouth breathing.

When enlarged adenoids do not resolve and complicate the medical picture, the otolaryngologist may perform a surgical adenoidectomy with or without concurrent tonsillectomy. Although this is a common childhood procedure, adenoidectomy can cause serious harm to speech in patients with cleft palate or velopharyngeal insufficiency, because the enlarged adenoids may be assisting with velopharyngeal closure. This occurs when children with (apparent) adequate velopharyngeal closure suddenly develop inadequate closure directly after adenoidectomy. In these cases, the adenoids were likely masking an undetected velopharyngeal gap or short soft palate. Hypernasal speech develops postsurgically because of the increased distance the soft palate (velum) must move to obtain adequate contact and closure with the posterior pharyngeal wall. Traditional adenoidectomy is therefore contraindicated in a patient with cleft palate or submucous cleft. A modification of adenoidectomy where only the choanal adenoids are removed is referred to as a superior adenoidectomy. This procedure does not appear to cause speech deterioration, as the adenoids are left intact at the level of velopharyngeal closure (Kakani, Callan, & April, 2000).

Tonsil hypertrophy causes similar symptoms to enlarged adenoids, with sleep apnea, snoring, bad breath, and recurrent tonsil infections being common symptoms. Although antibiotic use helps in the short term, tonsillectomy is the only long-term solution for chronic tonsil problems. Although removing the tonsils can change resonance somewhat, their removal does not cause velopharyngeal insufficiency and hypernasality. Because tonsils are located inferior to the horizontal plane of velopharyngeal closure, the tonsillectomy has virtually no effect on the velopharyngeal mechanism and should not be viewed as the same procedure as an adenoidectomy by a health professional.

## Laryngomalacia

Newborns with cleft and craniofacial anomalies have the same risk as other babies for developing laryngomalacia during the first 2 months of life. Laryngomalacia is identified initially by the presence of inspiratory stridor, due to "floppy" supralaryngeal structures, especially the epiglottis, that are drawn into the airway during inspiration. Laryngomalacia is confirmed when the otolaryngologist performs a direct laryngoscopy to observe the larynx and airway. The condition usually resolves by 1 year of age, as the airway grows and tissues stabilize, and rarely requires surgery. Laryngomalacia is often seen in association with gastroesophageal reflux disease (GERD), so antacid-type medications are often helpful for both conditions.

Tracheomalacia is much rarer than laryngomalacia and is demonstrated by expiratory stridor and wheezing during infancy, as a symptom of tracheal narrowing during exhalation. This problem may become evident after other surgery to the trachea, for example, after repair of a congenital tracheoesophageal fistula. Tracheomalacia is usually treated with positive air pressure and occasionally with surgery. Positive pressure is usually delivered using a mask that fits over the nose, or the nose and mouth. The mask is connected by tubing to a machine that delivers pressurized air. The pressure level can be set to whatever level is needed to distend the airways enough to keep them from collapsing. These positive pressure devices are referred to as CPAP (Constant Positive Airway Pressure) or BiPAP (Bilevel Positive Airway Pressure).

## Pharyngeal Flap

A final risk of airway obstruction in patients with cleft palate or craniofacial anomalies is due to pharyngeal flap surgery. When the flap remains too wide even after swollen tissues are healed, the lateral breathing ports may be too narrow or may become blocked easily. Speech resonance may sound normal or even hyponasal and be perfectly acceptable, but a wide pharyngeal flap can obstruct the airway and cause snoring, nasal congestion, slower physical growth, and sleep apnea (Liao et al., 2002). Diagnosis of sleep apnea in this situation usually requires a formal sleep study to determine whether apneic episodes are clinically significant. If so, the only treatment available is a surgical revision to narrow the pharyngeal flap and widen the lateral breathing ports.

# Feeding Problems

Early feeding problems are common in newborns with cleft palate. Most often, there is a necessary period of adjustment in response to the infant's inability to generate adequate and prolonged suck because of the cleft palate (Kaufman, 1991). The role of the otolaryngologist is to rule out any medical threat to feeding and swallowing so that infants with early feeding challenges will grow and develop normally.

Typically, babies born with an uncomplicated cleft lip or palate can be fed using specialized nipples and a variety of soft squeeze bottles designed specifically for use with these babies. The bottles allow milk to flow gently into the mouth when the caregiver squeezes, alleviating the need for a strong suck. Usually, once the milk is delivered into the mouth, normal swallow patterns are triggered. Although feeding appliances to obturate the cleft palate and help with neonatal feeding have been well described (Reid, 2004), they are not widely used because the appliances are difficult to fit and maintain in the newborn, and expertise in constructing them is not commonly available. Nearly all babies with cleft palate can be fed properly with a cleft feeding bottle. Babies with cleft palate tend to swallow more air and need to be burped more frequently. See Chapter 6 for Breen, Chibbaro, and Hopper's comprehensive description of feeding issues, nursing support, and counseling for parents and families.

Although many mothers would prefer to breastfeed their babies with cleft palates, this is rarely successful in providing adequate nutrition because the baby cannot suck enough milk before getting tired. If the mother can pump breast milk, that milk is still preferred as the best nutrition for an infant and can be used whenever possible in the cleft bottle. Some mothers may experience significant frustration and even depression arising from feelings of inadequacy if their babies cannot breastfeed. These negative reactions can be prevented with proper education, support, and counseling for the mother.

Babies with cleft palate who do not seem to adjust comfortably to these feeding adaptations or who demonstrate poor feeding and insufficient weight gain often have more critical, unrecognized airway difficulties. For example, occult anatomic abnormalities such as laryngeal cleft must be ruled out in infants who demonstrate symptoms of chronic aspiration following feeding. Problems with feeding and swallowing in infants always suggest a possible risk of airway threat or obstruction. When airway problems persist, infants will not feed by mouth, so weight gain deteriorates. For this reason, developmental growth and weight gain in cleft babies should be monitored closely in the early weeks, with a guideline of regaining birth weight by 2 weeks, followed by daily gains of 0.5–1.0 oz as an acceptable goal.

Fortunately, the timing of the cleft lip repair and healing period should not interfere at all with feeding by bottle or breast, which can usually continue within 24 hours of surgery. Care must be taken to clean the suture lines and monitor tissue swelling after lip repair. However, most surgeons prefer that babies be weaned off bottle feeding before repairing the secondary palate, so that palatal motion during sucking does not place too much tension on new suture lines in the soft palate (Cohen, Marschall, & Schafer, 1992).

Rarely, a baby with uncomplicated cleft palate will have ongoing problems with weight gain and adequate oral intake. The conservative approach is to try different cleft feeding bottles, nipples, and/or formulas; provide nursing support for the parents and caregivers; and monitor these attempts patiently, to give the baby time to be successful. On rare occasions, children with cleft palate will require short-term supplemental feeding with a nasogastric or even a gastrostomy feeding tube. These tubes place additional responsibility on parents, who must learn to care for the tubes and surrounding equipment. One potential problem is that after even a few months of tube feeding, some otherwise normal babies will develop an oral aversion to feeding by mouth, and will require months or years of oral feeding rehabilitation to achieve adequate nutrition by mouth rather than feeding tube (Byars et al., 2003). Whenever possible, the use of feeding tubes should be avoided.

## Hearing Problems

Ensuring that children have normal hearing during the first 5 years of life is crucial to normal speech and language development. The otolaryngologist has primary responsibility for monitoring the child's hearing health and advocating for audiology testing and (re)habilitation services, as needed, as well as treating ear disease through medical management or surgical interventions. Children with cleft palate or craniofacial anomalies are at larger risk for hearing loss due to possible interaction with other, unrecognized syndromes. Eustachian tube dysfunction is a known etiology of otitis media (middle ear infections). Because it is nearly universal in children born with cleft palate, all cleft babies are at risk for developing chronic middle ear effusions and conductive hearing loss, and most of these children will experience fluctuating hearing loss in the early years of life.

The eustachian tube is a conduit that angles medially from the middle ear space and inferiorly into the nasopharynx. This tube primarily allows air pressure in the middle ear to equalize with atmospheric air pressure in the nasopharynx (see Figure 15.2). This maintenance of equal pressure helps to keep the middle ear dry and healthy. If the pressure in the middle ear cannot equalize with atmospheric pressure, then a negative pressure vacuum effect will take place in the middle ear. Fluid cannot be reabsorbed under these conditions and will accumulate in the middle ear space and eventually become contaminated and infected.

Children born with cleft palate have a significant disadvantage that predisposes them to ear disease. Normal eustachian tube function relies on the tensor veli palatini muscles, which loop around the hamulus bone on the side of the palate and insert into the soft palate. When the tensor

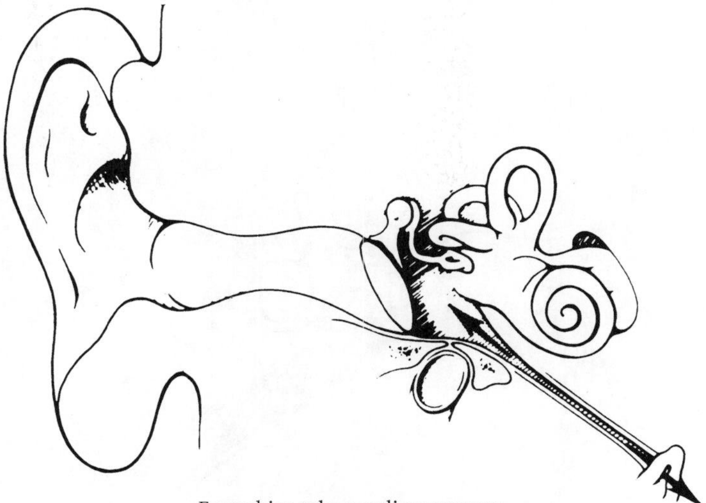


FIGURE 15.2. The eustachian tube connects the middle ear to the nasopharynx. Arrows indicate air movement through the tube.

veli palatini muscles contract, the eustachian tube opens wider (see Figure 15.3). In children with cleft palate, however, these muscles are inserted improperly and result in chronic eustachian tube dysfunction. Consequently, the eustachian tubes cannot dilate effectively to equalize air pressure or to drain fluid buildup in the middle ear. In the era before pressure equalization (PE) tubes, nearly 10% of children with cleft palate later developed cholesteatoma (benign growth) of the middle ear (Dominguez & Harker, 1988). Many of these children also developed permanent conductive hearing loss, even with reconstructive surgery. Today, most otolaryngologists believe that all children with cleft palate should have PE tubes placed before 1 year of age (Muntz, 1993). Some will place the tubes as early as the cleft lip repair (if a cleft lip exists) or anywhere from 4 to 12 months of age.

It is common for children with cleft palate to develop recurrent otorrhea (ear drainage) after PE tubes are in place. This outcome is due to continuing eustachian tube dysfunction and chronic middle ear effusions. These episodes of otorrhea can almost always be treated with topical antibiotic drops or by suctioning the ear during an office visit to the otolaryngologist. Systemic antibiotics or further surgical intervention are

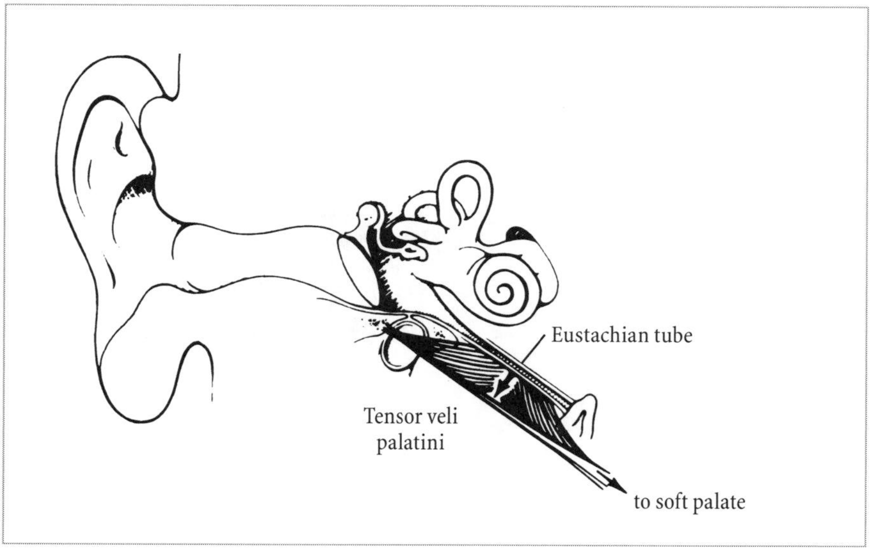


FIGURE 15.3. The tensor veli palatini muscle contraction (note arrow) dilates the eustachian tube to equalize middle ear pressure with atmospheric air.

rarely necessary, and the long-term benefits of good hearing health and healthy ears outweigh the inconvenience of intermittent otorrhea.

It seems intuitive that eustachian tube dysfunction would improve in children with cleft palate once the palatal muscles have been reapproximated during the cleft palate repair. However, multiple studies have shown that this is not the case, as cleft palate repair does not seem to reduce middle ear disease (Smith, DiRuggiero, & Jones, 1994). Fortunately, eustachian tube dysfunction seen in children with cleft palate seems to resolve itself by about age 5–7 years for most, regardless of the timing of the cleft palate repair. In some patients with clefts, the middle ear disease can persist into adulthood, requiring multiple sets of PE tubes and more advanced repairs of the tympanic membrane or middle ear ossicles.

With or without placement of PE tubes, some children will develop perforations in one or both of the tympanic membranes. These perforations usually cause a mild conductive hearing loss and allow contamination from the outer ear to enter the middle ear, where it may cause chronic infections. For these reasons, the perforation should be repaired when the otolaryngologist feels that the child has nearly outgrown the eustachian tube dysfunction associated with cleft palate. The tympanoplasty procedure (surgical repair of the eardrum) can usually restore normal hearing.

Children with isolated cleft palate do not have a significantly higher risk of sensorineural hearing loss than other children. Nonetheless, some of these children do have unrecognized syndromes, so all should be screened for hearing loss as early as possible. Fortunately, most states now conduct universal newborn hearing screenings to detect congenital losses. Annual hearing screenings are essential for babies and children with cleft palate throughout their early childhood and school-age years. This screening should be done by an audiologist and not only by primary doctors' offices or school screening programs. If sensorineural hearing loss is identified, the otolaryngologist will work closely with the audiologist to establish a plan for appropriate amplification, as described in detail by Carlstrom and Nelson in Chapter 9.

## Summary

Otolaryngology is a surgical specialty that diagnoses and treats diseases of the ear, nose, throat, head, and neck. Specific concerns that are common to babies and children with cleft palate or craniofacial anomalies are due to the unique anatomic differences of the head, neck, and upper airway in these populations. These structural defects have the potential to influence airway protection and obstruction, early feeding and swallowing abilities, hearing health, speech and voice production, and other developmental factors. Thus, the role of the otolaryngologist on the interdisciplinary team is to provide medical treatments or surgical repairs to manage these problems effectively.

## References

Altman, K. W., Wetmore, R. F., & Mahboubi, S. (1998). Comparison of endoscopy and radiographic fluoroscopy in the evaluation of pediatric congenital airway abnormalities. *International Journal of Pediatric Otorhinolaryngology, 44*(1), 43–46.

Bershof, J. F., Guyuron, B., & Olsen, M. M. (1992). G syndrome: A review of the literature and a case report. *Journal of Cranio-Maxillofacial Surgery, 20*(1), 24–27.

Byars, K. C., Burklow, K. A., Ferguson, K., O'Flaherty, T., Santoro, K., & Kaul, A. (2003). A multicomponent behavioral program for oral aversion in children dependent on gastrostomy feedings. *Journal of Pediatric Gastroenterology and Nutrition, 37,* 473–480.

Cohen, M. M., Jr. (1999). Robin sequences and complexes: Causal heterogeneity and pathogenetic/phenotypic variability. *American Journal of Medical Genetics, 84,* 311–315.

Cohen, M., Marschall, M. A., & Schafer, M. E. (1992, July 3). Immediate unrestricted feeding of infants following cleft lip and palate repair. *Journal of Craniofacial Surgery, 1,* 30–32.

Daskalogiannakis, J., Ross, R. B., & Tompson, B. D. (2001). The mandibular catch-up growth controversy in Pierre Robin sequence. *American Journal of Orthodontics and Dentofacial Orthopedics, 120,* 280–285.

Dominguez, S., & Harker, L. A. (1988). Incidence of cholesteatoma with cleft palate. *Annals of Otology, Rhinology and Laryngology, 97,* 659–660.

Drake, A. F., Davis, J. U., & Warren, D. W. (1993). Nasal airway size in cleft and noncleft children. *Laryngoscope, 103,* 915–917.

Heaf, D. P., Helms, P. J., Dinwiddie, R., & Mathew, D. J. (1982). Nasopharyngeal airways in Pierre Robin syndrome. *Journal of Pediatrics, 100,* 698–703.

Kakani, R. S., Callan, N. D., & April, M. M. (2000). Superior adenoidectomy in children with palatal abnormalities. *Ear, Nose and Throat Journal, 79,* 300, 303–305.

Kaufman, F. L. (1991). Managing the cleft lip and palate patient. *Pediatric Clinics of North America, 38,* 1127–1147.

Li, K. Y., Lo, L. J., Chen, K. S., Wong, K. S., & Chang, K. P. (2002). Robin sequence: Review of treatment modalities for airway obstruction in 110 cases. *International Journal of Pediatric Otorhinolaryngology, 65*(1), 45–51.

Liao, Y. F., Chuang, M. L., Chen, P. K., Chen, N. H., Yun, C., & Huang, C. S. (2002). Incidence and severity of obstructive sleep apnea following pharyngeal flap surgery in patients with cleft palate. *Cleft Palate-Craniofacial Journal, 39,* 312–316.

Mann, E. A., & Sidman, J. S. (1994, July). Results of cleft palate repair with the double-reverse Z-plasty performed by residents. *Otolaryngology–Head and Neck Surgery, 111,* 76–80.

Messner, A. H. (2003). Treating pediatric patients with obstructive sleep disorders: An update. *Otolaryngologic Clinics of North America, 36,* 519–530.

Mitchell, R. B., & Kelly, J. (2007). Behavioral changes in children with mild sleep-disordered breathing or obstructive sleep apnea after adenotonsillectomy. *The Laryngoscope, 117,* 1685–1688.

Muntz, H. R. (1993). An overview of middle ear disease in cleft palate children. *Facial Plastic Surgery, 9,* 177–180.

Myer, C. M., III, Reed, J. M., Cotton, R. T., Willging, J. P., & Shott, S. R. (1998). Airway management in Pierre Robin sequence. *Otolaryngology–Head and Neck Surgery, 118,* 630–635.

Prows, C. A., & Bender, P. L. (1999). Beyond Pierre Robin sequence. *Neonatal Network, 18*(5), 13–19.

Reid, J. (2004). A review of feeding interventions for infants with cleft palate. *Cleft Palate-Craniofacial Journal, 41,* 268–278.

Sidman, J. D., Sampson, D., & Templeton, B. (2001). Distraction osteogenesis of the mandible for airway obstruction in children. *Laryngoscope, 111,* 1137–1146.

Smith, T. L., DiRuggiero, D. C., & Jones, K. R. (1994). Recovery of eustachian tube function and hearing outcome in patients with cleft palate. *Otolaryngology–Head and Neck Surgery, 111,* 423–429.

Trenite, G. J., Paping, R. H., & Trenning, A. H. (1997). Rhinoplasty in the cleft lip patient. *Cleft Palate-Craniofacial Journal, 34,* 63–68.

Vegter, F., Hage, J. J., & Mulder, J. W. (1999). Pierre Robin syndrome: Mandibular growth during the first year of life. *Annals of Plastic Surgery, 42,* 154–157.

Warren, D. W., Drake, A. F., & Davis, J. U. (1992). Nasal airway in breathing and speech. *Cleft Palate-Craniofacial Journal, 29,* 511–519.

Wei, J. L., Mayo, M. S., Smith, H. J., et al. (2007). Improved behavior and sleep after adenoidectomy in children with sleep disordered breathing. *Archives of Otolaryngology—Head & Neck Surgery, 133,* 974–979.

CHAPTER 16

# Orthodontic Diagnosis and Treatment During Growth and Development

*Bryan J. Williams and Richard R. Bevis*

In addition to describing the discipline of orthodontics and the education and training required, Williams and Bevis outline some general principles of orthodontic treatment for patients with cleft lip and palate. The orthodontist needs to closely monitor each patient's facial, dental, and jaw growth and development because this can directly affect what can and cannot be accomplished with appliance therapy alone. The authors discuss the phases of orthodontic treatment relating to stages of dental and skeletal development from infancy to adulthood.

1. The authors emphasize the importance of minimizing time spent in orthodontic treatment phases and the value of coordinating with other disciplines. Defend their views.
2. Some research is cited indicating favorable facial form and development of the maxilla when clefts have gone unrepaired for several years. What information would persuade you to encourage early palatal closure?
3. Define *cephalometry.* Why is it important to orthodontists in diagnosis and treatment planning?
4. Describe the rationale for presurgical orthopedics and early bone grafting. What are the disadvantages?
5. What are the treatment goals and objectives in the early mixed dentition stage? Later mixed dentition stage? Permanent dentition?
6. What do Williams and Bevis say about intraoral expansion appliances and speech production? What are some questions the speech-language pathologist, treating the child with an expansion appliance in place, might ask the orthodontist?

The American Association of Orthodontists defines orthodontics/dentofacial orthopedics as the dental specialty that includes the diagnosis, prevention, interception, and correction of malocclusion, as well as neuromuscular and skeletal abnormalities of the developing or mature orofacial structures. The role of the orthodontist in the treatment of persons with cleft lip and palate must include all elements of this definition plus special interest in, knowledge about, and commitment to the study of facial form and functional development of patients with clefts and craniofacial anomalies. The orthodontist who treats these special patients must develop broader knowledge, including a basic knowledge of the key issues for the other specialties involved in the team care of these children. For the clinical orthodontist, the treatment of patients with clefts is both similar to and different from treating patients without clefts.

Currently, the additional training for the specialty of orthodontics beyond the doctorate of dental surgery (DDS) degree is a minimum of 2 years, but most commonly requires a 3-year program of study. Orthodontic specialty training programs include several thousand hours of didactic instruction and supervised clinical activity. The orthodontic resident must master anatomical sciences, including embryology, histology, head and neck anatomy, and cellular biology. Other courses typically include biometrics, mechanics of tooth movement, cephalometrics (measurement of oriented head radiographs), and surgical orthodontics (orthognathic surgery). The resident must become proficient in assessing and influencing dentofacial growth and development. Training also covers abnormal development, including syndromes of the head and neck, discrepancies of facial and jaw growth, and psychological aspects of facial difference. The orthodontist must master the biophysics of tooth movement, including the mechanical and physical response of the bone as the teeth are moved.

The management of patients with cleft lip and palate should also be an integral part of orthodontic specialty training. The current reality, however, is that the extent of training in craniofacial patient evaluation and treatment during orthodontic specialty training programs can vary widely across programs. Given the specialized orthodontic care needed for patients with craniofacial anomalies, craniofacial orthodontics is gradually being recognized as a subspecialty and is moving toward fellowship-level training.

Outcomes hinge on the dynamic principles of team care, and the orthodontist must learn to work with the patient and family in close association with other health care professionals as a part of a cleft palate and craniofacial team. Each team member should have some knowledge of the diagnostic procedures, primary concerns, and general treatment principles of other team specialties, as this is important in better overall care (see Chapter 1 by Moller).

The orthodontic concerns and treatment of patients with cleft palate are well documented in the literature (Aduss & Figueroa, 1990; Berkowitz, 1977; Evans, 2004; Kuijpers-Jagtman, 2006; Ross, 1987; Vargervik, 1981, 1983; Vig & Turvey, 1985). Successful management demands a team effort, with the timing of various treatments closely correlated with the patient's physical and psychological growth and development. The best learning tool in stimulating innovative and efficient treatment approaches is to be an active member of a cleft palate team. The team approach assures not only the most favorable treatment timing, but also the expeditious and effective achievement of overall treatment goals. All treatment decisions should be made with clear respect for the burden of care for the patient and family and with full appreciation that each patient is unique (see Chapter 2 by Aspinall).

## General Principles of Orthodontic Treatment

Although each patient has a unique overall situation and differing needs for orthodontic intervention, some general principles or guidelines can be applied to all patients with cleft lip and palate:

1. Carefully monitor each patient's skeletal growth and dental development (see Appendix 16A for figures showing child and adult teeth).
2. Coordinate orthodontic treatment to the most favorable growth and development stages, including the development of speech.
3. Coordinate the timing of orthodontic treatment with other treatments to yield stable, long-lasting results.
4. Maintain a "global perspective" and, consistent with favorable outcomes, minimize the phases of orthodontic treatment and the patient's total time in orthodontic treatment.

The overall goal should be to utilize the most effective and efficient treatments to achieve the best possible outcome when adulthood is reached. The orthodontist should have the goal of using the fewest possible stages of orthodontic treatment. Also, each treatment phase should be as short as possible, to minimize the effects of appliance wear on the patient's oral health, speech and oral function, physical comfort, and future cooperation. Prolonged orthodontic treatment not only can be harmful for oral health but also can, over time, cause burnout on the part of the patient as well as generate significant inconvenience and financial burdens for the family. Burnout precipitated by prolonged treatment that is not essential will be a barrier to success when later the patient has orthodontic treatment needs that are essential to the quality of the overall outcome. A principle that holds for treatment of all patients, but is especially applicable to the orthodontic management of a patient with cleft palate, is to never do comprehensive treatment too early, when the treatment may either interfere with normal growth or be completed before the completion of the pubertal growth spurt.

Beneficial orthodontic treatment can be performed in the very young (i.e., newborns), throughout the mixed dentition, and into adulthood with dramatic and rewarding results. Both removable and fixed orthodontic appliances are useful in obtaining the treatment goals established by the interdisciplinary team. Comprehensive pretreatment record review and periodic treatment planning conferences are required with all the professionals who are, or will be, involved with the patient's dental and medical care.

Finally, specific orthodontic diagnostic and treatment procedures must be cooperatively formulated with other team members who have to deal with the direct consequences of any orthodontic treatment. For example, early removable orthodontic appliances may present short-term hazards for speech, but be very beneficial for speech articulation in the long run. Therefore, specific treatment plans and the timing of treatment must be discussed and coordinated with other disciplines to yield an optimal outcome.

## The Orthodontist's Role on the Cleft Palate Team

The orthodontist is the professional on the team who has not only the greatest knowledge of facial growth and development but also the best ability to assess and monitor it over time. Therefore, the orthodontist's major role on the team is to follow the orofacial growth and development of each patient and to develop an accurate prediction of final outcome from an aesthetic and functional standpoint. The final aesthetic and functional occlusion is based on the culmination of multiple treatment planning sessions and specific treatment interventions from infancy to adulthood. The individual growth and development of each patient is an ever-changing composite of the soft and hard tissue changes with multiple tooth and dental arch variables. The team must rely on the orthodontist for periodic evaluation and prediction of growth and development and for providing orthodontic treatment that is appropriately associated with the patient's physical and behavioral growth and development.

On smaller, less established teams, the orthodontist may be the only dental professional and therefore may need to monitor the patient's basic dental health and provide guidance in this regard for the patient and family. In these smaller team environments, as necessary, the orthodontist should connect the patient with appropriate dental professionals in the surrounding community. On larger teams, there will be direct dental or pediatric dental participation on the team, and it is important that the orthodontist and the dentist or pediatric dentist meet early in the patient's treatment to evaluate and discuss tooth development, morphology, positions, and bone support in or near the alveolar cleft. Subsequently, the orthodontist is involved with the team surgeons in determining the benefits and timing of alveolar bone grafting and oronasal fistula closure. Reconstructive surgery involves both soft and hard tissue alterations in the lip, palatal, and pharyngeal areas, as well as nasal modifications. The majority of these surgical procedures occur early and affect dental arch form and jaw development to some degree; however, with advancements in surgical techniques, severe effects on dental and jaw growth and development are now uncommon. Timing of interventions is important for all team members, and the orthodontist's timing and selection of treatment procedures can be crucial for the rest of the team. Orthodontic decisions and treatment actions as the child is growing can influence the need for and type of later treatments, such as prosthodontic management of missing teeth (see Chapter 18 by Leeper, Charles, and Sills). Communication with the speech-language pathologist is very important. A dialogue about the timing and effect on speech of either removable or fixed appliance treatment is important in the development of a plan for the best treatment approach. The team social worker and/or psychologist should be involved in decisions regarding early versus late treatment options. The psychological health and cooperation of both the patient and the family must be considered before any treatment can begin. Also, the overall burden of care must be considered, and the psychological support members of the team are most valuable in assessing this, as well as providing resources and emotional support for the family. Of utmost importance in final treatment outcome is the patient's overall oral and dental health. Without excellent cooperation and support of the patient's dentist and a rigorous home oral health maintenance program, treatment will be compromised and goals will not be met. All team members can participate in emphasizing the importance of oral health maintenance and its impact on the overall outcome of treatment.

## Growth and Development in the Cleft Palate Patient

In Chapter 5, Gorlin and Baylis discuss in more detail the embryology and formation of the primary and secondary palate. The discussion in this chapter is more superficial. Growth in the primary palate (upper lip, premaxilla) starts embryologically with a proliferation from the first branchial arch, called the maxillary process. The process grows medially from lateral to the stomodeum to near the medial nasal process. Veau (1938) proposed that cleft lips are the result of failure of mesodermal penetration of the epithelial walls formed during the uniting of facial processes. Tondury (1961) similarly explained cleft formation as a disturbance and incomplete formation of the epithelial wall based on defective growth of a nasal swelling (e.g., of the lateral nasal process). Stark (1954) felt that clefting is the result of reduced amounts of mesoderm in the tissue within the cleft area.

Whereas the primary palate begins development at 4–5 weeks in the embryo, the secondary palate (hard and soft palate) begins formation at 7–8 weeks. The secondary palate develops in three stages after a medial extension of the maxillary process grows vertically into two palatal shelves. The three stages involve a movement of the shelves from a vertical to a horizontal position by (1) shelf growth, (2) shelf elevation, and (3) shelf merging. A failure of any of the three stages or a combination of effects will cause various degrees of clefting of the palate.

The maxilla is further altered by continuing growth after birth. Early surgical intervention will stabilize the maxilla and round out the upper arch form, but may constrict and slow down future anterior-posterior, transverse, and vertical growth. The cleft maxilla with no surgical intervention may not have any inherent tendency for growth deficiency. A study from Sri Lanka of 28 unoperated males with cleft lip and palate over age 13 reported similar maxillary growth compared with Sri Lankan children without clefts of the same age group (Mars, James, & Lamabadusuriya, 1990). However, in another report, these same adolescents were found to have severe speech disorders (Sell & Grunwell, 1990).

The assessment of skeletal and dental growth patterns is of fundamental importance for all orthodontists, but especially for those who focus on the care of patients with clefts and craniofacial anomalies. The cranial portion of the skull completes growth relatively early, and normal facial growth proceeds in a downward and forward direction away from the skull base. In general terms, there are two time periods of accelerated facial growth. The first is between ages 7 and 9 years and is less substantial than the prepubertal growth spurt, which is of much greater velocity and overall impact on facial morphology.

In general, there are three major patterns of facial growth (see Figure 16.1). For patients with clefts, it is common to see some level of underdevelopment of the maxilla and midface. In more severe situations, the individuals have a lack of fullness in the midface, creating a concave facial profile, and an underbite (negative overjet, anterior crossbite) or Class III occlusal relationship. When there is severe restriction of maxillary development, these problems with growth can become evident at an early age. Figures 16.2 and 16.3 demonstrate the cephalometric tracing

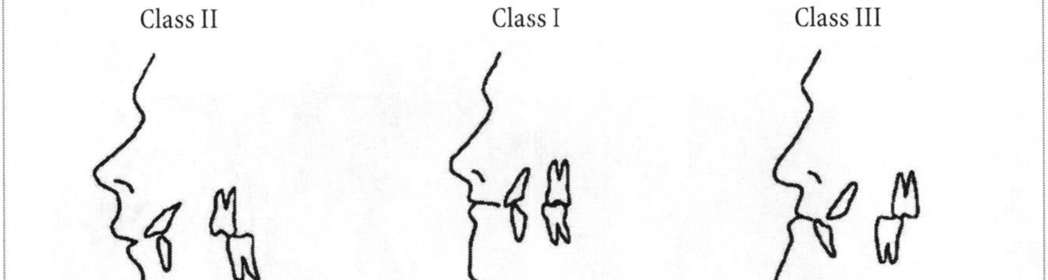


Figure 16.1. Patterns of facial and skeletal growth: (A) convex profile with retrognathic mandible and Class II dental relationship; (B) straight profile with orthognathic mandible and Class I dental relationship; (C) concave profile with prognathic mandible and Class III dental relationship.

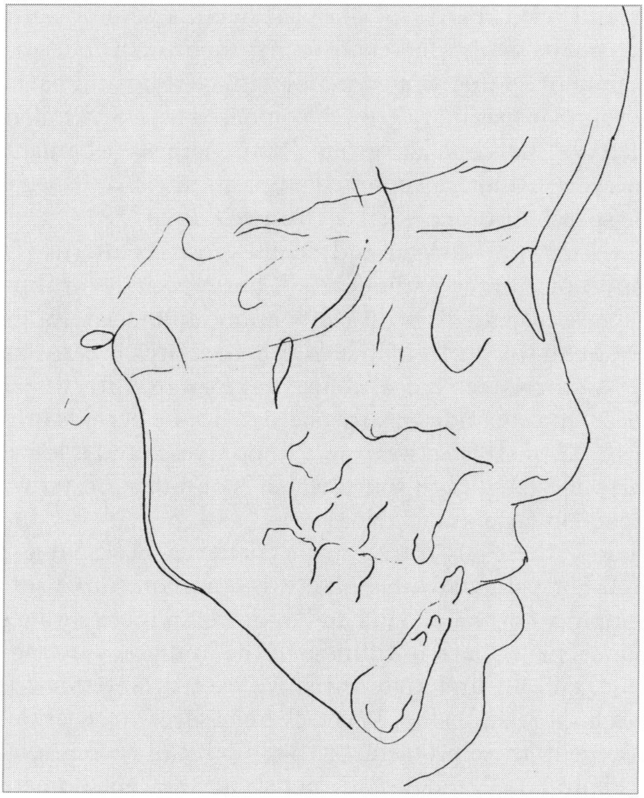

FIGURE 16.2. Cephalometric tracing for 3½-year-old female with cleft palate and severe midfacial/maxillary growth deficiency.

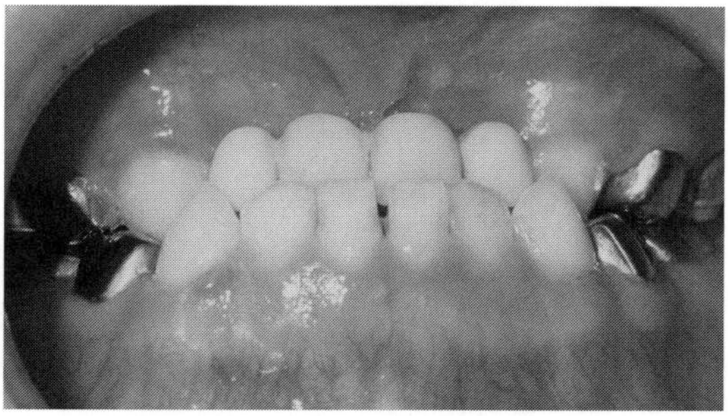

FIGURE 16.3. Intraoral view of severe Class III malocclusion.

and occlusion of a patient with cleft palate who is only 3½ years old and is already demonstrating a Class III growth pattern.

Evidence of severe maxillary growth restriction at an early age is a poor prognostic indicator for future growth and points to an eventual need for combined surgical and orthodontic management when growth is complete. The orthodontist tracks skeletal and facial growth through serial cephalometric tracings with sequential superimposition on the cranial base. In Figure 16.4, serial superimposition of cephalometric tracings in a male from 6 years 7 months to 10 years 2 months of age demonstrates significantly less maxillary than mandibular development. The mandibular growth is normal in this patient, but the maxillary underdevelopment is significant and impacts the facial profile as well as the occlusion. This maxillary underdevelopment commonly occurs in multiple dimensions and, in addition to anterior-posterior midfacial growth deficiency, many children with clefts have maxillary transverse deficiency resulting in crossbites of the posterior dentition. As the child moves into the prepubertal growth spurt, one would expect the differential in amount of growth between the two jaws to increase as the overall rate of growth increases.

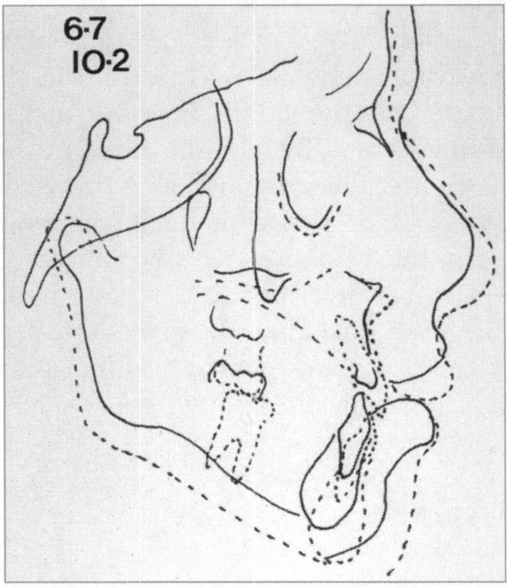


FIGURE 16.4. Superimposition of cephalometric tracing showing growth of a male patient with a cleft palate from 6 years 7 months to 10 years 2 months of age.

The quest of craniofacial orthodontics in the care of children with clefts is to find overall treatment approaches that minimize negative impacts on facial growth. Outcomes should be assessed using objective measurement criteria, which involve both assessment of diagnostic models as well as cephalometric and facial analysis (Mars, Plint, Houston, Bergland, & Semb, 1987; Prahl-Anderson & Ju, 2006). The orthodontist's knowledge of facial growth and development and ability to assess the growth objectively are invaluable in the evaluations. which help in defining team treatment approaches with the least impact on facial growth. To establish an approach for overall patient management, each team must weigh the burden of care for all interventions and especially assess the impact of type and timing of surgical interventions on facial growth and development, as well as speech and other areas.

## Monitoring and Recording Growth and Development

### Skeletal Patterns

Future arch discrepancies requiring orthognathic surgical treatment may become apparent as early as the toddler years when skeletal patterns are evaluated in the young patient. By the time of early mixed dentition, the child's skeletal pattern must be noted and documented, both to assess the current state and to serve as a baseline documentation that will aid in future treatment planning. In settings with a centralized cleft and craniofacial team where patients travel from outlying communities, members of the interdisciplinary team, including the orthodontist, often must communicate findings and treatment plans to health professionals providing care to the patient in the local community.

### Orthodontic Records

In general terms, orthodontic diagnostic records include photographs, radiographs, and orthodontic study models of the teeth and supporting tissues. Significant patient cooperation is required to secure complete records of optimum quality. This may not be possible with children who are preschool age or who have developmental delay. The first set of records obtained may not be a complete or ideal set, and for the preschool child the records may often be limited to some photographs and limited radiographs. However, it is important that an attempt be made to obtain at least a portion of the records for the preschool child. Early information, such as number, status, and position of developing teeth, is important not only to the orthodontist, but also to other members of the team in planning future treatment. Most children of school age are able to manage having a full set of records taken. Optimally, every child with a cleft should have complete records early in the mixed dentition stage of development.

Figure 16.5 demonstrates a complete set of records, including

1. Full-face and profile photographs
2. Complete set of intraoral photos, including occlusals
3. Lateral and posterior-anterior cephalometric radiographs (tomographic radiographs may also be useful in some patients)
4. Panoramic radiograph of the jaws and teeth
5. Selected intraoral radiographs
6. Plaster casts or models of each arch with good peripheral extension
7. Full medical and dental history in conjunction with complete intraoral and functional examination of the patient

Accurate models and standardized radiographs, as the child grows and develops, are essential in optimal treatment planning. Models or impressions of the teeth in the upper and lower arches should be obtained periodically. Care should be exercised in extending the peripheries of the impressions and subsequent models to allow for more accurate overall assessment and, when surgery is planned, more accurate model surgery (see Chapter 17 by Swift). Because errors in predicting the type and extent of surgery can occur when the wrong occlusal wax bite registration is taken, this registration should be recorded carefully.

Patients with cleft palate or craniofacial conditions with canted or asymmetrical occlusal planes, facial asymmetries, or open bites are definite candidates for face-bow transfers to a jaw movement articulator. Checking bites and remounting are very important in certain orthognathic surgical procedures, which are described in more detail by Swift in Chapter 17.

As mentioned previously, cephalometrics is a science that both orthodontists and oral and maxillofacial surgeons must understand. Since lateral cephalometric radiographs have been taken with a standardized

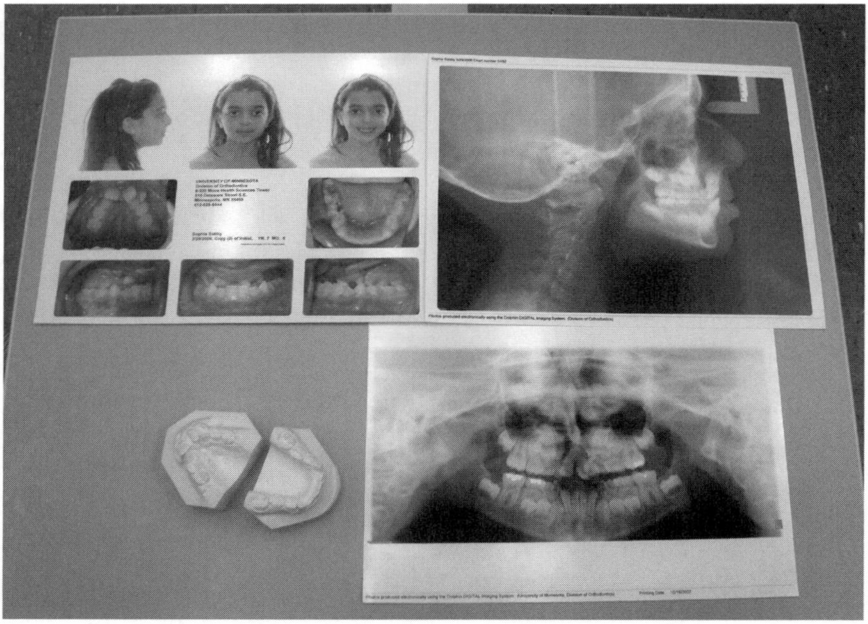

FIGURE 16.5. A typical set of complete orthodontic records, including models, photos, and full-mouth and cephalometric radiographs.

approach for over 100 years and used extensively in orthodontics since 1931, there are norm values for a broad range of skeletal measurements and races. A lateral cephalometric radiograph is traced and analyzed either manually or through a computerized program. This allows an objective quantification of the patient's underlying skeletal pattern, as well as the ability to objectively track growth over time by superimposing sequential tracings. Accuracy in taking the cephalometric radiograph is important. The most common cephalometric radiograph is the lateral cephalometric radiograph taken in centric occlusion. Centric occlusion is defined as the place where the teeth first touch in the natural bite. The following is a checklist for making sure the radiograph is taken properly:

1. Properly position the head in a head-holding device called a cephalostat.
2. Make sure the head is in a normal position without strain on the spinal column.

3. Standardize the distance from the source and adjust the film cassette to the fixed distance.
4. Use the proper radiographic settings to ensure the proper contrast for accurate tracing.
5. Have the patient relax the facial muscles and hold the centric occlusion for the duration of the radiographic exposure.

Once a satisfactory lateral cephalometric radiograph has been obtained in centric occlusion, other radiographs can be added for specific information. For example, important information may be obtained in surgical mandibular advancement cases by taking a lateral radiograph with the lower jaw in the advanced position that simulates the planned forward surgical movement of the jaw.

PA (posterior-anterior) cephalometric views have gained renewed importance with recent advancements in orthodontics and oral surgery. These films are useful in analysis of facial asymmetry and assessment of vertical and transverse maxillary position. The tracing of the PA cephalometric radiograph shows details of the orbits, the nasal septum, and the maxillary and mandibular central incisors and molars. Soft tissue is more difficult to evaluate because of the limited amount shown on the perimeter of the radiograph. Tracings of the PA cephalometric radiographs may prove to be important for evaluating asymmetrical orthognathic surgical cases where special emphasis is on soft tissue planning.

Tomography is a procedure that results in a radiograph highlighting a specific thin layer or section of tissue through a narrow beam of focus. In orthodontics, it usually delineates certain sections of the maxilla or mandible, most notably the temporomandibular joint areas. Tomograms are helpful not only in diagnosis and treatment planning, but also in postoperative evaluations of maxillary and mandibular surgical corrections for the patient with cleft palate. PA tomograms of the nasal septum are also useful in maxillary surgery. A deviated septum found prior to surgery can be addressed appropriately during the surgery when the maxilla is downfractured.

Temporomandibular joint (TMJ) radiographs have found a place in all phases of maxillofacial treatment planning and postsurgical evaluations, and can be useful for the patient with cleft palate, especially when mandibular surgery is needed.

Other radiographs, such as the classic panoramic radiograph, serve as excellent screening films for tooth development and relative tooth positions in the mandible and maxilla. The maxillary sinuses and the mandibular rami are also demonstrated by the panoramic radiograph. Detailed dental diagnosis and evaluation require other dental radiographic projections that are taken with intraoral films, such as bitewings, occlusals, and periapicals. The maxillary anterior occlusal film is especially useful in planning for alveolar bone grafting. The details of bone support for the teeth adjacent to the cleft, the positions of teeth relative to the cleft, and the morphology of the alveolar cleft are well demonstrated (see Figure 16.6).

In the current era of digital technology, it is becoming commonplace to take digital orthodontic radiographs rather than use classic film-based technology. Digital radiographs have some distinct advantages, including more rapid processing, no chemicals for developing, less radiation exposure for the patient, and rapidly improving quality. Currently, other techniques for digital recording of diagnostic information are under development in many craniofacial centers. Computed tomography (CT) is commonly used for evaluation of hard tissue structures in patients with

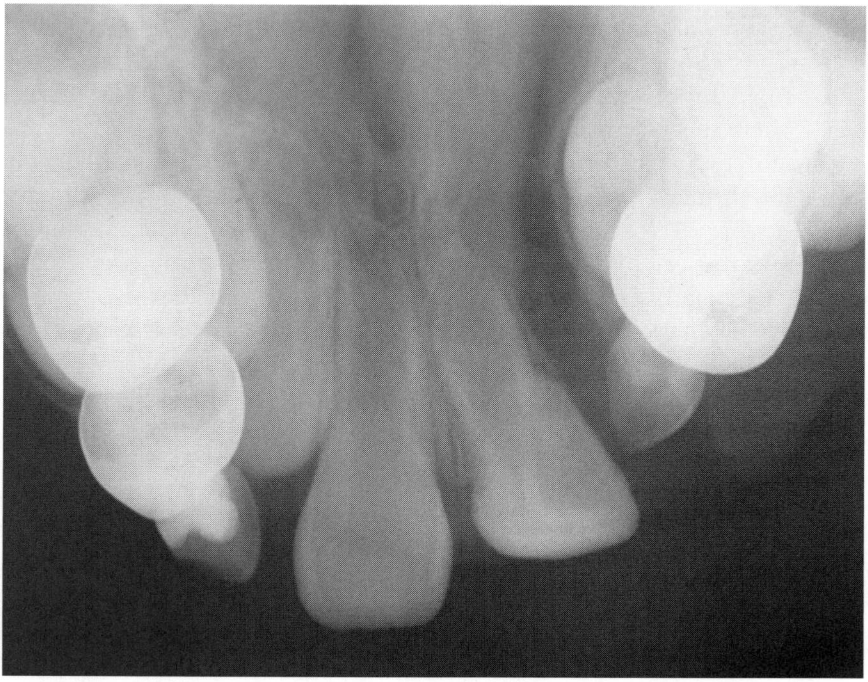

FIGURE 16.6. Maxillary occlusal radiograph of a patient with a unilateral cleft.

clefts and craniofacial anomalies. CT equipment is rapidly evolving to provide higher levels of detail, enable quicker scans, reduce radiation dosages, and reduce costs. Also, newer techniques that combine CT with digital photographic imaging allow visualization of the relationships between soft tissues and underlying osseous tissues.

## Orthodontic Treatment Phases

Although the orthodontist can provide important information regarding facial growth and development and overall clinical management for persons with craniofacial anomalies throughout the growing years, there are common times in the patient's development when active orthodontic treatment is needed for the best overall management of the patient. As mentioned previously, the team's treatment philosophy and treatment protocol will dictate certain orthodontic intervention times consistent with the orthodontic principle of coordinating treatment with growth and development. Active orthodontic treatment can be considered at the following times or phases of dental development: early infancy (early infant orthopedics), early mixed dentition, later mixed dentition, permanent dentition (adolescent), and adult (nongrowing). Although each of these is discussed separately, there are important transitional relationships that are unique for each patient.

### Early Infancy (Early Infant Orthopedics)

Much discussion and debate has occurred over many years regarding the benefits and drawbacks of early presurgical orthopedics, which involves orthodontically positioning the cleft maxillary segments prior to primary lip and palatal repair. It is important to understand that decisions regarding whether to do early infant orthopedics should not be made exclusively by the orthodontist. This procedure, which requires scientific evaluation and team-level discussion, should be considered only in the context of the overall treatment approach. In particular, the use of an early infant orthopedic appliance has to integrate well with and be of benefit in the approach to primary lip closure surgery and, when applicable, primary rhinoplasty (nasal surgery). In the very few centers where alveolar bone grafting is done early in infancy, early presurgical orthopedics is integrated into their approach because the alveolar segments must be aligned prior to the primary bone grafting. The majority of centers do more traditional secondary bone grafting, and the decision to adopt early infant orthopedics is based on its impact on initial soft tissue surgeries. For a more complete discussion of the history, rationale, and procedures, the reader is referred to sources that favor presurgical orthopedic procedures (Grayson, Cutting, & Wood, 1993; Grayson, Santiago, Brecht, & Cutting, 1999; Gruber, 1990; Hotz, Gnoinski, & Perko, 1986; Huebner & Marsh, 1990) and those that do not (Aduss & Figueroa, 1990; Berkowitz, 1977; Berkowitz, Mejia, & Bystrik, 2004; Bongaarts, Kuijpers-Jagtman, Van 't Hof, & Prahl-Anderson, 2004; Ross, 1987; Subtelny, 1990). Primary concerns regarding early infant orthopedics center around, first, whether the treatment may attenuate growth and, second, whether it really improves outcomes over the long term, especially in the face of the complexity and costs of some of the techniques for early infant orthopedics.

The rationale for early infant orthopedics is to improve, as much as possible, the position of the cleft maxillary segments before the primary lip repair (see Figure 16.7). The goal of primary lip repair is to connect the muscular elements (orbicularis oris) in the maxillary lip to provide natural lip function and appearance. Some professionals feel that appliance treatment facilitates more ideal primary lip surgery by reducing the gap between the edges of the cleft lip, and centers that utilize this approach feel it improves outcomes. Currently, very few craniofacial centers do primary bone grafting due to concerns regarding, and evidence demonstrat-

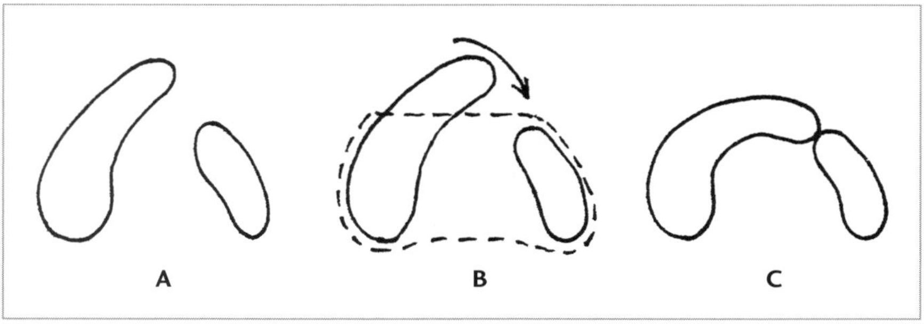


FIGURE 16.7. Diagram showing goal of early infant orthopedics for a patient with a unilateral cleft. (A) The relationship of the greater and lesser maxillary bony segments before lip surgery. (B) The prosthesis in place (dotted lines), holding the lesser segment stable (the arrow shows the direction of movement of the greater segment following lip repair). (C) The butt alignment of the segments.

ing, attenuation of overall maxillary growth. In centers that do not do early infant orthopedics, the rationale is that early appliance intervention does not reduce or eliminate the need for future orthodontic treatment or facilitate more favorable overall facial growth.

Recently, more attention has been directed to nasal morphology for infants with unilateral and bilateral complete clefts. Some early work demonstrated that ear deformities in infants could be successfully treated by careful application of pressure to the ear cartilage. An outgrowth of this work has been the development of an early infant orthopedic technique called nasoalveolar molding. This procedure was pioneered at the Craniofacial Center at New York University (NYU) (Grayson et al., 1993; Grayson et al., 1999). The technique initially involves the use of an intraoral molding appliance to align the arch segments and narrow the alveolar gap (see Figure 16.8). Once this is accomplished, the nasal component of the appliance is added, with the goal of lengthening and defining the columella and improving the contour of the nasal cartilages in advance of the primary lip and nasal surgical repair (see Figures 16.9, 16.10, and 16.11). In many cases, close alignment of the alveolar segments can allow the surgeon to do a primary gingivoperiosteoplasty, which can reduce the need for secondary alveolar bone grafting, although there are some concerns about the impact of this surgical procedure on growth. Nasoalveolar molding facilitates the primary lip and nasal surgery, and the team at NYU feels it improves both short- and long-term outcomes, although the burden of care for the family is significant. Ongoing research is needed to quantify the impact on long-term outcomes.

The orthodontist involved with a cleft and craniofacial team needs to be well versed in the overall protocol and treatment approach of the team and to be an active participant in evaluating outcomes, which is a critical step in determining the best approach to care of the patient with a cleft palate. The important considerations are what the most efficient and effective treatment is for each patient to ensure the best outcome in the long run, and whether the benefits outweigh the burden of care (time, effort, discomfort, family time attending appointments, etc.). Again, the discussion by Aspinall in Chapter 2 is relevant here.

## Early Mixed Dentition

Given the typical treatment protocol of the majority of cleft and craniofacial centers, the main focus in the early mixed dentition phase is directed

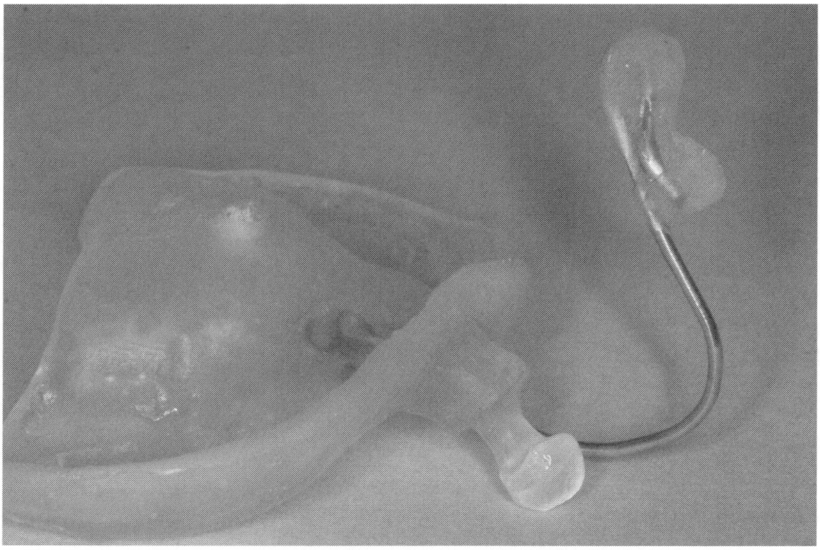

FIGURE 16.8. Nasoalveolar molding appliance for unilateral cleft.

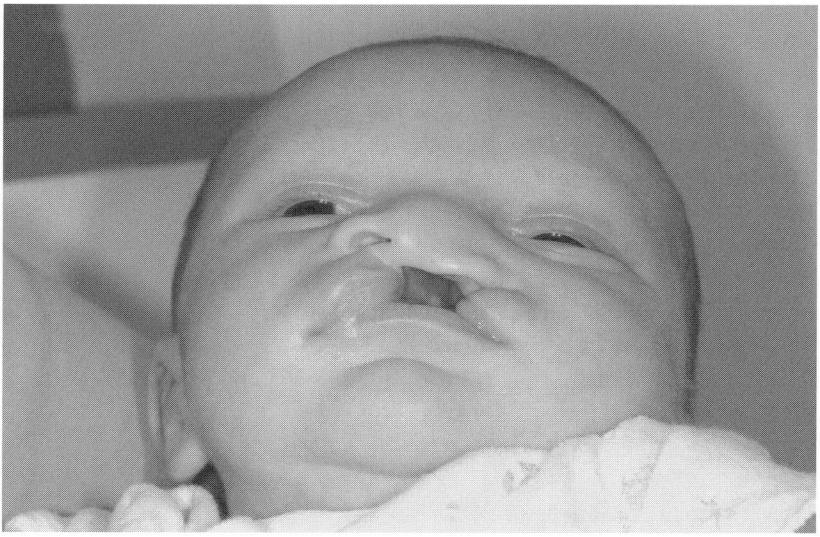

FIGURE 16.9. Infant with left unilateral complete cleft before nasoalveolar molding treatment.

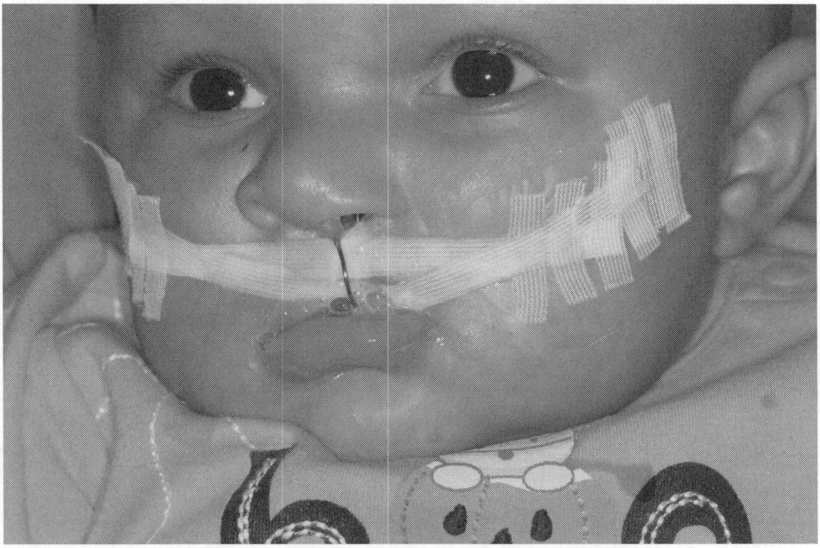

Figure 16.10. Infant with left unilateral complete cleft in later stages of nasoalveolar molding treatment.

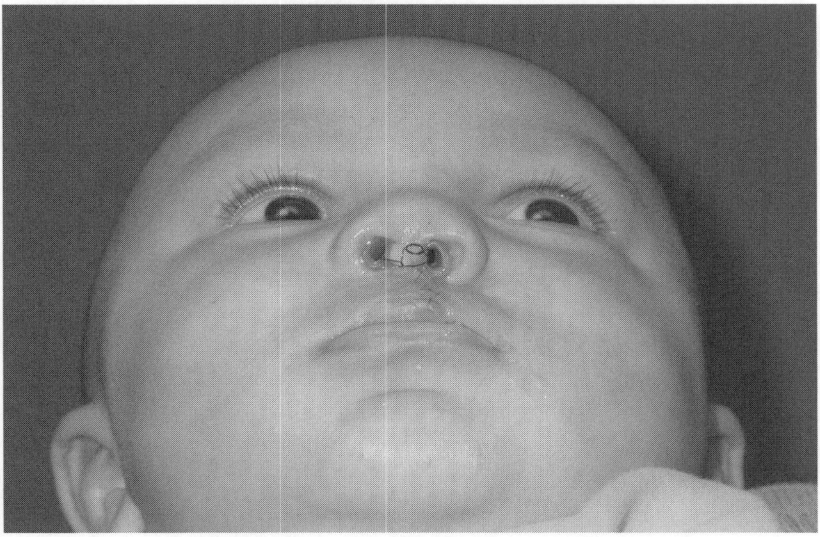

Figure 16.11. Infant with left unilateral complete cleft shortly after primary lip closure and primary rhinoplasty.

toward optimizing the alveolar bone graft procedures. There are a number of benefits to doing an alveolar bone graft to close the alveolar cleft, as Swift outlines in further detail in Chapter 17. The primary goals of secondary alveolar bone grafting from an orthodontic perspective are to reunify the alveolar ridge, stabilize it, and create an integrated dental arch with good bone support for eruption of teeth, future orthodontic movement, and prosthetic replacement of missing teeth if necessary.

The process surrounding alveolar bone grafting begins with a careful team evaluation and, in particular, discussion among the orthodontist, pediatric dentist, and oral and maxillofacial surgeon. One of the cornerstones of this evaluation is having comprehensive, high-quality diagnostic records, including excellent intraoral radiographs of the cleft area. Three primary questions must be discussed. First, the best timing for placement of the graft must be determined. In general terms, secondary alveolar bone grafts usually are done between 7 and 9½ years of age. However, and importantly, the specific timing is determined by the developmental status of the permanent teeth forming under the tissue in the area of the cleft. The permanent lateral incisor is often missing or malformed, in which case the timing is determined by the developmental status of the permanent canine. In most centers, the preference is for the unerupted canine root to be between one quarter and one half developed. In cases where the permanent lateral incisor is a viable tooth, the graft will be done earlier than when the canine is the key tooth.

Second, the dental members of the team must look carefully at all teeth (erupted and unerupted) in the area of the planned graft. The maxillary anterior occlusal radiograph is very useful in this evaluation. This film provides a clear view of the overall morphology of the cleft; it is important to realize that alveolar clefts are funnel shaped, with the narrow end of the funnel in the mouth and the wide end at the nasal floor. With a vision for optimal final occlusion, the dental members of the team must make decisions about the viability of individual teeth in the area of the cleft. Dental anomalies, including anomalies of tooth size, shape, position, and number (missing or extra teeth), are common in children with clefts. In many cases, teeth that are not essential for the overall occlusion and may interfere with the bone graft surgery or the healing of the graft should be extracted in advance of the orthodontic preparation for the graft (see Figure 16.12). Also, the overall occlusion must be evaluated as there may be a need to extract teeth in other areas of the mouth to alleviate arch crowding, and this may be an optimal time for these extractions as well.

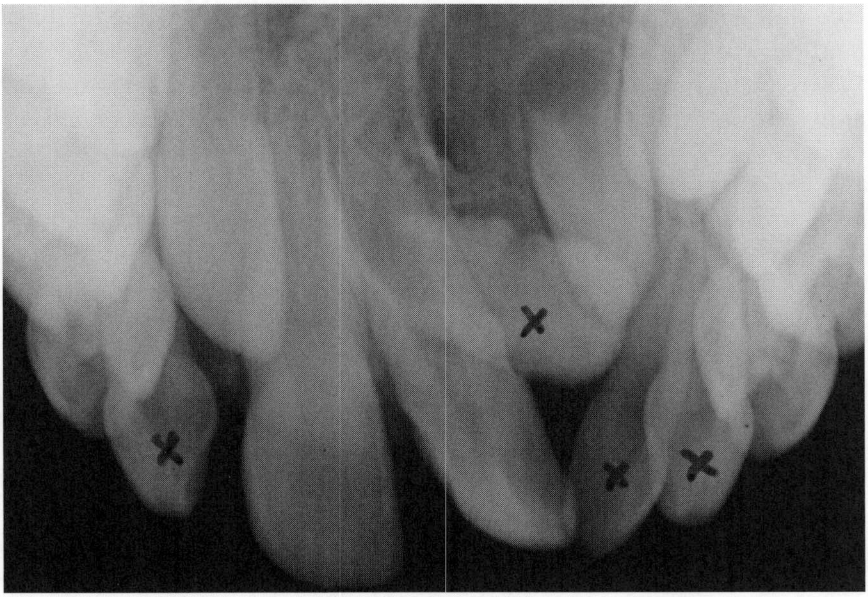

Figure 16.12. Maxillary occlusal radiograph with identification of teeth planned for extraction in advance of orthodontic preparation for alveolar bone graft.

Third, the nature of the orthodontic treatment needed in preparation for the graft must be planned. If the secondary palate (hard and soft) is intact, there may be no need for orthodontic preparation in advance of the graft since the maxillary transverse dimension is usually normal. In the majority of complete cleft cases (involving the primary and secondary palate), there will be maxillary transverse collapse and crossbite, so the orthodontic preparation focuses on arch expansion. It is preferable to have the correct transverse (side-to-side) maxillary relationship in advance of placing the bone graft, because it is more difficult to correct the transverse relationship after the graft has integrated. Communication between the orthodontist and the speech-language pathologist is important given that the orthodontic appliance necessary for expansion will at least temporarily affect speech.

Classically, when there is a cleft of the lip, alveolar ridge, and palate, the posterior arch segment collapses toward the midline. This narrowness is greater at the anterior or canine end of the segment. The expansion appliance that is commonly used is one of a variety of simple expanders

(W Arch, Quad Helix, etc.) (see Figure 16.13) that allow rotational expansion with greater expansion at the canine end of the segment. The W Arch is connected to bands on the first permanent molars and can either be soldered to the bands or have attachments that allow removal of the wire.

There are other types of expanders that require the family to turn an expansion screw, but these are rarely necessary for pre-bone graft expansion and are more commonly used in later stages of treatment. Commonly, there is significant malalignment of the anterior teeth, particularly the central incisor mesial to the alveolar cleft (see Figure 16.14). There is often early parental pressure to align the anterior teeth, but the orthodontist should have significant concern about moving teeth into areas where there is no bone support for the roots.

The orthodontist must either avoid anterior tooth movement at this stage of treatment or approach it with extreme caution to avoid potential for loss of teeth due to placing roots outside of bone support (see Figures 16.15 and 16.16). If roots of the erupted incisors adjacent to the cleft area are moved out of supporting bone, they will likely need to be extracted in advance of the graft. For the specifics of the surgical approach to alveolar bone grafting, see Chapter 17 by Swift.

The goals of alveolar grafting are to attain a complete seal between the mouth and nose and to have an alveolar ridge with enough fullness to support tooth eruption, further tooth movement, or the eventual placement of implants if teeth need to be replaced (see Figure 16.17). If the orthodontic and surgical aspects of the alveolar bone grafting are well managed, all future orthodontic treatment is greatly simplified and in

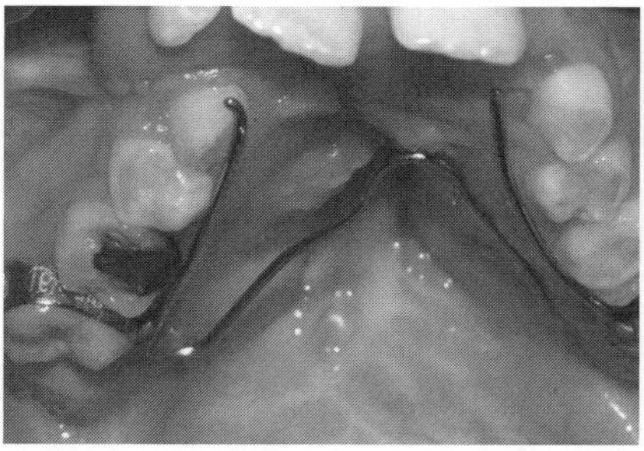

FIGURE 16.13. Simple W Arch Expander for preparation for alveolar bone graft.

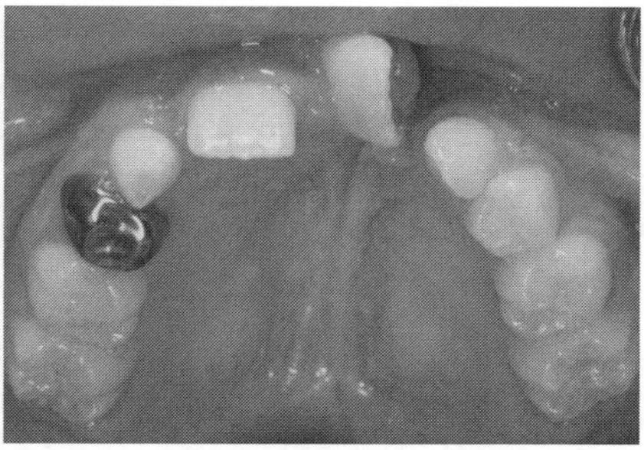

FIGURE 16.14. Intraoral occlusal photo showing severe rotation of central incisor adjacent to cleft of alveolar ridge.

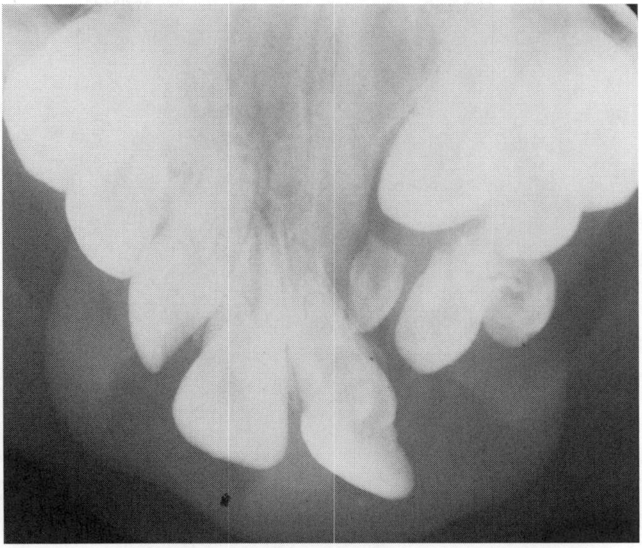

Figure 16.15. Initial maxillary occlusal radiograph showing very thin alveolar bone covering on cleft side of maxillary central incisor.

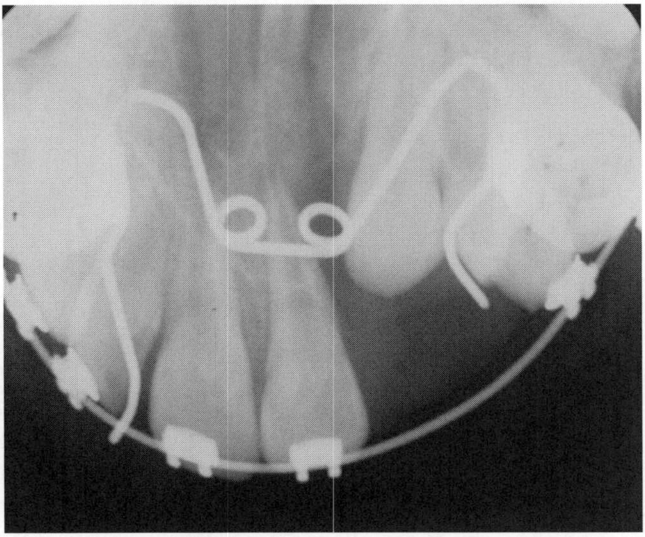

Figure 16.16. Maxillary occlusal radiograph showing loss of bone support for permanent central incisor due to orthodontic movement. Tooth had to be extracted before alveolar bone graft surgery.

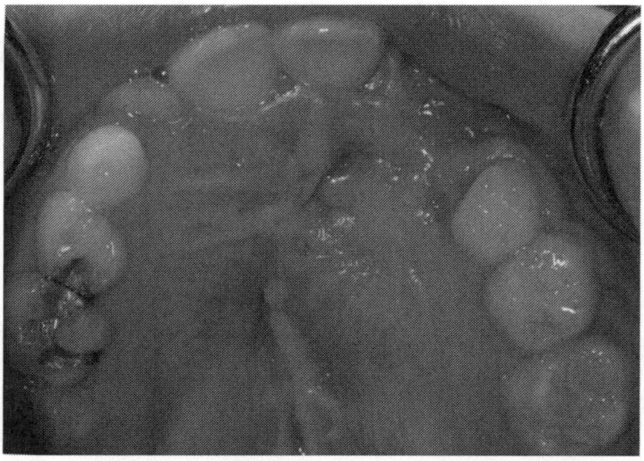

FIGURE 16.17. Maxillary arch showing good alveolar ridge fullness following alveolar bone grafting.

most respects the orthodontic treatment parameters become similar to those in patients without clefts.

In the child with severe skeletal discrepancy for whom orthognathic surgery is an eventual certainty, bone grafting may be delayed and later integrated with the orthognathic surgery. In these cases, the maxillary arch may be managed with segmental surgery to narrow or close the alveolar cleft and hence reduce the extent of the bone grafting. The specifics of this approach are based on close communication between the oral and maxillofacial surgeon and the orthodontist.

## Later Mixed Dentition

It is important to emphasize that after the graft is consolidated in the later mixed dentition, any orthodontic treatment should be targeted to specific orthodontic issues that can most efficiently be treated at this stage of development. Again, caution must be exercised to avoid prolonged treatment or treatment of orthodontic irregularities that can be more effectively treated at a later stage of development. The key orthodontic issues at the later mixed dentition stage of development are monitoring of the eruption of teeth through the bone graft, alignment of the maxillary anterior dentition when necessary, definitive assessment of the skeletal pattern, and definitive assessment and planning for the future management of missing teeth. If orthodontic treatment is indicated at this stage of development, it is limited treatment with specific goals and should not involve a full set of orthodontic appliances or prolonged treatment time.

Once the bone graft is in place and well consolidated, the overall occlusion should be reevaluated. In situations where there is severe malalignment of the maxillary anterior teeth, there are benefits to aligning the teeth at this stage. Not only does alignment improve aesthetics, self-image, and function, but movement of teeth into the area of the grafted bone helps to preserve the new bone because alveolar bone requires function in order to be maintained. Also, during the later mixed dentition phase, the eruption of the permanent canine teeth should continue to be monitored, especially as they are erupting through the bone graft(s) (see Figure 16.18). In cases with missing maxillary lateral incisors, careful planning is important to decide whether the missing tooth or teeth are going to be replaced with prosthodontic procedures, or if other teeth are going to be moved to take the place of the missing tooth or teeth. The orthodontist should be making these decisions in the late mixed dentition stage of development to set the treatment parameters for the patient's future orthodontic treatment.

Figures 16.19, 16.20, and 16.21 show intraoral views of a patient with a right-sided complete cleft who had a successful alveolar bone graft. The right lateral incisor is missing, and the left lateral incisor had been previously extracted. The maxillary right canine has erupted, but the central

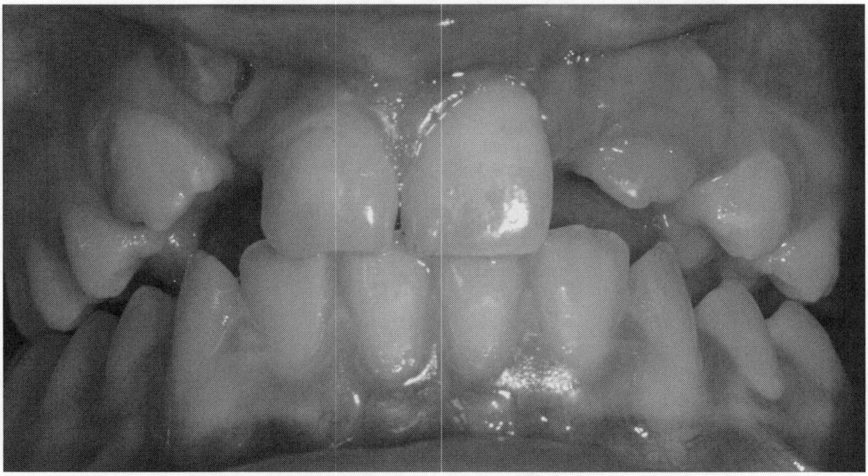

FIGURE 16.18. Maxillary permanent cuspids erupting through ridge after alveolar bone grafts in a patient with a bilateral complete cleft.

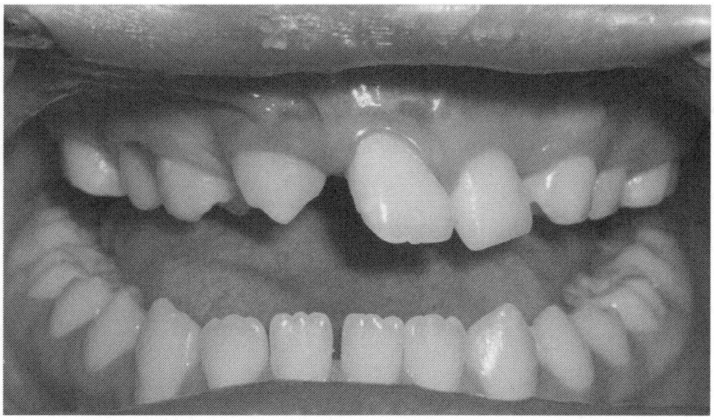

FIGURE 16.19. Male patient with complete right-sided cleft that had an alveolar bone graft. The right lateral was missing, and the left was extracted for symmetry and to address maxillary crowding. The midline is off to the left, and the left cuspid is blocked from erupting.

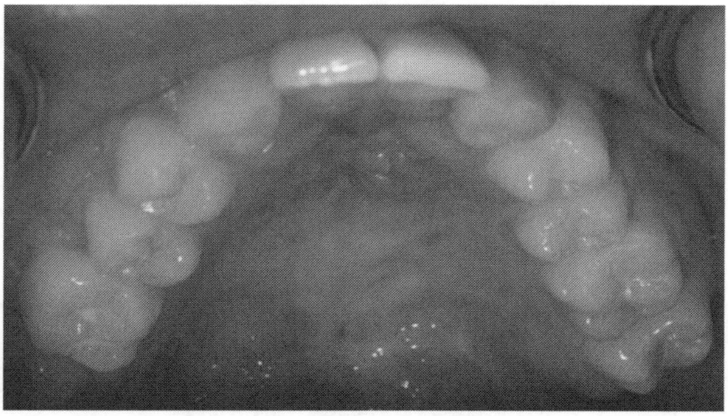

FIGURE 16.20. Occlusal view following limited orthodontics to align the incisors and open space for eruption of left cuspid.

incisors are off center, the maxillary left canine is blocked on the palate, and the left primary canine is over-retained. Limited orthodontics in the maxillary anterior area resulted in eruption of the palatally impacted left canine and improved anterior tooth alignment. The patient will need combined orthodontic and surgical management of his skeletal discrepancy and Class III malocclusion when growth is complete.

The patient's overall skeletal pattern should be evaluated carefully at this stage of development. It is of great value to have previous cephalomet-

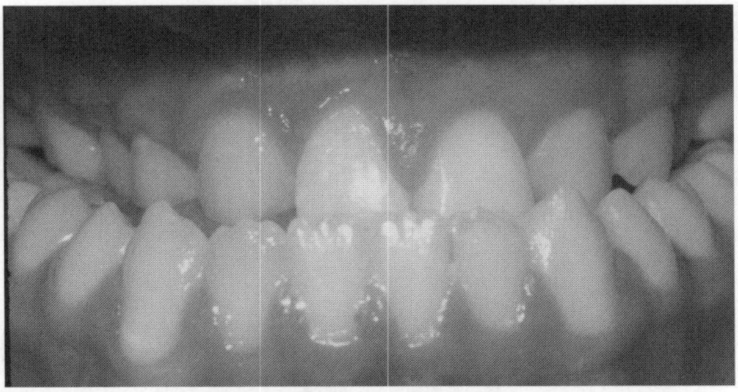

Figure 16.21. Frontal intraoral view of lateral incisors substituted for cuspids. When growth is complete patient will have surgical and orthodontic treatment to address the skeletal pattern and Class III malocclusion.

ric radiographs so the pattern of growth to date can be assessed through serial cephalometric superimposition. This record of previous growth is important in making an accurate projection for further growth. In some cases, there may be an anterior crossbite (Class III relationship). In situations where the Class III relationship is not related to a significant skeletal discrepancy, one can consider some orthodontic treatment to apply forward traction to the maxilla and maxillary dentition. In some cases, there may be an extreme discrepancy in jaw length with a severe maxillary and midfacial growth deficiency. Some of these children may have problems with chewing function, speech articulation, and/or psychological distress related to facial difference. In these cases, a coordinated plan may be developed that integrates orthodontics with surgery to progressively distract the maxilla and midface forward (see Figures 16.22, 16.23, and 16.24). For children with severe skeletal discrepancies, this may be done in the growing years, with a frank and open discussion with the patient and family that further jaw repositioning surgery and orthodontic treatment will be needed when growth is complete.

## Permanent Dentition—The Teenage Years

When the patient reaches the teenage years, the permanent teeth other than the third molars (wisdom teeth) are erupted, and it is critical to reevaluate all aspects of the facial, skeletal, and dental pattern. The most

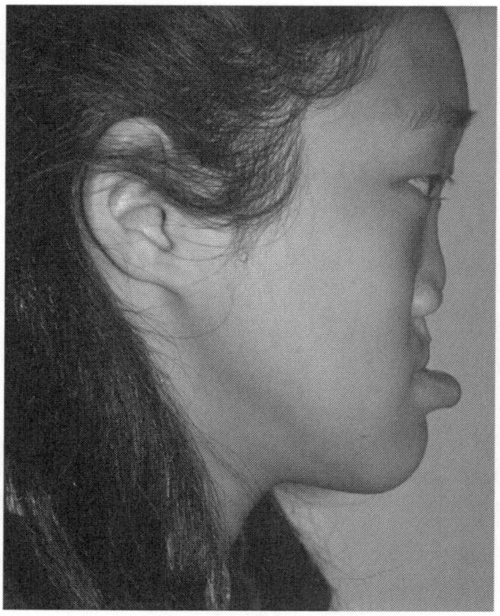

FIGURE 16.22. An 11-year-old patient with midline cleft, severe midfacial growth deficiency, and Class III malocclusion.

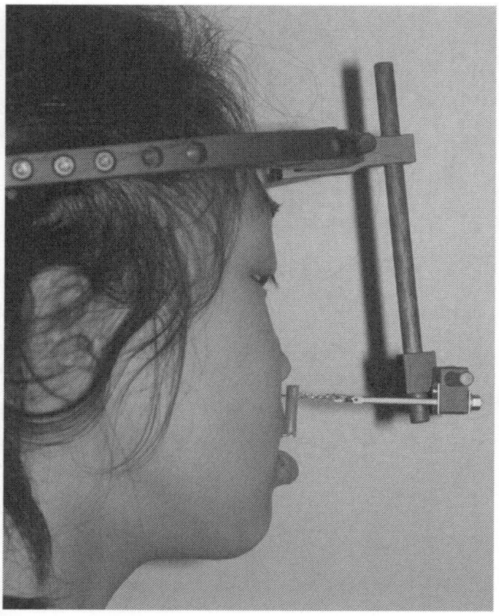

FIGURE 16.23. Patient postsurgery in active osteogenic distraction to move midface forward.

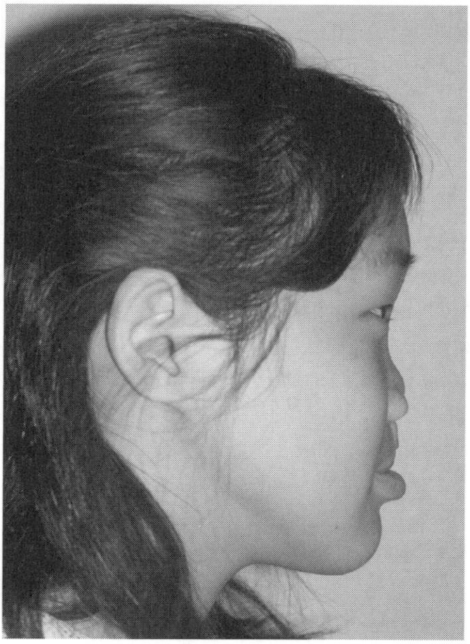

FIGURE 16.24. Profile after osteogenic distraction.

important determination is accurately defining the overall jaw development pattern. Also, it is important to recognize that the maximal pubertal growth spurt will occur between 12 and 13 years of age in girls and between 14 and 15 years of age in boys, although growth continues beyond the growth spurt. Girls' growth is generally complete between 17 and 18 years of age. Boys may not complete growth until 18–20 years of age. When the permanent dentition is erupted in the teenager, the team must make a definitive determination as to whether the underlying skeletal pattern will require surgical management when growth is complete. This determination will set the framework for the orthodontic treatment plan for the teenage years.

If the Class III malocclusion is mild, there are situations where orthodontic alignment of the teeth can correct the relationship. However, it is critical to realize that teeth should not be tipped off their boney bases in an attempt to cover up or mask a fundamental skeletal imbalance. This results in compromise in the final facial profile and inherent instability of the orthodontic result, as well as compromises in the periodontal support for teeth, resulting in decreased longevity of the dentition. In cases where orthognathic surgery will definitely be required when growth is complete, it may be wise to defer orthodontic treatment until it is time for the orthodontic preparation for the planned orthognathic surgery. Again, the overriding goal is to be as efficient as possible and, within the parameters of achieving a good outcome, to minimize the total time in orthodontics through the patient's lifetime.

In cases where growth is such that treatment goals can be addressed through orthodontic treatment without surgery in the teenage years, there are certain areas of focus for this stage of orthodontics. These relate to optimal eruption of permanent teeth, especially the maxillary canines; appropriately arranging spaces when missing teeth require replacement; aligning midlines; setting correct overjet-overbite relationships; and setting correct posterior transverse widths by managing posterior crossbite through expansion (see Figure 16.25).

Although partial fixed or removable appliances are sometimes used for teenagers, full fixed orthodontic appliances are usually necessary in the teenage patient with a cleft to align the erupting canines and bicuspids (premolars), as well as to coordinate the upper and lower arches with each other. When orthodontics alone can address the goals, orthodontic treatment in teenagers aims to establish a good working occlusion, as well as a balanced facial appearance. If the alveolar bone graft is successful, with the bone well integrated, and the facial growth is reasonably balanced,

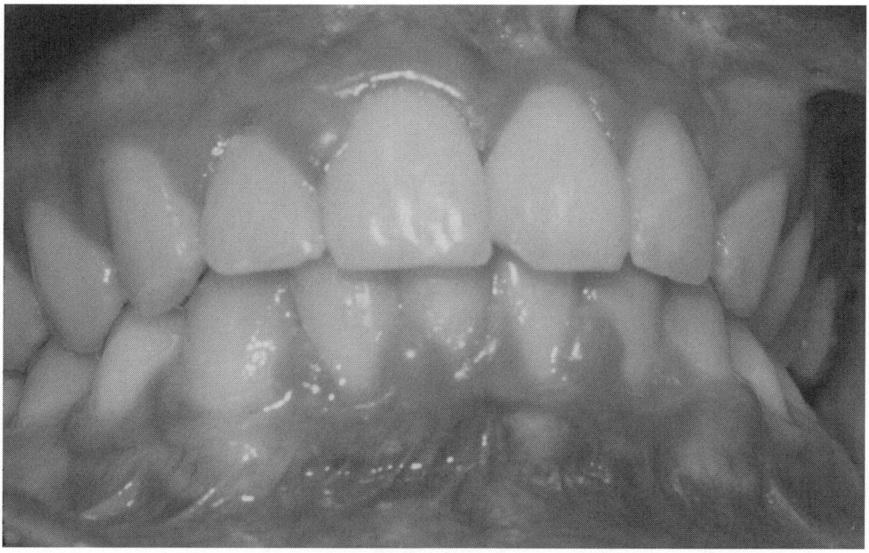

FIGURE 16.25. Frontal intraoral view following orthodontic treatment for a patient with a left complete cleft who had an alveolar bone graft and good growth.

then orthodontic decision making is straightforward. Given these parameters, the orthodontic treatment for a patient with a cleft can be managed in a similar fashion as orthodontic treatment for any patient.

In the majority of cases, the permanent canine(s) will erupt uneventfully through the grafted bone (El Deeb, Messer, Lehnert, Hebda, & Waite, 1982; Matsui, Echigo, Kimizuka, Takahashi, & Chiba, 2005). In rare instances, the permanent canine may require surgical uncovering and orthodontic traction to encourage eruption (see Figure 16.26). When orthodontic assistance is required to encourage canine eruption, it is usually done in the teenage years.

As part of definitive orthodontic treatment in the teenage years, maxillary orthodontic expansion may be required. When expansion is done at this stage of development, it is most commonly done with an expander that is fixed to the maxillary dentition at four points and has a midline screw device that is turned daily by the parent (see Figure 16.27). This is commonly called a rapid palatal expander (RPE) or Hyrax appliance. The RPE is often in the mouth for several months, and it is important for the orthodontist to discuss and coordinate the treatment with the team and the child's speech-language pathologist.

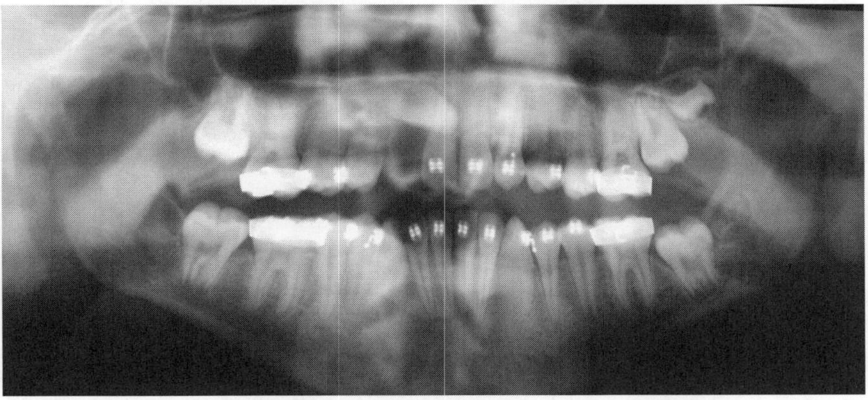

FIGURE 16.26. Panoramic radiograph showing impacted maxillary right cuspid in area of grafted alveolus requiring surgical uncovering and orthodontic traction to erupt tooth.

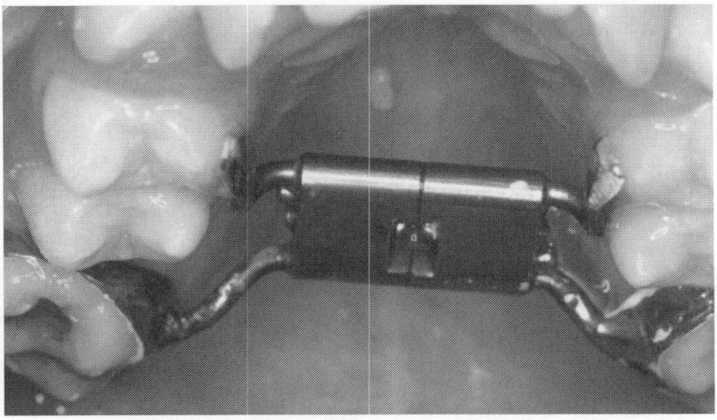

FIGURE 16.27. Rapid palatal expander or Hyrax appliance.

When definitive orthodontic treatment can be provided in the teenage years, the nature of the final occlusion must be carefully planned. When one or both maxillary lateral incisors are missing, there are two approaches to management. The options are (1) to orthodontically arrange the teeth to optimize spacing for prosthodontic replacement of the lateral incisor(s) or (2) to replace the lateral incisor(s) with a more forward positioning of the permanent canine(s). This decision making is complex and requires input from several team members, especially the prosthodontist and the oral and maxillofacial surgeon. Substituting permanent canines in the positions of the missing lateral incisors is more optimal in bilateral cleft situations where the tooth positions and aesthetics will be symmetric in the final occlusion. In addition, the size, morphology, and color of the permanent canines have an impact on the ability to achieve the best result with tooth substitution. When the decision is made to replace the lateral incisor(s) using implant-supported crown(s), it is critical to position the teeth orthodontically to optimize the space and root positions of adjacent teeth for proper implant positioning. Although the arches are often prepared for the implants in the teenage years, it is important to realize that the implant itself should not be placed until jaw growth is complete. Again, the reader is referred to Chapter 17 by Swift and Chapter 18 by Leeper, Charles, and Sills, which discuss implant-supported crowns in detail.

## Adult (Nongrowing) Orthodontic Treatment

As discussed previously, the time at which patients with cleft palate reach full maturity and facial growth varies between males and females. Growth of the female patient tends to finish at a much earlier age (16–17 years of age) than that of the male patient (18–20 years of age). Orthodontic treatment in the nongrowing years is primarily focused on coordination with definitive skeletal repositioning surgery to harmonize facial balance, occlusal function, and aesthetics. Also, when missing teeth are planned for replacement with implants, these implants cannot be placed until jaw growth is complete. In many of these cases, it is necessary to integrate some orthodontic treatment into the prosthodontic and oral surgical management plan.

Nowadays, it is extremely rare for a nongrowing patient who has not had previous team care to present to a cleft team. Adult patients who did not have the benefit of early integrated team care often present major challenges due to compromises in facial morphology, health of teeth, positions of teeth, and problems in periodontal support. It is difficult to achieve optimal results in the adult patient who has not had integrated care when young (see Figures 16.28, 16.29, and 16.30).

For the patient with a cleft palate who has been followed regularly by an interdisciplinary team over many years, the integrated orthodontic, oral surgical, and prosthodontic treatment for the nongrowing years has been previously planned. The most common surgical treatment involves advancing the maxilla to correct a lack of midfacial fullness and a

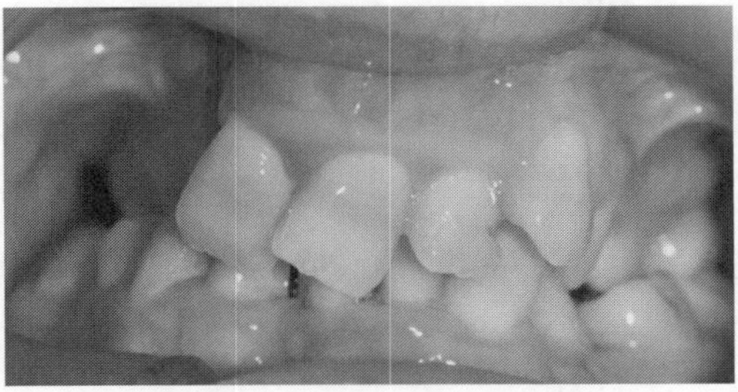

Figure 16.28. Frontal intraoral view of adult with unilateral cleft and severe malocclusion. There is severe malalignment of teeth as well as transverse collapse of the maxillary arch.

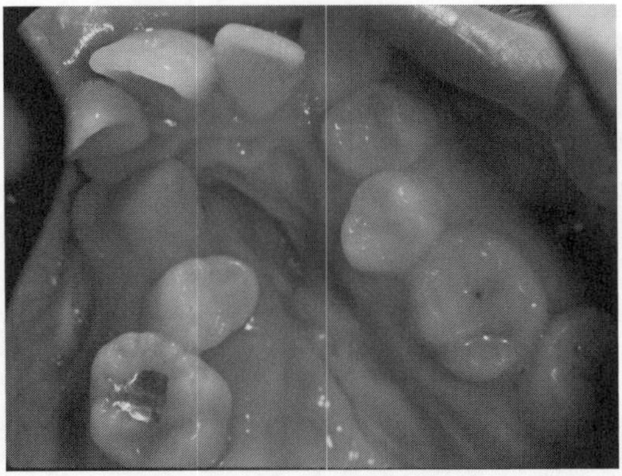

Figure 16.29. Occlusal view of the maxillary arch showing severe maxillary constriction and dental malalignment.

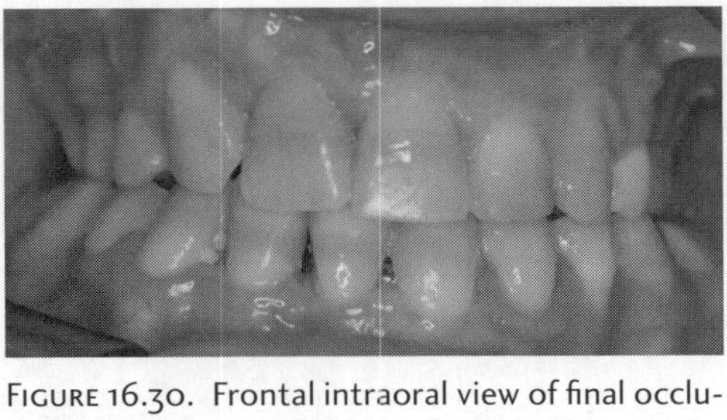

Figure 16.30. Frontal intraoral view of final occlusion with compromise that relates to the severity of the initial presenting situation. The patient did not have integrated team care but presented as an adult for care.

Class III malocclusion. (See Chapter 17 by Swift for more specifics regarding the surgical approaches.) Beyond the diagnostic and treatment planning process, the orthodontist's role is to provide orthodontic treatment that fully integrates with the surgical approach.

Traditionally, the first phase of the orthodontic treatment is called presurgical orthodontics. The goal of this phase is to decompensate the dentition and place the teeth in ideal position relative to their individual jaw structure. Commonly, when a patient has maxillary growth deficiency and a Class III malocclusion, the natural positions of the teeth are retroclined mandibular anterior teeth and proclined maxillary anterior teeth. The orthodontist must undo these compensations, which have adapted the tooth position to the jaw discrepancy. In many cases, the reverse overjet may become greater during the presurgical orthodontic phase of treatment. The goal is to have the teeth in a position that will provide an optimal fit when the jaw positions are surgically corrected. Also, optimal angulation of the anterior teeth is key to the ability to ideally position the jaws during the surgery. Once healing from the surgery is complete, the orthodontist continues with the postsurgical finishing phase of the treatment. The goal in this phase is to finalize the fine details of the tooth alignment to provide the best possible occlusal function with the new surgically created jaw positions (see Figures 16.31–16.36). In cases

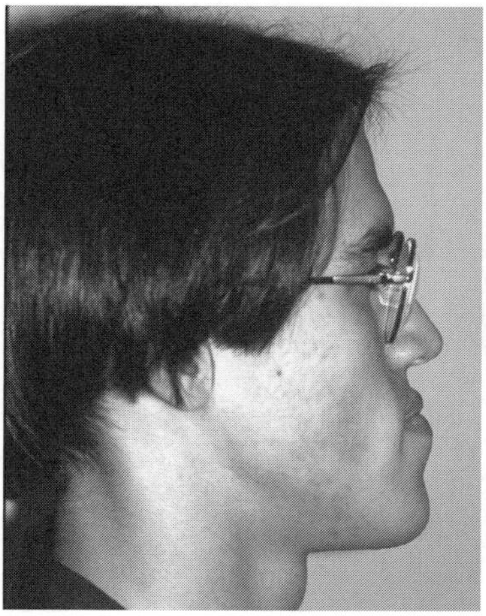

FIGURE 16.31. Presurgical facial profile for patient with cleft palate and severe midfacial growth deficiency.

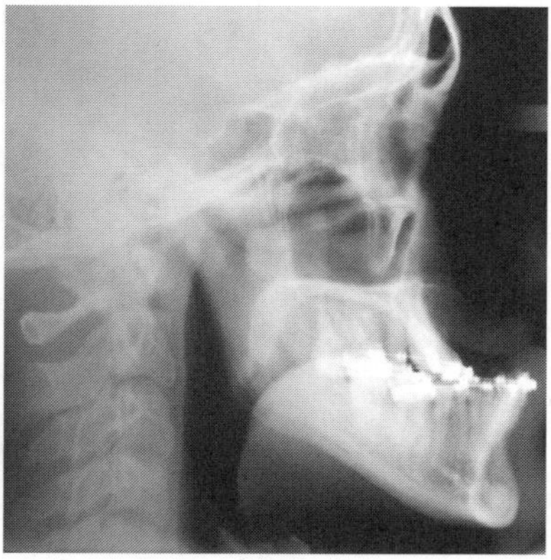

FIGURE 16.32. Presurgical cephalometric radiograph.

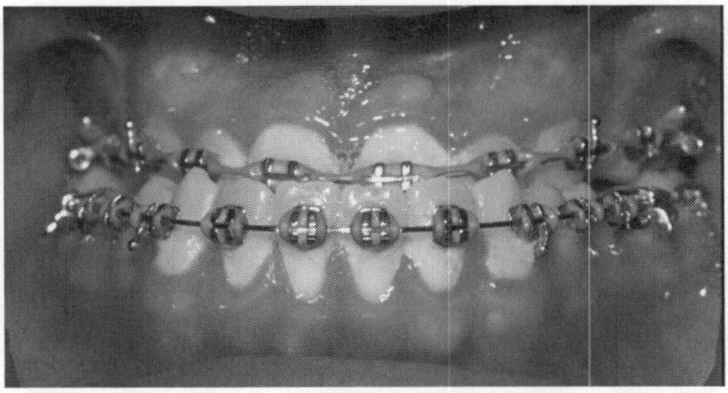

FIGURE 16.33. Presurgical Class III occlusion with orthodontic appliances in place.

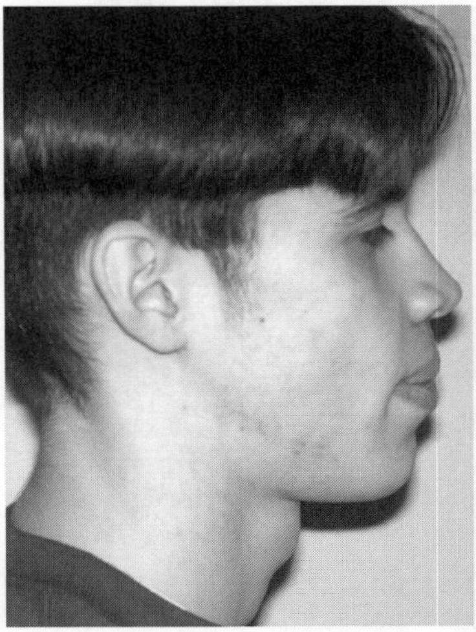

FIGURE 16.34. Final facial profile showing improved midfacial fullness and facial balance.

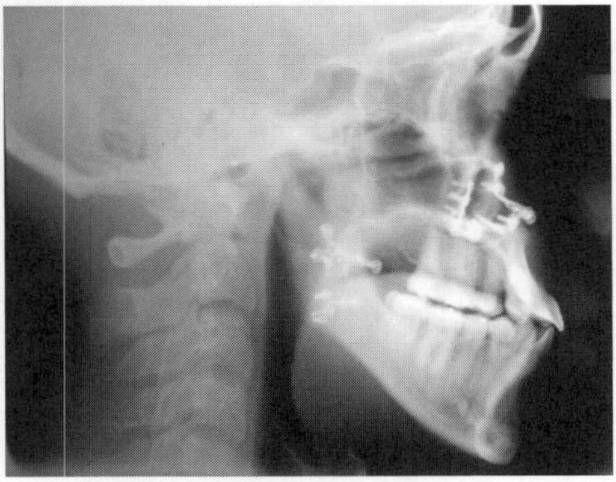

FIGURE 16.35. Final cephalometric radiograph.

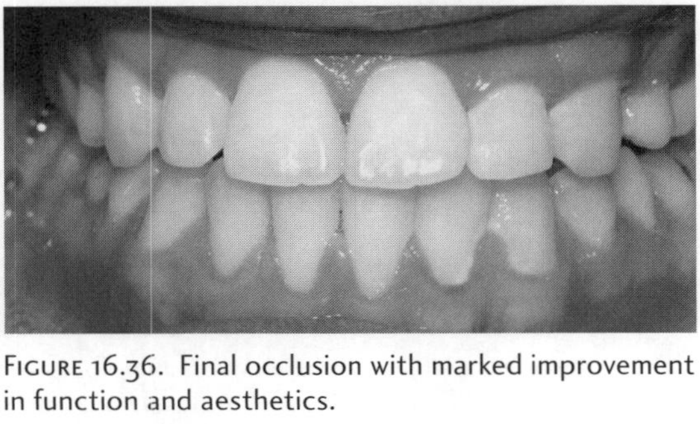

FIGURE 16.36. Final occlusion with marked improvement in function and aesthetics.

with missing lateral incisors, within certain parameters it is possible to move a posterior segment forward during the orthognathic surgery and in so doing close the space of the missing lateral incisor (see Figures 16.37 and 16.38).

In the adult nongrowing patient, it is important to monitor the periodontal supporting structures through the orthodontic and surgical treatment. Susceptibility to periodontal disease increases when a patient reaches adulthood, and adults lose more teeth from periodontal disease

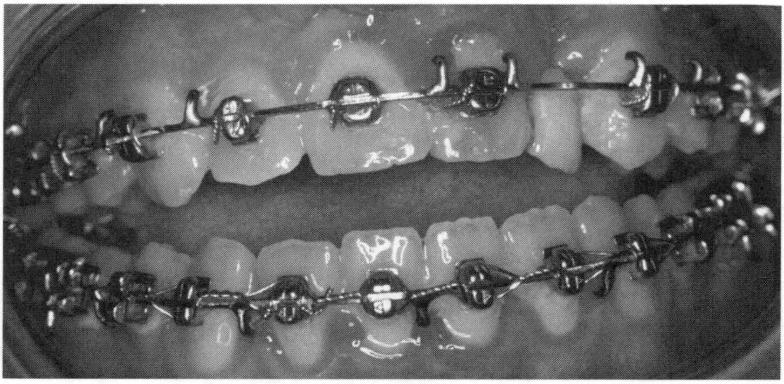

FIGURE 16.37. Intraoral photo of patient with a complete left-sided cleft who did not have an alveolar bone graft. The patient has a Class III malocclusion with an anterior open bite. Orthodontic preparation involves aligning arches in preparation for maxillary surgery that will address the jaw position as well as close the alveolar cleft.

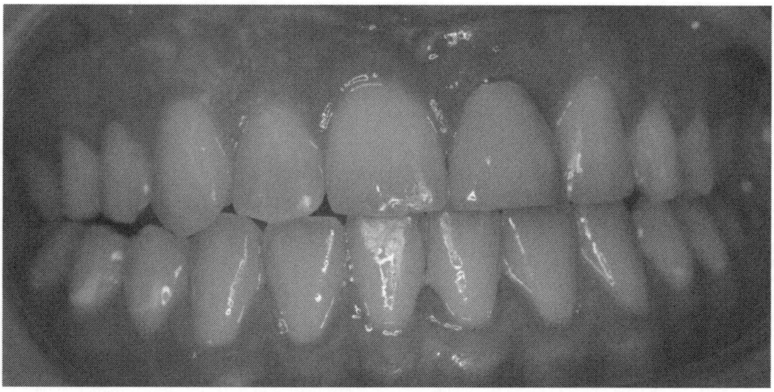

FIGURE 16.38. Final occlusion with mild compromise in the dental midlines but improved aesthetics and occlusal function.

than through dental caries. Team members can again reinforce the need for optimal oral hygiene throughout surgical orthodontic treatment for the patient with dentofacial disharmony secondary to cleft palate.

## Summary

The orthodontist plays a key role in the dynamics of craniofacial team function. The ideal team strives to improve, and improvement comes from objective assessment of outcomes and open dialogue among team members. The orthodontist is the member of the team who has a thorough understanding of facial growth and development and a skill set to objectively assess growth and the impact of treatment interventions. These skills are invaluable on an individual patient basis, but also important in the team's continued quest for excellence.

The orthodontist has significant cooperative treatment relationships with all team members, but particularly with other dental specialists and surgical and speech team members. These relationships with fellow professionals are immensely rewarding, in terms of both professional knowledge development and personal satisfaction. Any craniofacial orthodontist cannot adequately quantify the emotional boost that comes from working with a dedicated group of professionals to provide the patient with a result that is optimal for both function and aesthetics.

# APPENDIX 16A

# Child and Adult Teeth

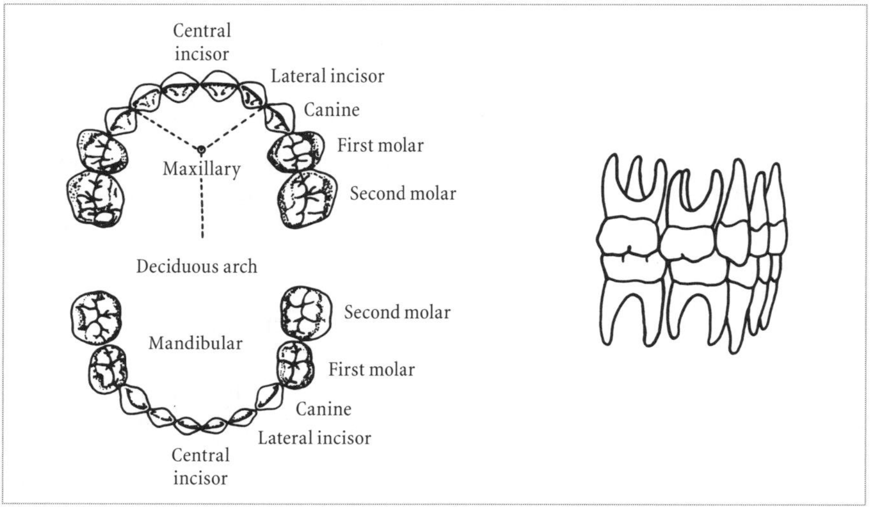


Child (deciduous) teeth and dental occlusion/bite.

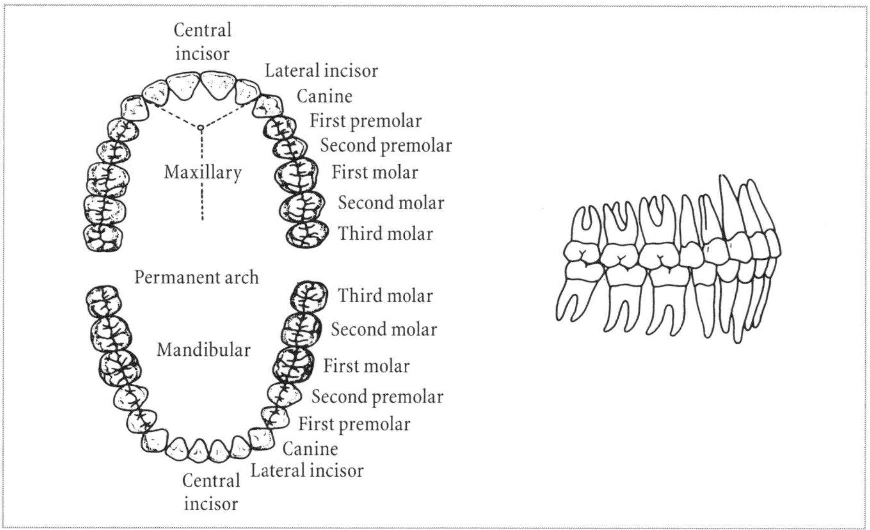


Adult (permanent) teeth and dental occlusion/bite.

# References

Aduss, H., & Figueroa, A. (1990). Stages of orthodontic treatment in complete unilateral cleft lip and palate. In J. Bardach & H. Morris (Eds.), *Multidisciplinary management of cleft lip and palate.* Philadelphia: Saunders.

Berkowitz, S. (1977). Cleft lip and palate research: An updated state of the art. Section III: Orofacial growth and dentistry. *Cleft Palate Journal, 14,* 288–301.

Berkowitz, S., Mejia, M., & Bystrik, A. (2004). A comparison of the Latham-Millard procedure with those of a conservative treatment approach for dental occlusion and facial aesthetics in unilateral and bilateral complete cleft lip and palate: Part 1. Dental occlusion. *Plastic and Reconstructive Surgery, 113,* 1–18.

Bongaarts, C. A. M., Kuijpers-Jagtman, A. M., Van 't Hof, M. A., & Prahl-Andersen, B. (2004). The effect of infant orthopedics on the occlusion of the deciduous dentition in children with complete unilateral cleft lip and palate. *Cleft Palate-Craniofacial Journal, 41,* 633–641.

El Deeb, M., Messer, L. B., Lehnert, M. W., Hebda, T. W., & Waite, D. E. (1982). Canine eruption into grafted bone in maxillary alveolar cleft defects. *Cleft Palate Journal, 19,* 9–16.

Evans, C. A. (2004). Orthodontic treatment for patients with clefts. *Clinics in Plastic Surgery, 31,* 271–290.

Grayson, B. H., Cutting, C. B., & Wood, R. (1993). Preoperative columellar lengthening in bilateral cleft lip and palate. *Plastic and Reconstructive Surgery, 92,* 1422–1423.

Grayson, B. H., Santiago, P. E., Brecht, L. E., & Cutting, C. B. (1999). Presurgical nasoalveolar molding in infants with cleft lip and palate. *Cleft Palate-Craniofacial Journal, 36,* 486–498.

Gruber, H. (1990). Presurgical maxillary orthopedics. In J. Bardach & H. Morris (Eds.), *Multidisciplinary management of cleft lip and palate.* Philadelphia: Saunders.

Hotz, M., Gnoinski, W., & Perko, M. (Eds.). (1986). *Early treatment of cleft lip and palate.* Bern, Switzerland: Hans Huber.

Huebner, D. V., & Marsh, J. L. (1990). Alveolar molding appliances in the treatment of cleft lip and palate infants. In J. Bardach & H. Morris (Eds.), *Multidisciplinary management of cleft lip and palate.* Philadelphia: Saunders.

Kuijpers-Jagtman, A. M. (2006). The orthodontist: An essential partner in CLP treatment. *B-ENT* (Suppl. 4), 57–62.

Mars, M., James, D., & Lamabadusuriya, S. (1990). The Sri Lankan cleft lip and palate project: The unoperated cleft lip and palate. *Cleft Palate Journal, 27,* 3–10.

Mars, M., Plint, D. A., Houston, W. J., Bergland, O., & Semb, G. (1987). The Goslon yardstick: A new system of assessing dental arch relationships in children with unilateral clefts of the lip and palate. *Cleft Palate Journal, 24,* 312–322.

Matsui, K., Echigo, S., Kimizuka, S., Takahashi M., & Chiba, M. (2005). Clinical study on eruption of permanent canines after secondary alveolar bone grafting. *Cleft Palate-Craniofacial Journal, 42,* 309–313.

Prahl-Anderson, B., & Ju, Q. (2006). Quality improvement of cleft lip and palate treatment. *Angle Orthodontic, 76,* 265–268.

Ross, R. B. (1987). Treatment variables affecting facial growth in complete unilateral cleft lip and palate. *Cleft Palate Journal, 24,* 5–77.

Sell, D., & Grunwell, P. (1990). Speech results following late palatal surgery in previously unoperated Sri Lankan adolescents with cleft palate. *Cleft Palate Journal, 27,* 162–168.

Stark, R. B. (1954). The pathogenesis of harelip and cleft palate. *Plastic and Reconstructive Surgery, 13,* 20.

Subtelny, J. D. (1990). Orthodontic principles in treatment of cleft lip and palate. In J. Bardach & H. Morris (Eds.), *Multidisciplinary management of cleft lip and palate.* Philadelphia: Saunders.

Tondury, G. (1961). On the mechanism of cleft formation. In S. Pruzansky (Ed.), *Congenital anomalies of the face and associated structures.* Springfield, IL: Thomas.

Vargervik, K. (1981). Orthodontic management of unilateral cleft lip and palate. *Cleft Palate Journal, 18,* 256–270.

Vargervik, K. (1983). Growth characteristics of the premaxilla and orthodontic treatment principles in bilateral cleft lip and palate. *Cleft Palate Journal, 20,* 289–302.

Veau, V. (1938). Hasenschanten menschlicher Keimlinge auf der Stufe. *Zeitschrift fur Anatomie and Entwickelungsgesch, 108,* 459–493.

Vig, K. W., & Turvey, T. A. (1985). Orthodontic surgical interactions in the management of cleft lip and palate. *Clinics in Plastic Surgery, 12,* 735–748.

# CHAPTER 17

# Oral and Maxillofacial Surgery

## Management of the Alveolar Cleft and Jaw Discrepancies

*James Q. Swift*

Swift discusses the discipline of oral and maxillofacial surgery and the education and training required. In addition to surgical training and skills, having a thorough knowledge and understanding about dental structures and occlusion places the oral and maxillofacial surgeon in an important role to diagnose, evaluate, and repair the alveolar cleft and the maxillary and mandibular jaw discrepancies, as well as perform other procedures beneficial for patients with cleft lip and palate. Swift discusses these procedures and emphasizes the importance of interdisciplinary analysis, planning, and treatment for optimal outcome.

1. Swift discusses the surgical repair of the alveolar cleft. What are two benefits of repairing an alveolar cleft with a bone graft?
2. At what age, or what stage of dental growth and development, does Swift prefer to graft the alveolar cleft? What are some reasons? What autologous bone do Swift and others consider to be the best and why?
3. As Swift describes, correction of maxillary and mandibular jaw discrepancies can be done utilizing conventional Le Fort I surgery or distraction osteogenesis (DO). When might the oral surgeon consider using DO? What does Swift say are disadvantages of DO compared to conventional surgery?
4. What are some possible positive and negative speech sequelae of surgically advancing the maxilla?
5. What is the primary reason for more difficult surgical orthognathic correction of jaw discrepancies in patients with clefts as compared to patients without clefts?

6. Describe the roles of the oral and maxillofacial surgeon, orthodontist, and prosthodontist in replacement of a missing maxillary lateral incisor in a patient who had a previous bone graft to repair the alveolar cleft.

The effective and complete management of individuals with congenital clefting of the lip, alveolus (dental ridge), and palate requires reconstruction of all anatomic structures involved. Requisites for normal oral function include an intact lip, intact palate, intact dental alveolus, and intact dentition. The usual sequence of surgical repair begins with the lip and continues with the posterior palatal repair to facilitate feeding, speech development, and cosmesis, usually within the 1st year of life.

The clinician managing individuals with clefts must recognize that further, or secondary, reconstructive surgery is important to the overall goal of establishing acceptable, or as close to normal as possible, structure and function of all anatomic units affected by the cleft. Surgery subsequent to the cleft lip and palate repair is not performed at any prescribed time interval but is based on growth, development, functional impairment, and appearance of the child or adult (Liao & Mars, 2005). Decisions for treatment may occur at any time between 1 year of age and skeletal maturity, at which time there is no significant potential for further facial growth (Li, Shi, Song, Zuo, & Zheng, 2006; Shetye, 2004). Furthermore, the interdisciplinary team approach has the best chance for optimal outcome. Table 17.1 shows the ages, treatment specialists involved, and rationales for oral and maxillofacial treatments following initial cleft lip and palate repair. Although there are other secondary treatments that may be beneficial, dependent on speech performance, as well as additional lip and nasal surgeries for function and cosmesis, Table 17.1 highlights the interventions related to the dentition and upper and lower jaws that are typically performed to establish the best possible outcome. By comparing this table with Table 14.1 in Chapter 14 by Buckley and Landis, the reader can see that the oral and maxillofacial surgeon works closely with the orthodontist and prosthodontist or restorative dentist in each treatment (see also Chapter 16 by Williams and Bevis and Chapter 18 by Leeper, Charles, and Sills). It is important to understand that proper management of the patient requires the least number of surgeries necessary to completely repair the sequelae of the congenital cleft.

**Table 17.1**
**Ages at Which Treatment Involving the Oral and Maxillofacial Surgeon Should Be Considered**

| Age (years) | Treatment | Specialists involved | Rationale |
|---|---|---|---|
| 3–12 | Alveolar cleft grafting, closure of oral-nasal fistula(e) | • Orthodontist<br>• Prosthodontist<br>• Speech pathologist<br>• Oral and maxillofacial surgeon (OMS) | Graft must be accomplished before teeth adjacent to the cleft erupt into the cleft area; speech considerations |
| | Determination about prognosis/extraction/retention of supernumerary, primary, and permanent teeth adjacent to the cleft | • Orthodontist<br>• Prosthodontist<br>• OMS | Teeth that are dysmorphic, hypoplastic, and/or hypocalcified may not be useful for dental reconstruction |
| 6–8 | Orthodontic treatment, which may include maxillary transverse expansion | • Orthodontist<br>• Prosthodontist<br>• OMS | Expand for grafting; align and level in preparation for orthognathic surgery and/or eventual dental reconstruction |
| 13–16 | Dental alignment and leveling; temporary dental reconstruction | | |
| 16–18 | Correction of skeletal maxillary hypoplasia, if indicated | • Orthodontist<br>• Prosthodontist<br>• OMS<br>• Speech-language pathologist<br>• Plastic and reconstructive surgeon | Potential speech effects of orthognathic surgery; orthodontic leveling and alignment, desired dental arch relationships, plan for prosthodontic reconstruction and canine position |
| 18 | Implant therapy:<br>• Augmentation grafting<br>• Placement of implant<br>• Prosthodontic crown | • Orthodontist<br>• Prosthodontist<br>• OMS<br>• Plastic and reconstructive surgeon | Before debanding, teeth must be aligned appropriately for implant reconstruction |

Oral and maxillofacial surgery (OMS) is a specialty of dentistry. A dentist matriculates into an advanced education program in oral and maxillofacial surgery after obtaining a dental degree (DDS or DMD). The training program or residency is 4 years in length, during which time the dentist gains experience and training in patient management, medicine, anesthesia, general surgery, and oral and maxillofacial surgery. Many OMS residency training programs also offer a medical degree (MD) as a component of OMS training.

The dental- and surgical-based knowledge and skills acquired by oral and maxillofacial surgeons enable them to provide surgical reconstruction of the alveolus and restoration of the dentition. These professionals are also well trained in orthognathic surgery techniques. Some oral and maxillofacial surgeons choose to focus on management of patients with clefts and craniofacial anomalies. They become involved with interdisciplinary management teams to provide the best possible outcomes for the patients with clefts.

This chapter focuses on those areas of cleft management for which the skills of the oral and maxillofacial surgeon are most beneficial:

- Reconstruction of the cleft alveolus
- Orthognathic surgery to correct skeletal facial dysmorphia
- Dental implant placement to replace missing teeth associated with clefting
- Other adjunctive procedures

## Reconstruction of the Cleft Alveolus

The alveolus is the component of the maxilla that contains and provides support for the dentition. In an individual with a complete cleft of the primary palate (unilateral), the alveolus fails to fuse, resulting in an absence of bony and soft tissue (gum) continuity. In most situations, there is a residual communication between the oral cavity and the nasal cavity, commonly called an oral-nasal fistula (see Figure 17.1). This opening allows passage of fluids, debris, and bacteria between the oral cavity and the nasal cavity. In cases where the fistula is wide and occurs behind the teeth, nasal air emission may be detected during speech production. The individual may also complain of regurgitation of oral fluids into the na-

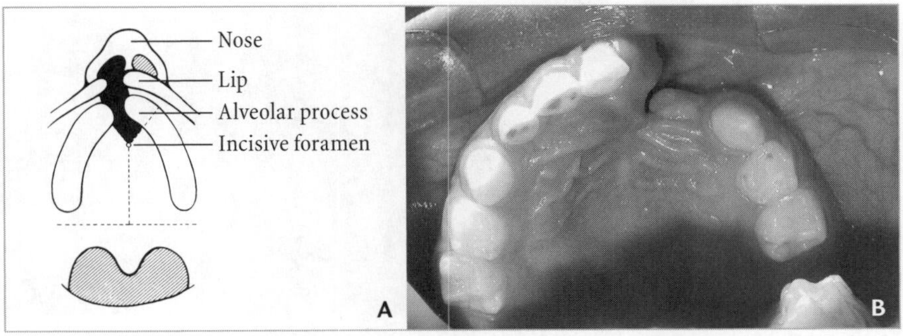


Figure 17.1. (A) Diagram of unilateral right cleft of the primary palate—palatal aspect. (B) Clinical photo of unilateral left cleft of the primary palate—palatal aspect.

sal cavity and out of the nares on some occasions. Because of the lack of bony continuity of the maxillary alveolus, there is resultant mobility of the two maxillary dental segments when mastication and tooth contact occur. The goal of alveolar cleft grafting is to repair the structure and appearance of the alveolus and dentition such that it appears there was no cleft in the area.

In the bilateral cleft alveolus, the premaxillary or central bony segment is typically very mobile, easily displaced a few millimeters with lateral pressure (see Figure 17.2). This segment must be stabilized with grafting to limit mobility and provide the stability necessary for mastication and dental reconstruction.

Some clinicians recommend primary or early repair of the cleft alveolus, typically by performing a rib graft or a procedure called a gingivoplasty, which is a technique used to close the opening by a series of transpositional flaps (Savaci, Hosnuter, Tosun, & Demir, 2005). Although positive outcomes have been described for very young patients, in most situations the repair of the cleft alveolus is delayed until a later age. Additionally, some clinicians advocate the use of oral appliances to control the development of the maxillary alveolus. This technique requires that the appliances be refabricated to accommodate for growth and is not frequently utilized in the management of individuals with clefts (Grayson & Maull, 2004; Renkielska, Wojtaszek-Slominska, & Dobke, 2005; Rosenstein, Grasseschi, & Dado, 2003).

The most commonly employed technique to repair the alveolar cleft is surgical closure of the oral-antral communication via reconstruction of the alveolar bone defect with free autologous (the patient's own) bone

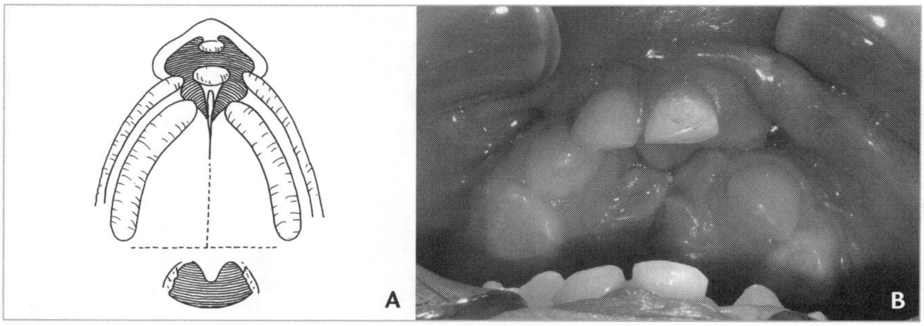


FIGURE 17.2. (A) Diagram of bilateral cleft of the primary palate—palatal aspect. (B) Clinical photo of bilateral cleft of the primary palate—palatal aspect.

transfer. This technique has been shown to be dependable and reliable and to provide a successful outcome.

The timing of the alveolar cleft reconstruction is dependent upon several factors. Proper timing facilitates surgical success. The decision to proceed with alveolar cleft reconstruction is best made by members of the integrated cleft palate team. Each clinician considers several variables to determine the most opportune time to proceed. The variables include age, dental occlusion, transverse maxillary dental arch width, existing and developing dentition adjacent to the cleft, and, in some cases, speech.

The orthodontist managing the patient must be well informed and involved in the decision making as to when to reconstruct the cleft alveolus (Scheuer, Holtje, Hasund, & Pfeifer, 2001). The restorative dentist providing prosthodontic care to the cleft patient must also be informed and involved to make decisions regarding the prognosis of developing teeth (see Chapter 16 by Williams and Bevis).

I believe that alveolar cleft repair is best implemented at the earliest age possible after eruption of the primary dentition and a radiographic determination that the permanent teeth are developing in the area of the cleft. Smaller individuals have less bone available to harvest for the cleft repair but usually have an adequate amount. However, the ideal time for bone graft reconstruction for any particular patient can range from 3 to 12 years of age.

Transverse maxillary deficiency, clinically manifested by posterior dental crossbite, may result from fibrosis associated with the palate repair or may be a component of the clefting phenomena. This is not uncommon. In cases of incomplete clefting with the secondary palate being unaffected, the occurrence of transverse deficiency and posterior crossbite is less likely.

The dentition adjacent to the cleft also affects the timing of alveolar reconstruction. The permanent central and lateral incisors are expected to erupt between 6 and 8 years of age. If a permanent tooth erupts into the cleft before grafting, it becomes difficult, if not impossible, to obtain the optimum bone volume in the grafted cleft to support the tooth. The prognosis for retention of that tooth for the long term is guarded. The graft should be placed prior to eruption of permanent teeth into the cleft.

The timing of alveolar reconstruction sometimes creates a dilemma and a difference of treatment protocol between the orthodontist and the surgeon providing the cleft alveolus repair. Orthodontic expansion of the maxilla generally is not time-consuming. Expansion can occur rapidly because the maxillary bony segments are not fused because of the original cleft. However, expansion requires orthodontic anchorage in the posterior maxilla. If there is a need to wait for the eruption of the maxillary first permanent molars to provide anchorage for expansion, the teeth approximating the cleft alveolus may erupt into the cleft. This may result in the loss of a permanent tooth. Some orthodontists will provide maxillary expansion utilizing the primary dentition as anchorage, which allows for earlier repair.

In many situations, the teeth approximating a cleft alveolus may be hypoplastic (small) or dysmorphic (misshapen or malformed) and, as such, nonrestorable or expendable. It is also common to find supernumerary or extra teeth approximating the cleft alveolus. However, the prognosis of an unerupted tooth may be difficult to determine. The dentist providing restorative care and prevention may be able to help make a determination regarding prognosis, which, in turn, would help in determining the timeframe for the grafting procedure.

It has been reported that the optimum time for grafting the alveolar cleft is when the approximating canine tooth root is two thirds formed and not yet erupted into the cleft (El Deeb, Messer, Lehnert, Hebda, & Waite, 1982; Troxell, Fonseca, & Osbon, 1982). This approach could delay the grafting procedure until age 10 or later. If the central or lateral incisors have already erupted into the cleft at this point, they may not be salvageable.

Another reason for early secondary cleft repair is that the maxillary central incisors approximating the cleft alveolus are often malposed. For these teeth to be properly aligned for appearance and function, the oral and maxillofacial surgeon must reconstruct the alveolus prior to orthodontic alignment. If the roots of the teeth approximating the cleft are moved into the cleft before surgical reconstruction, the tooth roots may become exposed in the cleft, resulting in tooth loss or an inability to gain adequate bone volume with a subsequent grafting procedure. As noted previously, the repair of the cleft alveolus establishes continuity of the maxillary dental arch. The graft also provides support for the alar base of the nose and the upper lip.

Once the decision is made to repair the alveolar cleft, the procedure is accomplished under general anesthesia in the operating room environment. A source of autologous bone must be identified. Several options are available, including proximal tibia, rib, cranium, mandible, and iliac crest of the hip. Generally, particulate cancellous marrow bone is preferred. Cortical grafts or block grafts can provide continuity to the defect and must be stabilized to integrate. The stability that may be rendered with the use of a cortical graft is rarely necessary. A problem with cortical grafts is that they may restrict tooth eruption. There has been research investigating the use of alloplastic, allogeneic, and xenogeneic materials as bone graft substitutes. Bone morphogenic protein has also been considered as a bone graft substitute but at this time is not indicated for alveolar cleft reconstruction (Chin, Ng, Tom, & Carstens, 2005).

The iliac crest is preferable. It provides an adequate quantity of particulate cancellous marrow bone. The bone is milled to uniform size and compressed in order to provide the greatest number of cells possible to the site. Also, harvest of the anterior iliac crest allows two surgical teams to work simultaneously, which reduces total surgical time.

The unilateral cleft alveolus should be completely examined under anesthesia. Local anesthesia is injected prior to the surgical incision. A shoulder roll facilitates visibility of the palatal component of the cleft. The surgeon must confirm or deny the presence of an oral-nasal fistula before incisions are made, as it will affect the approach. This is done with a nerve hook or lacrimal duct probe. Once the size and location of the fistula is determined, incisions are made on both sides of the cleft through gingiva and mucosa to the bony alveolus and along the facial gingival crevice. Vertical releasing incisions are made in the molar region to facilitate anterior flap rotation to cover the graft site. Similar incisions are made on the palate without the releasing incisions.

The mucosal and gingival tissue approximating the cleft is dissected away from the cleft. On the anterior and posterior margins of the cleft where there may not be a bone margin, the mucosal tissue is undermined, taking care not to perforate into the nasal cavity. The fistula is dissected away from the alveolar bone margins and pushed into the nasal cavity (see Figure 17.3). Once this tissue is freely dissected so as not to interfere with the bone graft placement, the fistula is closed using inverted resorbable sutures. The palatal tissue flaps are then reapproximated and sutured (see Figure 17.4). Any teeth interfering with the closure are removed. Any teeth destined to be extracted by the orthodontist or dentist are also removed.

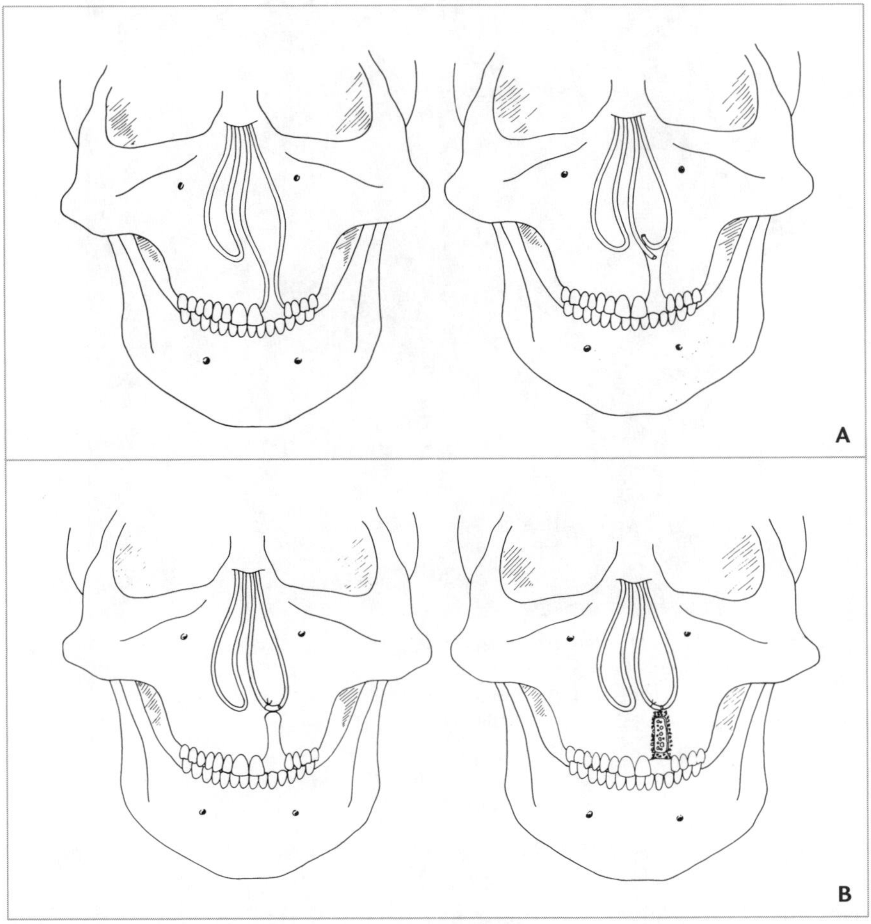


Figure 17.3. Schematic drawings demonstrating steps in closure of unilateral cleft and placement of bone grafts. *Note.* From "Residual Alveolar and Palatal Clefts," by D. E. Waite and R. B. Kersten (1980), in W. H. Bell, W. R. Proffit, and R. P. White (Eds.), *Surgical Correction of Dentofacial Deformities,* Vol. 2, Philadelphia: Saunders. Copyright by W. B. Saunders. Reprinted with permission.

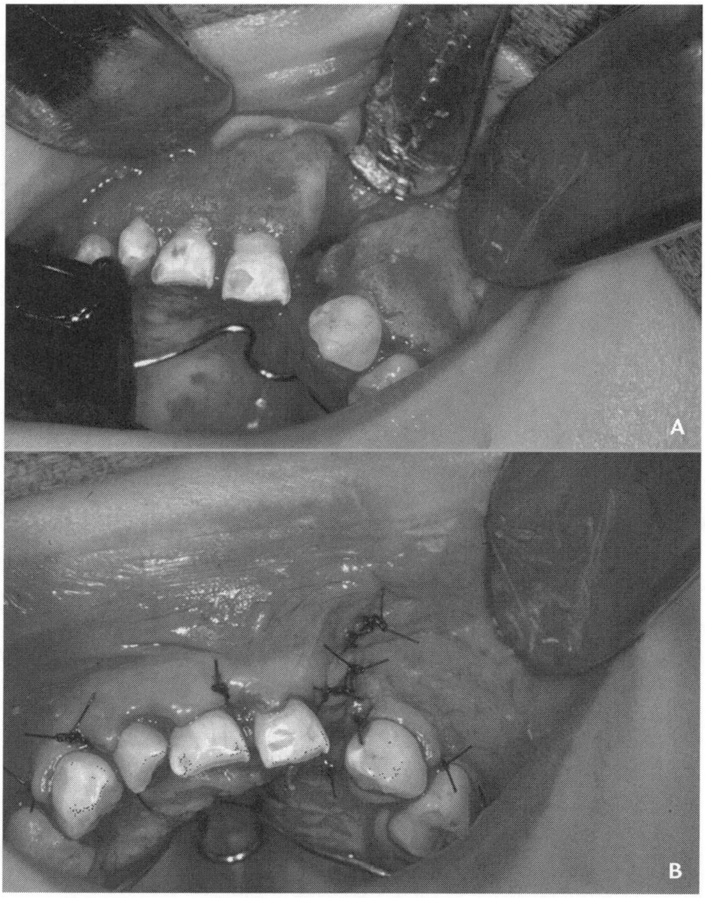


FIGURE 17.4. (A) Exposed alveolar cleft, nasal side closed and prepared for placement of autogenous bone graft. (B) Surgical closure after graft placement. Note that the gingivae (gum tissues) have been advanced and that the papillae do not "line up" with the teeth.

The bone graft is then placed into the cleft alveolar defect and packed into position. The facial gingival and mucosa flaps are then positioned over the grafted alveolus. Aggressive flap mobilization is desired. Tension of the flaps is assessed. If the flap tension will restrict passive closure, the flaps are released by submucosal dissection and careful scoring of the periosteum. Advancement of the lateral facial flaps allows for attached keratinized gingival tissue to be transposed over the cleft site. This will allow the permanent teeth erupting in the area of the cleft to erupt into gingival as opposed to mobile mucosa, thereby enhancing the periodontal health of the tooth. Rotation of mucosal "finger" flaps, while providing coverage for the bone graft, results in mobile mucosa approximating teeth. This may necessitate the need for keratinized tissue grafting at a later date to maintain the periodontal health and appearance of teeth erupting into the cleft site. The vertical labial component of the cleft is closed last. This type of closure, commonly called the "four-corner" flap closure, may result in the dental papillae being malpositioned. This is of little consequence, as the papillae will regenerate (Figure 17.5). Figure 17.6 shows a unilateral alveolar cleft (A) before grafting and (B) 6 months after after grafting, with tooth erupting through the graft. Figure 17.6C is a radiograph showing the tooth in the graft site.

The bilateral cleft alveolus is much more difficult to manage surgically. The premaxilla is usually quite mobile due to the bony discontinuity of the alveolus. This mobility can be magnified by contact with the mandibular dentition on oral function. It is desirable to stabilize the premaxillary segment with a splint, orthodontic appliances, or some other means to enhance healing and consolidation of the bone grafts (Bitter, 2001).

The premaxillary segment in bilateral clefts receives its blood supply to some degree from the labial mucosa. It is important to recognize that this blood supply should not be compromised in bilateral alveolar cleft

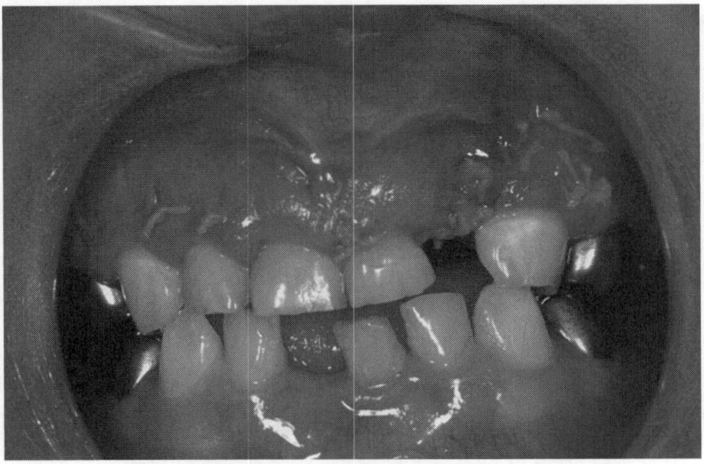

Figure 17.5. One week following grafting and closure. Fistula has been repaired and papillae have conformed to the interdental spaces.

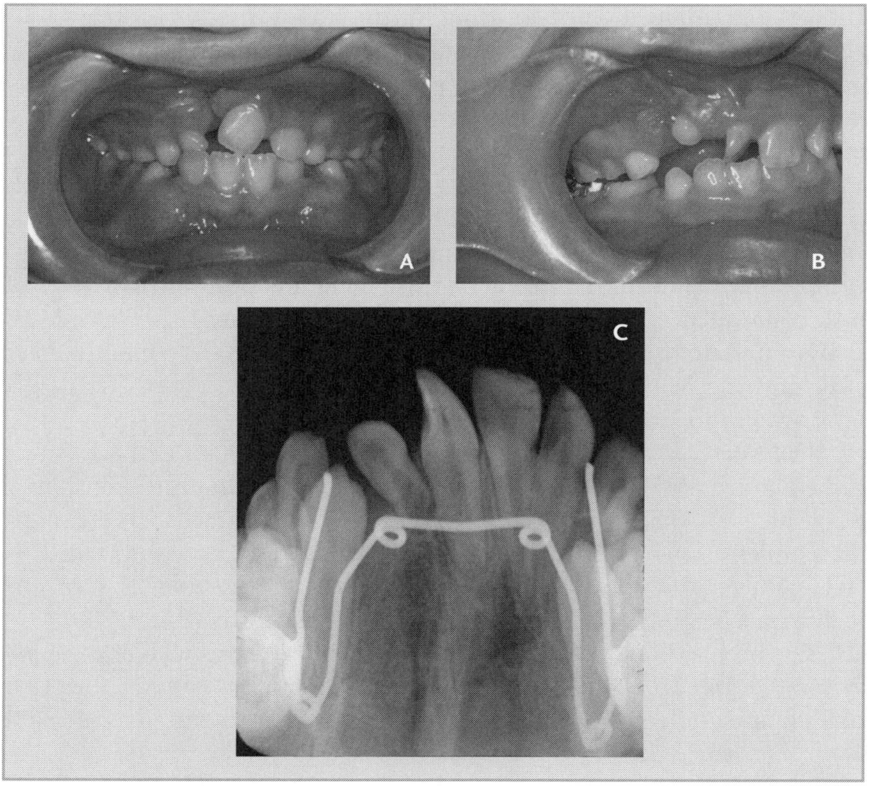


FIGURE 17.6. (A) Unilateral cleft alveolus with malocclusion and tooth malposition prior to grafting with particulate cancellous marrow autologous bone. (B) Six months after healing. Tooth is erupting into the grafted alveolar site. Note preservation of attached gingival on the labial surface of the alveolus. (C) Occlusal radiograph of erupting tooth. Although small and misshapen, it will serve as a functional tooth.

repair. The lateral facial flaps can be extended further toward the midline when compared to those in unilateral cleft repairs.

Closure of the oral-nasal fistula on the palatal side of the bilateral alveolar cleft presents some challenges, because it is difficult to visualize. Because most clefts are small in this area, it is difficult to provide nasal-sided closure. The palatal tissue on the premaxillary segment should also be preserved to minimize the possibility of devascularization of the premaxilla (see Figure 17.7).

In some situations, the premaxilla is malpositioned in relation to the posterior alveolus and dental segments. The malposition may be the result

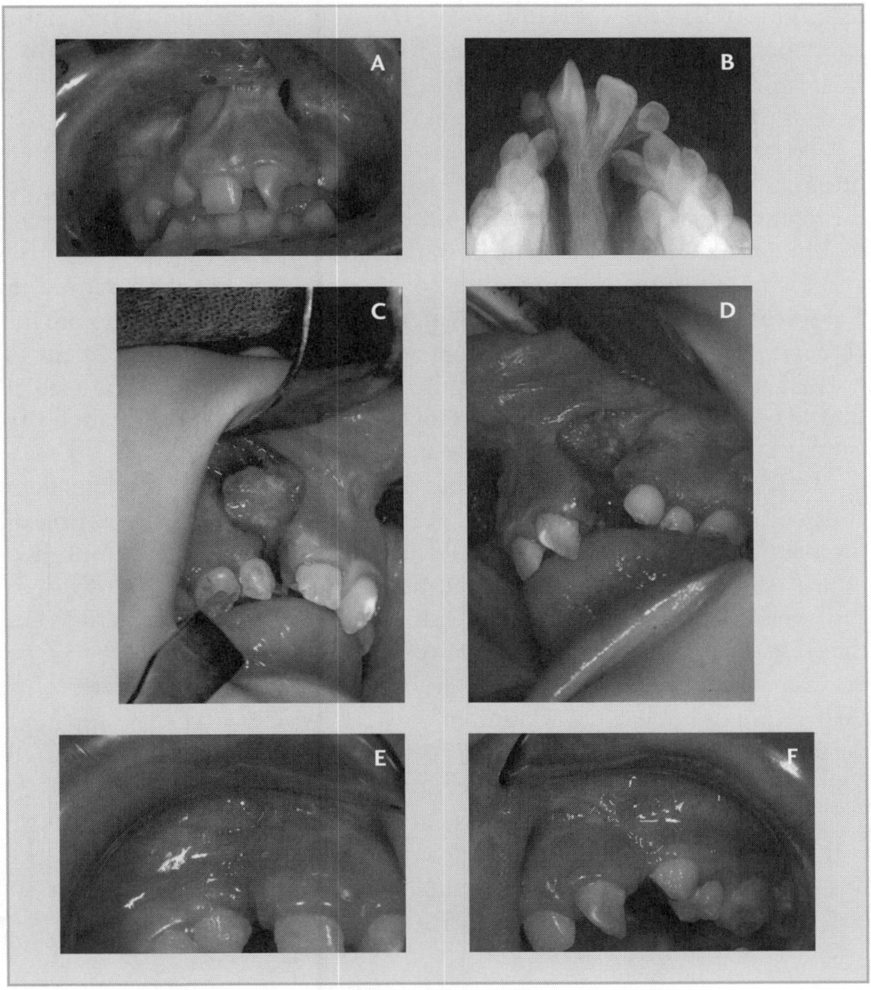


Figure 17.7. (A) Bilateral alveolar clefts. (B) Maxillary occlusal radiograph showing bilateral alveolar clefts. Note lack of bony continuity between premaxilla and both maxillary lateral segments. (C) Exposed alveolar cleft on right side. (D) Exposed alveolar cleft on left side. (E) Repaired right alveolus, approximately 3 months postoperatively. (F) Repaired left alveolus, approximately 3 months postoperatively.

of fibrosis in the vestibular area associated with the previous cleft lip and palate repairs. A decision must be made regarding the potential surgical repositioning of the premaxillary segment by the orthodontist and the surgeon. If it is necessary to reposition the premaxilla, a rigid fixation technique must be devised to stabilize the grafted segments. Orthodontic appliances, a surgical splint, or rigid fixation appliances may accomplish this. Failure to adequately stabilize may result in a very mobile premaxilla and failure of the grafting procedure.

Postoperatively, supportive care is provided. The patient is instructed not to create nasal or oral pressure that may force bacteria or debris into the graft. An elastic tape may be placed across the upper lip to prevent or limit hematoma. Overnight hospitalization is usual for pain control and for monitoring ambulation and oral intake. Sutures are removed in 2–3 weeks, if nonresorbable sutures are used. Postoperative home care includes chlorhexadine rinses, adequate oral hygiene, and advancement to normal activity as tolerated. If a stabilization splint or appliance is used, it should be maintained for at least 2 months, and possibly longer if mobility is suspected on postoperative follow-up.

Orthodontic tooth movement in the grafted area can be implemented approximately 3 months after the grafting procedure. Repositioning of the maxillary central and/or lateral incisors is most often accomplished to facilitate function, to prevent traumatic occlusion of the lower teeth to the upper teeth, and for appearance. If the maxilla has been expanded in the transverse dimension prior to surgery, a retainer or appliance may be necessary to maintain the expansion. Imaging may be used to determine ossification or bone consolidation of the graft, which will not be apparent for up to 6 months to 1 year after grafting. Teeth erupting into the grafted cleft will maintain alveolar bone vertically and horizontally.

An alveolar cleft grafting procedure and protocol as described above will result in alveolar continuity, closure of communication between the nose and the mouth, and eruption and function of the permanent maxillary dentition (Hynes & Earley, 2003).

## Orthognathic Surgery to Correct Facial Skeletal Dysmorphia Associated with Cleft Lip, Palate, and Alveolus

Individuals with congenital cleft lip, alveolus, and palate with the usual subsequent surgical treatment have a higher rate of midfacial or maxillary hypoplasia compared to those not affected by clefting (Posnick & Ricalde, 2004). The clinical presentation is skeletal malocclusion with Class III molar and canine relationships with reverse overjet or incisor crossbite (see Figure 17.8). The restriction of midfacial and maxillary anterior and inferior growth may be due to many factors, including a "bandeau" effect of a repaired cleft upper lip, a posterior tethering of the maxilla by a pharyngeal flap done to improve velopharyngeal closure for speech, a lack of development of anterior teeth and the maxillary alveolus, or a sequela of the congenital cleft phenomena. Approximately 30% of adolescent patients with clefts seen by the University of Minnesota Cleft Palate Team present with some degree of Class III skeletal malocclusion and would benefit from correction to establish optimal occlusion. This type of malocclusion is frequently associated with functional impairment, including speech articulation distortions and difficulty with effective mastication of food. There is also undesirable cosmetic appearance, resulting from a relative prognathism due to midfacial hypoplasia and normal mandibular projection.

There is debate as to when and how to determine if inherent facial growth is complete. Utilization of hand and wrist radiographic images to assess closure of epiphyseal plates to determine completion of growth is questionable. Serial sagittal radiographic images allow comparison of skeletal landmarks over time, but cannot determine, definitively, if growth of the maxilla or mandible is complete. Some clinicians believe that the correction of Class III skeletal malocclusions should be delayed until definitive completion of facial skeletal growth, because further growth, particularly of the mandible in the late teen years, can result in a recurrence or

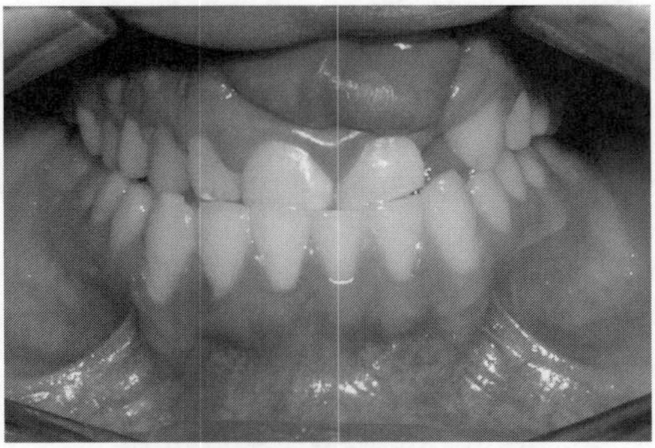

Figure 17.8. Residual Class III malocclusion after alveolar reconstruction with autogenous bone grafts. This individual will need orthodontics and orthognathic surgery for optimal functional correction.

relapse of the corrected malocclusion. Since it is impossible to determine via objective assessment when growth is absolutely complete, performing orthognathic surgery in the teen years is acceptable.

Waiting for eruption of all permanent teeth (with the exception of third molars) allows orthodontic management of the dental components of malocclusion. Although tooth eruption may be delayed in the individual with clefting, all permanent teeth are usually erupted in the early teen years. Orthodontic treatment goals at that time are leveling and aligning dental arches. Consideration must be given to the axial inclination of the anterior teeth with the mandibular plane and skull base to delineate if the malocclusion may be treated orthodontically only or both orthodontically and surgically. (See Chapter 16 for Williams and Bevis's descriptions of the goals of orthodontic intervention at various stages of growth and development.)

Again, the integrated team approach to management of the malocclusion must involve the orthodontist, the surgeon, and in many situations the restorative or prosthetic dentist. When one team member proceeds with a limited treatment, the result may be a retreatment that requires additional time, cost, and tolerance by the patient. Orthodontic-only correction of a Class III malocclusion in a patient with a cleft may result in compromised cosmetic and functional outcome.

Orthodontic leveling and alignment takes 12–24 months to complete in most cases. If the orthodontic therapy is initiated when all permanent teeth are erupted, the average patient with maxillary hypoplasia will be ready for correction at approximately 15–16 years.

Full facial evaluation, in frontal and lateral planes, must be performed to facilitate the decision regarding which surgical procedure should be employed. To determine the surgical procedure(s) that will have the most optimal outcome, the following should be assessed: the nasofrontal angle, nasal projection, infraorbital and zygomatic projection, nasolabial angle and upper lip prominence, tooth and gingivae exposed at rest and while smiling, and the magnitude of the reverse overjet.

An assessment of speech articulation and resonance characteristics must be done prior to any orthognathic surgery. Velopharyngeal function must be addressed because surgical anterior repositioning of components of the midface may contribute to velopharyngeal inadequacy (VPI), resulting in nasal air emission and excessive nasality. Although this complication occurs infrequently, it must be considered and explained to the patient and family (Chanchareonsook, Samman, & Whitehill, 2006). Close collaboration with the speech-language pathologist will help to minimize this complication. It is possible that a surgical procedure to correct induced VPI may be necessary following midface advancement (Janulewicz et al., 2004; Phillips, Klaiman, Delorey, & MacDonald, 2005).

The surgical treatment objective is then finalized with consideration of the patient's desires, the opinion of the other care providers, the clinical examination, and radiographic and photographic images. The magnitude of maxillary hypoplasia occurring in patients with clefting and subsequent repair tends to be greater than in individuals with hypoplasia without clefts. Sagittal hypoplasia greater than 1 cm is not unusual in persons with clefts. It is impossible to determine before surgery the amount of maxillary mobility and potential advancement that may be accomplished. Therefore, it is reasonable to plan maxillary advancement of various magnitudes and intervals, but also with a plan to surgically position the mandible posteriorly to make up the difference on the maxillary advancement and the reverse overjet (see Figure 17.9). Surgical splints with 5-mm intervals of movement are constructed so as to maximally advance the maxilla. After maxillary stabilization, the mandible may need to be posteriorly positioned utilizing a bilateral sagittal split ramus osteotomy with rigid fixation to achieve the best occlusion. This may result in a compromised surgical outcome when the lateral profile is considered, but this technique allows the surgery to be accomplished in one procedure.

When it is anticipated that anterior movement of the maxilla will be greater than 1 cm, consideration can be given to the use of distraction osteogenesis (DO) (Cheung, Chua, & Bendeus, 2004). This technique allows anterior maxillary repositioning over time, achieving surgical moves

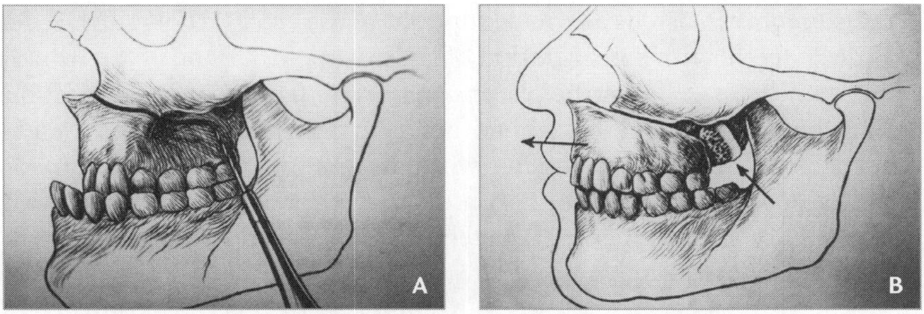


Figure 17.9. (A) Schematic drawing showing cutting the lateral maxillary bone with a surgical drill. Notice the maxilla in a retruded position as related to the mandible. (B) Schematic drawing showing advancing the maxilla into the desired occlusion and placing bone graft between the posterior maxillary surfacial and the pterogoid plate (marked by posterior arrow).

of greater than 2 cm. DO fixation hardware can be applied to the midface from a completely transoral approach or by the use of a head frame attached to the cranium as seen in the series of photographs in Figure 17.10 of a patient who underwent a distraction approach. The disadvantages of DO include a longer treatment time; somewhat unsightly and stigmatizing external hardware if the cranial head frame is used; and difficulty controlling the vectors of movement of the maxilla, which can result in residual malocclusion. This malocclusion may be corrected with a mandibular setback procedure after consolidation of the maxillary surgery and orthodontic preparation for mandibular surgery.

The conventional surgical approach to correcting the maxillary hypoplasia associated with cleft lip, palate, and alveolus utilizes a Le Fort I technique in which the osteotomy cuts are made closer to the orbits than with conventional Le Fort I. Ocular complications including blindness have been associated with maxillary osteotomy in patients with repaired clefts. A horizontal incision superior to the mucogingival junction is made for access to the piriform aperture and anterior maxillary wall. Some clinicians utilize limited incisions with vertical components to maintain a vascular pedicle to the maxilla. Dissection is challenging due to scarring from prior surgical lip, alveolar, and palate repair. The piriform aperture is asymmetric, extending inferiorly and laterally on the cleft side compared to the unaffected side. Separation of the nasal mucosa from the nasal floor is also a challenge on the side of the cleft due to the cleft and subsequent repair. Sharp dissection of the nasal mucosa from the nasal floor is often employed. The technique for bilateral clefting is comparable to unilateral clefts when performing orthognathic surgery. (See Figure 17.11 for photographs taken before and after maxillary advancement.)

Osteotomy incisions are made superior to the apices (root ends) of the maxillary teeth, with consideration of the thickness of bone of the frontal process of the maxilla for the placement of rigid fixation for stabilization after repositioning. The horizontal anterior maxillary osteotomy is extended as far superiorly as possible without impinging on the infraorbital nerve to augment the infraorbital projection that will be obtained with the maxillary advancement. The lateral nasal walls and nasal septum are separated from the caudal maxilla.

After the Le Fort I osteotomies are complete, the maxilla is downfractured. This is facilitated by inserting spreader instruments in the anterior osteotomies in the area of the piriform aperture. Because of the previous posterior soft tissue palate repair, there is fibrosis in the posterior aspect of

(*Text continues on page 594*)

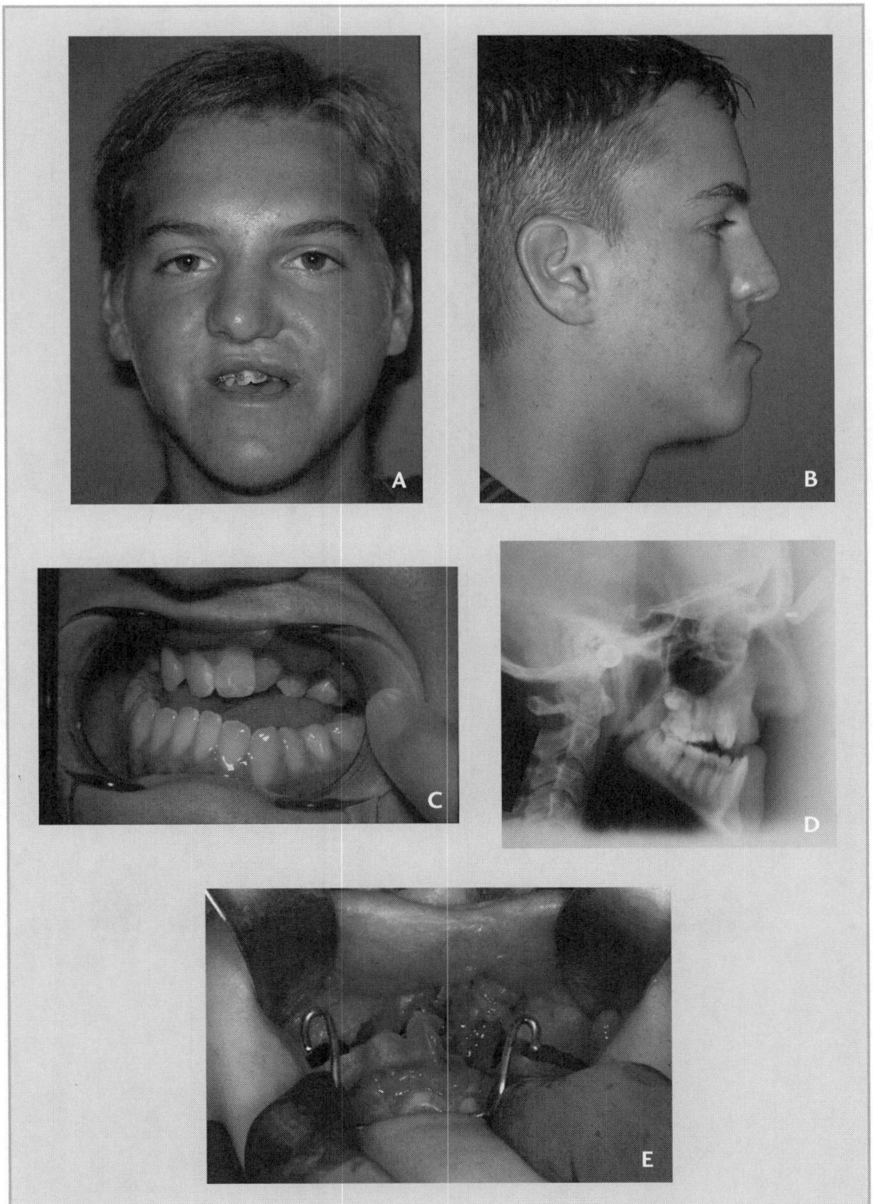


Figure 17.10. (A) Patient with repaired primary and secondary clefts with severe malocclusion (full face). (B) Profile view. (C) Malocclusion. (D) Lateral preoperative cephalogram. (E) LeFort I osteotomy with distraction appliance in place.

(*continues*)

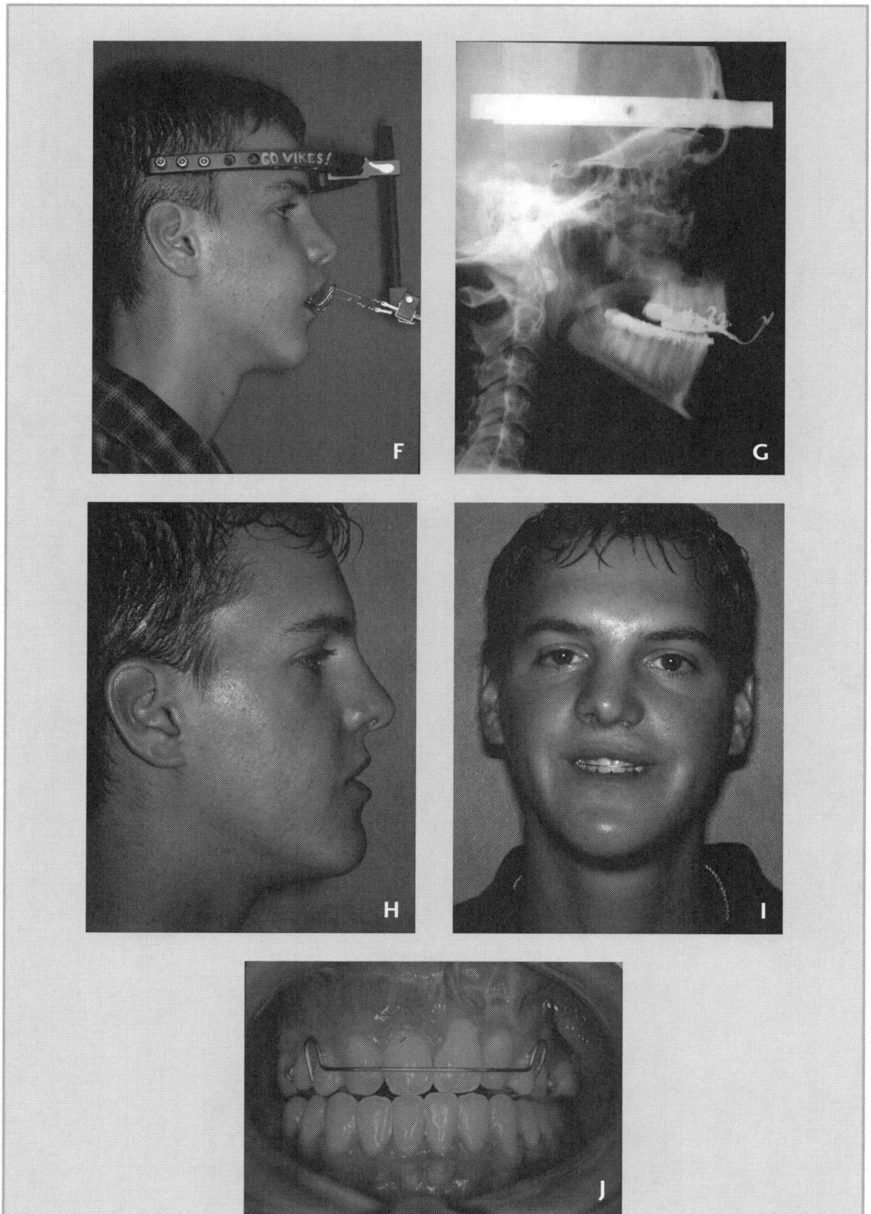


FIGURE 17.10. (*continued*) (F) Profile view with external distractor in place. (G) Lateral cephalogram after distraction. (H) Profile view after distraction. (I) Full face view after distraction. (J) Final dental occlusion.

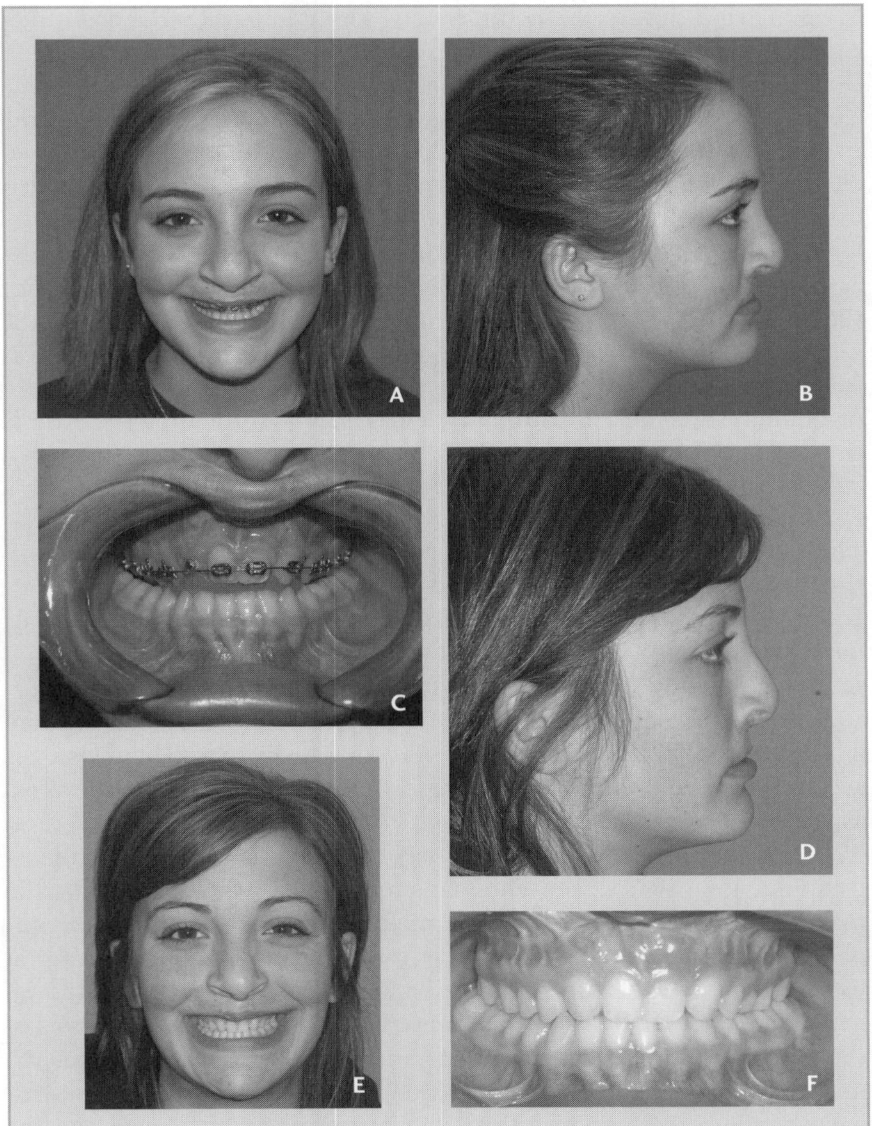


Figure 17.11. (A) Patient after bilateral cleft repair, after orthodontic preparation for orthognathic surgery to treat severe Class III malocclusion. Note the anterior open bite. (B) Profile view, showing the upper jaw is behind the lower jaw. Advancing the upper jaw will treat the malocclusion. (C) This malocclusion makes it difficult to chew and speak because the teeth do not meet. (D) Postsurgical profile after maxillary advancement. (D) Postsurgical profile after maxillary advancement. (E) Postsurgical full face view. (F) Final dental occlusion.

the maxilla in the area of the tuberosity. This complicates the downfracture compared to the Le Fort I technique utilized in the noncleft patient.

The maxilla is then mobilized using disimpaction forceps. Extreme care must be taken with the forceps, as unintentional fractures of the maxillary alveolus are possible. Once the maxilla is mobilized, the occlusal splint is applied to the maxilla, and the maxilla is positioned anteriorly. If the maxillary teeth can be made to interdigitate with the mandibular teeth, maxillomandibular fixation (MMF) is applied. If the maxilla cannot be repositioned into the splint, it can be further mobilized with the disimpaction forceps. Instruments may also be inserted between the maxillary tuberosities and the pterygoid plates posteriorly to provide anterior traction to the maxilla. A wire may be placed around the maxillary orthodontic appliance or through the nasal spine (providing the bone is thick enough) to provide additional anterior traction. Once positioned into the splint, MMF is applied.

In most cases, the maxillary movement will be anterior and inferior. There are few, if any, bone interferences with moves in these directions. Rigid fixation plating is then applied in the piriform aperture area, bilaterally. In many situations, additional bone plates are applied in the zygomatic buttress region, posteriorly. It is important to use bone plates and screws that solidly engage the bone to prevent relapse.

After stabilization, MMF is removed. The dental occlusion is checked and rechecked. If the interdigitation of teeth is easily repeatable, closure is accomplished with nasal alar base repositioning and closure of the labial aspect of the upper lip.

With the utilization of distraction osteogenesis (DO), the surgical technique is similar to conventional surgery (Le Fort I) except that the maxilla is not repositioned at the time of surgery. DO stabilization appliances are placed on the maxillary teeth and the cranium (extraoral technique) or on the superior maxilla and bilateral zygomas (intraoral technique). The maxilla is then advanced at 1 mm per day. The vectors of the movement are more easily altered with the external device. Once the maxilla is advanced to the final position, it is left for a period of time for consolidation, or alternative final stabilization is accomplished and the device is removed (Kumar et al., 2006).

Postsurgical supportive care is comparable to that for patients without clefts undergoing Le Fort I osteotomy. The patient is instructed not to create nasal or oral pressure that may force bacteria or debris into the graft. An elastic tape may be placed across the upper lip to prevent or limit hematoma. Overnight hospitalization is usual for pain control and for monitoring ambulation and oral intake. Sutures are removed in 2–3 weeks, if nonresorbable sutures are used. Postoperative home care includes chlorhexadine rinses, adequate oral hygiene, and advancement to normal activity as tolerated.

Orthodontic treatment may be continued approximately 6 weeks following maxillary advancement. Because of greater relapse potential due to the posterior scarring of the maxilla secondary to previous cleft palate repair or pharyngeal flap, the postoperative occlusion must be closely monitored. If surgical or orthodontic relapse occurs, mandibular osteotomy with posterior repositioning is the procedure of choice to achieve the best possible outcome.

Any cosmetic or functional reconstructive surgical procedures to correct lip and especially nasal deformities in the cleft patient should be delayed until completion of orthognathic surgical procedures. Procedures performed to the nose or lip prior to the establishment of a stable facial skeletal base may not be advisable, as the outcome may be altered following maxillary and/or mandibular repositioning. To facilitate the best possible outcome, there must be frequent communication and collaboration between the oral and maxillofacial surgeon and the surgeon providing the facial plastic and reconstructive surgical procedures to the lip and nose. See Chapter 14 by Buckley and Landis for further discussion about timing issues in planning final nasal reconstruction.

## Dental Implant Placement to Replace Missing Teeth Associated with Clefting

Final dental reconstruction for the cleft patient may be accomplished after skeletal maturity and establishment of the optimum dental occlusion by orthodontics and/or orthognathic surgery (Takahashi et al., 1997). Treatment options available for dental reconstruction include conventional prosthodontics, such as fixed partial dentures (dental bridges), resin-bonded dental restorations, removable partial dentures, veneers, and tooth replacement with dental implants. The restorative dentist or prosthodontist managing the patient must be actively involved in planning treatment for this phase of the reconstruction. See Chapter 18 by

Leeper, Charles, and Sills for detailed discussion of the prosthodontic treatment for persons with cleft lip and palate.

If there has been failure of tooth development in the cleft site (hypodontia), or if the tooth that has erupted into the grafted cleft alveolus is diminutive, hypoplastic, dysmorphic, or otherwise nonrestorable, replacement consideration is most frequently given to dental implants and subsequent restoration with a dental crown. Dental implant reconstruction allows tooth replacement without altering the shape, form, or structure of adjacent teeth. If a tooth adjacent to the missing tooth is also hypoplastic, dysmorphic, diminutive, or periodontally unstable, it may not be able to serve as a satisfactory abutment for dental bridging. Evaluation of the adjacent dentition must be made to determine the potential success of a conventional dental restoration technique.

If a space is maintained or created orthodontically for a missing tooth or teeth, over time there may be atrophy of the alveolus in the area of the cleft. If the alveolus is grafted at an early age to allow tooth eruption, and the tooth is subsequently lost, alveolar atrophy is an expectation (Fukada, Takahashi, & Iino, 2003).

Final dental restoration is delayed until age 18 or later, as it is more likely that skeletal maturity has been achieved. Because an implant performs comparable to a tooth that is ankylosed (fixated in bone), subsequent active or passive tooth eruption or vertical alveolar growth will cause a relative retrusion of the implant-supported replacement tooth, resulting in a short tooth adjacent to longer teeth.

If there is insufficient bone to support an implant in the site of the missing tooth, conventional dental prosthodontic treatment may be considered. However, if implants are desired in the presence of atrophy of the alveolar bone, additional bone grafting can be performed to augment the edentulous site to allow accommodation for an implant.

The alveolar augmentation can be accomplished with a cortical bone graft in an outpatient clinical setting. This procedure may be provided with the use of moderate or deep sedation if desired. The graft can be harvested from either the symphysis or the ramus area of the mandible. A graft of $1 \times 1.5$ cm will usually suffice. The atrophic alveolus is augmented horizontally. The site may be prepared by creating a box form to mortise (stabilize) the graft into the recipient site to provide for enhanced stability. The graft is secured into position with at least two bone screws. Rigid fixation and stability is crucial. After placement, the edges of the graft must be smoothed. The covering gingival/mucosal flap must be released and extended with undermining and periosteal release to prevent dehiscence of the wound. This graft should be allowed to heal for 3 months prior to implant placement.

After the graft has healed, the surgical site is re-evaluated and an implant system is selected. The surgical approach allows exposure of the grafted alveolus. The fixation screws are removed. The implant osteotomy is performed with rotary instrumentation. Care must be taken with osteotomes for site preparation, as overzealous use may result in fracture and separation of the block graft. The implant of desired size and width is inserted. Depending on insertion torque, occlusion, implant size, and site, the implant may be left exposed (one stage) or be provisionally restored. This decision should be made by the restorative dentist or prosthodontist, who should determine the implant stability necessary for the prosthodontic technique employed. After implant integration, the final restoration is fabricated and placed. Figure 17.12 shows the sequence of the implantation approach for a missing lateral incisor.

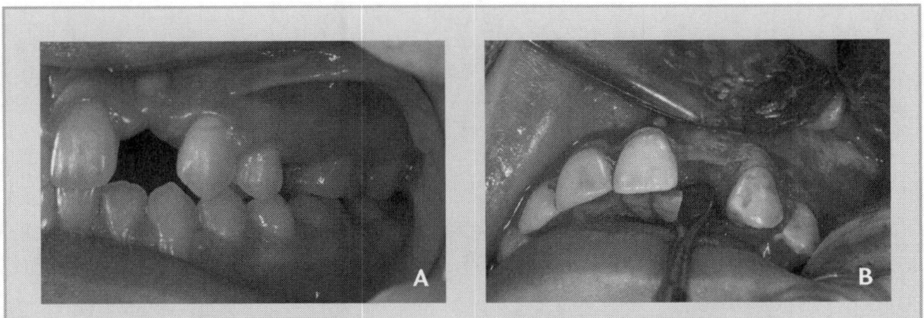


Figure 17.12. (A) Preoperative spacing and missing tooth due to clefting. (B) Surgical exposure of the implant site. Notice the absence of bone. (C) Bone graft is placed and stabilized with screws. (D) The crown is fixed to the implant.

(*continues*)

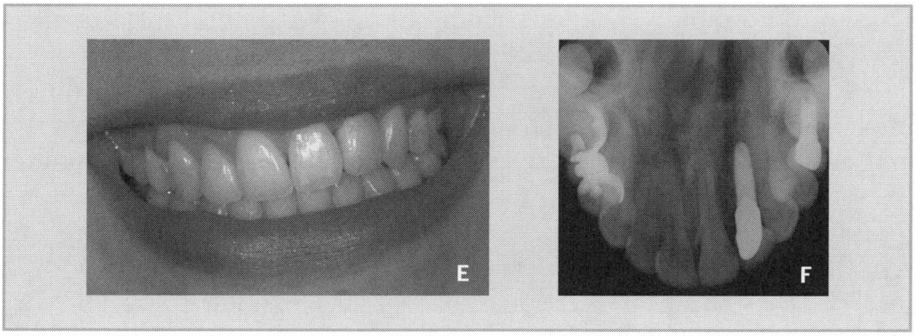


FIGURE 17.12. (*continued*) (E) When this person smiles, it is difficult to tell which tooth is supported by an implant. (F) Final radiograph shows the implant next to natural teeth.

## Other Adjunct Procedures

Some additional surgical procedures may be necessary for complete reconstruction. They include the possibility of gingival grafting on the facial surfaces of teeth or in the area of implants, to provide optimal periodontal support for teeth in the area of the cleft. In addition, if there is limited lip mobility due to fibrosis of the upper lip and absence of a labial vestibule for the same reason, a vestibuloplasty to deepen the sulcus can be performed utilizing tissue grafts. The upper lip may be lengthened with mucosal transposition flaps. Areas around implants or prosthodontic reconstructions can be augmented with connective tissue grafts to facilitate cosmetic outcome.

## Conclusion

The oral and maxillofacial surgeon provides surgical procedures for individuals with congenital cleft lip, palate, and alveolus. The procedures may be provided from a very young age to skeletal maturity and beyond. Key features of successful surgical outcomes are critically dependent on frequent and regular interdisciplinary team evaluations and thoughtful, frequent collaboration by health care providers. With this type of treatment approach, orofacial defects due to congenital clefting can be successfully repaired with minimal sequelae and few of the stigmata traditionally associated with clefts and the subsequent surgical repair.

## References

Bitter, K. (2001). Repair of bilateral cleft lip, alveolus and palate: Part 3. Follow-up criteria and late results. *Journal of Craniofacial Surgery, 29,* 49–55.

Chanchareonsook, N., Samman, N., & Whitehill, T. L. (2006). The effect of craniomaxillofacial osteotomies and distraction osteogenesis on speech and velopharyngeal status: A critical review. *Cleft Palate-Craniofacial Journal, 43,* 477–487.

Cheung, L. K., Chua, H. D., & Bendeus, M. (2004). Distraction or osteotomy for the correction of maxillary cleft deformities: Which is better? *Annals of Australian College of Dental Surgery, 17,* 57–63.

Chin, M., Ng, T., Tom, W. K., & Carstens, M. (2005). Repair of alveolar clefts with recombinant human bone morphogenetic protein (rhBMP-2) in patients with clefts. *Journal of Craniofacial Surgery, 16,* 778–789.

El Deeb, M. E., Messer, L. B., Lehnert, M. W., Hebda, T. W., & Waite, D. E. (1982). Canine eruption into grafted bone in maxillary alveolar cleft defects. *Cleft Palate Journal, 19,* 9–16.

Fukada, M., Takahashi, T., & Iino, M. (2003). Dento-alveolar reconstruction of a missing premaxilla using bone graft and endosteal implants. *Journal of Oral Rehabilitation, 30,* 87–90.

Grayson, B. H., & Maull, D. (2004). Nasoalveolar molding for infants born with clefts of the lip, alveolus, and palate. *Clinics in Plastic Surgery, 31,* 149–158.

Hynes, P. J., & Earley, M. J. (2003). Assessment of secondary alveolar bone grafting using a modification of the Bergland grading system. *British Journal of Plastic Surgery, 56,* 630–636.

Janulewicz, J., Costello, B. J., Buckley, M. J., Ford, M. D., Close, J., & Gassner, R. (2004). The effects of Le Fort I osteotomies on velopharyngeal and speech functions in cleft patients. *Journal of Oral and Maxillofacial Surgery, 62,* 308–314.

Kumar, A., Gabbay, J. S., Nikjoo, R., Heller, J. B., O'Hara, C. M., Sisodia, M., et al. (2006). Improved outcomes in cleft patients with severe maxillary deficiency after LeFort I internal distraction. *Plastic and Reconstructive Surgery, 15,* 1499–1509.

Li, Y., Shi, B., Song, O. G., Zuo, H., & Zheng, O. (2006). Effects of lip repair on maxillary growth and facial soft tissue development in patients with a complete unilateral cleft of lip, alveolus and palate. *Journal of Craniomaxillofacial Surgery, 34,* 355–361.

Liao, Y. F., & Mars, M. (2005). Long-term effects of lip repair on dentofacial morphology in patients with unilateral cleft lip and palate. *Cleft Palate-Craniofacial Journal, 42,* 526-532.

Phillips, J. H., Klaiman, P., Delorey, R., & MacDonald, D. B. (2005). Predictors of velopharyngeal insufficiency in cleft palate orthognathic surgery. *Plastic and Reconstructive Surgery, 115,* 681–686.

Posnick, J. C., & Ricalde, P. (2004). Cleft-orthognathic surgery. *Clinics in Plastic Surgery, 31,* 315–330.

Renkielska, A., Wojtaszek-Slominska, A., & Dobke, M. (2005). Early cleft lip repair in children with unilateral complete cleft lip and palate: A case against primary alveolar repair. *Annals of Plastic Surgery, 54,* 595–597.

Rosenstein, S. W., Grasseschi, M., & Dado, D. V. (2003). A long-term retrospective outcome assessment of facial growth, secondary surgical need, and maxillary lateral incisor status in a surgical-orthodontic protocol for complete clefts. *Plastic and Reconstructive Surgery, 111,* 1–13.

Savaci, N., Hosnuter, M., Tosun, Z., & Demir, A. (2005). Maxillofacial morphology in children with complete unilateral cleft lip and palate treated by one-stage simultaneous repair. *Plastic and Reconstructive Surgery, 115,* 1509–1517.

Scheuer, H. A., Holtje, W. J., Hasund, A., & Pfeifer, G. (2001). Prognosis of facial growth in patients with unilateral complete clefts of the lip, alveolus and palate. *Journal of Craniomaxillofacial Surgery, 29,* 198–204.

Shetye, P. R. (2004). Facial growth of adults with unoperated clefts. *Clinics in Plastic Surgery, 31,* 361–371.

Takahashi, T., Fukuda, M., Yamaguchi, T., Kochi, S., Inai, T., Watanabe, M., et al. (1997). Use of an osseointegrated implant for dental rehabilitation after cleft repair by periosteoplasty: A case report. *Cleft Palate-Craniofacial Journal, 34,* 268–271.

Troxell, J. B., Fonseca, R., & Osbon, D. B. (1982). A retrospective study of alveolar cleft regrafting. *Journal of Oral and Maxillofacial Surgery, 40,* 721–725.

Waite, D. E., & Kersten, R. B. (1980). Residual alveolar and palatal clefts. In W. H. Bell, W. R. Proffit, & R. P. White (Eds.), *Surgical correction of dentofacial deformities* (Vol. 2). Philadelphia: Saunders.

# CHAPTER 18

# Prosthodontic Management of Maxillofacial and Palatal Defects

*Herbert A. Leeper, Jr., David H. Charles, and Paul S. Sills*

Leeper, Charles, and Sills discuss prosthodontic issues and procedures applicable not only to persons with cleft lip and palate, but to individuals with other oral problems as well. They define the discipline of prosthodontic dentistry, state the training involved to become this type of specialist, and espouse the opportunities for cooperative efforts between speech-language pathologists and prosthodontists. They list several oral and patient factors that influence prosthesis design and detail a physiological systems approach to assessment and management. Finally, the authors focus on specific oral problems and their clinical management.

1. What do the authors mean by the dual role of the "prosthetic speech appliance"?
2. The authors emphasize the importance of prosthodontists and speech-language pathologists working together. Describe a clinical situation in which cooperative efforts between the speech-language pathologist and prosthodontist would be ideal.
3. What do the authors mean by a physiological assessment of the speech-producing mechanism? How can this be helpful in determining a management strategy?
4. In the authors' focus on evaluation of velopharyngeal function, they describe a multidimensional approach. What dimension is readily available to the speech clinician in any work setting?
5. What are some of the existing dental hazards to articulation? Anterior appliances? What is known about speakers' adaptations to oral-facial defects and to speech prostheses?
6. What are some conditions in which prosthodontic treatment rather than surgical treatment might be indicated for soft palate defects?

7. Describe what is meant by a prosthesis reduction program. Describe the procedures typically used.

Many disorders of speech are associated with maxillofacial defects, particularly those involving maxillary and palatal regions. Etiologies of these defects can generally be classified as developmental, such as in cleft lip and palate, or acquired, due to oral cancer, neurologic disease, or structural injury. Regardless of the cause, the presence of the defect may influence speech by changing the resonance properties of the vocal tract through the inappropriate coupling of the nasal cavity or by changing the capacity to impound, direct, or constrict the vibrated flow of air for articulation.

Mastication, deglutition, and speech can be improved through the close technical interaction and cooperation between the disciplines of speech-language pathology and prosthodontics (Kuehn & Moller, 2000; McGrath & Anderson, 1990; Wolfaardt, Wilson, Rochet, & McPhee, 1993). Prosthodontics is a branch of dentistry concerned with restoration and maintenance of oral function, comfort, appearance, and health of the patient, including restoring natural teeth and replacing missing teeth. A prosthodontist is a dental specialist with advanced training in prosthetic dentistry. Specialty training in prosthodontics generally consists of a 2- or 3-year postgraduate university-based education. Maxillofacial prosthodontics is a subdivision of this specialty that covers the restorative rehabilitation of patients with extensive oral-facial deformities. A maxillofacial prosthodontist requires an additional 1–2 years of study, usually acquired in a hospital-based setting. Because of the nature of palatal defects, the planning and fabrication of prosthetic speech appliances usually requires more specialized clinical training and skill than is needed for routine removable partial dentures.

This chapter focuses on the general treatment considerations for individuals with cleft palate and craniofacial anomalies, including select factors that influence the speech prosthesis design. We have included management guidelines for patients with hard palate defects, soft palate defects, and velopharyngeal dysfunction. Although the focus of the chapter is on defects that are common to the cleft palate condition, other congenital and acquired conditions affecting these structures and functions are discussed.

# The Prosthetic Speech Appliance

The phrase "prosthetic speech appliance" refers to a hybrid dental device that serves a dual role in replacing oral structures, usually teeth and supporting mucosa, while assisting in speech rehabilitation. A pure speech appliance, such as a palatal lift, fulfills no dental replacement function. Both appliances share components in common with removable dentures. A removable denture replaces both dental and oral tissues and may be inserted or removed from the mouth by the patient. Removable dentures may be partial, replacing some missing teeth, or complete, replacing all of the teeth. Acceptable removable partial dentures must be secured in the mouth and resist movement under normal oral functions. To achieve this stability, partial denture clasps encircle selected abutment teeth to resist forces that dislodge the denture. Supporting elements, called rests and bases, resist forces directed toward the teeth and underlying soft tissues. Vertically oriented denture components, called bracing elements, resist laterally directed forces (McGivney & Carr, 2000). (See Figure 18.1.)

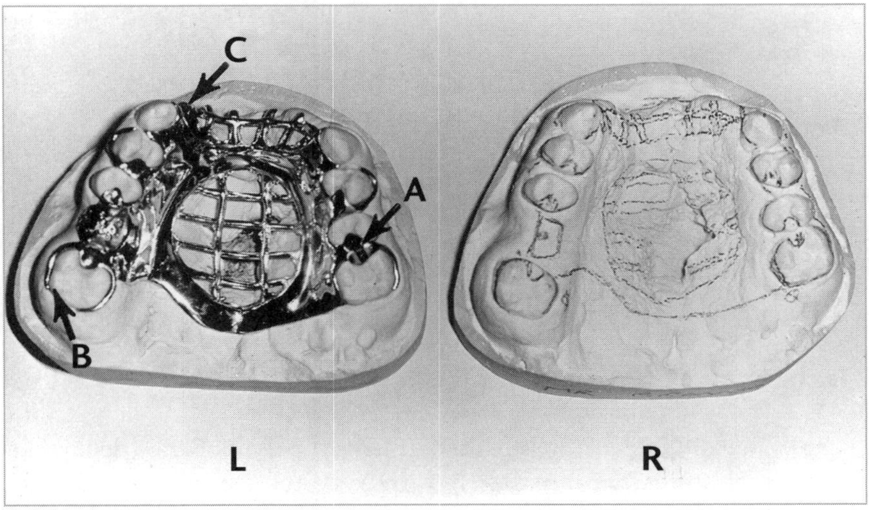


FIGURE 18.1. Left: Maxillary cast metal partial denture framework on a master model illustrating (A) supporting elements, (B) clasping elements, and (C) bracing elements. Right: Diagnostic model showing proposed framework design.

Effective prosthetic speech appliances incorporate these basic features of partial denture design. A maxillary prosthetic speech appliance commonly consists of a palatal base structure to which other components connect. The size, location, and nature of the palatal defect determine the type of component attaching to the base. For cleft defects limited to the hard palate, an obturator usually forms part of the base of the prosthesis. The term *obturator* is used in this chapter to suggest complete or partial obturation of an opening. However, posteriorly located defects involving the soft palate, due to clefts or other sources of velopharyngeal inadequacy, require a posterior "tail" section added to the maxillary base. This extension supports either an obturator in the nasopharyngeal space to compensate for short soft palate length or a palatal lift, which elevates soft palate tissue to compensate for lack of soft palate mobility range or timing. Thus, the location and type of palatal defect directly influences the eventual form or design of the prosthetic speech appliance. For openings of the hard palate (e.g., as a result of palatal surgical excision or palatal fistulae following cleft palate repair), complete obturation is required. For velopharyngeal closure problems, partial obturation of the velopharyngeal space is required, and this pharyngeal section has commonly been called a *speech bulb.*

## Factors Influencing Prosthetic Therapy for Maxillary Defects

Several factors influence the design of the prosthetic speech appliance and the treatment outcome. These can be divided into oral factors and patient factors.

### Oral Factors

A major factor influencing prosthetic therapy is the patient's dental status. Dental status encompasses a variety of tooth-related conditions. These conditions act alone or together to affect prosthesis design. Healthy mouths pose few problems for construction of prosthetic speech appliances, whereas mouths in poor health complicate therapy and threaten the prognosis for successful treatment. The types of dental conditions and the influence they exert on a prosthetic speech appliance design are described briefly.

## Number and Location of Existing Teeth

For completely dentate patients, multiple tooth surfaces offer a wide range of possible locations for retentive and supporting elements, generally simplifying the speech appliance design. Partially dentate conditions increase the complexity of appliance design and retention, especially when many teeth are missing. Entirely tooth-supported designs generally exhibit greater stability than do those that rely on support from both teeth and underlying mucosa of the palate and edentulous alveolar ridges. Artificial teeth are included in all partially edentulous designs, thus improving appearance as well as function.

At times, the original location of the teeth may be unsuitable for function or aesthetics. In many cases, orthodontic treatment adjusts tooth position and arch alignment to facilitate prosthesis construction (Chierici, 1979; Shiere, Fox, & Perry, 1962). When tooth malposition precludes conventional removable partial denture therapy, partial or complete overdentures may provide an effective treatment option. An overdenture is a hybrid removable prosthesis, which covers some or all of the remaining teeth and shares features common to both complete and partial dentures. Overdentures allow greater flexibility for artificial tooth placement for both function and aesthetics.

When all of the teeth are missing, a modified complete denture may serve as a speech prosthesis. In these situations, the retention of the complete denture may be poor due to an inadequate retentive seal about the peripheral tissues. Denture adhesives may provide the only means for adequate prosthesis retention.

## Condition of Existing Dentition

Existing teeth must be free of cavities or restored to an acceptable contour prior to instituting prosthetic therapy. Routine alloy and composite restorations are frequently sufficient for treating cavities. However, if large tooth defects require significant repair, full crown coverage must often be employed.

## Occlusal Relationships

Occlusal relationships refer to the manner in which the opposing teeth intercuspate or mesh. Close intercuspation may prevent ideal placement of rests and clasp units.

### Periodontal or Gum Conditions

The periodontium consists of the ligamentous tissue attaching teeth to bone and the mucosa surrounding the teeth. Periodontal disease attacks the tooth-bone attachment and, in its most destructive form, causes tooth loss. Mouths severely affected by this disease may exhibit teeth that are unstable and therefore unsuitable for prosthesis support or retention. In such cases, the prosthesis design must be modified to avoid overstressing periodontally compromised teeth.

### Oral Hygiene

All removable prostheses attract dental plaque that places teeth and gums at greater risk for cavities and gum disease. This risk increases dramatically with xerostomia or dry mouth. Dry mouth may be drug or radiation induced, occur as a result of pathosis (e.g., Sjogren's syndrome), or result from surgical removal of the salivary glands. Individuals wearing removable prostheses must maintain effective plaque control to ensure a favorable prognosis. Patients with xerostomia usually require additional preventive measures, including topical fluoride applications to reduce the risk of tooth decay.

## Patient Factors

Patient factors also play an important role in the design of the prosthetic speech appliance and in the treatment outcome. Age and health are particularly important factors.

### Age

Transitional types of prostheses best serve young patients who require speech appliances but who have incompletely developed oral structures. Transitional prostheses differ from permanent designs in that the base is made of acrylic resin instead of cast metal. Acrylic bases lack the strength and long-term stability of the metal casting, but can be modified easily to accommodate the patient's oral growth and cost less if replacement becomes necessary.

### Health

Patients with various disabling conditions or cognitive delays require careful evaluation to determine their capacity to insert and remove the prosthetic speech appliance. Some individuals may require assistance with routine oral hygiene procedures such as tooth brushing and flossing to prevent the loss of teeth to gum disease or decay.

# Team Approach to Defect Management

## Interdisciplinary Therapeutic Concepts

Decisions about the prosthetic management of individuals with maxillofacial defects are complex and must be made in the best interests of each patient. Planning the sequence of treatment, the timing of treatment revisions, and the projected outcomes requires the collaborative opinions of the team prosthodontist, orthodontist, oral and maxillofacial surgeon, dentist, and speech-language pathologist (Bohle et al., 2005; Kuehn & Moller, 2000).

In many situations, the prosthodontist and the speech-language pathologist work together to establish the need for a temporary or permanent prosthesis for speech purposes. The prosthodontist is responsible for deciding how to achieve optimal dental-occlusal relationships of the prosthesis for aesthetics and mastication and must also consider replacing missing teeth in either a fixed or removable form. When a prosthetic speech appliance is created to improve speech production, the prosthodontist should design it in collaboration with the speech-language pathologist. The two professionals often coevaluate the patient to ensure that the prosthesis design for the maxillary-alveolar region will not adversely affect speech sound production. Similarly, using visual images of the velopharyngeal port via nasendoscopy, measures of nasal air escape, and perceptual judgments of nasal resonance, the speech-language pathologist may advise the prosthodontist to increase the size of the obturator (speech bulb) or add vertical height or posterior extension to a palatal lift to improve resonance balance for patients with soft palate defects. (In Chapter 12, Glaze discusses the use of flexible nasendoscopy to further guide the prosthodontist in speech prosthesis fit to achieve optimal velopharyngeal closure.) This professional collaboration between the prosthodontist and speech-language pathologist arises from mutual respect for interdisciplinary contributions, as well as shared professional information about the basic anatomical, physiological, and aesthetic information about the oral-pharyngeal mechanism. (See Chapter 1, where Moller describes characteristics of effective interdisciplinary team members.) Professionals working together use common vocabularies and can exchange information easily, thus improving patient management. This interdisciplinary process also provides an excellent training model for young preprofessionals who view the interaction during teaching rounds (Sharry, 1976).

## Initial Prosthodontic Assessment

At the initial meeting with the patient, the prosthodontist must conduct a thorough examination of the hard and soft tissues, supported by appropriate radiographs. This diagnostic evidence provides information needed to determine dental factors affecting the prosthetic treatment plan and prognosis. At this appointment, preliminary impressions may be made of both jaws. Plaster diagnostic models are recovered from the impressions (see Figure 18.2). The models are then mounted on a dental articulator. Mounted models permit a clear view of tooth relationships, which is a necessary preliminary step in designing the prosthesis. In addition, the prosthodontist studies the maxillary model to choose the optimal location for prosthesis components.

## Prosthetic Clinical Procedures

Once the patient has accepted the treatment plan, a series of dental procedures must be accomplished to fabricate the prosthetic speech appliance. These procedures are needed to construct a permanent metal framework, which is the basis for most types of removable prosthetic speech appliances (see McGivney & Carr, 2000, for detailed procedures). Other clinical procedures needed to treat select palatal defects are discussed later.

1. Teeth are prepared by reshaping their surfaces as necessary to accommodate the design of the partial denture base.
2. Full arch impressions are made of the prepared teeth and soft tissues. Existing palatal clefts must be temporarily occluded to prevent impression material from flowing into the defect (Figure 18.2A).
3. A master model (cast) made from the impression serves as a base on which the metal framework is constructed (Figure 18.2B).
4. The fit of the metal framework (Figure 18.2C) must be verified in the mouth. Minor adjustments of the framework are usually

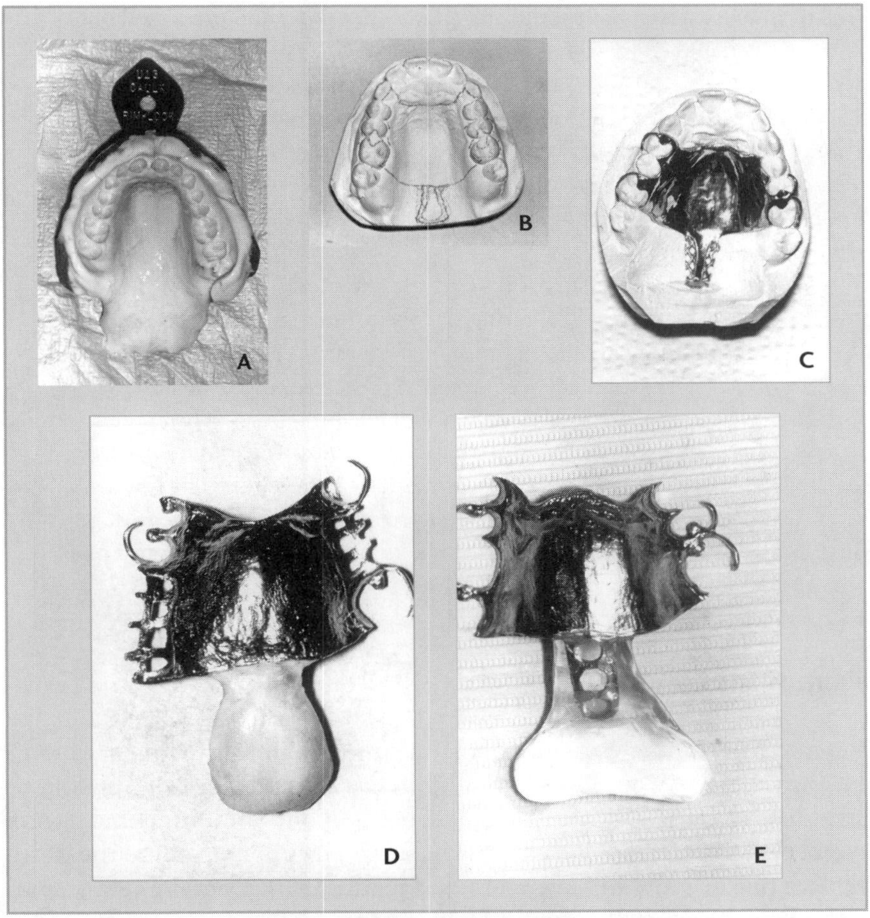


FIGURE 18.2. Dental procedures for fabrication of prosthetic speech appliances from a variety of patients: (A) full arch impression, (B) diagnostic model, (C) metal framework on master cast, (D) wax technique for functional impression of palatal tissue, and (E) posterior section in permanent acrylic resin as a completed speech prosthesis.

needed to ensure optimal fit. Once fitted, temporary acrylic resin is adapted to that portion of the metal framework associated with the defect. The acrylic resin forms a base to which other impression materials can be added to capture the anatomical form of the defect. The defect impression is converted to permanent acrylic resin by routine dental laboratory procedures (Figure 18.2D). This step may be delayed until the artificial teeth are set and processed onto the metal framework.

5. Artificial teeth are positioned for optimal aesthetics and function, and to achieve appropriate dental occlusion, which contributes to prosthesis stability. With large defects, it may be impossible to create a fully stable prosthesis. When tooth placement is completed, the prosthesis is completed by routine dental laboratory procedures (Figure 18.2E).
6. The prosthodontist ensures that the completed prosthesis fits the patient comfortably and that the occlusion is accurate. Pressure areas on the oral mucosa must be located and eliminated. Several office visits are usually required to correct minor tissue irritations, which are common with all newly made prostheses. The patient must also receive direct instructions for inserting and removing the prosthesis, as well as guidelines for care and use. The importance of ongoing dental care and prosthesis maintenance must be stressed, and a regular dental recall schedule (e.g., every 6 months) should be arranged.

## Dental Implants

Advances in the area of dental implants offer expanded treatment options for partially and completely edentulous patients who require prosthetic speech appliances. A dental implant consists of one or more artificial teeth connected to a small metal core that is surgically implanted into the jaw to replace one or more missing teeth (see Figure 18.3). Dental implants pioneered over the past decade allow prosthodontists to achieve excellent sup-

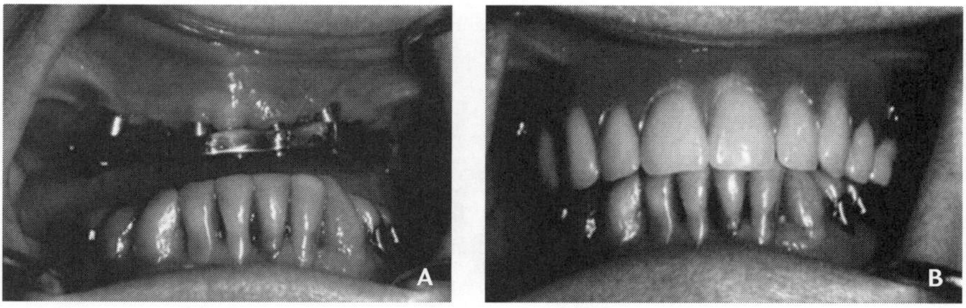


FIGURE 18.3. (A) Metal core and bar of dental implant, surgically implanted into bone. (B) Artificial teeth in place, attached to dental implant.

port and retention (Eckert & Desjardins, 2000; Markt, 2001; Roumanas, Nishimura, Davis, & Beumer, 1997; Weischer, Schettler, & Mohr, 1997). The improvement in prosthesis stability minimizes destructive forces that are usually associated with all removable appliances, thus reducing the potential for remakes.

The metal core of the dental implant, which is usually made from titanium or titanium alloys, is cylindrical in shape and approximately the size of tooth roots. Anchored in the jawbone, it connects to a separate intraoral component (abutment) of varying designs. For a patient with many missing teeth, several implants may be used to support and retain the speech prosthesis. Retention is usually achieved either by individual ball and socket-like attachments or through connection of the abutments to a bar, to which the prosthetic speech appliance is fastened. In addition to retention and support, these attachments allow patients to remove the appliance for care and maintenance. Although expensive, implants dramatically improve stability for speech devices in patients with missing teeth.

## Principles of Speech Assessment

The speech-language pathologist's role is to evaluate the patient's speech using perceptual, acoustical, and physiological measurements. A systematic evaluation of each speech subsystem (i.e., respiratory, laryngeal, velopharyngeal, articulatory) will allow the clinician to develop a thorough description of the type and severity of the speech problem. Information gained about articulatory precision in patients with primarily hard palate defects (e.g., oral-nasal fistulae) must be compared to concerns about the airflow through a potentially incompetent velopharyngeal mechanism (posterior defects) to discern the relative and sometimes overlapping contributions of anterior anomalies versus velopharyngeal defects.

Our approach to prosthetic management is based on a physiological evaluation of speech production in individuals with disordered anatomical and physiological characteristics, such as cleft lip and palate. The goal is to determine the severity and type of involvement of each functional valve in the speech system, including the diaphragm, abdomen, rib cage, larynx, velopharyngeal port, tongue, jaw, and lips (Netsell & Daniel, 1979; Rosenbek & Netsell, 1985). Such an approach should allow the clinician to select a management strategy based on knowledge of how each valve interacts with the others in conversational speech. Although we emphasize the velopharyngeal and oral articulatory valves, a competent evaluation of the orofacial complex always requires a comprehensive examination of all coordinating structures in the human speech subsystems, from the diaphragm to the lips. (See Chapter 10 for Moon's comprehensive description of the physiological evaluation of speech.)

Motor speech research has demonstrated that changes in speech articulatory and resonatory valves influence speech production patterns beyond the oral and velopharyngeal cavities. For example, altering performance of the velopharyngeal valve can yield subsequent changes in laryngeal tone and respiratory action, as well as measurable differences in speech muscle activity. These broader crossover effects illustrate the impact that changes in one subsystem (e.g., velopharyngeal valving) can produce on the coordinated subsystems of motor speech control. Indeed, research suggests that these speech subsystems (i.e., respiration, phonation, articulation, or resonance) do not operate independently (Folkins, 1985; Hamlet, Geoffrey, & Bartlett, 1976; Hamlet & Stone, 1974, 1978; Hamlet, Stone, & McCarty, 1978; Tachimura, Hara, & Wada, 1995; Witt et al., 1995).

## Existing Oral or Dental Conditions and the Effects on Speech

Children with abnormal anterior dental occlusal structures may face special challenges to speech sound development following surgical or prosthodontic changes in the size, shape, and position of the oral structures. Dental defects associated with clefts of the primary palate (e.g., congenitally missing lateral incisors, anterior and posterior crossbite, Class III malocclusion, malpositioned teeth) add an additional burden to the patient who is learning (or the speech-language pathologist who is teaching) correct articulatory patterns (Moller, 1994). Even though emphasis is placed upon the maxillary segments of the oral cavity, mandibular aspects of oral function for prosthetic design, occlusal factors, and cosmesis should also be considered during the speech evaluation. Because the jaw and tongue are an integral part of the functioning of the oral mechanism, the relationships between the upper and lower jaws must be considered before and following prosthetic management. Although variations in design of the maxillary and mandibular components of the prosthesis may certainly affect mastication, deglutition, and articulation (Bloomer, 1971;

Garber, Speidel, & Siegel, 1980; Lawson & Bond, 1969; Palmer, 1974; Starr, 1979), these variations do not generally inhibit correct articulation or mastication, thanks to the remarkable adaptability of the human organism to variations in structure, especially for eating and speaking.

## Anterior Palatal Portion of the Appliance

In speech prostheses for individuals with orofacial anomalies, emphasis is often restricted to the posterior or velopharyngeal component. In addition to problems with oral-nasal coupling, other problems of neurological integrity, oral sensation, jaw relationships, tooth alignment, tongue function, abnormal size and shape of the hard palate, and lip deformities may also contribute to the speech characteristics of the patient with cleft lip and palate.

The factors that may affect sound production following the placement of the appliance into the anterior region of the oral cavity include (a) position of the anterior teeth, (b) alterations in the vertical dimension (interdental space), (c) alterations in the occlusal plane level (an imaginary line drawn from the tips of the anterior teeth to the posterior teeth, (d) confinement of intraoral space (thick alveolar ridge of the dental appliance), (e) problems with anterior overbite (excessive overlap of the upper and lower teeth), (f) increased lingual flange size of the appliance (mandibular denture base overextension), and (g) chronic displacement or loosening of the anterior portion of the appliance (noted as appliance dropping or "clattering" against lower teeth). Each of these factors may cause distortions or substitutions of speech sound elements (particularly fricative and sibilant sounds) that are separate from the types of sound errors related to posterior velopharyngeal valving problems. In some patients, both anterior and posterior openings between the oral and nasal cavities occur and must be managed concurrently.

## Structural Position of the Anterior Teeth

Variations in position of the teeth or portions of the alveolar ridge typically relate to defective /s/ phoneme production. If the upper anterior teeth and alveolar gum ridge are positioned anteriorly, there may be a slight whistle to the /s/ production or a variation of the /ʃ/ sound. If the upper anterior incisors are situated too far posteriorly, the tongue tip may lateralize the /s/ sound as a compensatory effort. Further, if a dental appliance is placed over a hard palate defect, resulting in excessive thickness, a total blockage of the midline air channel may affect fricatives /s, z, ʃ/ and affricatives /tʃ, ʤ/.

If the lower incisors are positioned posteriorly and the tongue tip moves upward, certain speakers produce an interdental /θ/ for /s/ sound substitution. Some individuals move the mandible forward as a compensation, which makes the sound more /s/-like, but this channels the airstream upward rather than downward and may affect its quality. A thick alveolar ridge around dental appliances typically causes only minor problems, such as anterior or superior posturing of the tongue.

## Altered Vertical Dimension (Interdental Space)

Because of anterior malocclusion or placement problems with a dental appliance, an individual may face either increased or decreased vertical height. If the vertical dimension is increased, the palatal arch will be higher than normal. This condition may cause distortion (weak production) of the linguapalatal sounds /s, z, ʃ/ and affect bilabial /p, b/ and labiodental /f, v/ sound production because the lower lip may not be able to reach the upper lip as quickly or as firmly. There may also be a change in oral resonance because of the increased tongue-palate gap. If the vertical dimension is reduced, the tongue tip and blade will be nearer to the palate due to the smaller oral cavity space. This typically causes lateralization of /s/, /z/ and /ʃ/, with a subsequent loss of sound power and lower oral resonant frequency characteristics for these sounds. To compensate, some individuals may make a lingual seal on the upper posterior molars, causing further lateralization and more posterior posturing of the tongue.

## Altered Occlusal Plane

The occlusal plane level is an imaginary line drawn through the tips of the anterior teeth to the posterior teeth. The level of the occlusal plane affects tongue function. In this condition, the sides of the tongue may have to be raised further above the normal plane of occlusion to achieve a seal for correct sibilant sounds such as /s/ and /z/ and may produce a /θ/ for /s/ sound substitution. This upward change in tongue blade position may affect oral resonance characteristics and thus reduce the airway channel space. This distortion is particularly apparent in cases where an anterior prosthesis, partial denture, or complete dentures have been inserted. With a lowered occlusal plane, some individuals may adopt a higher tongue tip position for /s/ and /z/ because it is easier to produce.

## Confined Intraoral Space

When the alveolar ridge is too thick or the upper posterior teeth are positioned too far lingually, a lack of space for the tongue may force the tongue forward. This may result in tongue fronting of the /s/ sounds in conversational speech. A forward shifting of the mandible may also occur, but this compensatory movement typically exaggerates the tongue fronting for sibilants /s/ and /z/. With excessive buccal (cheek) placement of teeth, particularly in individuals with dentures, the tongue may spread out to obtain a seal, thus causing a reduction in the air channel and a lateralization of /s/ or a variation of the /ʃ/ sound production. When the lower posterior teeth are malpositioned, the tongue may be displaced superiorly. When the teeth are positioned too far lingually and the tongue tip is placed forward, a /θ/ for /s/ substitution may result. For patients who wear only lower dentures, this malpositioning may dislodge the speech appliance.

## Problems with Anterior Overbite

When the vertical overlap of the upper and lower front teeth exceeds 3 mm, the mandible may have difficulty adjusting to the restricted anterior oral space. Thus, in the more closed condition, the /s/ and /z/ sounds become more distorted or "muffled." Oral resonance for vowels, diphthongs, and other voiced consonants may also be distorted. With a reduced overbite, an end-to-end bite or open bite may occur and a distorted /s/ sound typically results. This generally occurs from the broad channeling of the airstream over the lower incisors.

## Oversized Appliance Base

As a result of a primary surgical procedure to repair the cleft or secondary alveolar bone grafting, the dental base may be more than a few millimeters thick. The reduction in oral cavity size may cause the tongue to overshoot targets for fricatives and affricates, resulting in a stop for fricative substitution. Once the base is reduced, the fricative substitution should be reduced to a minor distortion, typically either a fronted or lateralized sound, until the patient adjusts to the space and develops a more precise channel for air escape.

## Increased Lingual Flange Size

Excessive overextension of the lingual flange of a mandibular denture may restrict superior movement of the tongue for speech sounds. If the anterior portion is excessive, movement to and from low tongue position (rest and low vowels) to the alveolar ridge for /l/, /t/, and /d/ and even for /ʃ/, /tʃ/, and /ʤ/ may be interrupted. Similarly, posterior lower overextension may cause problems for linguavelar sounds such as /k/ or /g/ or /ʒ/. A general indistinct sound production and a reduction in movement to and from one sound to another may result. In addition, the excessive size may cause the tongue to pull the denture loose, causing "clattering" of the denture during speech production.

## Chronic Displacement of Anterior Appliance

Persistent denture or appliance displacement occurs when retentive clasps loosen, teeth move, or the vertical dimension is inaccurate. These problems may also indicate excessive pressure (velopharyngeal muscular force) on the posterior portion of a compound appliance (speech obturator), causing anterior displacement. In addition, change in base shape because of bone or soft tissue resorption may create looseness. None of these conditions are acceptable to the patient, prosthodontist, or speech-language pathologist. Some patients may refuse to wear an ill-fitting appliance. Others will simply hold the prosthetic appliance in place with the back of the tongue or by clenching the teeth together, which reduces the articulatory transition rate and sound precision, particularly for sibilants. Immediate attention to resolve these problems is essential for patient compliance.

## Anterior Oral-Nasal Fistulae

Openings between the oral and nasal cavities occur in a small percentage of patients with clefts of the lip, alveolus, or hard palate. While they may occur anywhere inside the anterior nares, in the buccal-nasal sulci, or along the hard palate, a large number are found in the area of the incisive foramen (see Figure 18.4). Although some can be closed surgically, others may be excessively large or the region may be too scarred to allow successful surgical closure. These fistulae may affect speech adversely, especially when they exist in conjunction with velopharyngeal incompetence (VPI). Shelton and Blank (1984) suggested that even small oral-nasal fistulae can cause significant problems with speech. In these cases, the clinician must determine the separate contribution of each orifice (front or back) to speech performance. By closing the anterior oral-nasal fistulae temporarily, the clinician can assess the effect of VPI with and without the anterior problem present. Several techniques have been offered to assess changes in resonance balance, nasal air emission, and articulatory precision. The first technique (Bless, Ewanowski, & Dibbel, 1980) promotes covering the anterior opening with soft dental wax. Another group of clinicians recommend using a medical-grade adhesive to cover the hole (Reisberg, Fold, & Dorf, 1985). Even chewing gum may be used to obturate the fistula temporarily, if care is taken to ensure that the fistula is cleaned following the examination, to avoid subsequent infection and tissue irritation.

A useful assessment protocol includes speech sounds produced on the alveolar ridge area (e.g., /t, d, s, z/) in conjunction with high vowels (e.g., /i, u/) in syllables, words, and phrases. These contexts require the speaker

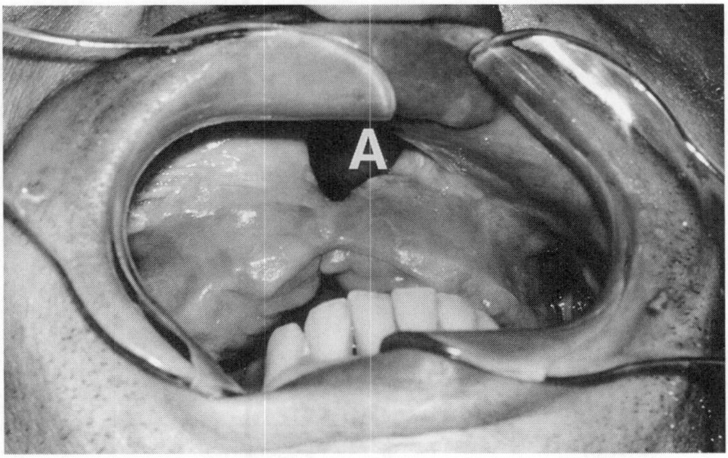


FIGURE 18.4. An edentulous maxilla with an oral-nasal fistula demonstrating a labial defect (A).

to produce a seal around the alveolar ridge to create intraoral air pressure and demand velopharyngeal port closure.

Once the speech-language pathologist has determined the impact of the anterior oral-nasal fistula on speech, the prosthodontist should determine what type of appliance should be used (e.g., temporary or permanent, fixed or removable) to close the defect and clarify what impact the anterior prosthesis has on any velopharyngeal closure problems in speech. Therefore, speech testing with and without the anterior prosthesis is a necessity when designing the total prosthesis.

# Specific Defect Management

## Anterior Oral Defects (Hard Palate Clefts and Oral-Nasal Fistulae)

Defects of the maxilla may occur as a result of destructive inflammatory conditions, ablative tumor surgery, and trauma (Bohle et al., 2005). Included in this group of maxillary defects are clefts of the hard palate and oral-nasal fistulae (see Figure 18.5). Such defects cause fluid and food leakage into the nasal cavity, impaired mastication, hypernasality, nasal

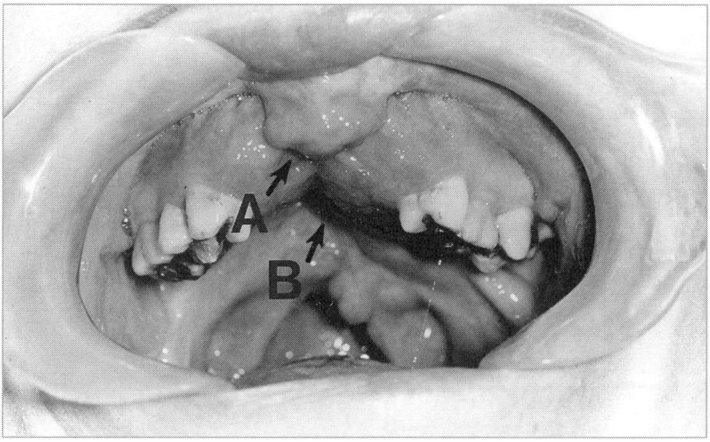


FIGURE 18.5. An anterior oral-nasal defect showing oral-nasal defect (A) and hard palate cleft (repaired) (B).

air emission, and other articulatory problems that decrease speech intelligibility. Prosthetic appliances may obturate space resulting from lost tissues and thereby minimize these hazards to speech intelligibility. With hard palate defects, prostheses attempt to create an effective seal at the perimeter of the palatal opening and replace missing teeth anteriorly. Effective obturation will prevent inappropriate air and fluid leaks between the nasal and oral cavity. In most situations, it is neither possible nor desirable to completely fill the defect, especially when it is very large, as bulky obturators are difficult to retain securely. To decrease mass and weight, the obturator may be hollow or the nasopharyngeal surface may be left open, simulating a "topless box" (Oral, Aramany, & McWilliams, 1979). Even so, the retentive clasps of the prosthesis must be of sufficient strength and number to prevent dislodgement. Some tooth contours do not allow good clasp retention and may require modification. Contouring material can be bonded to the lower tooth margin, creating a broader rim that will hold a retention clasp in place (Sills & Leeper, 1984).

## Soft Palate Defects

In most cases, congenital clefting of the soft palate can be successfully repaired with surgery. However, prosthodontic treatment should be considered in cases where unusually large clefts exist; acquired surgical defects remain; severe velopharyngeal inadequacy is present; or medical, psychosocial, or religious reasons prohibit surgery (Mazaheri, 1976; Shiere et al., 1962). Patients with soft palate defects generally exhibit hypernasality, nasal air emission, and decreased speech intelligibility. Individuals demonstrating good velopharyngeal movement usually adapt more readily to the prosthetic speech appliance (Blakeley, 1960, 1964; Wong & Weiss, 1972). These patients need an appliance that closes the velopharyngeal port, without inhibiting correct anterior articulation.

The prosthetic speech appliance for soft palate defects typically consists of three sections: maxillary, palatal, and nasopharyngeal (see Figure 18.6). In edentulous patients, the complete upper denture serves as the maxillary section. If the edentulous maxilla lacks sufficient retentive capacity to support the additional weight of the posterior sections, adhesives must be used to help retain the prosthesis. Without adhesives the patient may be unable to chew or speak adequately.

For infants and toddlers, the prosthesis for soft palate defects may serve as a feeding aid and later as an aid for early speech development. For

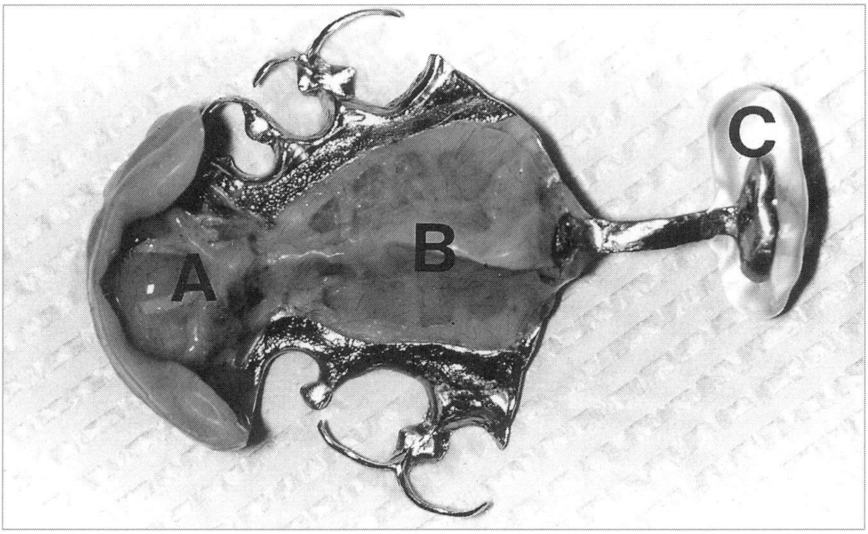


FIGURE 18.6. Example of maxillary speech appliance comprising three sections: (A) maxillary, (B) palatal, and (C) nasopharyngeal.

young children, the palatal appliances must be adjusted and refit every 1–2 months to accommodate the growing oral cavity and erupting teeth. In older childhood and adolescents, a combination of an orthodontic and palatal obturator may be necessary. As the patient ages and as dental or occlusal abnormalities change, a palatal prosthesis can be added to partial or complete dentures to maintain oral-nasal separation and to provide adequate potential for speech production.

## Speech Considerations

Although prosthodontic devices, such as obturators, speech bulbs, and palatal lift appliances, are designed to reduce the size of the velopharyngeal port, their effectiveness is most useful for increasing the efficiency of the valve. Indirectly, the appliance acts to improve articulation by increasing aerodynamic and acoustical power (Warren, 1986). These changes in velopharyngeal closure should improve listener judgments of voice quality (Counihan & Cullinan, 1970) and overall speech intelligibility (Schneiderman & Mann, 1978). The size and location of the cleft and the condition of the tissues surrounding it govern the design of the velopharyngeal and pharyngeal sections of a device. Obturators for defects of the entire soft palate take their shape from movements generated by the lateral and posterior pharyngeal walls during speech trials and, if possible, based on visual impressions made during flexible nasendoscopy.

The obturator section is constructed in acrylic resin and relies on an internal metal framework for support and connection to the anterior base section. The internal metal frame provides scaffolding on which impression materials (thermoplastic waxes, self-curing resins) are sequentially layered to achieve the most physiologically acceptable obturator form. The obturator should be located at the level of greatest pharyngeal wall movement and need not extend more than 10 mm vertically (Curtis & Beumer, 1979). Soft palate obturators positioned too low may produce gagging and restrict normal tongue movements, whereas those placed too high may occlude the nasopharynx and cause problems of nasal airway patency. Ideally, the nasopharyngeal section should be located in the nasopharynx region at the level of the normal palatal closure (Curtis & Beumer, 1979). Passive contact must exist between the acrylic of the obturator and the mucosa of the velopharynx and pharynx. During swallowing and coughing, the palatal extension and nasopharyngeal section should not be displaced. Nasopharyngeal obturators that incorporate a polished, convex superior surface and a concave palatal surface minimize accumulation of mucus and provide adequate tongue space for swallowing and speech purposes.

At the delivery (insertion) stage, movements similar to those used to obtain the impression are used to identify areas where the internal surface of the obturator presses on the mucosa. After the initial prosthesis placement, several appointments must be anticipated for retentive clasp adjustments and buffing or polishing to reduce the obturator's size slightly to achieve optimal comfort and function.

## Partial Soft Palate Clefts

Partial soft palate clefts occur in surgically resected palates (e.g., following oral or pharyngeal cancers) or incompletely repaired palates. Short, taut residual soft palates are common surgical sequelae and, when present, should not be covered by the prosthesis. In these cases, the nasopharyngeal section obturates only the palatal defect and avoids the adjacent tissues. Lifting of the residual soft palate may be required when dealing with long or immobile soft palate tissues (Subtelny, Sakuda, & Subtelny, 1966). Tissues adjacent to the cleft seldom exhibit full movement or elevation. Thus, the obturator should extend from the midline defect bilaterally to the lateral pharyngeal walls to sufficiently close the gap (Curtis & Beumer, 1979). Some patients experience delays in initiating definitive prosthetic treatment until surgically resected tissues heal. For cancer patients, radiation therapy may further prolong the healing period, sometimes up to 6 months (Leeper & Gratton, 1999).

## Procedural Considerations with Speech Appliances

Rosen and Bzoch (1958) suggested that the posterior portion of the speech appliance be adjusted until the patient can produce voiceless stops, such as /p/ or /t/, or voiceless fricatives, such as /s/, /ʃ/, or /f/, without audible nasal air emission. The patient also must have enough nasal airway patency to produce acceptable /m/, /n/, or /ŋ/ sounds without hyponasal voice quality. High intraoral air pressure oral consonants and high vowels, such as /i/ and /u/, should be combined in syllables or words and placed into longer contexts (e.g., phrases). They should be repeated with greater or less stress, and produced at faster and slower than normal speaking rates to evaluate articulatory and phonatory changes following speech appliance fitting. Again, flexible nasendoscopy is useful as a relatively noninvasive technique for observing changes in the velopharyngeal port during connected speech trials conducted during prosthetic fitting (Riski, Hoke, & Dolan, 1989).

Patient adjustments to the insertion of a speech appliance have been of interest to a number of investigators (Blakeley, 1960, 1964, 1969; Blakeley & Porter, 1971; Mazaheri & Mazaheri, 1976; Shelton et al., 1971; Subtelny et al., 1966; Weiss, 1971; Weiss & Louis, 1972; Wong & Weiss, 1972). The underlying premise has been that certain subjects develop posterior and lateral pharyngeal wall action with prosthesis wear, thus prompting the mechanism to achieve better velopharyngeal closure than was evident before the prosthesis was placed. These apparent gains in tissue closure allow the prosthodontist to systematically reduce the size of the bulb while still maintaining acceptable speech quality. In reports of patients who successfully increased velopharyngeal closure after prostheses were placed, researchers measured subjective and objective reductions in hypernasality despite reduced obturator size. Wong and Weiss (1972) suggested several features that appeared to predict positive prosthesis training outcomes: (a) Younger patients did better than older patients, (b) females did better than males in reducing nasalization, (c) family and patient compliance appeared to assist in developing velopharyngeal action, and (d) patients with longer veli and greater pharyngeal wall action were more often able to undergo speech bulb reduction. Although the number of patients in each of the listed studies was not large, between one quarter and one third of the sampled population could accommodate speech bulb reduction while maintaining speech and resonant quality.

The important factor in obturation or palatal lift reduction in patients with velopharyngeal inadequacy is the ability of the velopharyngeal musculature to adapt to the "foreign body" placed in the defect area. In the case of the lift, the musculature reacts by pulling (lifting) away from the object, hence enhancing closure, or in the case of the obturator, there is an increase in lateral-posterior pharyngeal wall and velar closure against the speech bulb. This increased activity by the surrounding musculature allows the speech-language pathologist to note changes in perceptual, acoustical, and physiological activities associated with speech production, such as reduced hypernasality, reduced nasal air emission, and reduced velopharyngeal port orifice area.

Most appliance reduction programs have focused on the long-term changes in the muscular adaptation of the velopharyngeal complex. Changes in the amount of velopharyngeal closure must be monitored from week to week during an ongoing speech management program. Careful measurement procedures designed to note subtle changes in perceptual, acoustical, visual, or aerodynamic activity are essential in determining how much material may be taken away from the obturator or palatal lift. Reduction of the dental material in the posterior region is usually accomplished by using visual (nasendoscopy), aerodynamic (air pressure/flow), and perceptual judgments (reduced hypernasality, nasal air emission) criteria. Generally, contact paste is placed on the bulb or lift and fitted in the oral cavity by the prosthodontist. A series of speech tasks (syllables, words), including production of high pressure consonants in high vowel environments produced at slowly increasing rates of speech, seem to satisfy the requirements. In some cases, patients have been able to withdraw from wearing their lifts or speech bulbs following a reduction therapy program. Usually, these adaptations occur over a fairly long period (14–16 months) and demand close attention to the subtle alterations in the appliance as well as the resultant speech output changes. There is little consensus on the usefulness of these appliance reduction programs, likely due to the inherent individual differences in patients who receive speech prostheses. New instrumental techniques for analyzing small changes in the acoustical and physiological events associated with speech production in patients wearing prosthetic appliances should provide better information concerning which patients make changes, the optimal time period for change, and which speech management programs are the most effective.

Design considerations of speech appliances have related primarily to position of the posterior pharyngeal portion of the appliance in the nasopharynx. Early clinical procedures used the area at or near Passavant's ridge as a place of closure. Aram and Subtelny (1959), Fletcher, Haskins, and Bosma (1960), Lloyd, Pruzansky, and Subtelny (1957), and Mazaheri and Millard (1965) reported that, in general, inferior-superior placement of the speech bulb had little or no effect on resonance as long as sufficient closure was present to obtain close approximation. Lateral dimensions appeared as important as vertical dimensions for the maintenance of adequate resonance balance. Clearly, individual differences in each patient's anatomical defect and physiological action must be considered when fabricating and modifying posterior speech bulb appliances. Functional assessment should include physiological, acoustical, and perceptual measurements of speech performance observed prior to and following speech appliance insertion. By combining input from both the speech-language pathologist and the prosthodontist, an appliance that functions properly for mastication, deglutition, and speech can be successfully developed for the patient.

## Velopharyngeal Incompetence in Speakers Without Clefts

Individuals who exhibit hypernasality, excessive nasal emission of air, and decreased speech intelligibility due to traumatic injuries, stroke, neuromuscular disease, brain tumors, or other idiopathic conditions resulting in velopharyngeal incompetence may also benefit from speech prostheses (Gonzalez & Aronson, 1970; Kipfmueller & Lang, 1972; LaVelle & Hardy, 1979; Marshall & Jones, 1971; Mazaheri & Mazaheri, 1976). When the soft palate structure is normal, a palatal lift prosthesis may reduce hypernasality and increase overall speech intelligibility by elevating the soft palate to the pharyngeal wall (Gibbons & Bloomer, 1958). When the soft palate is elevated, the size of the velopharyngeal valve is decreased, restoring oral-nasal resonance balance and increasing speech intelligibility. Similar measures are used to assess the efficiency of the palatal lift appliance as for other speech prostheses, including audio-perceptual judgments, flexible nasendoscopy, and acoustical and aerodynamic measures.

## Treatment Considerations for Palatal Lifts

In addition to the patient's dental status, several other factors may affect the design of the lift section of the palatal lift and the individual's accommodation to it. These factors include (a) palatal vault contour, (b) pharyngeal size and form, (c) displacement characteristics of the soft palate, (d) distance between the border of the soft palate and the posterior pharyngeal wall, (e) degree of symmetrical muscular activity of the velum, (f) sensitivity of the gag reflex, and (g) position, size, shape, and activity range of the tongue. Each factor must be considered carefully for the individual with velopharyngeal inadequacy; thus, each patient's lift appliance will have a unique design (Leeper & Sills, 1986).

## Structural Features Peculiar to the Palatal Lift

Tissue pressures exerted on the palatal lift exceed those experienced by simple removable partial dentures. The speech prosthesis must be designed to distribute these forces widely and uniformly to the retaining and supporting structures. To provide the needed strength, the components of the maxillary and palatal sections should be made as a one-unit metal casting. To achieve adequate support for the soft palate, the lift or palatal section is shaped and developed to provide the best possible velopharyngeal closure assistance for a given patient. For some individuals, a narrow palatal section may be sufficient (see Figure 18.7A), and for others, a wide palatal section is required (see Figure 18.7B). The lift may be augmented

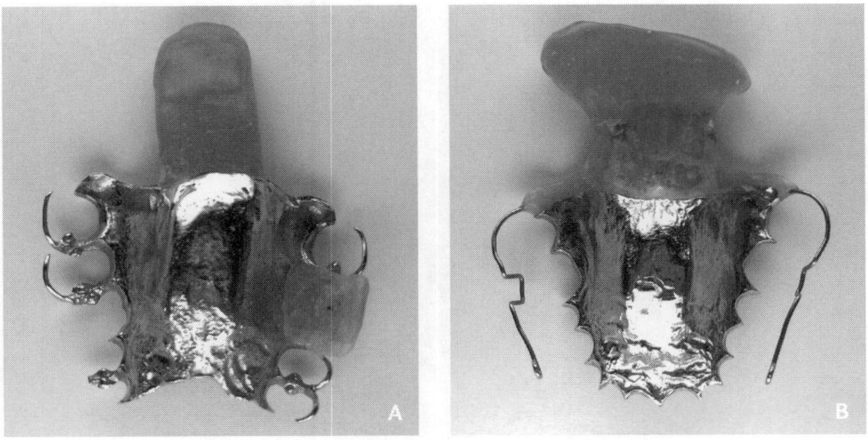


FIGURE 18.7. Examples of palatal lift speech appliances showing (A) narrow palatal section and (B) wide (butterfly) palatal section.

by an obturator in those individuals presenting with short palates. A clear acrylic resin lift portion provides good visual access to the underlying tissues, which is helpful when adjusting or modifying the lift (Sills & Leeper, 1984). Palatal lifts may also be used with individuals who are edentulous in the upper arch (Sato, Sato, Yoshida, & Tsuru, 1987).

## Meatal Obturators

An older method for treatment of velopharyngeal incompetency employs the use of a meatal obturator (see Figure 18.8). Unlike the palatal lift, which relies on muscular activity of the velopharyngeal structures for effect, the meatal obturator simply impedes (blocks) nasal airflow in the nasopharynx. Positioned above and behind the hard palate terminus, the meatal obturator acts as a barrier that regulates nasal airflow. Airflow control is achieved by reducing the lateral borders of the obturator, or by drilling one or more holes through the posterior portion. The remaining components of the meatal obturator resemble similar maxillary prosthetic speech appliances. Some prosthodontists prefer meatal obturators because they may weigh less than palatal lifts and are thought to reduce gagging. The nasopharynx impression technique for the meatal obturator is more demanding than that for the palatal lift and requires several sequential impressions to acquire the appropriate configuration (Sharry, 1976).

## Prosthetic and Speech Team Management of the Patient

Once the framework has been produced according to the treatment plan, acrylic resin tray material is adapted to the lift extension portion of the

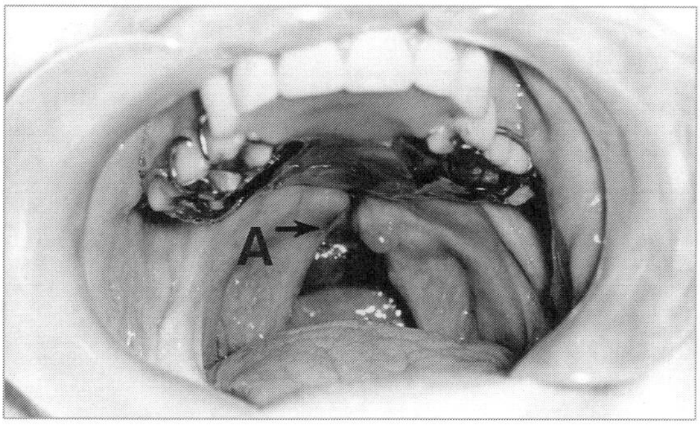


FIGURE 18.8. Example of a meatal obturator (in situ), partially obscured by terminus of velum.

framework extending onto the soft palate. The lift impression is made initially by using a low-fusing thermoplastic material with the soft palate elevated to make contact with the posterior pharyngeal wall. The impression is extended to achieve the degree of lift required, based on the objective clinical evaluation of speech production tasks discussed previously (Leeper & Sills, 1986; Muntz, D'Antonio, Gay, & Marsh, 1985). When the desired velopharyngeal closure is achieved, the tissue surface of the thermoplastic material is reduced approximately 1 mm, and a final wax impression is taken. Often, it is prudent to build up the lift portion over several appointments to compensate for functional tissue adaptation, avoid unnecessary tissue irritation, and improve patient tolerance.

During this modification process, the speech-language pathologist and prosthodontist work together to evaluate the effectiveness of the palatal lift. Lift configuration is influenced by (a) depth of the oropharynx, (b) width of the posterior pharyngeal wall, (c) degree of palatal movement during phoneme production, (d) extent of the lateral pharyngeal wall port openings, (e) degree of hyper- or hypotonic palatal pharyngeal muscles, and (f) sensitivity of the gag reflex.

The prosthodontist must accommodate the lift to the physiological constraints placed on it by tissue displacement, whereas the speech-language pathologist is interested in obtaining the best resonance balance possible. If the lift does not produce sufficient closure, hypernasality or nasal air emission will persist. If too much closure is observed, nasal production becomes oralized (e.g., /b/ for /m/ substitutions) and hyponasal resonance results. The prosthodontist can increase or reduce the surface of the lift by trimming or adding to the thermoplastic material, accordingly. Once fit is optimal, the patient wears the lift continuously except when eating or sleeping. As experience and confidence increase, the lift can be worn during meals. However, it should never be worn 24 hours a day, as this practice frequently leads to mucosal inflammations, such as papillary hyperplasia. A rest period of 6–8 hours per day with the prosthesis out of the mouth is recommended. During this time period the prosthesis must be stored wet, preferably in water-based denture disinfectant solutions or commercial cleansers, to prevent possible shrinkage of the acrylic resin created by dehydration.

### Assessment of Modifications

Sills and Leeper (1984) evaluated the records of 14 patients with dysarthria and accompanying velopharyngeal incompetence who wore palatal lift prostheses. On average, significant changes from premanagement (no lift condition) to postmanagement (lift inserted condition) demonstrated decreased nasal airflow, increased respiratory effort (intraoral air pressure, subglottal air pressure), and decreased estimated velopharyngeal orifice areas for plosive and fricative syllable contexts and oral phoneme sentence contexts. Also, lateral cephalometric X-ray measures confirmed decreased velopharyngeal gap size for sustained /u/ and /s/ phonemes and a corresponding slight increase in intrinsic length (velar stretch) of the velum following lift placement. These physical findings correlated well with listener judgments of decreased hypernasality and with slight improvement in whole-word articulatory precision. These data add support to palatal lift research reported by Gonzalez and Aronson (1970), LaVelle and Hardy (1979), Shaughnessy, Netsell, and Farrange (1983), and Aten, McDonald, Simpson, and Gutierrez (1984), who found decreased velopharyngeal port size, decreased hypernasality and nasalization, and improved speech intelligibility following palatal lift management.

Although decreased hypernasality or reduced nasal air emission should be expected following placement of a palatal lift, certain well-learned but abnormal articulatory patterns (e.g., velar, pharyngeal, or glottal substitutions for tongue fronted sounds) may persist. The clinician should continue to address correct articulatory placements to reduce aberrant distortions or substitutions under these better conditions of reduced nasality. (See Chapter 11 for Trost-Cardamone's description of articulation treatment.)

# Long-Term Management

## Dental

Continual dental evaluation is crucial to the postdelivery success of maxillary prosthetic speech appliance treatment (McGivney & Carr, 2000). Patients wearing such prostheses cannot always be relied upon to monitor their dental status and must therefore return for regular dental examinations. Minimally, an annual checkup should be mandatory, with more frequent recalls as required. Of particular concern is the health of the supporting oral structures and the mucosa, and the physical condition of the prosthesis. Typically, the teeth may become more prone to caries and periodontal disease. Clasped abutment teeth must be observed for increased mobility and, when present, the cause corrected. Mucosa bordering the acrylic resin portion frequently exhibits inflammation that must be controlled. Finally, prostheses must be inspected for wear or damage, and the appropriate adjustment made.

Refitting (relining) the acrylic resin portion of the prosthetic speech appliance to accommodate changes in the underlying mucosal surfaces must be anticipated. The peripheral seal of obturators must be maintained for effective air and fluid control. Eventually, however, the prosthesis will require replacement, as some of the materials have a limited life span. In general, 10 or more years of service from one prosthesis should be considered satisfactory.

## Speech

Many individuals seen for prosthetic management may be referred from other hospital or rehabilitation units in the area. Because most will return to their "home" unit for ongoing speech therapy, it is imperative that good communication exist between the prosthetic team and that home unit. Communication may be enhanced by providing in-service training for the speech professionals in those units, covering topics such as (a) criteria for successful prosthodontic management, (b) technical characteristics of the appliance, (c) modification procedures, (d) timing of modifications, (e) continuing evaluation procedures, and (f) long-term care of the appliance and oral environment. Written progress reports concerning each step in the process should be forwarded to the referring unit or professionals.

Because each prosthetic device is uniquely fit for each individual, minor alterations to the anterior or posterior components are often necessary. Slight changes in soft or hard tissue environments may cause the appliance to lose its retentive characteristics, or the wearer may begin to adapt to the posterior segment, as evidenced by speech improvement, and need to have some of the acrylic removed (reduced). In any case, information from the home unit may be useful in describing problems with the appliance to the team's prosthodontist and speech-language pathologist. Important indices of prosthesis fit derive from speech quality (hypernasality/hyponasality), nasal air emission, aerodynamic activity through the velopharyngeal system (orifice area estimation), structural movement of the velum and the lateral and posterior pharyngeal walls (nasendoscopy, videofluoroscopy), and overall speech intelligibility. Re-evaluation using a standard protocol allows the attending professional to note positive or negative changes in the patient's performance following alterations made to the appliance. Modifications to the appliance may occur over an 8-month to 2-year period, depending on the type of defect, the impact of various medical and behavioral treatments, and the age and compliance of the individual involved.

## Summary

In this chapter, we have attempted to outline procedures for the assessment, fabrication, and modification of prosthetic appliances for anterior and posterior oral defects. Each team of professionals must work together to develop an effective treatment plan that considers oral function and speech performance as integrated treatment goals. The collaboration between the prosthodontist and speech-language pathologist enhances prosthetic care and offers the patient with oral structural defects or velopharyngeal dysfunction the best opportunity for improved communication.

## References

Aram, A., & Subtelny, J. D. (1959). Velopharyngeal function and cleft palate prosthesis. *Journal of Prosthetic Dentistry, 9,* 149–158.

Aten, J. L., McDonald, A., Simpson, M., & Gutierrez, R. (1984). Efficacy of modified palatal lifts for improving resonance. In M. R. McNeil, J. C. Rosenbek, & A. E. Aronson (Eds.), *The dysarthrias: Physiology, acoustics, perception, management* (pp. 331–342). San Diego: College Hill Press.

Blakeley, R.W. (1960). Temporary speech prosthesis as an aid in speech training. *Cleft Palate Bulletin, 10,* 63.

Blakely, R. W. (1964). The complementary use of speech prostheses and pharyngeal flaps in palatal insufficiency. *Cleft Palate Journal, 1,* 194–198.

Blakely, R. W. (1969). The rationale for temporary speech prosthesis in palatal insufficiency. *British Journal of Disorders of Communication, 4,* 134–139.

Blakely, R. W., & Porter, D. R. (1971). Unexpected reduction and removal of an obturator in a patient with palate paralysis. *British Journal of Disorders of Communication, 6,* 33–36.

Bless, D. M., Ewanowski, S. E., & Dibbel, D. G. (1980). A technique for temporary obturation of fistulae. *Cleft Palate Journal, 17,* 297–300.

Bloomer, H. (1971). Speech defects associated with dental malocclusions and related abnormalities. In L. Travis (Ed.), *Handbook of speech pathology and audiology* (pp. 715–766). New York: Appleton-Century-Crofts.

Bohle, G., III, Rieger, J., Huryn, J., Verbel, D., Hwang, F., & Zlotolow, I. (2005). Efficacy of speech aid prostheses for acquired defects of the soft palate and velopharyngeal inadequacy—Clinical assessments and cephalometric analysis: A Memorial Sloan-Kettering Study. *Head and Neck, 27,* 195–207.

Chierici, G. (1979). Cleft palate rehabilitation. In J. Beumer, T. A. Curtis, & D. N. Firtell (Eds.), *Maxillofacial rehabilitation: Prosthodontic and surgical considerations* (pp. 292–310). St. Louis, MO: Mosby.

Counihan, D. T., & Cullinan, W. L. (1970). Reliability and dispersion of nasality ratings. *Cleft Palate Journal, 7,* 261–270.

Curtis, T. A., & Beumer, J. (1979). Speech, palatopharyngeal function, and restoration of soft palate defects. In J. Beumer, T. A. Curtis, & D. N. Firtell (Eds.), *Maxillofacial rehabilitation: Prosthodontic and surgical considerations* (pp. 244–291). St. Louis, MO: Mosby.

Eckert, S. E., & Desjardins, R. P. (2000). The impact of endosseus implants on maxillofacial prosthodontics. In T. D. Taylor (Ed.), *Clinical maxillofacial prosthodontics: Quintessence of dental technology* (pp. 145–153). Hanover Park, IL: Quintessence.

Fletcher, S. G., Haskins, R. C., & Bosma, J. F. (1960). A movable bulb appliance to assist in palatopharyngeal closure. *Journal of Speech and Hearing Disorders, 25,* 249–258.

Folkins, J. W. (1985). Issues in speech motor control and their relation to the speech of individuals with cleft palate. *Cleft Palate Journal, 22,* 106–122.

Garber, S. R., Speidel, T. M., & Siegel, G. M. (1980). The effects of noise and palatal appliances on the speech of five-year-old children. *Journal of Speech and Hearing Research, 23,* 853–863.

Gibbons, P., & Bloomer, H. A. (1958). The palatal lift: A supportive-type aid. *Journal of Prosthetic Dentistry, 8,* 362–369.

Gonzales, J. B., & Aronson, A. E. (1970). Palatal lift prosthesis for treatment of anatomic and neurologic palatopharyngeal insufficiency. *Cleft Palate Journal, 7,* 91–104.

Hamlet, S., Geoffrey, V. C., & Bartlett, D. M. (1976). Effect of a dental prosthesis on speaker-specific characteristics of voice. *Journal of Speech and Hearing Research, 19,* 639–650.

Hamlet, S. L., & Stone, M. (1974). Reorganization of speech motor patterns following prosthodontic changes in oral morphology. In G. Fant (Ed.), *Proceedings of the Speech Communication Seminar.* Stockholm: Royal Institute of Technology.

Hamlet, S. L., & Stone, M. (1978). Compensatory alveolar consonant production induced by wearing a dental prosthesis. *Journal of Phonetics, 6,* 227–248.

Hamlet, S. L., Stone, M., & McCarty, T. (1978). Conditioning prostheses viewed from the standpoint of speech adaptation. *Journal of Prosthetic Dentistry, 40,* 60–66.

Kipfmueller, L. J., & Lang, B. R. (1972). Treating velopharyngeal inadequacies with a palatal lift prosthesis. *Journal of Prosthetic Dentistry, 27,* 63–72.

Kuehn, D. P., & Moller, K. T. (2000). Speech and language issues in the cleft palate population: The state of the art. *Cleft Palate-Craniofacial Journal, 37,* 348-1–348-35.

LaVelle, W. E., & Hardy, J. C. (1979). Palatal lift prosthesis for treatment of palatopharyngeal incompetence. *Journal of Prosthetic Dentistry, 42,* 308–315.

Lawson, W. A., & Bond, E. K. (1969). Speech and its relation to dentistry. *The Dental Practitioner, 19,* 150–156.

Leeper, H. A., & Gratton, D. G. (1999). Oral prosthetic rehabilitation of individuals with head and neck cancer. *Journal of Speech-Language Pathology and Audiology, 23,* 117–133.

Leeper, H. A., & Sills, P. S. (1986). Prosthetic and speech management of patients with velopharyngeal incompetence. *Human Communication Canada, 10*(5), 5–20.

Lloyd, R. S., Pruzansky, S., & Subtelny, J. D. (1957). Prosthetic rehabilitation of a cleft palate patient subsequent to multiple surgical and prosthetic failures. *Journal of Prosthetic Dentistry, 8,* 216–230.

Markt, J. C. (2001). An endosseus, implant-retained obturator for the rehabilitation of a recurrent central giant cell granuloma: A clinical report. *Journal of Prosthetic Dentistry, 85,* 116–120.

Marshall, R. C., & Jones, R. N. (1971). Effects of a palatal lift prosthesis on the speech intelligibility of a dysarthric patient. *Journal of Prosthetic Dentistry, 25,* 327–333.

Mazaheri, M. (1976). Indications and contraindications for prosthetic speech appliances in cleft palate. *Plastic and Reconstructive Surgery, 30,* 663–669.

Mazaheri, M., & Mazaheri, E. H. (1976). Prosthetic aspects of palatal elevation and palatopharyngeal stimulation. *Journal of Prosthetic Dentistry, 35,* 320–327.

Mazaheri, M., & Millard, R. T. (1965). Changes in nasal resonance related to differences in location and dimension of speech bulbs. *Cleft Palate Journal, 2,* 167–175.

McGivney, G. P., & Carr, A. (2000). *McCracken's removable partial denture prosthodontics* (10th ed.). St. Louis, MO: Mosby.

McGrath, C. O., & Anderson, M. W. (1990). Prosthetic treatment of velopharyngeal incompetence. In J. Bardach & H. L. Morris (Eds.), *Multidisciplinary management of cleft lip and palate* (pp. 809–815). Philadelphia: Saunders.

Moller, K. T. (1994). Dental-occlusal and other oral conditions and speech. In J. E. Bernthal & N. W. Bankson (Eds.), *Child phonology: Characteristics, assessment, and intervention with special populations* (pp. 3–28). New York: Thieme.

Muntz, H. R., D'Antonio, L. L., Gay, W. D., & Marsh, J. (1985, May 26–31). *The use of fiberoptic nasendoscopy for fitting palatal lift prostheses and the management of velopharyngeal dysfunction.* Paper presented at the XIII World Congress of Otorhinolaryngology, Miami Beach, FL.

Netsell, R., & Daniel, B. (1979). Dysarthria in adults: Physiologic approach to rehabilitation. *Archives of Physical Medicine and Rehabilitation, 60,* 502–508.

Oral, K., Aramany, M. A., & McWilliams, B. J. (1979). Speech intelligibility with buccal flange obturator. *Journal of Prosthetic Dentistry, 41,* 323–328.

Palmer, J. (1974). Analysis of speech in prosthodontic practice. *Journal of Prosthetic Dentistry, 31,* 605–614.

Parel, S. M., Branemark, P.-I., & Janson, T. (1986). Osseointegration in maxillofacial prosthetics. *Journal of Prosthetic Dentistry, 55,* 490–494.

Reisberg, D. J., Fold, H. O., & Dorf, D. S. (1985). A technique for obturating palatal fistulas. *Cleft Palate Journal, 22,* 286–289.

Riski, J. E., Hoke, J. A., & Dolan, E. A. (1989). The role of pressure flow and endoscopic assessment in successful palatal obturator revision. *Cleft Palate Journal, 26,* 56–62.

Rosen, M. S., & Bzoch, K. R. (1958). The prosthetic speech appliance in rehabilitation of patients with cleft palate. *Journal of the American Dental Association, 57,* 203–210.

Rosenbek, J. C., & Netsell, R. (1985). Treating the dysarthrias. In J. C. Rosenbek (Ed.), *Seminars in speech and language: Current views of dysarthria.* New York: Thieme-Stratton.

Roumanas, E. D., Nishimura, R. D., Davis, B. K., & Beumer, J. (1997). Clinical evaluation of implants retaining edentulous maxillary obturator prostheses. *Journal of Prosthetic Dentistry, 77,* 184–190.

Sato, Y., Sato, M., Yoshida, K., & Tsuru, H. (1987). Palatal lift prostheses for edentulous patients. *Journal of Prosthetic Dentistry, 57,* 204–208.

Schneiderman, C. R., & Mann, M. (1978). Air flow and intelligibility of speech of normal speakers and speakers with a prosthodontically repaired cleft palate. *Journal of Prosthetic Dentistry, 39,* 193–199.

Sharry, J. J. (1976). Curriculum curtailment in prosthodontic education. *Journal of Prosthetic Dentistry, 35,* 469–471.

Shaughnessy, A. L., Netsell, R., & Farrange, J. (1983). Treatment of a four-year-old with a palatal lift prosthesis. In W. R. Berry (Ed.), *Clinical dysarthria* (pp. 216–230). San Diego: College Hill Press.

Shelton, R. L., & Blank, J. L. (1984). Oronasal fistulas, intraoral air pressure, and nasal air flow during speech. *Cleft Palate Journal, 21,* 91–99.

Shelton, R. L., Lindquist, A. F., Chisum, L., Arndt, W. B., Youngstrom, K. A., & Stick, S. L. (1971). Effect of prosthetic speech bulb reduction on articulation. *Cleft Palate Journal, 13,* 127–137.

Shiere, F. R, Fox, A., & Perry, C. C. (1962). Removable partial prosthesis for the cleft palate patient. *Dental Clinics of North America,* pp. 837–849.

Sills, P. S., & Leeper, H. A. (1984). *An investigation of changes in speech behaviour using a palatal lift prosthesis* (Final report). Toronto: Ontario Ministry of Health.

Starr, C. D. (1979). Dental and occlusal hazards to normal speech production. In K. R. Bzoch (Ed.), *Communicative disorders related to cleft lip and palate* (pp. 90–99). Boston: Little, Brown.

Subtelny, J. D., Sakuda, M., & Subtelny, J. D. (1966). Prosthetic treatment for palatopharyngeal incompetence: Research and clinical implications. *Cleft Palate Journal, 3,* 130–158.

Tachimura, T., Hara, H., & Wada, T. (1995). Oral air pressure and nasal air flow rate and levator veli palatini muscle activity in patients wearing a speech appliance. *Cleft Palate-Craniofacial Journal, 32,* 382–389.

Warren, D. W. (1986). Compensatory speech behaviors in cleft palate: A regulation/control phenomenon. *Cleft Palate Journal, 23,* 251–260.

Weischer, T., Schettler, D., & Mohr, C. (1997). Titanium implants in the zygoma as retaining elements after hemimaxillectomy. *International Journal of Oral Maxillofacial Implants, 12,* 211–214.

Weiss, C. E. (1971). Success of an obturator reduction program. *Cleft Palate Journal, 8,* 291–297.

Weiss, C. E., & Louis, H. (1972). Toward a more objective approach to obturator reduction. *Cleft Palate Journal, 9,* 157–160.

Witt, P. D., Rozelle, A. A., Marsh, J. L., Marty-Grames, L., Muntz, H. R., Gay, W. D., et al. (1995). Do palatal lift prostheses stimulate velopharyngeal neurotransmitter activity? *Cleft Palate-Craniofacial Journal, 32,* 469–475.

Wolfaardt, J. F., Wilson, F. B., Rochet, A., & McPhee, L. (1993). An appliance-based approach to the management of palatopharyngeal incompetency: A clinical pilot project. *Journal of Prosthetic Dentistry, 69,* 186–195.

Wong, L. P., & Weiss, C. E. (1972). A clinical assessment of obturator-wearing cleft palate patients. *Journal of Prosthetic Dentistry, 27,* 632–639.

# About the Authors

**Karlind T. Moller, PhD,** is a speech-language pathologist and director and coordinator of the Cleft Palate/Craniofacial Clinics at the University of Minnesota School of Dentistry, where he has served for over 30 years. He has academic appointments as professor in the Department of Developmental and Surgical Sciences in the School of Dentistry and adjunct professor in the Department of Speech-Language-Hearing Sciences at the University of Minnesota. He received his PhD from the University of Minnesota in 1970 and was awarded a National Institute of Dental Research Special Research Fellowship in the School of Dentistry from 1970 to 1972. His teaching and scholarship have focused on interdisciplinary care, speech production and physiology in persons with cleft palate, and the impact of dental and occlusal conditions on speech. Dr. Moller has published articles, chapters, and books on speech, cleft palate, and interdisciplinary care. He is a past-president of the Minnesota Speech-Language-Hearing Association and its Foundation, and has served on the Board of Directors of the Cleft Palate Foundation and Executive Council of the American Cleft Palate-Craniofacial Association. He is a Fellow of the American Speech-Language-Hearing Association and holds honorary membership in the Omicron Kappa Upsilon Dental Society and the International College of Dentists. In 1997, he received the School of Dentistry Century Club Outstanding Professor Award.

**Leslie E. Glaze, PhD,** is a speech-language pathologist specializing in voice disorders, cleft palate, and alaryngeal speech and is an adjunct assistant professor in the Department of Speech-Language-Hearing Sciences at the University of Minnesota. She received her MA from the University of Kansas and her PhD from the University of Wisconsin–Madison. Dr. Glaze has participated in the Cleft Palate/Craniofacial Clinics at the University of Minnesota as speech-language pathologist and clinical supervisor. She has served two terms as coordinator of the American Speech-Language-Hearing Association's Special Interest Division 3 on Voice and

Voice Disorders and is former president of the Minnesota Speech-Language-Hearing Association. She is coauthor or coeditor of three textbooks and has contributed several chapters and articles in the areas of voice, cleft palate, and alaryngeal speech. She is a Fellow of the American Speech-Language-Hearing Association.

**Cassandra L. Aspinall, MSW, LICSW,** is a medical social worker who has been on staff at Seattle Children's Hospital and Regional Medical Center for over 20 years, focusing on the Craniofacial Center in the last decade. She received both her bachelor's and master's degrees at the University of Washington, where she is a Clinical Assistant Professor. She conducts interdisciplinary training in advocacy and patient- and family-centered care and serves as a practicum instructor for advanced social work graduate students. Her research areas include adolescent quality of life and how it is impacted by facial differences and family access to complex dental and orthodontic treatments in the community. She has been a long-term member of the hospital Ethics Committee, is an on-call ethics consultant, and received a Certificate in Health Care Ethics from the University of Washington in 1997. On a personal note, she was born with a bilateral cleft and has 3 children, the youngest of whom has a cleft lip and palate.

**Adriane L. Baylis, PhD,** is a speech-language pathologist and cleft lip and palate specialist at the Masters Family Speech and Hearing Clinic at the Children's Hospital of Wisconsin in Milwaukee, Wisconsin. She received her BA degree from Marquette University in Milwaukee and her MA and PhD in speech-language-hearing sciences from the University of Minnesota. She served as a speech-language pathologist at the University of Minnesota School of Dentistry Cleft Palate, Craniofacial and Speech Prosthesis Clinics from 2001 to 2007. Her research interests include velopharyngeal anatomy and physiology and biofeedback speech treatment approaches for patients with Velocardiofacial and DiGeorge syndromes (22q11.2 deletion). She has coordinated the Upper Midwest VCFS/DiGeorge Syndrome Community (www.vcsfconnect.org) and the Twin Cities VCFS/DiGeorge Family Support Group and remains actively involved in the Upper Midwest VCFS/DiGeorge Community. She has presented nationally and internationally on applications of speech prostheses to management of velopharyngeal closure and speech and language issues in Velocardiofacial and DiGeorge syndromes. She received a New Century Scholars Doctoral Dissertation Award from the American Speech-Language-Hearing Foundation in 2005 and a Minnesota Speech-Language-Hearing Foundation Scholarship Award in 2004.

**Richard R. Bevis, DDS, PhD,** is a clinical professor at the University of Minnesota School of Dentistry in the Cleft Palate-Craniofacial Program. He received his DDS, advanced orthodontic training, and PhD in anatomy from the University of Minnesota. He was on the faculty in the Division of Orthodontics for many years and is currently in private practice in the Twin Cities area. Dr. Bevis has received research training awards from the National Institute of Dental Research (NIDR) and has published articles and presented nationally and internationally on orthodontic management. He has served as an orthodontist on the interdisciplinary team at the University of Minnesota for over 30 years.

**Mary L. Breen, RN, MS,** is the clinical nurse specialist and coordinator for Children's Craniofacial and Reconstructive Plastic Surgery Center at Dell Children's Medical Center of Central Texas, a position she has held for the past 6 years. She received her BA in history from the University of Texas, her BS in nursing from the University of Texas Medical Branch (UTMB), and her MS in nursing from the University of Oklahoma. Previously, she served for 15 years as coordinator for the cleft and craniofacial teams at Children's Medical Center of Dallas and for 2 years at the UTMB Child Health Center in Galveston. Currently, she conducts prenatal counseling, newborn hospital visits, and feeding assessments; performs preoperative preparation; and coordinates the multidisciplinary cleft team. She also organized and coordinates the parent support group. She is a member of the Sigma Theta Tau Nursing Honor Society and the American Cleft Palate-Craniofacial Association, where she was a member of the Executive Council in 1999–2000. She has been a contributor to nursing and medical textbooks and has lectured to various audiences on the care of children with cleft lip and palate.

**Marie-Claire Buckley, MD,** is an assistant professor of plastic surgery in the Department of Surgery at the University of Minnesota Medical Center. She completed her medical training at the Mayo Medical School, followed by a residency in general surgery at Downstate SUNY and another in plastic surgery at the University of Minnesota. She completed a craniofacial surgical fellowship at the Primary Children's Hospital of the University of Utah. Dr. Buckley participated in several medical trips to developing nations to perform surgical repairs of the cleft lip and palate. She has been a member of the University of Minnesota Cleft Palate/Craniofacial Anomalies teams since 2002.

**Jane E. Carlstrom, MA, AuD,** is an audiologist and clinical specialist in the Department of Speech-Language-Hearing Sciences at the University of Minnesota. She received her MA in audiology at the University of Iowa and her AuD from the University of Florida. She has been audiologist on the cleft palate and craniofacial teams at the University of Minnesota for 25 years and has served as audiologist on a cleft palate surgical team in Guatemala for the past 10 years. She has held numerous leadership positions with the Minnesota Speech-Language-Hearing Association and is a recipient of MSHA Honors of the Association.

**Kathy L. Chapman, PhD,** received her BS and MS degrees from Texas Tech University in speech-language pathology and a PhD in audiology and speech sciences from Purdue University. She began her academic career at the University of Montana and then moved to Case Western Reserve University, where she also served as department chair. Dr. Chapman is currently an associate professor in the Department of Communication Sciences and Disorders at the University of Utah. She has taught courses in language and phonological disorders in young children, cleft palate, and research methods. Her early research focused on children with specific language impairment and, more recently, on language and phonological development in young children with cleft palate. She is especially interested in the impact of clefting on the developing speech sound system. Dr. Chapman has numerous data-based articles and presentations related to these areas of study. She was the coinvestigator on a multicenter longitudinal study of speech and language development of young children with cleft palate from 6 to 39 months of age. Dr. Chapman has served on numerous editorial boards and was associate editor for the *American Journal of Speech-Language Pathology.*

**David H. Charles, DDS, MS,** participated on the maxillofacial treatment team at the University of Western Ontario with coauthors Leeper and Sills. His academic responsibilities at Western included serving as chair of the Division of Prosthodontics, chair of Dental Biomaterials, and assistant dean of clinical affairs. He received his DDS from McGill University in Montreal. After graduation, he served 8 years with the Canadian Armed Forces Dental Services, the last 4 being at the Canadian Forces Dental Services School, where his responsibilities included patient care and clinical and laboratory training in prosthodontics. He later joined the Faculty of Dentistry at The University of Western Ontario in the Division of Prosthodontics. While at Western, he obtained his MS degree in clinical research design and biostatistics at the University of Michigan. He also maintained a private practice at the Dental Department at the University Campus London Health Sciences Centre. Dr. Charles retired in 2004 as professor emeritus.

**Patricia D. Chibbaro, RN, MS, CPNP,** has served for 20 years as the pediatric nurse practitioner in the Craniofacial, Cleft Lip/Palate and Microtia Programs at the Institute of Reconstructive Plastic Surgery, New York University Medical Center. She earned her MSN in parent-child nursing and her certificate as a pediatric nurse practitioner from the University of Colorado Health Sciences Center in Denver. Her 30 years in nursing have been devoted to the special care needs of pediatric patients, including pediatric oncology patients at Sloan Kettering Cancer Center, Denver Children's Hospital, and Bellevue Hospital in New York. She has also served as an adjunct clinical instructor in pediatrics at Hunter College School of Nursing and is currently a preceptor for graduate nursing students at several training programs. In 1992, she received the Donna Pruzansky Memorial Fund Nursing Award from the American Cleft Palate-Craniofacial Association. She has presented frequently on the topics of prenatal counseling for couples with a cleft-affected fetus, nursing management of the infant undergoing NAM (nasoalveolar molding), and care of the distraction osteogenesis patient.

**Michele J. Eliason, PhD,** is an associate professor at the University of California, San Francisco's Institute for Health and Aging and also teaches at San Francisco State University. She received her PhD degree in educational and pediatric psychology from the University of Iowa. Her research over the last several years has focused on the effects of substance use and abuse in women and children. She was associate professor in the College of Nursing at the University of Iowa for 15 years, where she published on the cognitive and psychosocial aspects of cleft lip and palate.

**Robert J. Gorlin, DDS, DSc,** was a member of the University of Minnesota Cleft Palate and Craniofacial team for over 40 years. He received his early training from Columbia University, Washington University, and University of Iowa. His lifework was devoted to oral pathology, cleft and craniofacial syndromes, and hereditary hearing loss. He was the author of over 600 publications and 14 texts. Dr. Gorlin was named a University of Minnesota Regents Professor and received numerous honorary degrees and memberships in professional organizations worldwide. These included Honors of the American Cleft Palate-Craniofacial Association; the Norton Ross Award for Excellence in Clinical Research and the Gold Medal Award, both from the American Dental Association; the Craniofacial Biology Research Award from the International Association for Dental Research; the Italian Premio Anni Verdi Award in Medical Genetics; and the American Society of Human Genetics Award for Excellence in Education. He was a Burroughs Wellcome Fellow of the Royal Society of Medicine and held honorary fellowships at the Royal College of Surgeons of Ireland and England, occupied the Spinoza Chair in the Netherlands, was a Nobel lecturer in Stockholm, and was elected Senior Fellow in the Institute of Medicine of the National Academy of Sciences. He received honorary DSc degrees from the University of Athens (Greece), the University of Copenhagen (Denmark), the University of Maryland, and the University of Minnesota. His book *Syndromes of the Head and Neck* is a quintessential text for craniofacial centers and clinicians. Dr. Gorlin died in August 2006.

**Virginia A. Hinton, PhD,** is associate professor in the Department of Communication Sciences and Disorders at the University of North Carolina–Greensboro. She received her bachelor's degree from the University of Tennessee–Knoxville, her master's degree from Northwestern University, and her PhD from the University of Iowa. All degrees are in speech-language pathology. Beginning in 1979, Dr. Hinton worked for 6 years as a speech-language pathologist and research assistant with the UNC–Chapel Hill Craniofacial Team. Her research focused on the upper airway characteristics of patients with a variety of facial differences. She has worked in academic settings and has continued to pursue both clinical and research interests in the area of oral-facial clefting. Dr. Hinton has published articles in the *Cleft Palate-Craniofacial Journal* and has presented at American Cleft Palate-Craniofacial Association (ACPA) annual meetings. In addition, she has served on several ACPA committees and currently chairs the Cleft Palate Foundation Scholarship Committee. Dr. Hinton has participated in international missions that focus on the care of patients with craniofacial differences.

**Gerrilyn M. Hopper, MHS,** is a registered dietitian and nutritionist. She graduated with honors with a BS in biochemistry and dietetics from Memorial University of Newfoundland, where her research focused on infant feeding. She then studied at the University of Toronto, where she completed a master's of health science in nutrition. She has worked as a clinical dietitian in various acute care settings, as well as a nutrition educator in the public and private sectors. Her research interests include behavior modification and nutritional assessment techniques. She has most recently been involved with the diet intervention arm of the national Women's Health Initiative Study. She currently resides in Seattle, Washington, with her husband and twin daughters.

**David L. Jones, PhD,** is professor in the Division of Communication Disorders at the University of Wyoming. Over the last 20 years, he has served on interdisciplinary cleft palate teams at the University of Iowa, Indiana University School of Medicine, and the State of Wyoming. His clinical specialty includes instrumental assessment of velopharyngeal function. He has numerous publications and presentations in the area of cleft palate. His research interests include outcomes of cleft palate treatment, the physiology of velopharyngeal function, and the production and perception of disordered nasalization. He has served on the Editorial Board of the *Cleft Palate-Craniofacial Journal*, the Board of Directors of the Cleft Palate Foundation, and the Executive Council for the American Cleft Palate-Craniofacial Association.

**George H. Landis, MD,** is adjunct clinical professor at the University of Minnesota Medical Center and the Cleft Palate/Craniofacial Program in the School of Dentistry. He received his undergraduate and medical degrees from the University of Arizona and completed general surgery and plastic surgery residency training at the University of Minnesota. He was in academic practice until 2001, when he entered private practice in the Minneapolis–St. Paul area. Dr. Landis has served on several medical/surgical trips to Peru and Guatemala and actively participates in the interdisciplinary cleft clinic team at the University of Minnesota. He has a broad-based practice of plastic surgery with a focus on cancer reconstruction and surgical management for cleft lip and palate.

**Herbert A. Leeper, Jr., PhD,** was a professor in the School of Communication Sciences and Disorders, University of Western Ontario, London, Ontario, Canada, where he taught courses in craniofacial disorders and resonance disorders. He received his doctorate from Purdue University in West Lafayette, Indiana. Dr. Leeper was cross-appointed to the Faculties of Medicine and Dentistry and collaborated in assessment, treatment, and research with Otolaryngology and Maxillofacial Prosthodontics. Prior to his untimely death in May 2001, he published widely about the characteristics and management of communication disorders related to cleft and craniofacial anomalies. He was a Fellow of the American Speech-Language-Hearing Association and received Honours of the Profession from the Canadian Association of Speech-Language Pathologists and Audiologists. He was a member of the American Cleft Palate Craniofacial Association and previously served on the Executive Council.

**Jerald B. Moon, PhD,** is associate professor in the Department of Speech Pathology and Audiology at The University of Iowa. He received a BSc and MClSc in communicative disorders from the University of Western Ontario and a PhD from Purdue University. He went to Iowa as a research scientist on a National Institutes of Health (NIH)–funded Cleft Palate Program Project and has taught and conducted research at Iowa ever since. He is an active member of the American Cleft Palate-Craniofacial Association and served as editor of the *Cleft Palate-Craniofacial Journal* from 1998 to 2008. He has authored or coauthored over 40 manuscripts and numerous book chapters in the area of cleft palate.

**Peggy B. Nelson, PhD,** is an audiologist and associate professor in the department of Speech-Language-Hearing Sciences at the University of Minnesota. She received her PhD from the University of Kansas. She has been an audiologist since 1982 and has worked with children in schools, family centers, and clinics. Her research focuses on hearing aid development and hearing loss and speech perception in noise in a variety of populations, including hard-of-hearing listeners and cochlear implant users. She is a member of the working group that developed the American National Standards Institute (ANSI) standards on Classroom Acoustics. She has received two Editor's Awards for her research articles published in the *American Journal of Audiology.* She is a Fellow of the Acoustical Society of America.

**Lynn C. Richman, PhD,** has been a faculty member in Pediatric Psychology, University of Iowa, College of Medicine, since 1973. He is currently professor and division director of Pediatric Psychology. He received his BA from Grinnell College and his MA and PhD from the University of Iowa. He has specialized in research and clinical service in the areas of learning disorders, attention-deficit/hyperactivity disorder, language disorders, and psychological aspects of cleft lip and palate. He has served on the Board of Directors and numerous other committees for the American Cleft Palate-Craniofacial Association. He has served as principal investigator on many National Institutes of Health (NIH) grants, and has served as a reviewer on numerous NIH study sections. He has been the Behavioral Sciences Section Editor for the *Cleft Palate-Craniofacial Journal.*

**Earl J. Seaver, PhD,** has served as an interdisciplinary team member of the Cleft Palate Clinic at the University of Illinois College of Medicine at Rockford since 1975. As a member of the faculty at Northern Illinois University, he has taught undergraduate and graduate classes, including a graduate course in craniofacial anomalies. He has served as vice provost at Northern Illinois University since July 2003. He received his bachelor's and master's degrees in speech pathology at Western Michigan University and a PhD in speech sciences at the University of Iowa. His numerous journal articles and professional presentations have focused on the improvement of speech therapy for children born with facial differences, including cleft lip and palate and other craniofacial anomalies. He serves as president of the Cleft Palate Foundation. Seaver is a Fellow of the American and Illinois Speech-Language-Hearing Associations and has received the Honors of the Illinois Speech-Language-Hearing Association.

**Helen M. Sharp, PhD,** is an assistant professor in the Department of Speech Pathology and Audiology at Western Michigan University with a joint appointment as an adjunct assistant professor in the College of Dentistry at the University of Iowa. She received her BSc in human kinetics from the University of Guelph, her MS in speech-language pathology from the University of Pittsburgh, and a PhD in speech and hearing science from the University of Iowa. She previously served as a staff speech-language pathologist and member of the craniofacial team at Loma Linda University Medical Center in California before returning to academics as a Fellow at the MacLean Center for Clinical Medical Ethics, University of Chicago, with joint affiliation at Oak Forest Hospital. Her interest in cleft and craniofacial conditions began as an undergraduate research assistant at the Hospital for Sick Children in Toronto. She has served on various committees for the American Cleft Palate-Craniofacial Association. She teaches cleft, craniofacial, and resonance disorders, clinical ethics and professionalism, and conducts research in measurement of patient-centered outcomes.

**James D. Sidman, MD, MSD, MEd,** is an associate professor in otolaryngology and pediatrics at the University of Minnesota. He graduated from Vassar College, and spent 2 years in the Peace Corps in Micronesia. He received his MD from Dartmouth Medical School and served in the National Health Service Corps as a general practitioner in rural Maine for 2 years before completing an otolaryngology residency at the University of North Carolina at Chapel Hill. He was a faculty member at the University of Connecticut, where he served as the acting chief of otolaryngology for 1 year. He started Pediatric ENT Associates in 2001 after practicing in the Twin Cities for 8 years. His special interests are in cleft lip and palate, airway reconstruction, and the treatment of facial paralysis. He has served on various committees for the American Academy of Otolaryngology, American Cleft Palate-Craniofacial Association, and American Society of Pediatric Otolaryngology, and as an oral board examiner for the American Board of Otolaryngology. He directs the Pediatric Otolaryngology Fellowship at Children's Hospital and the University of Minnesota and the Cleft and Craniofacial Team at Children's Hospital–Minneapolis.

**Paul S. Sills, DDS,** joined the Faculty of Dentistry, University of Western Ontario, and was chair of Removable Prosthodontics from 1977 until his retirement in 1991. He maintained a consultant and referral practice at the Department of Dentistry, London Health Sciences Centre, where he also held the chair of the Orofacial Rehabilitation Unit Team. After "retirement" he continued teaching prosthodontics as professor emeritus, instructing the undergraduate program until his death in 2004. He graduated from the University of Toronto, then completed a prosthodontic residency training program at Walter Reed Army Medical Center in Washington, D.C. He served with the Canadian Forces Dental Services until 1972. He received several teaching awards, including the prestigious 3M Teaching Award for the most outstanding teacher at the University of Western Ontario in 1989. Dr. Sills was a Diplomate of the American Board of Prosthodontics and held Fellowships in the American College of Prosthodontics, the International College of Dentists, and the American College of Dentists. He was past-president of the Canadian Academy of Prosthodontics and Association of Prosthodontists of Canada.

**James Q. Swift, DDS,** is professor and director of the Division of Oral and Maxillofacial Surgery at the University of Minnesota School of Dentistry. He is a graduate of the University of Iowa College of Dentistry and completed his oral and maxillofacial surgery residency training at the University of Oklahoma Health Sciences Center. Dr. Swift is currently president of the American Dental Education Association and former president of the American Board of Oral and Maxillofacial Surgery. He has also held various positions within the American Association of Oral and Maxillofacial Surgeons, American Dental Education Association, and American Dental Society of Anesthesiology and was a member of the Board of Directors of Fairview Health Services. He was named as a Fellow of the American College of Dentistry and the Century Club Outstanding Professor for the University of Minnesota School of Dentistry. Dr. Swift's research and clinical interests have focused on pain management, temporomandibular joint inflammatory mediators, dental implants, and cleft palate and craniofacial anomalies. He has been a member of the Cleft Palate and Craniofacial Anomalies Teams at the University of Minnesota for almost 20 years.

**Judith E. Trost-Cardamone, PhD, CCC-SLP,** is a professor in the Department of Communication Disorders and Sciences at California State University at Northridge, and consultant for the Ventura Cleft Palate Team. She received her BS, MA, and PhD degrees from Northwestern University. Her publications have focused on description, assessment, and treatment of cleft palate speech errors. She is nationally and internationally recognized for her clinical expertise and educational contributions. She is on the Professional Advisory Board of RSF-Earthspeak, a nonprofit organization devoted to developing affordable resources for cleft palate speech rehabilitation in developing countries around the globe. She is a Fellow of the American Speech-Language-Hearing Association, as well as member, historian, and past-secretary of the American Cleft Palate-Craniofacial Association.

**Bryan J. Williams, DDS, MSD, MEd,** is director of the Department of Dental Medicine at Children's Hospital and Regional Medical Center in Seattle, Washington. He is also an affiliate professor in the Departments of Pediatric Dentistry and Orthodontics at the University of Washington. He received his dental training at the University of Western Ontario and specialty training at the University of Washington, as well as a master's in education. With specialty training in both orthodontics and pediatric dentistry, he is a Diplomate of both the American Board of Orthodontics and the American Board of Pediatric Dentistry. He lectures nationally and internationally on pediatric behavior management, emergency management, cleft palate and craniofacial anomalies, and the care of children with complex medical and developmental problems. Currently, in addition to being department director, he is a staff orthodontist for the Craniofacial Team at Children's Hospital. His professional interests include dental care for children with complex medical problems, management of dentoalveolar trauma, and orthodontic management of children with cleft palate and other craniofacial anomalies.

# Author Index

# Subject Index